T0203166

BSAVA Manual of Canine and Feline Haematology and Transfusion Medicine

Second edition

Editors:

Michael J. Day†
BSc BVMS(Hons) PhD DSc DiplECVP FASM FRCPath FRCVS
Professor of Veterinary Pathology; School of Veterinary Sciences,
University of Bristol, Langford, Bristol BS40 5DU

and

Barbara Kohn
Dr.med.vet DipECVIM-CA
Professor of Small Animal Internal Medicine; Clinic of Small Animals,
Faculty of Veterinary Medicine, Freie Universität Berlin,
14163 Berlin, Germany

Published by:

British Small Animal Veterinary Association
Woodrow House, 1 Telford Way, Waterwells
Business Park, Quedgeley, Gloucester GL2 2AB

A Company Limited by Guarantee in England.
Registered Company No. 2837793.
Registered as a Charity.

First edition 2000
Second edition 2012
Reprinted 2019, 2020, 2021

Figure 5.1 was drawn by S.J. Elmhurst BA Hons (www.livingart.org.uk) and is printed with her permission.

Front cover main image courtesy of Daniel Chan.

A catalogue record for this book is available from the British Library.

ISBN 978-1-905319-29-9

Printed in the UK by Severn, Gloucester GL2 5EU – a carbon neutral printer
Printed on ECF paper made from sustainable forests

17095PUBS21

Other titles in the BSAVA Manuals series:

Manual of Avian Practice: A Foundation Manual
Manual of Backyard Poultry Medicine and Surgery
Manual of Canine & Feline Abdominal Imaging
Manual of Canine & Feline Abdominal Surgery
Manual of Canine & Feline Advanced Veterinary Nursing
Manual of Canine & Feline Anaesthesia and Analgesia
Manual of Canine & Feline Behavioural Medicine
Manual of Canine & Feline Cardiorespiratory Medicine
Manual of Canine & Feline Clinical Pathology
Manual of Canine & Feline Dentistry and Oral Surgery
Manual of Canine & Feline Dermatology
Manual of Canine & Feline Emergency and Critical Care
Manual of Canine & Feline Endocrinology
Manual of Canine & Feline Endoscopy and Endosurgery
Manual of Canine & Feline Fracture Repair and Management
Manual of Canine & Feline Gastroenterology
Manual of Canine & Feline Haematology and Transfusion Medicine
Manual of Canine & Feline Head, Neck and Thoracic Surgery
Manual of Canine & Feline Musculoskeletal Disorders
Manual of Canine & Feline Musculoskeletal Imaging
Manual of Canine & Feline Nephrology and Urology
Manual of Canine & Feline Neurology
Manual of Canine & Feline Oncology
Manual of Canine & Feline Ophthalmology
Manual of Canine & Feline Radiography and Radiology: A Foundation Manual
Manual of Canine & Feline Rehabilitation, Supportive and Palliative Care: Case Studies in Patient Management
Manual of Canine & Feline Reproduction and Neonatology
Manual of Canine & Feline Shelter Medicine: Principles of Health and Welfare in a Multi-animal Environment
Manual of Canine & Feline Surgical Principles: A Foundation Manual
Manual of Canine & Feline Thoracic Imaging
Manual of Canine & Feline Ultrasonography
Manual of Canine & Feline Wound Management and Reconstruction
Manual of Canine Practice: A Foundation Manual
Manual of Exotic Pet and Wildlife Nursing
Manual of Exotic Pets: A Foundation Manual
Manual of Feline Practice: A Foundation Manual
Manual of Ornamental Fish
Manual of Practical Animal Care
Manual of Practical Veterinary Nursing
Manual of Psittacine Birds
Manual of Rabbit Medicine
Manual of Rabbit Surgery, Dentistry and Imaging
Manual of Raptors, Pigeons and Passerine Birds
Manual of Reptiles
Manual of Rodents and Ferrets
Manual of Small Animal Practice Management and Development
Manual of Wildlife Casualties

For further information on these and all BSAVA publications, please visit our website:
www.bsava.com/shop

Contents

Contributors

Anthony C.G. Abrams-Ogg DVM DVSc DipACVIM(SAIM)
Associate Professor, Department of Clinical Studies; Small Animal Clinic Head,
Health Sciences Centre Teaching Hospital; Ontario Veterinary College, University of Guelph,
Guelph, Ontario N1G 2W1, Canada

Gad Baneth DVM PhD DipECVCP
Associate Professor of Veterinary Medicine; Koret School of Veterinary Medicine,
Hebrew University, PO Box 12, Rehovot 76100, Israel

Dorothee Bienzle DVM PhD DipACVP
Professor and Canada Research Chair in Veterinary Pathology; Department of Pathobiology,
University of Guelph, 419 Gordon St, Guelph ON N1G 2W1, Canada

Marjory B. Brooks DVM DipACVIM(SAIM)
Section Director, Comparative Coagulation Laboratory; Animal Health Diagnostic Center,
College of Veterinary Medicine, Cornell University, Ithaca, NY 14853, USA

James L. Catalfamo MS PhD
Comparative Coagulation Laboratory; Department of Population Medicine and Diagnostic Sciences,
Animal Health Diagnostic Center, College of Veterinary Medicine, Cornell University, Ithaca,
NY 14853, USA

Michael J. Day[†] BSc BVMS(Hons) PhD DSc DipIECVP FASM FRCPath FRCVS
Professor of Veterinary Pathology; School of Veterinary Sciences, University of Bristol, Langford,
Bristol BS40 5DU

Jane M. Dobson MA BVetMed DVetMed DipECVIM-CA(Onc) MRCVS
European and RCVS Specialist in Veterinary Oncology; Department of Veterinary Medicine,
University of Cambridge, Madingley Road, Cambridge CB3 0ES

Gillian Gibson VMD DipACVIM MRCVS
Axiom Veterinary Laboratories, The Manor House, Brunel Road, Newton Abbot, Devon TQ12 4PB

Anne S. Hale DVM
Advanced Veterinary Transfusion Solutions, 4983 Bird Drive, Stockbridge, MI 49285, USA

Andreas H. Hasler Dr.med.vet. DipACVIM(SAIM) DipECVIM-CA
Tierärztliches Überweisungszentrum, 4456 Tenniken, Switzerland

Shimon Harrus DVM PhD DipECVCP
Associate Professor of Veterinary Medicine; Koret School of Veterinary Medicine, Hebrew
University, PO Box 12, Rehovot 76100, Israel

Ann E. Hohenhaus DVM DipACVIM (Onc, SAIM)
Head of Jaqua Transfusion Medicine Service, Staff Veterinarian, Certified Veterinary Journalist;
Animal Medical Center, 510 East 62nd Street, New York, NY 10065, USA

Peter J. Irwin BVetMed PhD FANZCVS MRCVS
Associate Professor in Small Animal Medicine; School of Veterinary and Biomedical Sciences,
Murdoch University, South Street, Murdoch, WA 6150, Australia

Barbara Kohn Dr.med.vet DipECVIM-CA
Professor of Small Animal Internal Medicine; Clinic of Small Animals, Faculty of Veterinary Medicine, Freie Universität Berlin, Oertzenweg 19b, 14163 Berlin, Germany

Annemarie T. Kristensen DVM PhD DipACVIM DipECVIM-CA DipECVIM-Onc
Department of Small Animal Clinical Sciences, Faculty of Life Sciences, University of Copenhagen, Frederiksberg C, Denmark

Mary C. Lewis MSc DVM
Clinical Pathology Resident; Tufts Cummings School of Veterinary Medicine, North Grafton, MA 01536, USA

Caroline Mansfield BSc BVMS MVM DipECVIM-CA MANZCVS
Hill's Senior Lecturer in Small Animal Medicine; Section Head Small Animal Medicine; Faculty of Veterinary Science, University of Melbourne, Australia

Jennifer N. Mills BVSc MSc PhD DClinPath PGradDipEd
School of Veterinary Clinical Sciences, Murdoch University, Murdoch, WA 6150, Australia

Reinhard Mischke Dr.med.vet DipECVIM-CA
Professor of Veterinary Cytology and Laboratory Medicine; Small Animal Clinic, University of Veterinary Medicine Hannover, Bünteweg 9, 30559 Hannover, Germany

Joanna Morris BSc BVSc PhD DipECVIM-CA(Onc) FRCVS
European and RCVS Specialist in Veterinary Oncology; School of Veterinary Medicine, College of Medical, Veterinary and Life Sciences, University of Glasgow, Bearsden Road, Glasgow G61 1QH

Mathios E. Mylonakis DVM PhD
Assistant Professor of Companion Animal Medicine; Companion Animal Clinic, Faculty of Veterinary Medicine, Aristotle University of Thessaloniki, 11 Stavrou Voutyra St, 54627 Thessaloniki, Greece

Cynthia M. Otto DVM PhD DipACVECC
Associate Professor of Critical Care; Department of Clinical Studies – Philadelphia, School of Veterinary Medicine, University of Pennsylvania, 3900 Delancey St, PA 19104, USA

Jed A. Overmann DVM DipACVP
Assistant Clinical Professor, Clinical Pathology; Veterinary Clinical Sciences Department, 1352 Boyd Avenue, University of Minnesota, St. Paul, MN 55108, USA

Kostas Papasouliotis DVM PhD DipRCPath DipECVCP MRCVS
Diagnostic Laboratories, Langford Veterinary Sciences and School of Veterinary Sciences, University of Bristol, Langford, Bristol BS40 5DU

Roger Powell MA VetMB DipRCPath DipACVP FRCPath MRCVS
PTDS, Unit 2a, Manor Farm Business Park, Higham Gobion, Hertfordshire SG5 3HR

Alexandre Proulx DVM
Emergency and Critical Care Resident; Department of Clinical Studies – Philadelphia, School of Veterinary Medicine, University of Pennsylvania, 3900 Delancey Street, Philadelphia, PA 19104, USA

Virginia T. Rentko VMD DipACVIM
Medical Director; Cummings School of Veterinary Medicine, Tufts University, 200 Westboro Road, North Grafton, MA 01536, USA

Stephanie A. Smith DVM MS DipACVIM
Research Assistant Professor; College of Medicine, University of Illinois, Urbana, IL 61801, USA

Laia Solano-Gallego DVM PhD DipECVCP
Lecturer, Veterinary Clinical Pathology; Department of Pathology and Infectious Diseases, Royal Veterinary College, University of London, Hawkshead Lane, North Mymms, Hatfield, Hertfordshire AL9 7TA

Andrew Sparkes BVetMed PhD DipECVIM MRCVS
Veterinary Director, International Society of Feline Medicine; Taeselbury, High Street, Tisbury, Wiltshire SP3 6LD

Tracy Stokol BVSc PhD DipACVP (Clin Path)
Associate Professor in Clinical Pathology; Department of Population Medicine and Diagnostic Sciences, College of Veterinary Medicine, Cornell University, Ithaca, NY 14853, USA

Michael Stone DVM DipACVIM (SAIM)
Clinical Assistant Professor; Department of Clinical Studies, Cummings School of Veterinary Medicine, Tufts University, 200 Westboro Road, North Grafton, MA 01536, USA

Simon Tappin MA VetMB CertSAM DipECVIM-CA MRCVS
RCVS and European Veterinary Specialist in Internal Medicine
Dick White Referrals, Station Farm, London Road, Six Mile Bottom, Newmarket, Suffolk CB8 0UH

Séverine Tasker BSc BVSc(Hons) PhD DSAM DipECVIM-CA PGCertHE MRCVS
RCVS Recognized Specialist in Feline Medicine
European Specialist in Small Animal Internal Medicine
Senior Lecturer in Small Animal Medicine; School of Veterinary Sciences and Langford Veterinary Services, University of Bristol, Langford, Bristol BS40 5DU

Andrew Torrance MA VetMB PhD DipACVP DipACVIM DipECVCP MRCVS
RCVS Recognized Specialist in Clinical Pathology
TDDS, Unit G, Innovation Centre, Rennes Drive, Exeter University, Exeter EX4 4RN

Harold Tvedten DVM PhD DipACVP (Clin Path, Anatomical Pathology) DipECVCP
Department of Clinical Sciences, Faculty of Veterinary Medicine, Box 7054, Swedish University of Agricultural Sciences, SE 750 07 Uppsala, Sweden

Elizabeth Villiers BVSc FRCPath DipECVCP CertSAM CertVR MRCVS
European Specialist in Veterinary Clinical Pathology
Honorary Associate Professor in Veterinary Clinical Pathology, University of Nottingham
Dick White Referrals, Station Farm, London Road, Six Mile Bottom,
Newmarket, Suffolk CB8 0UH

Trevor Waner BVSc PhD DipECLAM
Israel Institute for Biological Research, PO Box 19, 74100 Ness Ziona, Israel

Christiane Weingart Dr.med.vet
Clinic of Small Animals, Faculty of Veterinary Medicine, Freie Universität Berlin, Oertzenweg 19b, 14163 Berlin, Germany

Douglas J. Weiss DVM PhD DipACVP
Emeritus Professor; Department of Veterinary and Biomedical Sciences, College of Veterinary Medicine, University of Minnesota, St. Paul, MN 55108, Minnesota, USA

Carrie White DVM DipACVIM
Staff; Department of Internal Medicine, Animal Medical Center, 510 East 62nd Street, New York, NY 10065, USA

Bo Wiinberg DVM PhD
Department of Small Animal Clinical Sciences, Faculty of Life Sciences, University of Copenhagen, Frederiskberg C, Denmark

Foreword

With the advent of automated haematology and serum biochemistry analysers, most clinics now do their own laboratory work in house. Clinical pathology, and specifically haematology, are achieving prominence in general practice. Most practitioners now want to 'get extra miles out of their analysers', in addition to evaluating the patient, blood and bone marrow smears, and additional diagnostics.

This Manual provides a wealth of clinically relevant information for the practitioner. It is very well organized, is easy to read, has excellent illustrations and tables, and it is written by world-renowned clinicians and clinical pathologists. Most of the chapters are written by individuals who have published extensively in those areas.

The chapters are succinct, and provide valuable, right-to-the-point information, easily applied to the clinical case the practitioner is reading about. In addition, they provide substantial background information for those who want to learn more about that particular topic.

I really like the novel approach of including infectious diseases commonly leading to blood disorders in a Haematology Manual. It makes it even more practical!

The transfusion medicine section is also well organized, and quite practical, and it is well covered in only five chapters. In brief, a book anybody interested in haematology should have.

C. Guillermo Couto DVM DipACVIM
The Ohio State University Veterinary Medical Center

Preface

It is now 11 years since the publication of the first edition of the *BSAVA Manual of Canine and Feline Haematology and Transfusion Medicine*. Although topics covered in this manual overlap with the content of manuals in clinical pathology and emergency medicine, the first edition of this book was sold out and there is a clear demand for the more in-depth coverage of haematology that is provided herein.

The basic principles of haematology are still the core of the second edition, but these have been updated to discuss new diagnostic procedures and laboratory equipment, as well as new treatment strategies. We have invited a number of new authors to contribute to this second edition – either providing a fresh perspective on previous content or introducing new elements to the Manual. There are new chapters on the anaemia of inflammation and neoplasia, on non-regenerative anaemia and on vascular thrombosis. In the years since publication of the first edition, the arthropod-transmitted infectious diseases of companion animals have become increasingly significant as they have extended their traditional endemic areas (e.g. within Northern Europe and North America) or have become important differential diagnoses in travelling pets. Most of these infectious diseases (e.g. leishmaniosis, babesiosis, monocytic ehrlichiosis and anaplasmosis) have fundamental effects on the haemopoietic system, and haematological analysis is part of the first-line of diagnosis. These diseases are covered in detailed individual chapters. Another area in which there have been significant advances since the first edition is feline haemoplasmosis, and a completely revised chapter provides the latest information on these infectious agents.

The section on transfusion medicine has been reorganized and expanded in the second edition. Canine and feline blood groups are now discussed separately, together with the newly available in-practice diagnostic techniques for their identification. Canine and feline blood transfusion practice is also now considered in separate chapters and there is a new chapter on the use of blood substitutes.

The second edition of this manual has been made possible through the excellent and timely contributions of the chapter authors who are all internationally recognized specialists from Europe, North America, the Middle East and Australia. We are grateful to all of you for providing chapters and corrected proofs on time and for responding rapidly to our questions. Our thanks for their support and encouragement are also due to members of the BSAVA Publishing Team, who have led us through the production process.

Michael J. Day†
Barbara Kohn
November, 2011

1

Introduction to haematological diagnostic techniques

Roger Powell and Andrew Torrance

Introduction

The major innovations in small animal haematology in the last few years have been the introduction and wide application of laser-based counting systems, flow cytometry, immunolabelling and digital imaging. Notwithstanding these innovations, haematology remains a specialist discipline and the comments and acumen of a skilled veterinary clinical pathologist are the most useful and important contribution to the diagnostic investigation of haematological disease.

Haematological techniques are an essential part of the diagnostic process. The haematological profile includes measurement of haemoglobin (Hb), haematocrit (Hct) or packed cell volume (PCV), red cell indices (mean corpuscular volume (MCV), mean corpuscular haemoglobin (MCH), mean corpuscular haemoglobin concentration (MCHC)), total cell counts (platelets, red blood cells (RBCs) and white blood cells (WBCs)), differential WBC counts and comments by a veterinary haematologist on the morphology of the erythrocyte, leucocyte and platelet populations.

Microscopic examination of a blood smear alone may reveal the diagnosis in many haematological diseases. In diseases of other systems, interpretation of the haematological profile in conjunction with biochemistry, urinalysis, history and physical findings directs the clinician in the selection of subsequent, ultimately diagnostic, imaging and sampling techniques. Dogs and cats exhibit a wider range of haematological pathology than other species, making diagnostic haematology particularly important in small animal medicine.

Blood sampling

To be of diagnostic value, a sample of blood must truly reflect the impact of disease processes on the blood cells and platelets. The composition of blood is changing constantly, and there is a rapid response to physiological phenomena such as splenic contraction or demargination of neutrophils. These processes are readily induced by stressing the patient at the time of sampling and will produce physiological alterations that may confuse interpretation of the haematological profile. Stress-induced neutrophilia may be mistaken for an inflammatory leucogram in cats, and an increased PCV associated with splenic contraction may be mistaken for dehydration in dogs. Sedatives and analgesics have profound haematological effects, which mask disease processes and include spurious non-regenerative anaemia, neutropenia and lymphopenia. Physiological effects such as age can also play a significant role, with a more prominent lymphocytosis being common in young cats stressed during sampling. This is in part related to splenic contraction, but is also because young animals naturally have relatively higher lymphocyte counts than older ones. Each time a blood sample is taken for haematological examination it is therefore only a snapshot of what is occurring at that time. The cell counts and possibly morphology may change within hours, and certainly in days, so close serial monitoring often provides vital prognostic information.

Physical damage to blood constituents during collection is the most common and frustrating cause of poor blood samples. The fragility of erythrocytes and the aggregability of platelets are quite unpredictable and vary between individuals and pathological processes.

These problems can be minimized by using consistent, excellent technique. The slow flow and application of variable vacuum, which occurs during collection of blood from a peripheral vein, tests the resilience of blood cells and encourages platelet aggregation. Extraction with consistent vacuum from a large central vein is less damaging and therefore preferable. Jugular venepuncture is easy in dogs and cats (Figure 1.1), is often less stressful than the use of peripheral veins and undoubtedly yields the most reliable results. Evacuated tubes and syringes are equally efficient in skilled hands, but should not be used together. Samples are ruined when blood is extracted with a syringe and needle and the needle is pushed through the cap of an evacuated tube. Blood cells are then forced through the lumen of the needle under pressure twice, and damage results. When blood has been collected into a syringe, the needle should be removed and the blood gently pushed into an open tube containing the appropriate anticoagulant. The tube should then be capped and rolled gently to ensure adequate mixing.

The commonest anticoagulant of choice for the haematological profile is ethylenediamine tetra-acetic acid (EDTA) because it preserves cell morphology and creates the basis for cell sizes

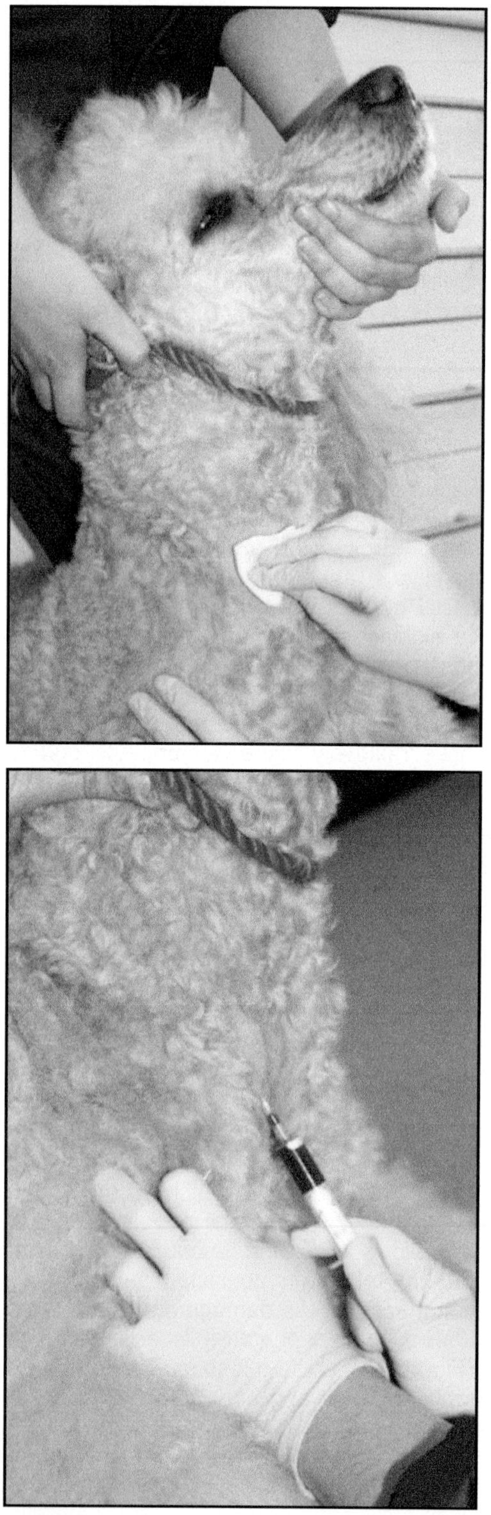

1.1 Jugular venepuncture in a dog, showing the restraint, positioning and site of access. (Courtesy of Jonathon Bray)

during automated analysis. Tubes contain either sodium (Na_2EDTA) or potassium (K_2EDTA, K_3EDTA) salts, which can variably influence cell morphology and size, especially with prolonged or excessive *in vitro* exposure due to sample storage, posting or poor filling (Hinchcliffe *et al.*, 1992). For example, under-filling will initially result in excessive red cell shrinkage, artificially reducing the PCV by up to 5%, although the calculated Hct may be unaffected because the cells are analysed in diluents, where their volume returns to normal before measurement (Cornbleet, 1983). However, given a 24-hour delay due to sample posting, under-filling will falsely elevate the MCV as the cells swell, causing an increased Hct and MCV, and a reduced MCHC. Tubes containing sodium citrate are used for coagulation tests. Both sodium citrate and EDTA prevent coagulation by complexing calcium, but sodium citrate is favoured for tests of coagulation because calcium binding is reversed more readily by addition of calcium. Heparinized blood is of little use for haematological examination because leucocyte staining is poor, cell sizes are very different, platelet clumping is more common and Wright's-stained smears develop a blue background, which impairs evaluation of morphology. Basic erythrocyte counts and indices, however, can be assessed in heparinized samples, but may need separate thresholds and parameters.

Basic quantification techniques

The measurement of PCV and cell counts can be performed manually by using microhaematocrit tubes and a haemocytometer.

Microhaematocrit

The microhaematocrit method for calculation of PCV is the simplest way to assess red cell mass manually. It is widely used in practice, intensive care units and haematology laboratories. The PCV is determined by centrifuging anticoagulated blood in a small capillary tube to separate cells from plasma. The PCV is calculated by dividing the length of the packed erythrocytes by the total length of the packed erythrocytes, buffy coat and plasma. Various simple devices (Figure 1.2) are available to perform this measurement, but only a ruler is required.

The minimal errors that occur with measurement of the microhaematocrit are usually associated with centrifugation. Microhaematocrit centrifuges operate at high speeds (11,500–15,000 rpm), which ensure adequate packing of erythrocytes. Multipurpose centrifuges may not rotate fast enough to pack the cells, and increased duration of centrifugation will not compensate for this. Adequate cell packing is achieved with 5 minutes of centrifugation at the appropriate speed. At a PCV above 50%, packing is not as complete after 5 minutes, leading to overestimation of red cell mass. In such cases an additional 5-minute period of centrifugation at an appropriate speed may be necessary. Over-filling the microhaematocrit tube by more than 75% of its length will also reduce the rate of packing and increase the centrifugation time. When the PCV is below 25%, the packing of erythrocytes will be tighter and may exaggerate the decrease in PCV, making the animal appear more anaemic than it really is. Similarly, under-filling the tube increases the force on the cells, increasing the packing, and underestimates

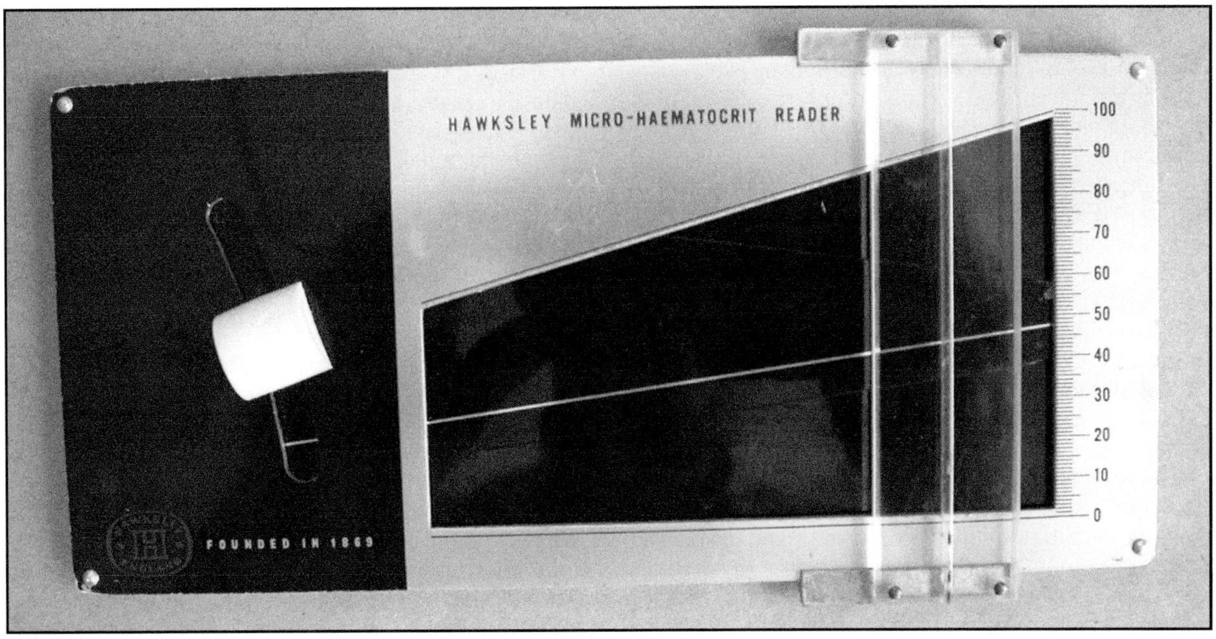

1.2 Reader with a sliding parabolic scale to facilitate measurement of the packed cell volume or microhaematocrit from a capillary tube.

the actual PCV. Small variations in PCV may also occur with different anticoagulants and incorrect filling or mixing of the original EDTA tube, an effect potentially exaggerated when an animal is anaemic, so the relative effects are greater. Certain breeds, such as some terriers, Dachshunds and sight hounds (e.g. Greyhounds), often have a relatively higher red cell mass (Hct/PCV, Hb and RBC) than other breeds.

Manual cell counts

Manual cell counts are done with an improved Neubauer-ruled haemocytometer, calibrated cover glass, disposable capillary pipette and plastic reservoir chamber containing a premeasured volume of diluent.

The haemocytometer is a transparent glass chamber that holds a cell suspension beneath the microscope for counting. The chamber is 0.1 mm deep and has a well defined space of known volume. The volume is subdivided by a grid of nine 1 mm^2 squares engraved on the base of the chamber. The central square of this grid is further subdivided into 25 squares of suitable size for counting RBCs at an appropriate dilution.

Blood is diluted to achieve an appropriate density of cells for counting with the diluent container. For erythrocyte counting the dilution is 1:200, for leucocytes 1:20 and for platelets 1:100. The total counts are then calculated using a correction factor that takes into account the counting volume and the dilution factors.

The count is performed in duplicate on different sides of the haemocytometer grid. The erythrocyte and leucocyte counts from the two sites should only vary by 20% and 10%, respectively, if performed correctly. If the two cell counts are consistent, the average of the two is multiplied by the conversion factor to obtain the count per litre.

Manual counts with a haemocytometer have a significant error compared with automated counts (± 20% on leucocyte counts). This is particularly important in monitoring changes in leucocyte number over time, for example a change of 20% can simply be an inter-count variation rather than a true alteration.

Automated quantification techniques

Measurement of red cells and leucocytes is now fully automated in laboratories and most practices. Improved haematology analysers also provide reliable information on red cell distribution width (RDW), which is an important index in the assessment of red cell regeneration. Some analysers can also provide red cell indices such as CH (cell haemoglobin mean), CHCM (cell haemoglobin concentration mean) and HDW (haemoglobin concentration distribution width), as well as extending such analysis to reticulocytes and platelets. However, such indices are yet to be fully evaluated clinically; their significance and usefulness is therefore unclear at present, especially in different species. Automated differential cell counting has improved with the advent of laser counting technology, but recent publications show that important morphological abnormalities are regularly missed if the blood smear is not examined by a veterinary haematologist (Becker *et al.*, 2008; Segev *et al.*, 2006). Differential leucocyte counts are best assessed visually because of the diversity of leucocyte patterns and morphology in dogs and cats. Automated differential counts should always be checked visually. Examination of a blood smear for the differential leucocyte count also provides an opportunity for the haematologist to comment on erythrocyte morphology and the presence of any abnormal cells. The diagnostic value of the haematological profile is seriously compromised when cell counts are interpreted without morphological examination, or vice versa (Segev *et al.*, 2006). Interpretive comments programmed into automated analysers are frequently irrelevant and can be extremely misleading (Becker *et al.*, 2008). The majority of analyser validation studies and software settings are based on studies of healthy cats and dogs, potentially using only one breed, and these do not translate to ill or diseased animals where the cell morphology is often altered.

Other factors affecting the quality of automatic counts include analyser type, sample damage, sample ageing, platelet aggregation and abnormalities in platelet size. The presence of microclots in damaged and poorly anticoagulated samples renders automated counts useless, and will also block the counting channels in some analysers. Damaged erythrocytes can fragment and lyse to form ghost cells; these will be miscounted as platelets and significantly reduce the RBC count. Platelets and white cells, especially if neoplastic and leukaemic, can lyse with prolonged *in vitro* storage, reducing numbers artificially.

Poor sample collection and sample ageing may result in platelet aggregation, and the platelet clumps may be counted as red or white cells, or missed altogether, leading to an erroneous platelet count. For this reason, it is always recommended that platelet counts are checked by manual estimation, and abnormal counts from automated cell counters should always be regarded with suspicion. Variations in platelet size may also lead to erroneous platelet counts. This was shown conspicuously in a study of breed-associated thrombocytopenia in Cavalier King Charles Spaniels (CKCSs) and related Norfolk Terriers in which manual platelet counts and automated counts were discordant. Affected dogs had a combination of large platelets (macrothrombocytes) and mild thrombocytopenia. The automated counts exaggerated the thrombocytopenia by counting macrothrombocytes as erythrocytes, thus artefactually decreasing the platelet count (Ecksell *et al.*, 1994; Gelain *et al.*, 2010). More recent studies of platelets in CKCSs have taken an innovative approach to the assessment of platelet numbers with the introduction of the concept of the 'thrombocrit' ('plateletcrit'). Analysers that work on the basis of centrifugation for separating cells (see buffy coat analysis, below) can measure a thrombocrit, which reflects platelet mass. CKCSs have giant platelets, but a normal platelet mass, and consequently their haemostasis is not affected by low platelet numbers.

Haemoglobin

Three methods for measuring Hb concentration are currently used by different analysers. The cyanmethaemoglobin method has been used as the international standard for many years, but the reagent contains potassium cyanide, which can cause problems with disposal and handling.

The oxyhaemoglobin method tends to underestimate total Hb because it only measures the oxyhaemoglobin fraction. This can cause problems with external quality control because the oxyhaemoglobin in samples converts to methaemoglobin with time. This is also a problem in samples from patients with significant methaemoglobinaemia.

Recently, the use of a less toxic reagent, sodium lauryl sulphate (SLS), has replaced the cyanmethaemoglobin method. The erythrocytes are lysed and Hb is converted to SLS–Hb by a four-step reaction and then quantified colorimetrically via a light-emitting diode. *In vitro* haemolysis, lipaemia and exogenous products such as Oxyglobin can falsely elevate the Hb measurement. Portable instruments that use two different wavelengths to measure azide methaemoglobin levels reduce the effect of these interferences.

Blood cell counts

Four major principles are currently used alone or in various combinations for automated analysis and counting by different types of analysers: conductivity by electrochemical blood gas instruments; quantitative buffy coat analysis (QBC); impedance cell counting by the Coulter principle; and electronic-optical counting using laser flow systems. These analysers have been designed for human blood analysis and then modified with varying success and accuracy for veterinary usage, primarily via software changes regarding cell discriminators.

Conductivity analysers

These electrochemical instruments, typically used for blood gas measurements, can also measure Hct and Hb. The conductivity of the blood is measured; conduction is reduced as the number of cells increases, so the Hct is inversely proportional to the conductivity. This relationship relies on red cell numbers being much greater than those of white cells or platelets, which may lead to significant positive bias if, for example, the white cell numbers increase significantly in inflammatory or leukaemic states. Similarly, the correlation assumes that other non-conducting elements, such as lipids and proteins, as well as conducting elements, are unchanged, which can be untrue in disease states. Some instruments correct the conduction value for concentrations of conducting electrolytes (sodium and potassium). Lipaemic samples falsely elevate the Hct, and altered proteins can artificially affect this measurement (e.g. hypoproteinaemia falsely decreases the Hct).

The Hb is calculated from this Hct via an assumed MCHC, typically 33 g/dl, using a conversion formula. If this assumption is incorrect for a particular animal, the resulting Hb value will also be wrong.

Quantitative buffy coat (QBC) analysis

White cell counts in these analysers are determined from the width and fluorescence of various cell layers in a buffy coat that is expanded artificially by a float. If the distinction between the bands is lost, as a result of haemolysis or lipaemia for example, this counting can be inaccurate or prevented. Whilst the width of the layer and degree of fluorescence reflect cell numbers (assuming normal sized cells), the differentiation of white cells is based on the variable fluorescence of white cells when stained with acridine orange (DNA fluoresces green, while RNA and lipoprotein fluoresce red). This differentiates mononuclear cells (lymphocytes and monocytes) from granulocytes (neutrophils and eosinophils). This variable fluorescence is very reliant on a lack of background interference and the presence of healthy normal cells. Often in disease, the size, nature and RNA content of the cells changes, and this discrimination is lost or inaccurate. Therefore, while these analysers generally give an accurate total white cell count, unless the animal is healthy, the differential count is often unreliable and misleading (Figure 1.3). The PCV is measured automatically, as with a manual PCV, and the MCHC is inversely proportional to the distance to which the float sinks in the red cell layer. The other red cell parameters are then calculated, including haemoglobin: Hb (g/dl) = PCV (%) × MCHC/100. Thus if the PCV is artificially altered by EDTA effects, the Hb calculation can also be affected.

Impedance counters

These analysers count cells using impedance; the cells are diluted in an electrolyte solution and then drawn through an aperture within an electrode. As each cell passes through, it creates a pulse of resistance: the more pulses, the more cells are present (Coulter principle). The size of each resistance (impedance) pulse equates to the size of the cell. Impedance counters must therefore be adjusted for each species so that the threshold size for each cell type is known. If there is overlap between two cell types, impedance counters can fail to distinguish the cells and ascribe them to the wrong type. In this fashion, the red cells are counted and only distinguished from platelets by the relative cell size (Figure 1.4).

This is true for many animal species, especially dogs. However, cats have smaller red cells and larger platelets, so the analyser can confuse platelets with red cells. Similarly, if a disease creates small red cells or very large platelets (e.g. iron deficiency or inflammation, respectively) this error can be exaggerated (Figure 1.5). Clumping of platelets caused by *in vitro* or sampling factors will reduce platelet numbers artificially, and will potentially falsely elevate red cell numbers or even white cell numbers, dependent on the size of the clump. This is particularly common in cats, *in vitro* clumping being the commonest cause of apparent thrombocytopenia in cats (Norman *et al.*, 2001), in which it can also falsely elevate the white cell numbers. Similarly, red cell agglutination in immune-mediated disease can falsely reduce the RBC whilst elevating the MCV artificially. White cell clumping can artificially reduce the WBC and can be a temperature-dependent *in vitro* phenomenon.

The white cells are also counted by impedance, but only after the red cells have been lysed in another solution. Different lysing solutions can be used to produce variable effects on white cells,

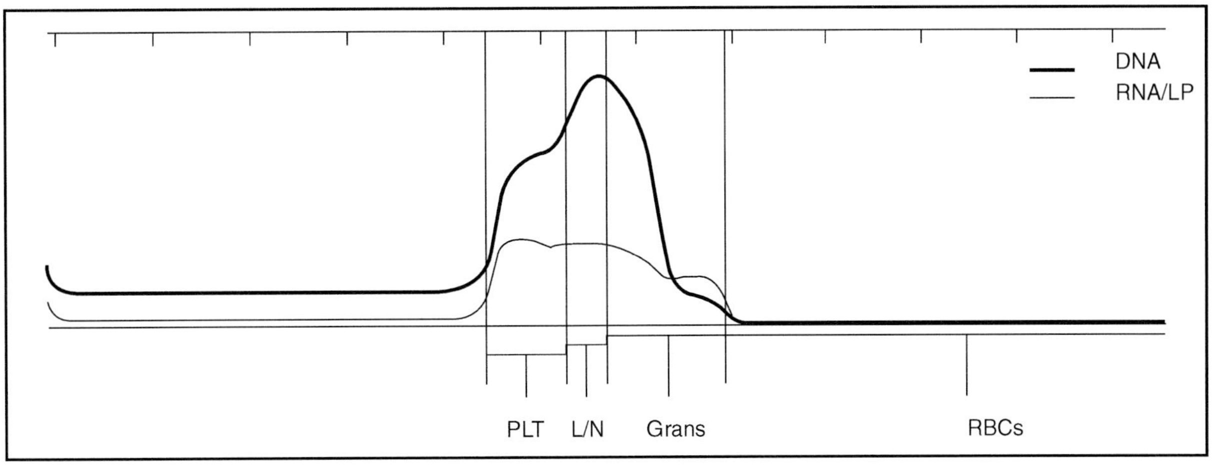

1.3 Buffy coat profile from a 1-year-old neutered male Labrador Retriever with pyrexia of unknown origin. The automated analysis reported significant eosinophilia (with no flags). Blood smear examination by a haematologist revealed significant lymphocytosis; the majority of these cells were granular lymphocytes that the analyser had misclassified as eosinophils ('Grans') owing to their granularity. The dog had an idiosyncratic and eventually self-resolving reaction to a booster vaccination.

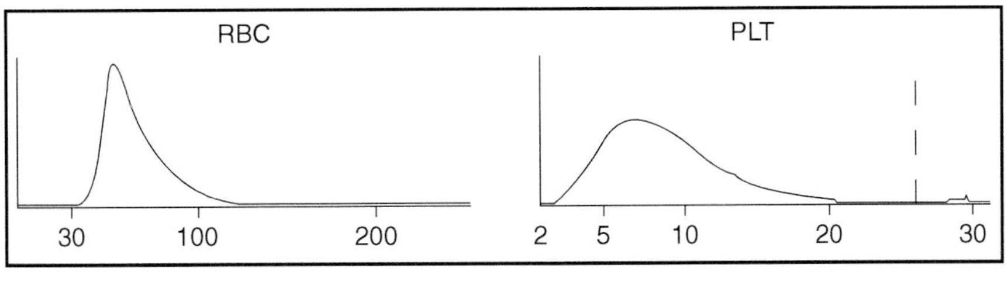

1.4 Impedance histograms for red cells (RBC) and platelets (PLT) in a healthy dog; the number of cells (*y* axis) is plotted against cell volume (x axis). There is good discrimination, the smallest red cells being just visible as a line over the 30 μm^3 mark.

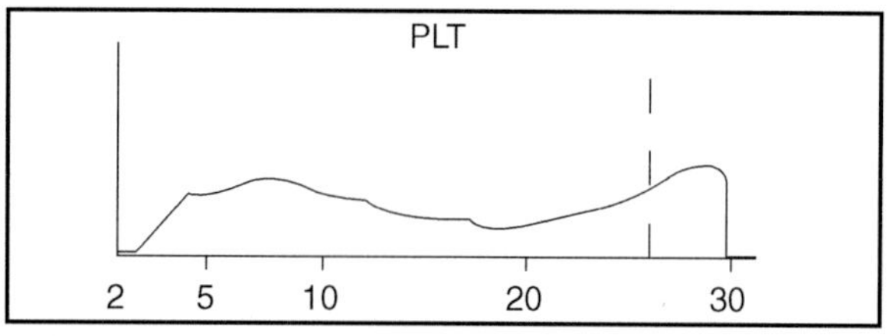

1.5 Dog with iron deficiency anaemia caused by gastrointestinal blood loss. The combination of microcytosis and thrombocytosis with macroplatelets prevents accurate automated differentiation because the platelet histogram (PLT) merges into the red cells on the right side, the set discrimination threshold (dotted line) not being applicable in this instance.

allowing white cell differentials to be produced automatically. Alkaline diluent, for example, will lyse neutrophils, monocytes and lymphocytes while leaving eosinophils intact, owing to the stability of eosinophil granules in alkaline conditions. The count is then performed on the eosinophil-rich sample.

This lysis strategy works primarily on anucleate cells, for example red cells, but some are resistant, especially immature nucleated red blood cells (nRBC). The analyser therefore 'assumes' that only white cells are present, which may not be true, especially in disease states. In this example, a nucleated red cell is counted as a mature lymphocyte. Therefore most impedance 'white cell counts' are in fact a nucleated cell count, so if nucleated red cells are present in significant numbers, the white cell count is artificially elevated and needs correcting. Newer and larger laser flow cytometers can inherently do this, but otherwise such discrimination relies on examination of the blood smear. The calculation is as follows:

$$\text{Corrected (true) white cell count} = \frac{100}{(\text{nRBC} + 100)} \times \text{nucleated cell count}$$

Laser flow cytometers

These are the basis for most commercial, larger and more expensive referral laboratory analysers. More recently smaller, cheaper and laser-based veterinary analysers have become available, but are inherently much more limited and much less accurate. In these analysers, a stream of single cells is passed through a laser beam, interrupting the light (equating to cell numbers) and also scattering the laser light in many directions. This scatter is both forwards (low angle – related to the size of the cell) and also to the side (high angle – related to the complexity or density of the cell). Therefore distinction of the many cell types is not only based on size but also on the density or complexity of the different cell types, which is much more variable and therefore discriminatory. For example red cells are much denser than platelets, so their distinction is much better. This scattering effect can again be enhanced by use of certain lysing solutions to leave only a few cell types for analysis. These analysers can also now use stains for cytoplasmic granules, such as peroxidase, to alter or highlight the characteristics of a cell under laser light (Figure 1.6). This combined analysis enhances the ability to identify cells accurately and

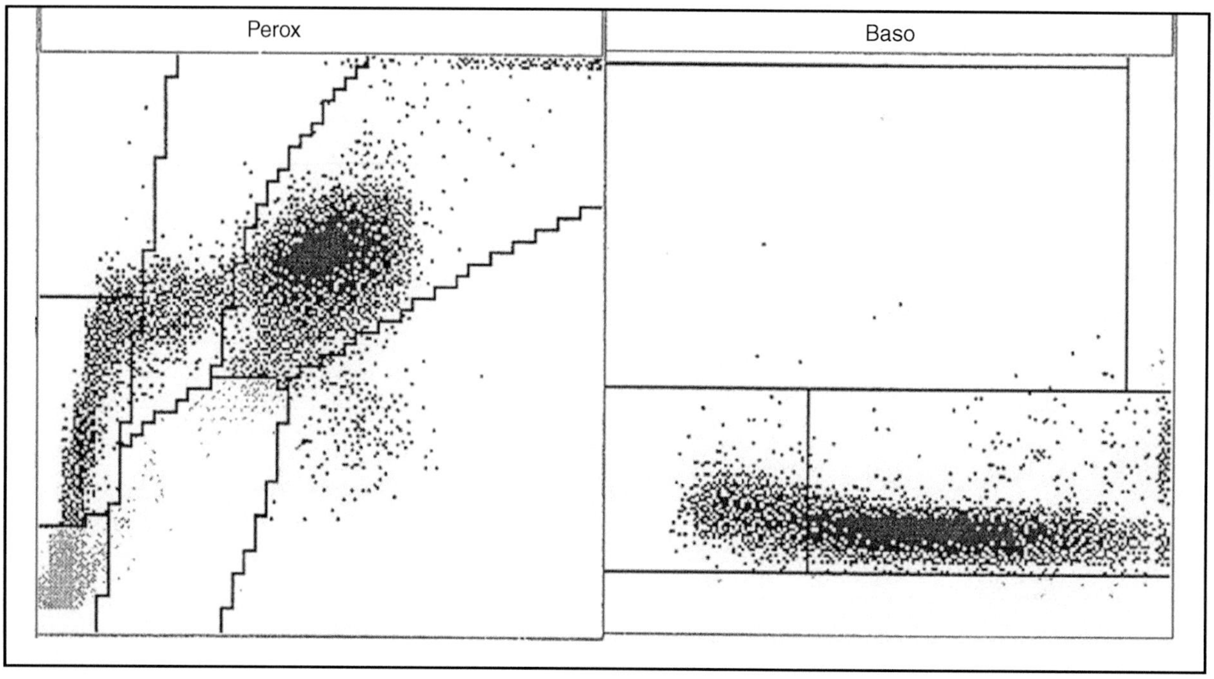

1.6 **(a)** Graphical display of white blood cells (WBCs) from a laser flow cytometer showing peroxidase staining (Perox; x axis) versus cell size (*y* axis). Each dot represents a cell, and the staggered lines show set thresholds for different cell types. **(b)** Graph showing particles after phthalic acid surfactant lysis for basophil (Baso) counting, showing nuclear configuration (*x* axis) and cell/nuclear size (*y* axis). While basophils are poorly identified in cats and dogs, the complexity of bare nuclei is also shown: mononuclear cells to the left, segmented cells to the right.

also allows more cell indices, such as CHCM, to be generated. Whereas the MCHC is calculated, the CHCM is generated from the mean of the actual measured Hb concentration within each erythrocyte as it passes through the laser beam. The CHCM is therefore much less affected by interference (e.g. by lipaemia) than MCHC. With the extra analysis and staining, such as oxazine 750 for RNA, reticulocytes and platelets can be similarly identified and assessed. This assessment can detect disease earlier than has been possible previously, such as iron deficiency in dogs via reticulocyte Hb content and reticulocyte volume (Steinberg and Olver, 2005). Nucleated red cells now become evident when there is a discrepancy between the cell counts obtained by the different methods. Cell clumping also becomes evident as a shifted population of cells. Leukaemic blast cells may be evident in certain regions, although identification of cell lineage and diagnosis rely on cell morphology in the smear or more detailed, but separate, immunophenotyping via fluorescent markers. Problems and pitfalls still remain, with basophils still not identified accurately and physiological differences (e.g. eosinophils in certain individuals or breeds such as Greyhounds) also being misidentified.

Once the cells have been counted and the sizes and Hb levels measured, the analysers calculate several red cell parameters on the basis of Wintrobe's formulas. The Hct, MCHC and MCH are calculated as follows:

Hct (l/l) = MCV (fl) × RBC (× 10^{12}/l)/1000

MCHC (g/dl) = Hb (g/dl)/Hct (l/l)

MCH (pg) = Hb (g/dl) × 10/RBC (× 10^{12}/l)

Graphical displays

When counting and assessing cells, all of the above methods, except conductivity, produce one or more graphical displays and histograms, both of cell size and also of various cellular constituents such as Hb. Using and visually assessing these displays enhances the information that is gained from the analysis, especially if extensive laser flow parameters and numbers are not available. While this does not replace the need to look at a fresh blood smear, it can identify potential artefacts and significant changes in cell populations that would otherwise be misdiagnosed or not identified when relying only on the numbers produced. For example, red cell indices are typically mean values, and significant changes must occur in the red cell population before the mean value changes (e.g. microcytosis in shunts and iron deficiency anaemia or hypochromic macrocytosis in regenerative anaemia; Figures 1.7 and 1.8). However, these displays commonly fail to detect morphological changes, such as those caused by toxicity in neutrophils, that would be evident in a blood smear to a trained haematologist.

An understanding of the types of automated analysis, as outlined above, each with associated caveats or possible artefacts, is more important as the severity of disease increases, because artefacts can be extreme and can also be seen in various combinations, especially if the disease is haematological (e.g. leukaemia). Much of the value of automated analysis relies on fresh blood; many of the parameters and features are obscured or lost with *in vitro* changes that occur over time (e.g. during sample transport). Whilst analyser cell counting is more reproducible because thousands of cells are counted, a fresh blood smear must always be examined to check that the analyser information is correct. Blood smear examination also allows assessment of cellular morphology that can provide additional valuable information about disease processes.

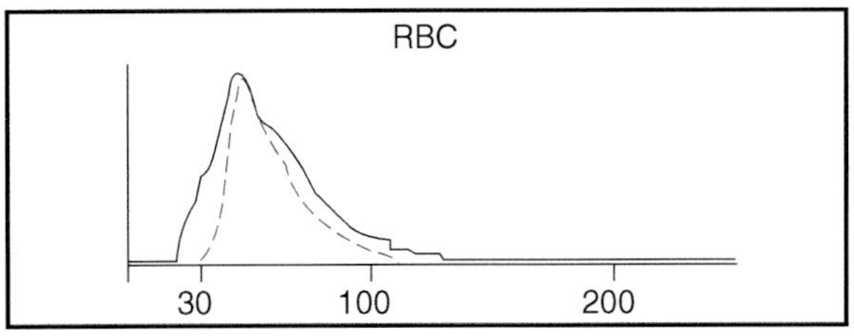

1.7 Impedance red blood cell (RBC) histogram of a dog with iron deficient regenerative anaemia (black line); a histogram from a healthy dog is also shown (dotted red line). The peaks are similar, and therefore the mean cell volume (MCV) was within reference limits, but the histogram clearly shows increased numbers of small cells (microcytosis) as well as macrocytosis caused by regeneration with polychromasia (reticulocytosis).

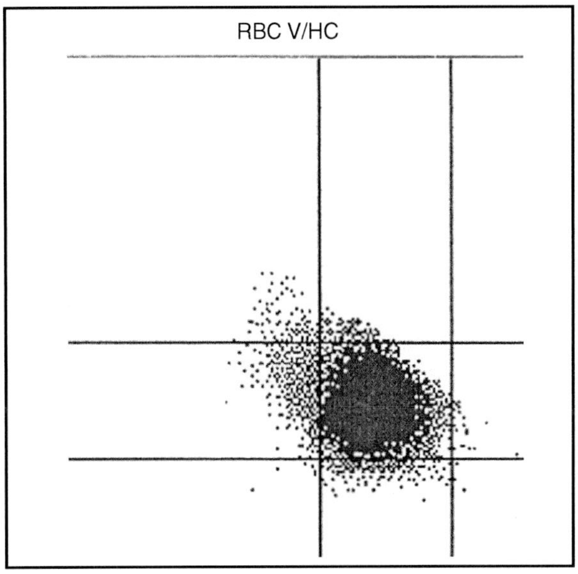

1.8 Red blood cell (RBC V/HC) scattergram from a resolving haemorrhagic anaemia, with haemoglobin concentration (*x* axis) plotted against red cell volume (*y* axis); the grid lines show set thresholds. In health, the majority of red cells fall in the central square, as seen here. Macrocytes would show in the top three rectangles and microcytes in the bottom three rectangles. Hypochromic red cells appear in the left three rectangles. Here, a slight shift up and to the left is evident, indicating immature red cells and a residual regenerative response. Prolonged effects of EDTA can mimic this pattern.

Blood smears

Whenever blood cannot be analysed within 2–3 hours it should be refrigerated at 4°C because erythrocyte swelling after 6–24 hours of storage at room temperature increases the PCV or Hct and MCV, so lowering the MCHC. These variables are unchanged for at least 24 hours in refrigerated blood. Samples sent to a laboratory by post can be expected to have artefacts caused by RBC swelling. The magnitude of these artefacts is unpredictable, and in many samples changes are minimal. Exposure to high or very low temperatures and damage during collection are highly detrimental to stored and transported blood samples. Samples must never be frozen as the thawing process completely destroys the cells.

Production of high quality blood smears (Figure 1.9) is a skill that can only be acquired with constant practice and is a matter of pride for most haematologists. Evenly spread blood smears are an absolute necessity for generating accurate and reproducible differential cell counts, as well as allowing detailed and reliable examination of cellular morphology. Veterinary surgeons are encouraged to submit a blood smear (fixed by air drying) to accompany the EDTA sample. Although these smears tend to have variable thickness (Figure 1.9) and are rarely used for differential cell counts, they can be extremely useful for distinguishing between changes in cell morphology caused by sample ageing and genuine diagnostic findings.

Staining

Blood smears are stained with Romanowsky stains such as Leishman's, modified Wright's or Giemsa. Staining must be consistent because the learned skills involved in morphological interpretation depend on examination of very large numbers of smears stained in exactly the same way. Staining can be done manually, but in laboratories with high turnover this becomes impractical. Automatic staining is consistent as long as blood smears are well made and homogeneous.

The Romanowsky stains are compound dyes that consist of a mixture of methylene blue and eosin, with several contaminating dyes that can alter staining characteristics. Methylene blue stains the acidic cell components such as nuclei and cytoplasmic RNA. Eosin is red and stains more basic components such as haemoglobin. The dyes are dissolved in methanol, which also acts as a fixative. Contamination of methanol with water will spoil the fixation and lead to loss of cell detail. The stain solutions must be kept free of water vapour in storage. This is a frequent cause of poor quality smears in laboratories where stains are made up in damp containers and not capped.

Diff-Quik style stains are simple haematological stains for use in practice. They are not strictly Romanowsky stains, but work on a similar principle, by using blue and orange dyes to give appropriate staining characteristics. The two dyes are in separate jars, and the intensity of blue and orange staining can be altered manually with the number of dips of the slide into each stain. Although easy and quick to perform, this method often results in a staining pattern that is very distorted, which can prevent colouring such as polychromasia being seen and falsely highlight certain white cell features.

All of these stains are finally rinsed off with either distilled water, or better, buffered water, because the pH of the dyes during staining is crucial in producing the required coloration. The use of tap water is not advised because its composition varies from day to day.

One further type of stain that is frequently used is 1% new methylene blue or brilliant cresyl blue. These are vital stains, which precipitate and dye the residual RNA in immature red cells, identifying them as reticulocytes. Blood anticoagulated with EDTA is mixed in equal parts with the dye and allowed to stand for 15–20 minutes. The blood is then resuspended and smeared for examination. The RNA within reticulocytes stains blue–black, whereas mature erythrocytes stain pale green.

Examination

Blood smears are scanned routinely without a cover slip with a ×10 or ×20 dry objective and then examined in detail at a higher magnification, using a ×40 dry or ×50 oil immersion objective. When using ×40 dry lenses, the cells will be slightly blurred if a cover slip (either mounted and glued or applied via a drop of thicker oil) is not used. Details of intracellular morphology, such as red cell parasites and toxic granulation, may require a ×100 oil immersion objective.

Routine differential leucocyte counts are based on at least 100 cells counted in a specific area of the smear. The area of the film selected is critical because differently sized cells spread at different rates, and the largest tend to be found in the tail and edges of the smear. The cells are counted in the body of the film (the monolayer) where the smear is

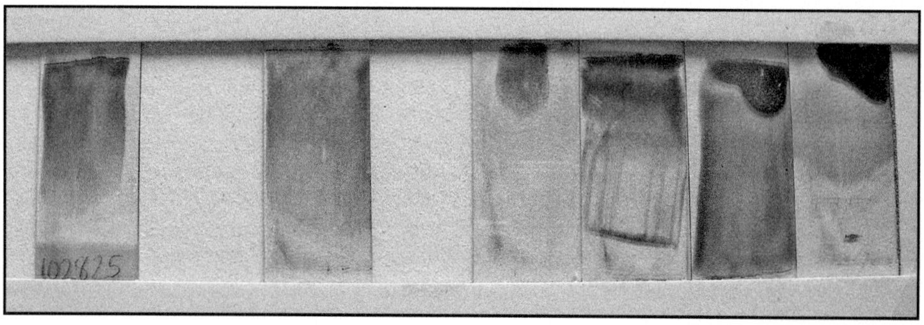

1.9 Several blood smears: the well made smear on the far left will allow accurate and reproducible examination and counting. Those to the far right can be used, but the cells may be altered and unevenly distributed, precluding accurate analysis.

one cell thick and where the individual cells are separated sufficiently to make individual cell morphology and abnormal aggregation clear (Figures 1.10 and 1.11). When counting, both the peripheral and the central areas should be included to prevent biased representation of either smaller or larger cells if only the centre or the periphery, respectively, is counted. The rest of the smear, including the tail, is then scanned for atypical or neoplastic cells, parasites and platelet clumps. The percentage differential leucocyte counts are multiplied by the total nucleated cell count to obtain the total differential counts.

Morphological comments on platelets, erythrocytes and leucocytes are recorded and graded subjectively (such as mild, moderate and marked) as an annotation to the haematological profile. Abnormal morphological features only may be noted.

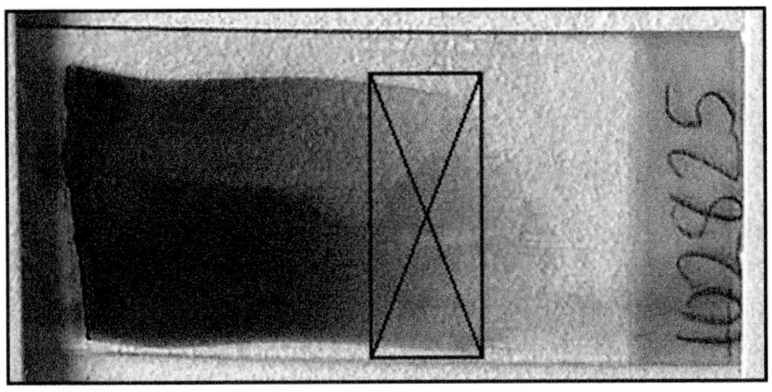

1.10 A good fresh blood smear: the hatched rectangular area shows the monolayer for examination of cell morphology and differential counts.

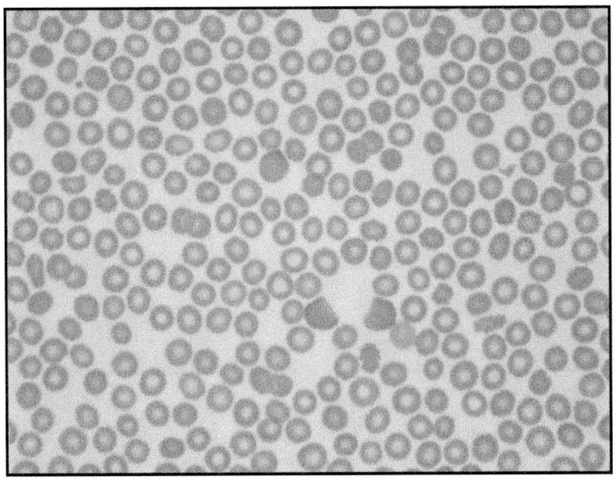

1.11 High power view of the monolayer area for accurate and reproducible morphological examination (original magnification ×500, modified Wright's stain).

Blood cell morphology and interpretation

Erythrocyte morphology

The size, colour, shape and stage of development of erythrocytes can all be assessed microscopically and they have great diagnostic significance. Please refer to the erythrocyte morphology index (EMI) page at the end of this chapter for images unless otherwise indicated. Healthy normal red cells are circular pale-centred discs, central pallor being much less prominent in cats (Figure 1.12; EMI 1 and 2). These cells are normochromic and normocytic.

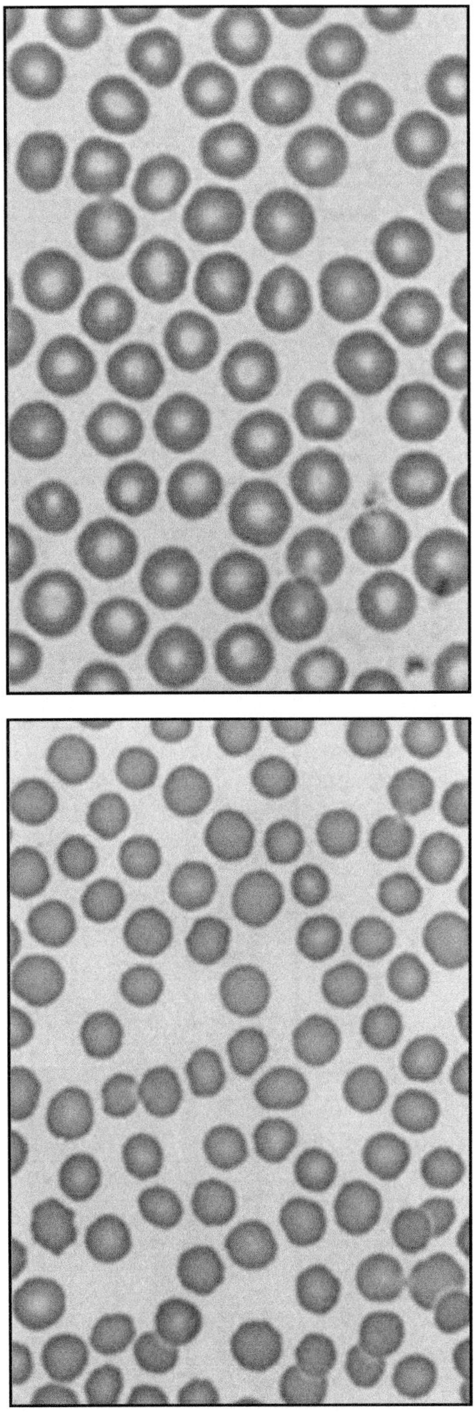

1.12 Healthy normochromic normocytic erythrocytes, canine above, feline below (original magnification ×500, modified Wright's stain).

Anisocytosis

Anlsocytosls Is a term applled when the erythrocytes in a smear are of variable, rather than consistent, volume or size (Figure 1.13). Subjective assessment and grading should correlate with the automated RDW, both being increased and evident before there is any change in the MCV. Anisocytosis is frequently seen in both regenerative and non-regenerative anaemias.

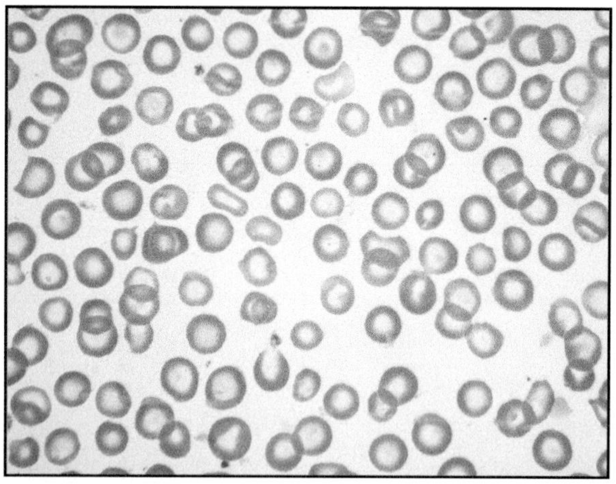

1.13 Anisocytosis, with normal, larger (macrocytic) and smaller (microcytic) red blood cells seen during regeneration with chronic haemorrhage (original magnification ×500, modified Wright's stain).

Macrocytes

Macrocytes are large erythrocytes, often equivalent in size to a mature neutrophil (Figure 1.14). They are often polychromatic (containing increased blue-staining RNA) immature erythrocytes and may be hypochromic. Breed-related normochromic macrocytosis is a normal finding in some Miniature Poodles. Abnormal numbers of macrocytes occur in damaged or aged samples as an artefact of erythrocyte swelling, especially if the sample tube is under-filled. They are produced in a regenerative response to blood loss or haemolysis. Normochromic macrocytes can be associated with feline leukaemia virus (FeLV) subgroup A infection in kittens and with myeloproliferative disorders of both dogs and cats.

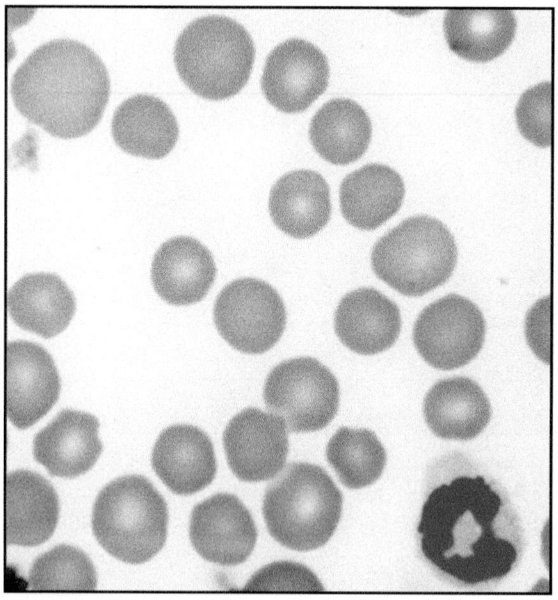

1.14 High power view showing a normochromic macrocyte (top left) in relation to a mature segmented neutrophil (bottom right), with the top of a polychromatic reticulocyte (bottom centre) (original magnification ×1000, modified Wright's stain).

Microcytes

Microcytes are small erythrocytes. They may be normochromic (normal Hb content) or hypochromic (reduced Hb content). Certain breeds such as Akitas, Shiba Inus, Chows and Shar Peis can naturally have unusually small erythrocytes that also can have a higher potassium content compared with those of other dog breeds.

Normochromic microcytes occur in anaemia of chronic inflammation. Hypochromic microcytes are important markers of altered iron metabolism and are present in dogs with iron deficiency and also in dogs with portosystemic shunts. The most common cause of iron deficiency in dogs is chronic occult blood loss from the gastrointestinal tract (Figure 1.15). The abnormality of iron metabolism in animals with portosystemic shunts is ineffective iron utilization, which leads to accumulation of iron in tissues, but reduced incorporation of iron into erythrocytes. The underlying abnormality is likely to be altered hepcidin production due to reduced functional hepatic mass. Hepcidin is the principal hormone involved in iron regulation and is synthesized and secreted by the liver.

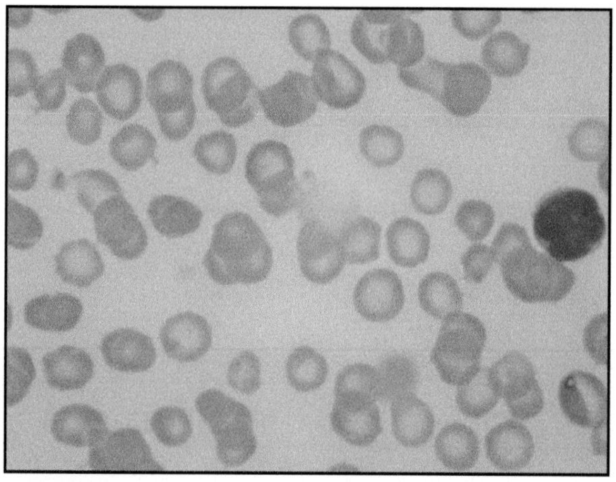

1.15 Microcytic hypochromic anaemia with polychromasia and anisocytosis in a dog with chronic gastrointestinal haemorrhage (original magnification ×500, modified Wright's stain).

Poikilocytosis

This is a generic term for any variation in erythrocyte shape. Erythrocytes are circular, so any uneven projections, cell fragments or loss of central pallor should be noted. Certain shapes can be seen in certain diseases; however, many shapes are not disease specific, but they do indicate processes or possibly artefacts that are significant and warrant further investigation. If many different shapes are seen (Figure 1.16), the general term poikilocytosis is used, but otherwise more specific terms are used, as below.

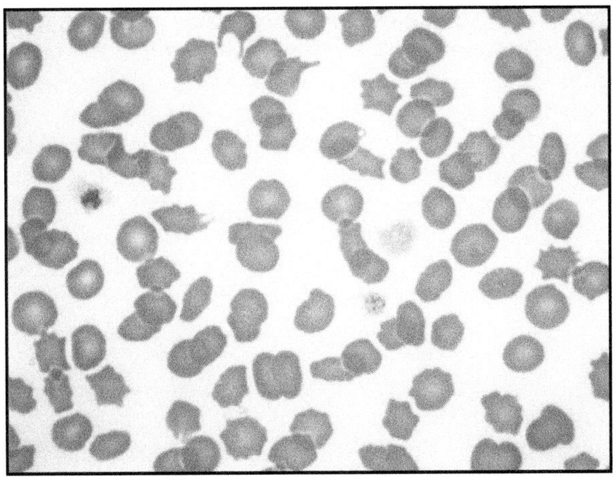

1.16 Poikilocytosis with several different non-circular and non-discoid shapes seen, including blister cells, pyknocytes, keratocytes and elliptocytes; no one specific form dominates (original magnification ×500, modified Wright's stain).

Echinocytes (Burr cells)

Echinocytes are regularly spiculated or scalloped erythrocytes, with evenly sized and distributed surface projections (EMI 5). They can be divided into three types (I, II and III), some being more specific for a particular disease process. They usually arise as an *in vitro* artefact caused by crenation during cell drying (types I and II).

Echinocytes that are not caused by crenation are seen in some dogs with lymphoma, chronic renal disease, glomerulonephritis or chronic doxorubicin toxicosis. Type III (regular multiple sharp fine projections) can be seen with snake envenomation, possibly owing to the action of phospholipases.

Spherocytes

Spherocytes are smaller and more densely stained spherical erythrocytes that lack central pallor (EMI 6). They adopt a spherical shape after a reduction in the cell membrane area (and hence surface area to volume ratio) caused by partial phagocytosis by mononuclear phagocytes. Feline RBCs have a lower MCV and less appreciable central pallor than canine RBCs, so spherocytes are rarely recognized in cats. The presence of spherocytes implies that the
erythrocytes have surface-bound antibody or complement, which is recognized by cell surface receptors on phagocytes. Spherocytes are less deformable than normal erythrocytes and consequently are osmotically fragile. The presence of spherocytes is a sensitive indicator of immune-mediated haemolytic anaemia (IMHA) in dogs.

Codocytes (target cells)

Codocytes are hat-shaped erythrocytes that, when viewed in two dimensions, have a dense centre surrounded by a clear area and a peripheral haemoglobin rim (EMI 7). This bizarre shape is adopted because of increases in the cholesterol to phopholipid ratio within the cell membrane. Reticulocytes have increased surface to volume ratio and can also appear as target cells in two dimensions, but this is not indicative of any underlying process other than the presence of red cell regeneration. Codocytes are commonly seen with regenerative responses and following corticosteroid therapy in dogs but may also be present in iron-deficiency anaemia, liver disease with cholestasis and after splenectomy in dogs.

Acanthocytes

Acanthocytes are irregularly spiculated erythrocytes with a few unevenly distributed surface projections of variable diameter and length (EMI 8). Similar to codocytes, acanthocytes may occur as a result of alterations in the cholesterol:phospholipid ratio of the cell membrane but can also be seen in association with RBC fragmentation. Acanthocytes are seen in dogs with diseases of capillary beds (microvascular angiopathies) such as splenic haemangioma/ haemangiosarcoma, diffuse liver disease or vasculitis.

Schistocytes

Schistocytes are irregular small erythrocyte fragments that result from mechanical trauma to circulating erythrocytes (EMI 9). They are markers of disseminated intravascular coagulation (DIC) and other microvascular angiopathies and are seen in patients with IMHA, thrombosis, splenic neoplasia, hypersplenism, glomerulonephritis, congestive heart failure, valvular heart disease, doxorubicin toxicosis and myelofibrosis.

Eccentrocytes

Eccentrocytes are erythrocytes in which oxidative damage causes fusion of opposing cell membranes on one edge of the erythrocyte. This has the effect of squeezing haemoglobin into a smaller volume. When viewed in two dimensions the fused membranes appear as a clear semicircle, whereas the compressed haemoglobin appears eccentric and darker than normal (EMI 10).

Eccentrocytes are a sensitive indicator of oxidative damage to blood cells in dogs. They may form following exposure to oxidative drugs but the most common cause of eccentrocytic anaemias in dogs is onion poisoning. Cats are more sensitive than dogs to oxidative erythrocyte damage, but this is more often manifested by the formation of numerous Heinz bodies than by eccentrocytes.

Erythrocyte inclusions

Erythrocyte inclusions of importance include parasites, Howell–Jolly Bodies, Heinz bodies and basophilic stippling.

Feline haemoplasmas: These organisms are highly pleomorphic and stain with variable intensity, appearing as chains, discs or rods on the surface of erythrocytes (EMI 11). They should not be confused with stain precipitate, which is more variable and refractile in nature. The presence of organisms within the blood is very variable and episodic, and

PCR testing is recommended if haemoplasmosis is suspected.

Babesia: *Babesia* spp. are intracellular basophilic tear-drop shaped to circular parasites of canine erythrocytes, which cause major morbidity in tropical and subtropical areas of the world (EMI 12). They are transmitted by various species of tick, particularly *Rhipicephalus sanguineus*. Canine babesiosis is not endemic in the United Kingdom, but cases have been documented since the introduction of the pet passport.

Heinz bodies: Heinz bodies are small, highly refractile bodies that stain poorly with Wright's stain and well with supravital stains. They are eccentrically located beneath the erythrocyte cell membrane or protrude through it (EMI 13). Heinz bodies are formed by irreversible precipitation of oxidatively denatured Hb. They are markers of oxidative damage, for example in paracetamol (acetaminophen) toxicosis in cats or in severe inflammatory states that involve the release of free radicals, such as feline pancreatitis.

Howell–Jolly bodies: Howell–Jolly bodies are purple- to black-staining, spherical and usually eccentric structures within the erythrocyte (EMI 14). They are remnants of the incompletely extruded metrarubricyte nucleus. They are seen with a regenerative response, but if this is not evident and numbers are increased, they usually reflect reticuloendothelial, particularly splenic, dysfunction or bone marrow disease.

Basophilic stippling

Basophilic stippling of erythrocytes and precursors (e.g. reticulocytes and metarubricytes) is characterized by the presence of punctate or reticulated basophilic granules (clumped ribosomes; EMI 15). Basophilic stippling can be seen with marked regenerative responses, or dysplastic regenerative responses in cats, and it occurs in lead poisoning where it can be associated with the presence of increased numbers of nucleated precursors, such as metarubricytes and rubricytes, but without the expected polychromasia.

Reticulocytes

The normal morphological response to blood loss is a regenerative pattern with many reticulocytes and fewer metarubricytes. In a normal Wright's or Giemsa-stained blood smear reticulocytes appear as large polychromatic cells (see Figure 1.11; EMI 3). When stained with new methylene blue, the reticulocytes show an internal reticulated pattern of RNA material and condensed organelles (EMI 16). A smear stained with new methylene blue or brilliant cresyl blue is used for the reticulocyte count, which is an objective index of the degree of regeneration.

In cats, reticulocytes show punctate (dots) or aggregate (clusters and lines) patterns of condensed organelles. This is a more prominent and significant feature of the maturation of reticulocytes in the cat. In feline regenerative responses, aggregate reticulocytes are released first. After a short maturation time of around 12 hours, the aggregate form becomes a punctate reticulocyte, which has a maturation time of 10–12 days. Aggregate reticulocytes therefore reflect active regeneration and equate to the degree of polychromasia in a smear, whereas punctate reticulocytes reflect recent cumulative regeneration, are not polychromatic and persist for a few weeks after a single episode of red cell loss.

Automated reticulocyte counting can be performed by some flow cytometers. With expensive analysers, the count can be accurate and very sensitive, especially in dogs, and may possibly be better and more reproducible than traditional reticulocyte counting in a smear when closely monitoring regeneration or identifying early iron deficiency. The usefulness of machine counts in cats for punctate versus aggregate discrimination is less clear and other inclusions (e.g. DNA and haemoparasites) may also stain and falsely elevate the count. Smaller cheaper flow cytometers do not perform as well, and do not always identify a significant regenerative response, with a negative proportional bias, the reproducibility also being variable (Becker *et al.*, 2008).

Nucleated red blood cells (nRBCs)

The nRBCs seen most frequently in the peripheral circulation are metarubricytes (EMI 4). These have a condensed pyknotic and more central circular nucleus with an equal volume of polychromatic (bluish staining) or normochromic (the colour of mature erythrocytes) cytoplasm. Rubricytes have a round viable nucleus that has a purple to black fractured texture, are larger than metarubricytes and are less commonly seen.

The presence of more than rare nRBCs in the circulation is always important. Metarubricytes appear during bone marrow regenerative responses to haemolysis or blood loss. They may also be liberated after extramedullary haematopoiesis in the reticuloendothelial system. They are typically present in dogs with splenic disease such as haemangiosarcoma and also occur in splenectomized individuals. The presence of earlier erythrocyte precursors (rubricytes and prorubricytes) in the circulation usually implies quite severe bone marrow or reticuloendothelial disease, but can occasionally be seen in association with very marked regenerative responses. Crucially they are seen at much lower frequency than their more mature counterparts, such that there is a pyramidal increase in numbers from rare rubricytes, frequent metarubricytes to common reticulocytes and mature erythrocytes.

Leucocyte morphology

Important morphological features of leucocytes include immaturity, abnormal cytoplasmic granulation and rarely infectious inclusions. Please refer to the leucocyte morphology index (LMI) page at the end of this chapter for images unless otherwise indicated.

Neutrophils

Mature neutrophils are 1.5–2 times the size of a red cell and have a long thin segmented/lobulated nucleus, with uneven but well defined nuclear margins and abundant, lightly eosinophilic to off-white, slightly granulated cytoplasm (LMI 1 and 2). Immature neutrophils are termed bands and are recognizable because the nucleus is elongated, but parallel sided and not lobulated (LMI 5). Metamyelocytes are larger than mature neutrophils and have a similar cytoplasm, but the nucleus is kidney bean shaped and not lobulated. Metamyelocytes can be difficult to distinguish from monocytes, because both potentially have reniform nuclei and blue cytoplasm. Crucially, metamyelocyte nuclei are dark purple and dense, similar to those of mature neutrophils, whereas monocytes have lighter, pink–purple and more open reticular chromatin (Figure 1.17).

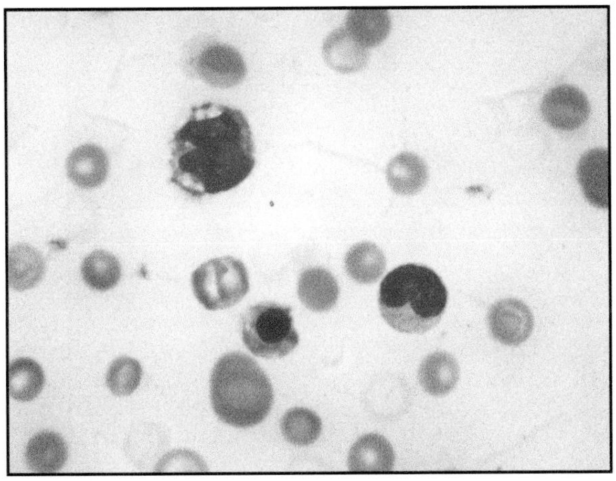

1.17 High power view showing an anaemic dog with anisocytosis and polychromasia. The three nucleated cells, clockwise from top left, are a monocyte, a metamyelocyte and a metarubricyte (original magnification ×500, modified Wright's stain).

The presence of immature neutrophils (band neutrophils and metamyelocytes) in the peripheral circulation is termed a 'left shift' and is either a response to increased neutrophil consumption by inflammatory and infectious processes or an abnormal increase in neutrophil production. When mature neutrophils greatly outnumber the immature forms and the mature neutrophil count is increased, the left shift is termed 'regenerative' and indicates that the immune system is coping with the inflammatory or infectious process. If the immature forms outnumber the mature forms, the left shift is termed 'degenerative', and is a poor prognostic sign. The combination of a low mature neutrophil count with a degenerative left shift is a grave prognostic sign, especially if persistent for more than 24 hours. The appearance of metamyelocytes in a left shift suggests a potent inflammatory or regenerative stimulus. If even earlier granulocyte forms appear, myeloproliferative disease and other disorders of bone marrow should be considered, as well as intense inflammation and neutrophil consumption caused by diseases such as gastrointestinal ulceration. This process will be compounded if drugs such as corticosteroids are involved. Regenerative left shifts are nearly always associated with systemic inflammation, except in unusual circumstances such as the administration of granulocyte/monocyte colony stimulating factor (GM-CSF). The observation that anaemias with marked regeneration (e.g. IMHA) are very frequently accompanied by a significant left shift has often been interpreted as a reflection of non-specific stimulation of the granulocyte cell line by mediators of RBC regeneration. There is continuing debate about this, but current research suggests that the left shift is actually associated with neutrophil consumption due to tissue damage and the systemic inflammatory response which either initiates, or is induced by, the haemolytic anaemia (McManus and Craig, 1999).

Occasionally, the regenerative response to an inflammatory stimulus is so excessive that enormously high neutrophil counts with a primitive left shift are generated. This is termed a 'leukaemoid response' and can be impossible to distinguish from myeloid leukaemia on morphological grounds alone.

'Toxic change' is a collective term for morphological features that develop in neutrophils as a result of disturbed or quickened cellular maturation in the bone marrow, often associated with marked inflammatory or septic processes or, more rarely, dysplasia with bone marrow disease. It can be seen in metamyelocytes, band neutrophils and mature segmented neutrophils, being seen commonly in overwhelming sepsis. The spectrum of toxic changes in canine and feline neutrophils correlates approximately with the severity and duration of the stimulus. One of the earliest changes is the presence of multiple irregular pale blue clumps called Döhle bodies (lamellar aggregates of rough endoplasmic reticulum) in the cytoplasm (LMI 6). As 'toxicity' becomes more severe, the cytoplasm becomes more deeply basophilic and develops a foamy appearance, but without discrete vacuoles (LMI 7). Intensely stained primary granules may also be apparent. Finally, the nucleus swells and the nuclear envelope appears ragged (LMI 8). Döhle bodies may be less useful for indicating disease severity or prognosis in cats than in dogs because they seem to be present earlier in the disease course or with milder clinical signs (Segev *et al.*, 2006). They are variously reported at low numbers in apparently healthy cats too, so they may not be specific or may possibly represent EDTA-induced artefactual effects.

Hereditary abnormalities of neutrophils occur occasionally in dogs and cats. Pelger–Huët anomaly has been reported in both species and is a failure of the normal nuclear maturation of neutrophils. The mature cells have a parallel-sided nucleus and mimic bands. Chédiak–Higashi syndrome has been reported in Persian cats and is characterized by poorly functioning neutrophils with giant eosinophilic intracytoplasmic granules. Large cytoplasmic vacuolation of neutrophils may be seen in storage disorders such as α-mannosidosis. Small irregular vacuoles due to *in vitro* degeneration should not be mistaken for this, and unlike storage diseases they are associated with coalescing nuclear lobes and loss of chromatin texturing.

Eosinophils

Eosinophils are 2–3 times the size of a red cell and have very recognizable morphology with bright pink–red uniformly stained granules in pale basophilic cytoplasm and a polymorphic nucleus, which is smoother, paler and less segmented than that of a neutrophil. Feline eosinophils usually have smaller, denser and more regular rod-shaped granules (LMI 10). Canine eosinophilic granules are much more variable in size and density, and may be single and large, while others have clear white cytoplasmic vacuolation because the granules do not stain (LMI 9). In some individuals and in certain breeds such as the Greyhound, eosinophils can be highly vacuolated with little to no identifiable pink–red granulation evident (Iazbik and Couto, 2008).

Basophils

Canine and feline basophils have rather unusual morphology and can easily be missed by inexperienced haematologists, often being mistaken for monocytes. The canine mature basophil is usually larger than a neutrophil and has a lobulated or strap-like nucleus. The cytoplasm is lightly basophilic with occasional large dark purple granules (LMI 11). Immature basophils tend to have more prominent granulation. Canine basophils can also be mistaken for highly toxic neutrophils, leading to errors in interpretation. Feline basophils have similar nuclear features, but as with feline eosinophils, have denser, smaller and more regular pale grey to lilac granules (LMI 12) that can be mistaken for eosinophil granules, especially if poorly stained.

Monocytes

Monocytes are the largest and most variable white cell and have amoeboid morphology (LMI 13–16). Monocytes can be differentiated from other large blood cells such as metamyelocytes by their blue ground-glass cytoplasm and, more crucially, their reticulated or ribbon-like, paler and pinker nuclear chromatin. The nuclear shape is variable, from convoluted to reniform, dumb-bell or C-shaped. Transformation of monocytes to active vacuolated and occasionally phagocytic macrophages in the circulation can be seen in severe chronic inflammatory processes such as bacterial endocarditis or IMHA.

Lymphocytes

Circulating lymphocytes have variable size and morphology. They can be small, medium or large, with nuclei varying from round to cleaved and convoluted. The most consistent features of lymphocytes are a coarsely clumped chromatin pattern and the presence of small quantities of basophilic cytoplasm.

The typical small lymphocyte has an eccentric round- or bean-shaped nucleus approximately the diameter of an RBC, with a thin rim of basophilic cytoplasm (LMI 3). Reactive lymphocytes are larger and have an increased volume of more basophilic cytoplasm than quiescent lymphocytes (Figure 1.18a and b). Larger granular lymphocytes in very low numbers are a normal finding (LMI 4). These have increased lightly basophilic cytoplasm containing

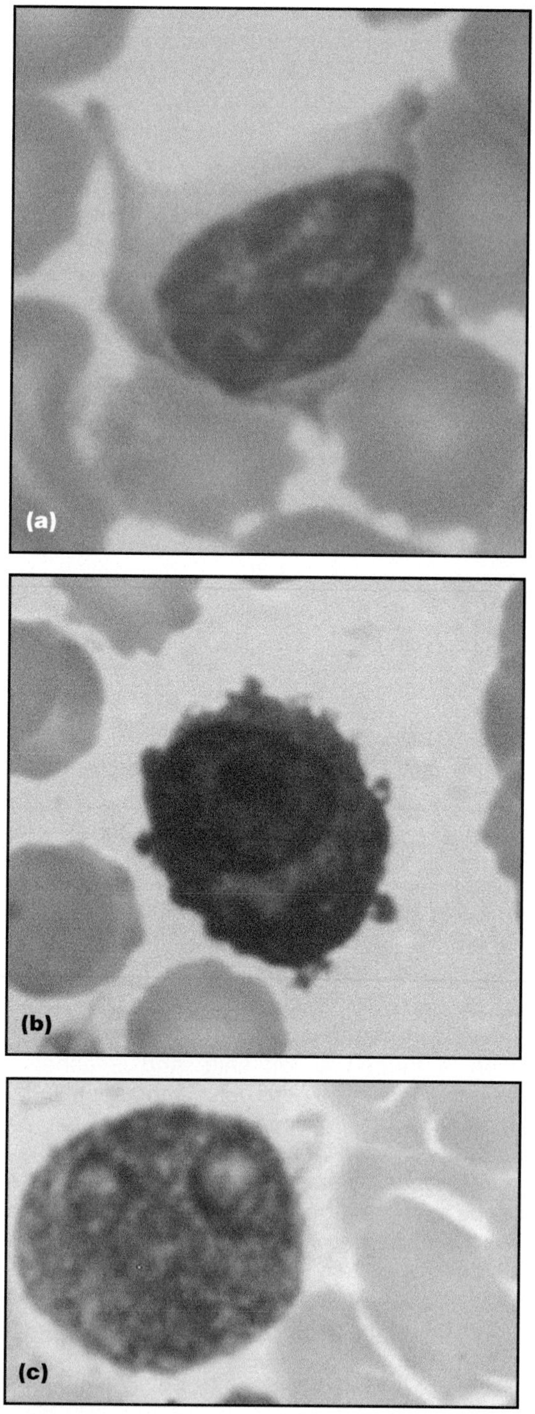

1.18 **(a)** Reactive lymphocyte with expanded amoeboid smooth dark blue cytoplasm. **(b)** Plasmacytoid lymphocyte with very dark blue cytoplasm and whiter perinuclear clearing. **(c)** Lymphoblast with irregular clumped chromatin, two prominent nucleoli and a small quantity of blue cytoplasm (All are ×1000 original magnification; modified Wright's stain).

small azurophilic granules and are cytotoxic T cells or natural killer (NK) cells. These and reactive lymphocytes, including rare large blastoid forms, are seen in younger diseased animals, especially those with systemic inflammation, and can be associated with a lymphocytosis.

Lymphoblasts are large lymphocytes that contain one or more prominent nucleoli (Figure 1.18c); their presence in the peripheral circulation is always of note and is usually associated with stage IV–V lymphoma or lymphoid leukaemia. Neoplastic lymphocytes can be fragile and are often damaged during preparation of the blood smear. The damaged cells are referred to as 'smear cells' or 'basket cells' and should be viewed with suspicion when observed in large numbers.

Platelet morphology

Platelets are anucleate structures, which have a lightly basophilic to pale pink granular staining pattern and are typically smaller than red cells (Figure 1.19a). Feline platelets are often more variable and larger (mean volume 17 fl) than canine examples (mean volume 11 fl). They have poorly defined cytoplasmic margins and often appear to have small hair-like projections from the surface. Giant platelets or macroplatelets, often larger than RBCs, occur in platelet regenerative responses and are a normal finding in some breeds, notably the Cavalier King Charles Spaniel (Figure 1.19b). Platelets (especially feline platelets) tend to form clumps in anticoagulants such as EDTA, which cause artefactually low automated platelet counts. The presence of platelet clumps in the tail of a blood smear is an indication that the automated platelet count will be erroneous. Unclumped platelets are normally scattered among the other blood cells in the smear.

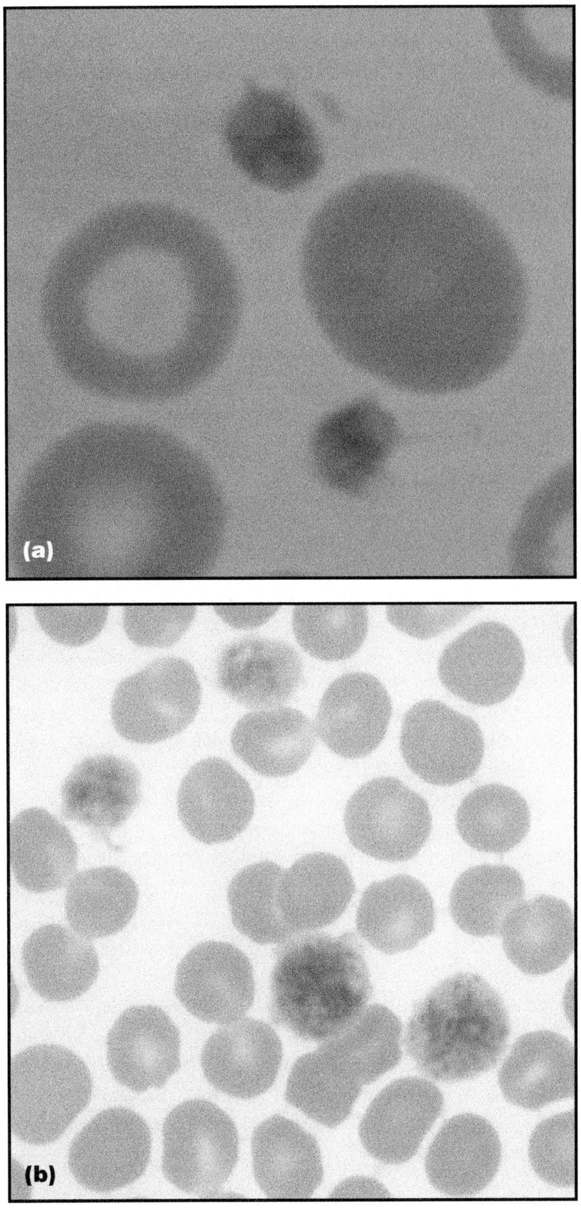

1.19 **(a)** Two platelets, top and bottom, with an irregular outline and fine pink irregular grainy cytoplasm (original magnification ×500, modified Wright's). **(b)** Four macroplatelets, similar in size or larger than red cells, from a Cavalier King Charles Spaniel (original magnification ×500, modified Wright's stain).

Interpreting the haematological profile

The standard haematological profile includes measurements of the variables listed previously. The profile must be interpreted as a whole, noting normal as well as abnormal values. A systematic approach to interpretation is important, aided by consistent presentation of the information. Data in an unusual format can lead to human error.

Erythrocyte variables

The Hb concentration must first be noted, because this is the most direct assessment of anaemia presuming no interfering factor such as lipaemia is evident. Then check the Hct. If the Hct is increased, compare with the erythrocyte numbers and MCV. Genuine erythrocytosis is unlikely if the erythrocyte numbers are within the reference range. Increased MCV is quite a common cause of an increased Hct and is typical of aged samples with erythrocyte swelling. Frequently, an increase in the Hct is due to relative haemoconcentration (splenic contraction) or dehydration.

Anaemia is present if the Hb concentration is below the reference range regardless of the erythrocyte numbers and the Hct, but in the majority of anaemias all three variables will be low. If anaemia is present, attempt to classify it by studying the MCV, MCHC and the comments on erythrocyte morphology. Many standard texts use the MCV as the primary index for the presence or absence of regeneration. This is surprising, because the MCV varies unpredictably with sample ageing, and many regenerative anaemias are not characterized by an MCV above reference intervals (see Figure 1.7). The presence or absence of polychromasia in the stained smear is a much more reliable index of regeneration. If there is polychromasia, then regeneration is present. The amount of polychromasia and the nRBC count usually reflect the adequacy of regeneration accurately, but in occasional cases a reticulocyte count will be needed to provide an objective index for monitoring regeneration. However, the presence of increased nRBCs alone with no polychromasia does not support appropriate regeneration, and is often seen with hepatosplenic or bone marrow disease.

It is customary to use the absolute reticulocyte count for the quantitative assessment of regeneration in dogs and cats. In cats the aggregate reticulocyte count is used to indicate current regeneration, whereas the punctate reticulocyte count is more indicative of the recent history of regeneration. Reticulocyte counts above 60 × 10^9/l in dogs and 50 × 10^9/l aggregate reticulocytes in cats indicate regeneration. The degree of regeneration is approximately proportional to the absolute count, and the adequacy of regeneration is interpreted in the context of the RBC variables and the clinical features of each case of anaemia. The adequacy of regeneration in any individual case may be assessed more objectively by using the reticulocyte production index (RPI), which is a ratio examining the reticulocyte count in relation to the HCT, but it is based upon human studies and has yet to be assessed properly in cats and dogs.

In most regenerative anaemias, the MCV is normal or high. One exception to this is the special situation of chronic blood loss in which the patient begins to become iron deficient. Such cases will have mixed erythrocyte morphology featuring increased polychromasia and also a progressively increasing percentage of microcytic cells. The MCV in such cases may be below the reference interval. In non-regenerative anaemias the MCV is usually normal or low. Rare cases of non-regenerative anaemia with increased MCV may be associated with myeloproliferative disease, especially FeLV-related disease in cats.

The MCHC is a calculated variable that expresses the mean Hb concentration per erythrocyte. Hypochromic anaemias may have a low MCHC. The MCH is a calculated variable that expresses the mean quantity of Hb per erythrocyte and, unlike the MCHC, does not take into account the volume of the erythrocyte. Thus microcytes will automatically have low MCH but may not be hypochromic. In such cases the MCHC will be normal.

Careful assessment of the morphology of the erythrocytes is of critical importance in the classification of anaemia. Morphological abnormalities such as the formation of spherocytes and eccentrocytes are highly sensitive indicators of underlying diseases such as IMHA and oxidative damage. The blood film examination also checks the interpretive validity of changes in the RBC indices; for example, if the MCHC and MCV are low the film should contain microcytic hypochromic erythrocytes. If not, significant numbers of macroplatelets may be present and the automated analyser may have miscounted these as red cells.

Erythrocyte morphology should also be noted when anaemia is not present. Polychromasia and nRBCs may indicate ongoing mild blood loss, which is balanced by erythrocyte production and therefore does not decrease the Hb concentration and PCV below the reference range. The presence of nRBCs in the absence of anaemia may also be an indicator of splenic or bone marrow disorders.

Automated platelet count

If the automated platelet count is low, the tail and sides of the blood film should be examined for the presence of platelet clumps, which are the commonest cause of pseudothrombocytopenia. The presence of large clumps is usually assumed to indicate a normal platelet count. When platelets are not clumped an average count of more than 10 per high power field (hpf, ×100) indicates adequate platelet numbers in dogs and cats. A useful film estimate of platelet numbers can be obtained by averaging 10 hpf and multiplying by 15–20. Macrothrombocytes may also cause erroneously low counts. Genuine thrombocytopenia alone is rarely considered to cause the classic signs of petechiation and ecchymoses unless the count is below 30 × 10^9/l. Concurrent disease may increase the risk of clinical bleeding, and screening for secondary coagulation defects is recommended if the platelet count is low and red cell fragments (schistocytes) are seen. Mild thrombocytopenia is non-specific and can be seen transiently with acute inflammation or infection, reduced marrow production producing variably low numbers. Immune-mediated thrombocytopenia (IMTP) is commonly associated with marked thrombocytopenia.

Thrombocytosis occurs relatively frequently in dogs and cats and may be due to several different processes. Mild thrombocytosis is often non-specific and associated with (established) inflammatory processes. Recently a correlation between persistent thrombocytosis and occult underlying neoplasia has been described (Snyder *et al.*, 2007). In dogs it is also a feature of the haematological pattern of iron deficiency, and erythrocyte variables should be checked carefully for evidence of hypochromia and microcytosis. Thrombocytosis is the first change seen in some cases of myeloproliferative disease.

Total leucocyte count

It is important to remember that the leucocyte count is actually a count of nucleated cells, and large numbers of nRBCs can produce an erroneously increased count. If a high percentage of nRBCs is present, the leucocyte count is corrected by the appropriate factor.

Differential leucocyte counts

Differential leucocyte counts should always be interpreted as total counts rather than percentage counts. Percentage counts should be regarded as a means to calculate the total counts and have little inherent interpretive value. Each differential leucocyte count should first be classified as normal, increased or decreased (e.g. absolute neutrophilia or neutropenia), then the overall leucocyte pattern can be assessed. The major patterns are the inflammatory leucogram, the stress leucogram, the leukaemoid response, various cytopenias and genuine leukaemias. Leucocyte counts and morphology must be assessed together.

Leucocyte patterns

Inflammatory leucogram

The classic inflammatory pattern is neutrophilia with a left shift and monocytosis. This pattern is typically seen in sepsis, severe localized infections and tissue necrosis. Neutrophilia with a left shift but no monocytosis often reflects a less well established or more acute inflammatory process. In longstanding inflammatory and/or infectious processes such as granulomatous disease and draining sinus tracts, the inflammatory pattern may evolve into a mature neutrophilia without a left shift but with monocytosis and lymphocytosis. Occasionally the only evidence for chronic inflammation is monocytosis. Regenerative and degenerative left shifts and leukaemoid responses are discussed above. The presence or absence of the morphological signs of neutrophil 'toxicity' is critical in patients with inflammatory leucograms because toxicity is considered a marker for the presence of underlying bacterial infection. Toxicity is also a significant prognostic factor.

Absolute eosinophilia is an inflammatory pattern with several different associations. Eosinophilia can be seen as an adjunct to neutrophilia, left shift neutrophilia and monocytosis in non-specific inflammatory processes, particularly in cats. Other causes of eosinophilia include hypersensitivity, parasitism, eosinophilic diseases and paraneoplastic eosinophilia, which may occur in various neoplastic diseases including lymphoma and systemic mastocytosis. Eosinophilic diseases of importance in dogs include eosinophilic bronchitis and enteritis. The cat shares these diseases, with the addition of the eosinophilic granuloma complex.

Stress leucogram

Stress leucograms are associated with the influence of stress hormones such as catecholamines and glucocorticoids. During acute stress, (young) cats may develop lymphocytosis and/or neutrophilia as result of catecholamine release. Lymphopenia may develop subsequently as a result of corticosteroid release during chronic stress. Dogs are less prone to catecholamine-induced haematological responses than cats, but are more sensitive to glucocorticoids. The canine stress leucogram has several patterns. Perhaps the most common pattern is absolute eosinopenia, followed by lymphopenia and then a combination of both. Less frequently, dogs can develop massive mature neutrophilia in response to glucocorticoids, and this response may mimic a chronic inflammatory pattern. It is quite common for dogs to have combined inflammatory and stress leucograms (e.g. neutrophilia with a left shift, monocytosis, lymphopenia and eosinopenia). Conversely, without endogenous corticosteroids the opposite can be seen, especially in dogs, with hypoadrenocorticism not uncommonly being associated with a mild eosinophilia and/or lymphocytosis, or at least, unremarkable lymphocyte and eosinophil counts in a clinically stressed dog.

Cytopenias

The stress leucogram, described above, is the most common cause of lymphopenia and eosinopenia. Persistent neutropenia is a significant haematological finding. The short intravascular life span of neutrophils (7–14 hours) makes them early markers of bone marrow dysfunction. The combination of non-regenerative anaemia, thrombocytopenia and granulocytopenia is termed pancytopenia and is invariably associated with severe bone marrow disease, assuming no iatrogenic factors such as general anaesthesia are present. Cytopenias that involve any two cell lines should also be regarded as suspicious of bone marrow disease.

Neutropenia is a feature of acute viral infections (e.g. parvovirus or distemper). Non-specific reversible neutropenia occurs quite commonly in dogs with gastroenteritis and is probably associated with margination of neutrophils in the gastrointestinal tract in response to the presence of local enterotoxins. Neutropenia can also be seen in patients with severe degenerative left shifts caused by overwhelming infectious or inflammatory processes. In such cases the neutrophils often exhibit toxic morphology. Cobalamin deficiency can also create only a neutropenia, and this may be hereditary in certain breeds such as Border Collies.

Leukaemia

Acute or immature leukaemia can usually be differentiated from an inflammatory response by the presence of blast cells in the peripheral circulation, although occasionally leukaemoid responses may also have blast cells. Genuine leukaemia may present with monotonous leucocyte morphology, often with inappropriate numbers of cells at each stage of maturation (Figure 1.20). Examination of a

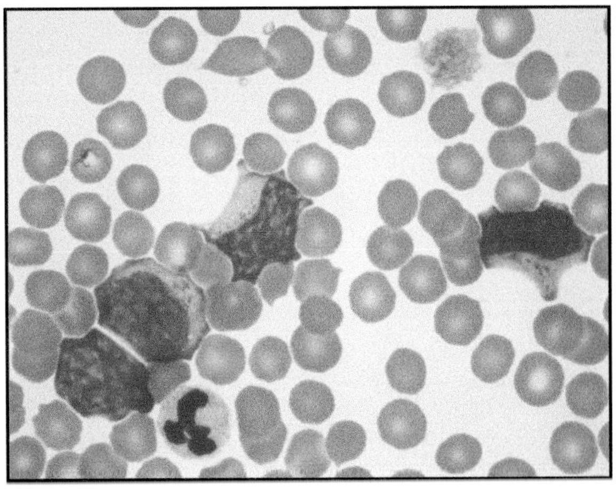

1.20 High power view showing mild red cell anisocytosis, a macroplatelet (top right), mature neutrophil (centre lower left) and four azurophilic granular leukaemic lymphoblasts in an acute lymphoid leukaemia (original magnification ×500, modified Wright's stain).

fresh blood film is crucial in the diagnosis of leukaemias, which automated analysis will often not identify. However, some types, such as chronic granulocytic leukaemia, can be indistinguishable from a leukaemoid response on the basis of standard haematological features alone.

The advent of immunophenotyping in veterinary medicine is set to transform diagnosis and treatment of haematopoietic neoplasms such as leukaemia, as it has in human medicine. Immunophenotyping of blood cells in whole EDTA blood or bone marrow uses various combinations of fluorescent dye markers to highlight cell membrane or cytoplasmic CD (cluster of differentiation) markers. The pattern of expression allows the cell of interest to be identified, providing more prognostic information and guiding therapy. At present this technique is only available for specially fixed or very fresh material, and only a few institutes offer it commercially. These factors mean that currently it remains primarily a research tool, especially given that the associated significance and resulting clinical information is yet lacking in veterinary medicine.

Conclusion

Whilst automated analysers are widely available, fresh blood film examination remains essential for the proper practice of small animal medicine. In order to maximize the information obtained from only a few hundred microlitres of blood, it is necessary to understand both the automated analysis and the implications of changes in blood film morphology. Placing this information in the context of the animal, clinical history and pathophysiology prevents misdiagnosis and allows appropriate therapy.

References and further reading

Becker M, Moritz A and Giger U (2008) Comparative study of canine and feline total blood cell count results with seven in clinic and two commercial laboratory haematology analysers. *Veterinary Clinical Pathology* **37**, 373–384

Cornbleet J (1983) Spurious results from automated haematology cell counters. *Laboratory Medicine* **14**, 509–514

Eksell P, Haggstrom J, Kvart C and Karlsson A (1994) Thrombocytopenia in the Cavalier King Charles Spaniel. *Journal of Small Animal Practice* **35**, 153–155

Gelain ME, Tutino GF, Pogliani E and Bertazzolo W (2010) Macrothrombocytopenia in a group of related Norfolk terriers. *The Veterinary Record* **167**, 493–494

Giger U (2000) Haematology and immunology. In: *Textbook of Veterinary Internal Medicine, 5th edn*, ed. SJ Ettinger and EC Feldman, pp. 1784–1857. WB Saunders, Philadelphia

Hinchcliffe RF, Bellamy GJ and Lilleyman JS (1992) Use of the Technicon H1 hyprochomia flag in detecting spurious macrocytosis induced by excessive K_2-EDTA concentration. *Clinical and Laboratory Haematology* **14**, 268–269

Iazbik MC and Couto CG (2008) Morphological characterisation of specific granules in Greyhound eosinophils. *Veterinary Clinical Pathology* **34**(2), 140–143

Jain NC (1993) Examination of the blood and bone marrow. In: *Essentials of Veterinary Haematology, 1st edn*, ed. NC Jain, pp. 1–19. Lea and Febiger, Philadelphia

Latimer KS (1995) Leukocytes in health and disease. In: *Textbook of Veterinary Internal Medicine, 4th edn*, ed. SJ Ettinger and EC Feldman, pp. 1892–1929. WB Saunders, Philadelphia

McManus P and Craig L (1999) Correlation between leukocytosis and necropsy findings in canine immune mediated haemolytic anemia (IMHA) patients. *Veterinary Pathology* **36**, 484

Norman EJ, Barron RCJ, Nash AS and Clampitt RB (2001) Prevalence of low automated platelet counts in cats: comparison with prevalence of thrombocytopaenia based on blood smear estimation. *Veterinary Clinical Pathology* **30**(3), 137–140

Segev G, Klement E and Aroch I (2006) Toxic neutrophils in cats: clinical and clinicopathological features, and disease prevalence and outcome – a retrospective case control study. *Journal of Veterinary Internal Medicine* **20**(1), 20–31

Snyder LA, Neel JA and Grindem CB (2007) Thrombocytosis in dogs: a retrospective study. *42nd Meeting of the ASVCP*, November 10–14, 2007, Savannah, Georgia, p.736

Steinberg JD and Olver CS (2005) Haematologic and biochemical abnormalities indicating iron deficiency are associated with decreased reticulocyte haemoglobin content (CHr) and reticulocyte volume (rMCV) in dogs. *Veterinary Clinical Pathology* **34**(1), 23–27

Tvedten H (1994) The complete blood count and bone marrow examination: general comments and selected techniques. In: *Small Animal Clinical Diagnosis by Laboratory Methods, 2nd edn*, ed. MD Willard, H Tvedten and G Turnwald, pp.11–31. WB Saunders, Philadelphia

Tvedten H and Weiss D (1999) The complete blood count and bone marrow examination: general comments and selected techniques. In: *Small Animal Clinical Diagnosis by Laboratory Methods, 3rd edn*, ed. MD Willard, H Tvedten and G Turnwald, pp.14–37. WB Saunders, Philadelphia

Weiser MG (1995) Erythrocyte responses and disorders. In: *Textbook of Veterinary Internal Medicine, 4th edn*, ed. SJ Ettinger and EC Feldman, pp. 1864–1891. WB Saunders, Philadelphia

Erythrocyte and leucocyte morphology indices ▶

Erythrocyte morphology index (EMI)

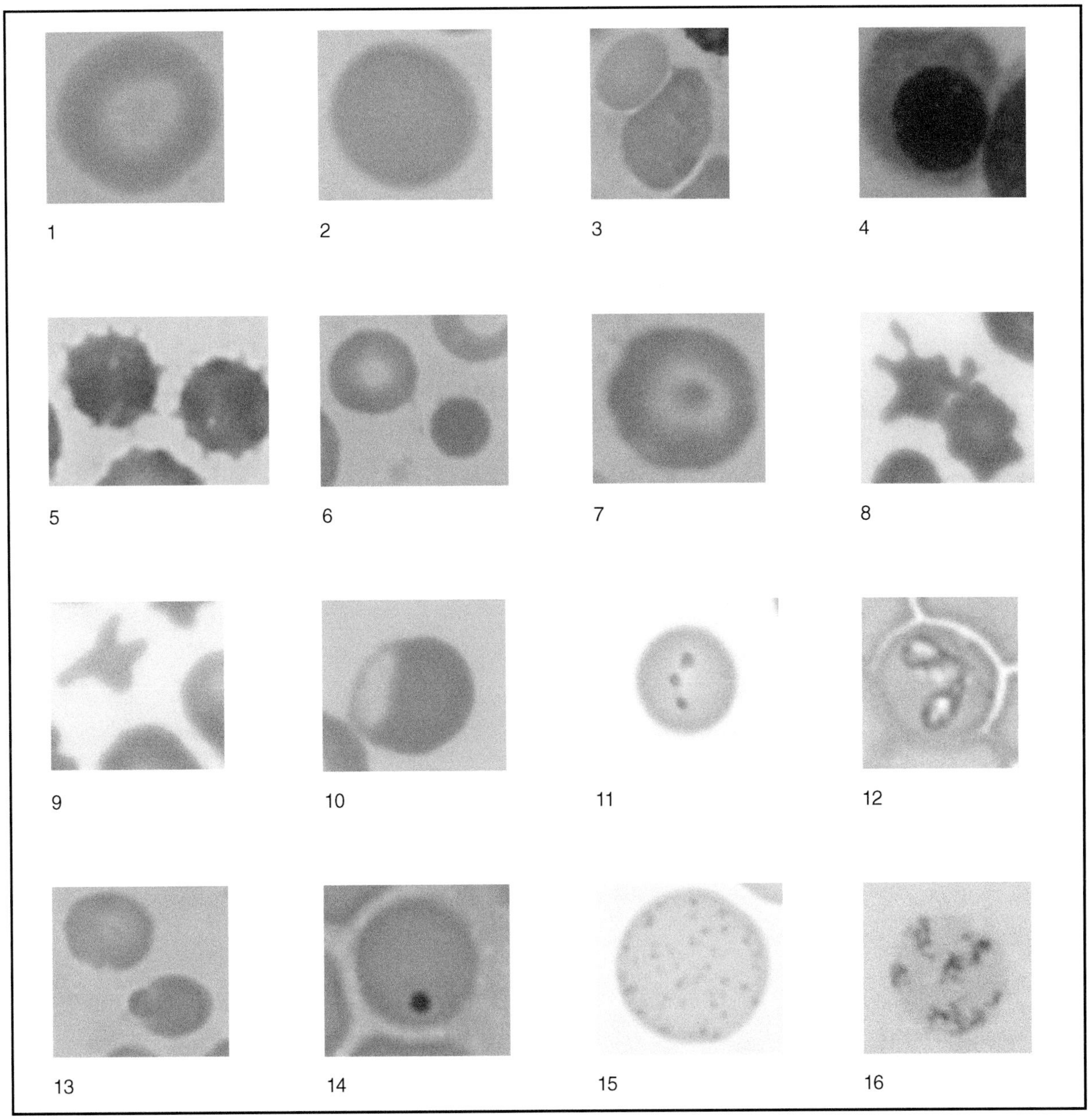

1. Normal canine erythrocyte
2. Normal feline erythrocyte
3. Reticulocyte (right)
4. Metarubricyte
5. Echinocytes
6. Spherocyte (right)
7. Codocyte (target cell)
8. Acanthocyte (left)
9. Schistocyte (top left)
10. Eccentrocyte
11. Haemoplasma
12. *Babesia*
13. Heinz body (right)
14. Howell–Jolly body
15. Basophilic stippling
16. Reticulocyte – aggregate (new methylene blue)

Leucocyte morphology index (LMI)

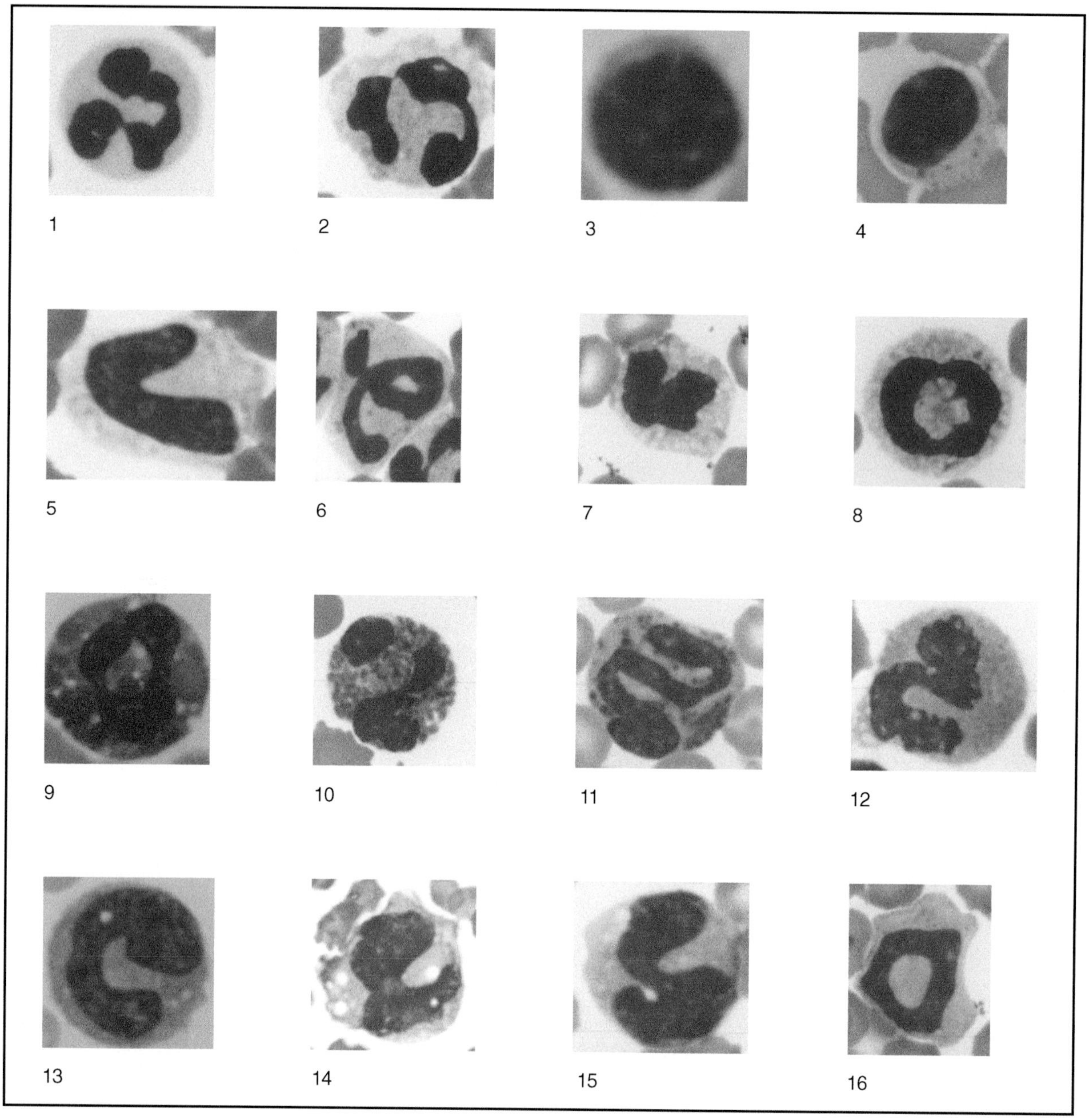

1. Neutrophil: segmented dark purple necleus, cream cytoplasm
2. Neutrophil: segmented dark purple nucleus, off white-pink cytoplasm
3. Lymphocyte: circular smudged dark nucleus, minimal smooth blue cytoplasm
4. Lymphocyte: circular smudged dark nucleus, blue cytoplasm, pink granules
5. Band neutrophil: parallel sided dark purple nucleus, cream-blue cytoplasm
6. Toxic neutrophil: irregular indistinct blue dots (Dőhle bodies), blue cytoplasm
7. Toxic neutrophil: foamy blue cytoplasm with Dőhle bodies
8. Toxic neutrophil: foamy cytoplasm, toxic (pink) granules, annular nucleus
9. Eosinophil – dog: blue cytoplasm, irregular, variable orange-pink globules
10. Eosinophil – cat: blue cytoplasm, regular, denser orange-pink rods
11. Basophil – dog: blue cytoplasm, irregular, variable purple granules
12. Basophil – cat: blue cytoplasm, denser, regular paler lilac granules

13–16. Monocytes: paler irregular chromatin, very variable nuclear shape, grey-blue-pink hue cytoplasm and variable clear white vacuoles

2

Collection and interpretation of bone marrow samples

Dorothee Bienzle

Introduction

The bone marrow is a complex and highly specialized organ within the central cavity of bone. It continuously produces large numbers of progeny cells that function to supply oxygen, defend against microbial agents, seal breaks in the vasculature and initiate wound healing. To meet such diverse roles, bone marrow is highly organized to assure orderly maturation of cells for release at precise moments of functional maturity. Haemopoietic tissue is in a unique dynamic equilibrium with the requirements of the animal for erythrocytes to supply oxygen to tissue, for leucocytes to function in inflammation, and for haemostasis by platelets; and it adjusts continually and rapidly to variable demands. Daily production of more than a billion blood cells from bone marrow means it is among the most mitotically active tissues, and even relatively brief impairments in production have distinct and severe clinical manifestations. Accordingly, lack of functional marrow is incompatible with life.

The bone marrow space is shared by haemopoietic and adipose tissue, with expansion and contraction of bone marrow cells reciprocated by changes in adipocytes. In young animals, most of the bone marrow space is comprised of haemopoietic cells; however, with increasing age haemopoietic cells are concentrated in the marrow of the axial skeleton (i.e. flat bones, vertebrae and sternebrae). Chronic haemopoietic stress (e.g. hypoxia or shortened lifespan of erythrocytes or platelets) will induce extramedullary haemopoiesis, most often in the spleen. Other cells in the bone marrow include stromal, endothelial, nerve and histiocytic cells that provide growth factors, blood supply, neurogenic stimuli and removal of damaged cells.

Indications for bone marrow examination

A haemogram or complete blood count (CBC) is part of the routine evaluation of most sick small animal patients. Abnormalities that are detected may be appropriate responses to a disease in another tissue, such as eosinophilia noted in some allergic responses, or regenerative anaemia secondary to blood loss or immune-mediated haemolytic anaemia (IMHA). Where deviations from reference values cannot be accounted for, further investigation is required. In general, when haematological abnormalities in an animal cannot be correlated with an apparent disease process, a bone marrow sample should be evaluated. Figure 2.1 outlines specific indications for examination of the bone marrow.

Persistent and unexplained changes in one or more blood cell type:
- Non-regenerative anaemia, leucopenia, thrombocytopenia
- Polycythaemia without dehydration; leucocytosis, thrombocytosis

Abnormal or atypical cells in circulation:
- Rubricytosis without regenerative anaemia
- Immature granulocytes in the absence of inflammation or infection
- Mast cells, macrophages or unidentifiable cells

Hyperproteinaemia, monoclonal gammopathy:
- Myeloma, plasma cell tumours, ehrlichiosis

Suspected systemic infection or metastatic disease:
- Fungal infection, leishmaniosis, ehrlichiosis, histoplasmosis
- Metastatic carcinoma, mast cell tumour

Hypercalcaemia, fever of unknown origin

2.1 Indications for examination of bone marrow.

The decision to examine bone marrow is usually based on findings on the CBC or on potential involvement of the marrow in a systemic disease process. Contraindications for the procedure are few and can be addressed with special precautions: particular attention should be paid to sterile procedures in neutropenic or immunosuppressed patients, and soft tissue trauma should be minimized in animals with haemostatic deficiency. Although marked thrombocytopenia may seem to be a contraindication for bone marrow biopsy, clinically significant bleeding is rare, presumably because of containment of the clot in the bone cavity. Sedation, analgesia or anaesthesia should be tailored to the temperament of the patient; sedation can be omitted completely in debilitated animals. Once an indication for examination of the bone marrow has been established, the procedure can be performed in essentially all patients.

Collecting a bone marrow sample

Types of sample

Two types of bone marrow sample can be collected: an aspirate of the non-adherent bone marrow elements or a solid core of tissue consisting of bony trabeculae, fat and haemopoietic tissue. Aspirates (the appearance is similar to 'thick blood') are smeared and are best for identifying cell types and infectious agents, assessing cell maturation and evaluating iron stores. Core biopsy samples require fixation and processing (Weiss, 1987). Only core samples yield architectural information about the bone marrow, such as overall cellularity and the presence and extent of myelofibrosis, primary or metastatic tumours, and bone lesions. If bone marrow cannot be aspirated, it may be due to the presence of myelofibrosis, and then the diagnosis depends largely on examination of the tissue core. Inability to aspirate bone marrow may also indicate improper needle placement. If bone lysis is identified on radiographs, then those sites should be sampled. Ideally, bone marrow evaluation should include cytological and histopathological assessment, but sometimes a diagnosis can be established solely from cytological evaluation.

Biopsy needles

Figure 2.2 shows some types of needle commonly used for collecting biopsy specimens. The large Jamshidi-type needles may be used for aspiration as well as biopsy. The smaller needles are less expensive, but can be used only for bone marrow aspiration. Given that solid cortical bone must be penetrated when collecting a bone marrow sample, it is important to use appropriate and sharp needles. A 13 gauge, 6–9 cm (2–3.5 inch) combination aspiration/biopsy needle, or a 16–18 gauge, 2.5–5 cm (1–2 inch) aspiration needle is adequate for most small animal patients, and the disposable types may be sterilized and re-used.

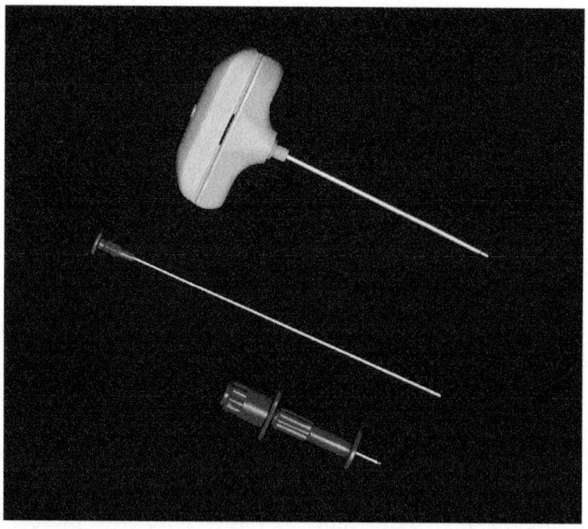

2.2 Bone marrow core biopsy needle (top) with stylet (middle) and disposable aspiration needle (bottom).

Active haemopoietic tissue is distributed equally throughout the body and many sites are suitable for collection of samples. In elderly animals the diaphysis of long bones consists predominantly of fat, hence sampling the axial skeleton such as the pelvis will provide a better yield. The marrow of the proximal humerus is also very accessible and remains haemopoietically active for longer than that of the diaphysis. In medium to large dogs, the sternum and costochondral junction are readily aspirated for cytological evaluation of cells and infectious agents (e.g. *Leishmania* spp.), but core samples cannot be obtained from these sites. For the purposes of this chapter, landmarks for aspirating the bone marrow of the pelvis, sternum, proximal humerus and femur will be described. Operator familiarity with a particular site is likely to be just as important as the actual origin of the sample.

Biopsy techniques

The biopsy site is clipped and prepared for surgery. In the sedated awake patient (of docile temperament or debilitated), a small area of skin and the periosteum at the chosen site are infiltrated with local anaesthetic containing adrenaline (epinephrine), with a 25 gauge needle. A small skin incision is made with the tip of a hypodermic needle or with a scalpel blade, and the bone marrow needle is inserted through the skin. The needle, with stylet firmly in place to yield a smoothly sharp tip, is positioned against bone and then advanced gradually into the marrow cavity using a back and forth and 'drilling' motion and steady pressure.

The iliac crest is palpated by placing the animal squarely in sternal recumbency with the hind legs folded under the gluteal muscles, which elevates the iliac crest (Figure 2.3), or having the animal stand squarely. The wing of the ilium is concave relative to the lateral aspects; therefore, the needle is best introduced slightly below the crest and at an angle, directed ventromedially (Figure 2.3). The ilium may also be aspirated anywhere else where it is clearly palpable, but because the bone is slightly concave, the needle may 'slip' if the angle is too small. Ideally, the angle should be 20–45 degrees relative to the ilial surface. For needle placement into the femur the

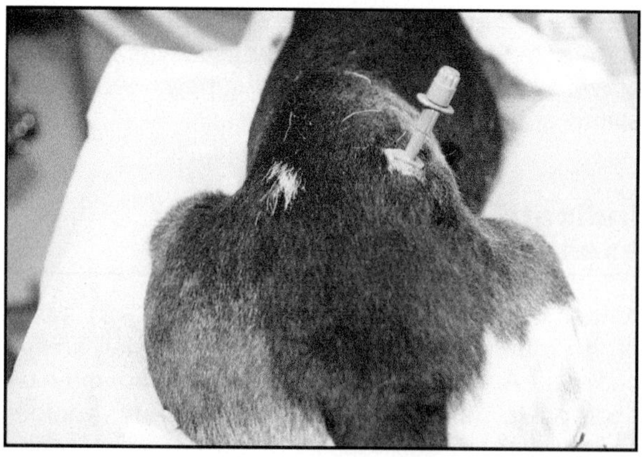

2.3 Aspiration needle firmly seated in the wing of the ilium of a dog in sternal recumbency.

animal should be in lateral recumbency. The greater trochanter is palpated and the needle inserted just medial to the trochanter and parallel to the shaft of the femur.

Samples from the head of the humerus are collected by placing the animal in lateral recumbency, palpating the greater tubercle and inserting the needle on the flat surface of the craniolateral aspect in a slightly 'downwards' direction (Figure 2.4a). The scapulohumeral joint must be avoided, and an approximately 45 degree angle with even force helps to avoid 'slippage' of the needle along the bone surface. Once the needle with stylet is seated properly in bone it should feel as if they are 'cemented in place' and the entire bone or small animal follows movement of the needle placed in the bone.

The sternum is best accessed for bone marrow aspiration with the animal standing or seated on its hindlimbs. The most anterior sternebra is palpated in the midline and in front of the scapulohumeral joint, and a 16–18 gauge aspiration needle is gradually drilled into the bone in a slightly downward and lateral to medial direction (Figure 2.4b).

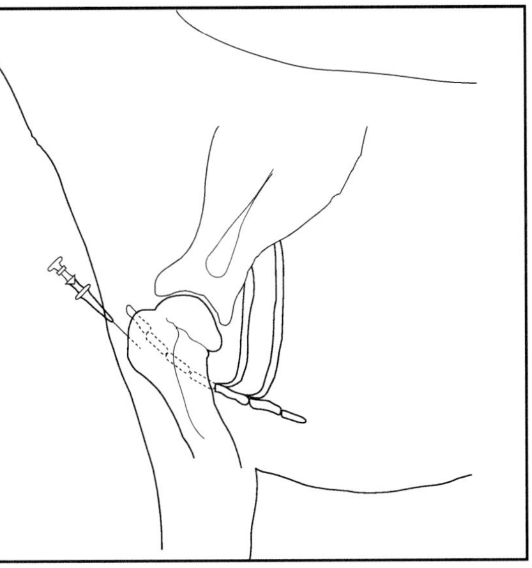

(a)

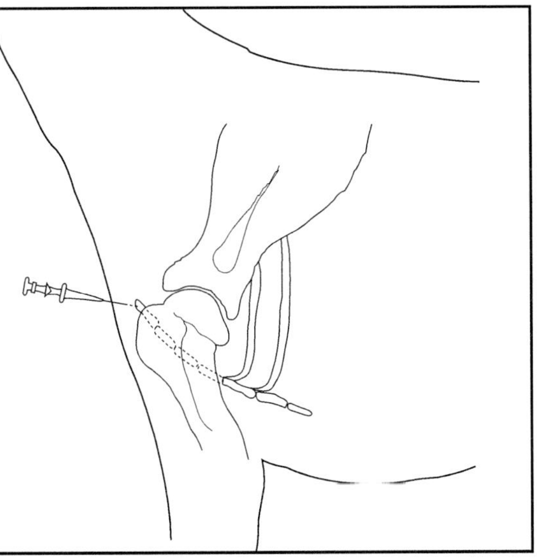

(b)

2.4 Placement of bone marrow aspiration needle in humerus **(a)** and sternum **(b)**.

Smear preparation from marrow aspirates

As bone marrow samples clot quickly, all equipment for preparing smears and preserving the biopsy sample should be ready before a sample is collected: six to eight glass slides, a 3 ml tube with ethylenediamine tetra-acetic acid (EDTA) anticoagulant, absorbent paper, sterile gloves on a sterile field, aspiration and biopsy needles and a jar with fixative.

For aspiration, once the needle is firmly seated in the marrow cavity, the stylet is removed (Figure 2.5), and a 12 ml syringe is attached firmly to the needle hub and negative pressure is applied. Bone marrow (which normally resembles thick blood) should appear in the hub of the syringe after a few moments of suction (Figure 2.6). When about 0.5 ml of bone marrow has been collected, the pressure is released, the syringe is detached and the stylet replaced in the aspiration needle, which has remained in the bone marrow. One large drop of bone marrow is placed on each of about five glass slides (Figure 2.7). The goal of preparing bone marrow smears is to concentrate the marrow components and to remove much of the contaminating blood. Therefore, the slides are tilted sideways to 45

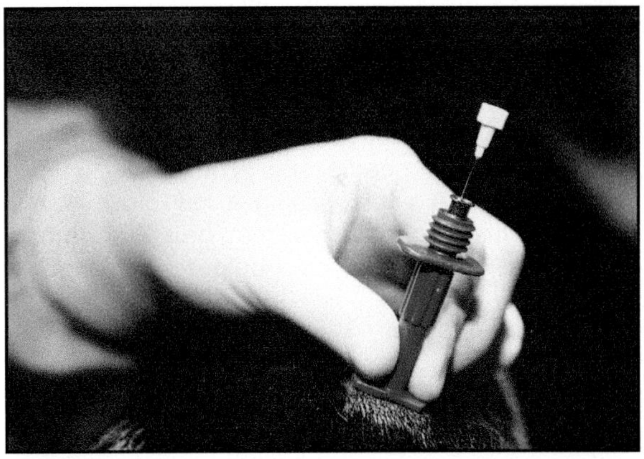

2.5 Needle cap removed and stylet withdrawn.

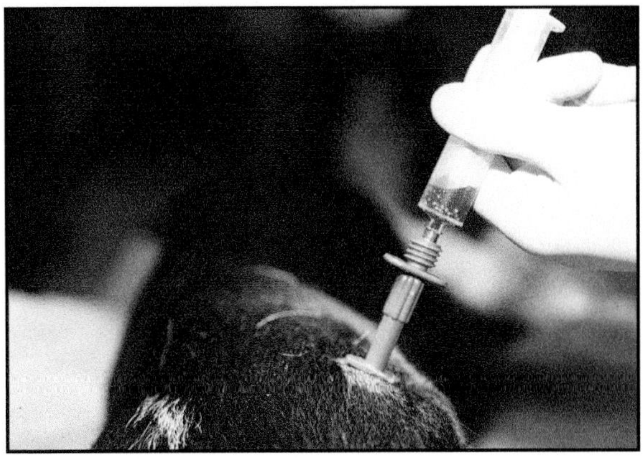

2.6 The syringe is attached, and several forceful aspirations yield thick sanguineous fluid.

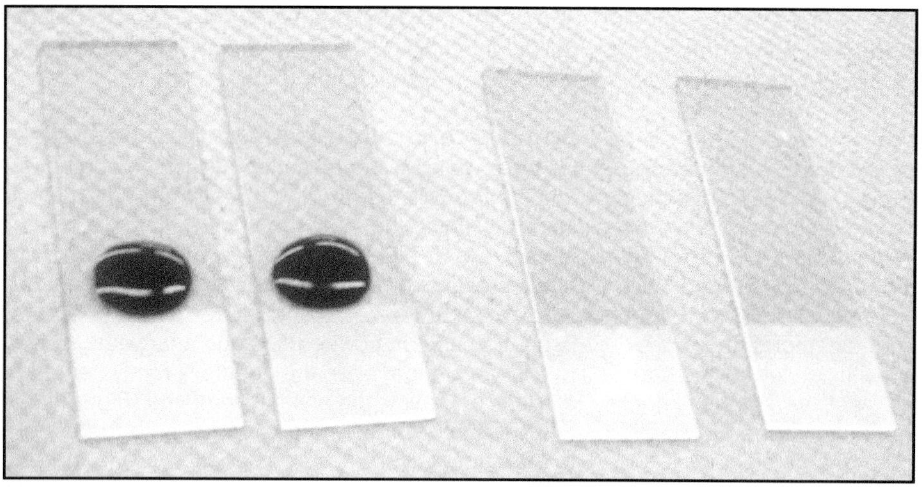

2.7 Thick drops of bone marrow are placed near the frosted edge of several glass slides.

degrees to allow excess blood to run off on to the absorbent paper, leaving the marrow particles, which are adherent to the glass (Figure 2.8). A clean glass slide is backed into the remaining bone marrow and the marrow is allowed to spread along the edge of the spreader glass slide, which is then pushed forward swiftly to produce a thin smear with a 'feathered' edge. Two further smears are prepared by removing excess blood in the same manner, laying a clean glass slide at right angles on top of the remaining drop of marrow (Figure 2.9) and gently pulling the slides apart ('squash preparation'). It is essential for good cell preservation that all smears be air-dried quickly. Because bone marrow clots quickly, speed is essential and preparation of all smears should take less than 1 minute. Alternatively, the sample can be anticoagulated by prior rinsing of the bone marrow needle and syringe with a 10% solution of EDTA and retaining a few drops in the needle, or the whole aspirate may be placed immediately in a 3 ml EDTA tube before preparing the smears.

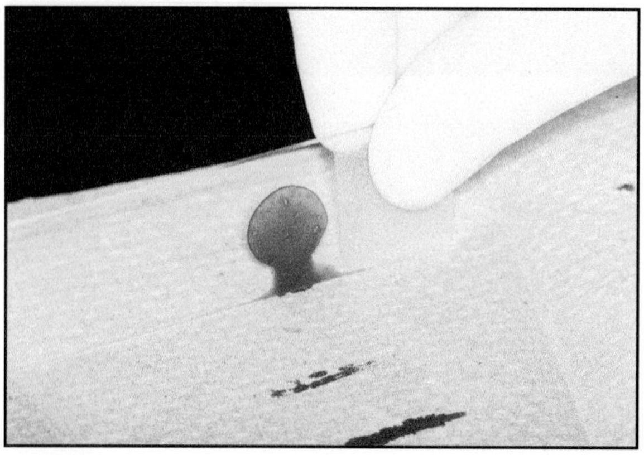

2.8 The slides are tilted to allow blood to run off on to absorbent tissue paper, leaving marrow particles attached to the glass.

A satisfactory aspirate is characterized by the presence of small granules, which are particularly visible after excess blood has been drained off the slide. These are the marrow particles. Small fat globules are frequently noted and are a normal component of bone marrow aspirates. An inability to aspirate bone marrow is often caused by bone fragments occluding the needle, particularly if the stylet was not precisely in place when the needle was drilled through bone. Alternatively, the needle may have become lodged in cortical bone. Retracting the needle a small distance may sometimes permit sample collection. If not, the needle should be removed, inspected for blockage and clots and re-inserted, with the stylet firmly in place, at a different site. Myelofibrosis or certain tumours of the bone marrow may preclude successful aspiration, yielding hypocellular smears despite a hypercellular marrow.

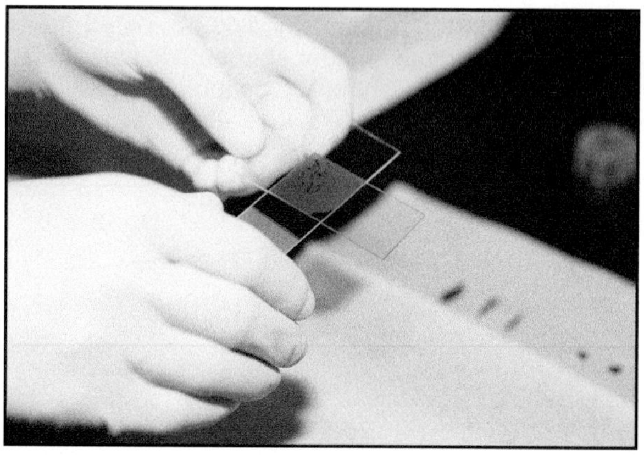

2.9 Slides are prepared by laying a glass slide at right angles across the remainder of the bone marrow drop, pulling the slides apart, and rapidly drying them in air.

The air-dried smears may be either submitted to a laboratory for staining and evaluation by a pathologist or stained directly. Romanowsky-type stains are most commonly employed, but 'quick' versions will yield adequate staining in many instances. Smears of bone marrow are generally so densely cellular that two staining cycles are required for adequate cell penetration.

Performing a core biopsy

Given that the marrow architecture becomes distorted in the immediate vicinity of an aspirate, it is important either that the biopsy specimen is collected prior to aspiration, the needle is completely redirected after aspiration, or another site is sampled. The biopsy needle is inserted into bone in the same manner as for an aspirate. Again, the needle, with stylet in place, is seated firmly in cortical bone. The stylet is then removed and the needle is advanced with a gentle 'drilling' motion and steady pressure. The sharp edge of the biopsy needle cuts a cylinder of tissue consisting of thin bony spicules with interspersed marrow. Once the needle has been advanced about 2.5 cm (a little less in cats and small dogs and more in large dogs), the needle is rotated and moved swiftly sideways a few times to 'break off' the distal part of the core, and is then gradually retracted. Biopsy needles have tapered tips to retain the core inside the lumen of the needle as it is withdrawn. To retrieve the specimen with minimal distortion, the blunt-ended probe part of the biopsy needle should be inserted in a retrograde fashion and the core should be carefully pushed from the tapered end backwards to the hub of the needle (Figure 2.10). Inability to obtain a core biopsy specimen may be because the core did not dislodge from the stromal or bony elements of the marrow cavity. In that case re-sampling with more vigorous effort to break off the distal core is necessary. Special biopsy needles with internal 'retainers' that may be activated in order to keep the core within the needle during retraction are also available (e.g. Goldenberg Snarecoil™ needles).

If it was not possible to obtain an aspirate, the core may be gently rolled on a glass slide for a cytological imprint, and then placed in buffered formalin or freshly prepared B-5 fixative. Formalin provides adequate fixation, but B-5 fixative is preferred by many haematopathologists (Naresh *et al.*, 2006). An adequate bone marrow core should be at least 1.5 cm long, but preferably more than 2.0 cm (Figure 2.11). If only a small sample is obtained, a second core specimen should be collected. Bone marrow smears should be kept separate from formalin jars because formalin vapours alter the staining characteristics of cells. All slides and biopsy samples should be labelled and submitted to the laboratory.

In conclusion, a complete submission for examination of bone marrow consists of an accurate history, three to six cytology smears, a bone marrow core, a copy of a recent CBC or concurrent blood sample for a CBC, and possibly an EDTA tube with additional bone marrow fluid. The history should include details of drug administration, physical and laboratory findings and previous or current illness.

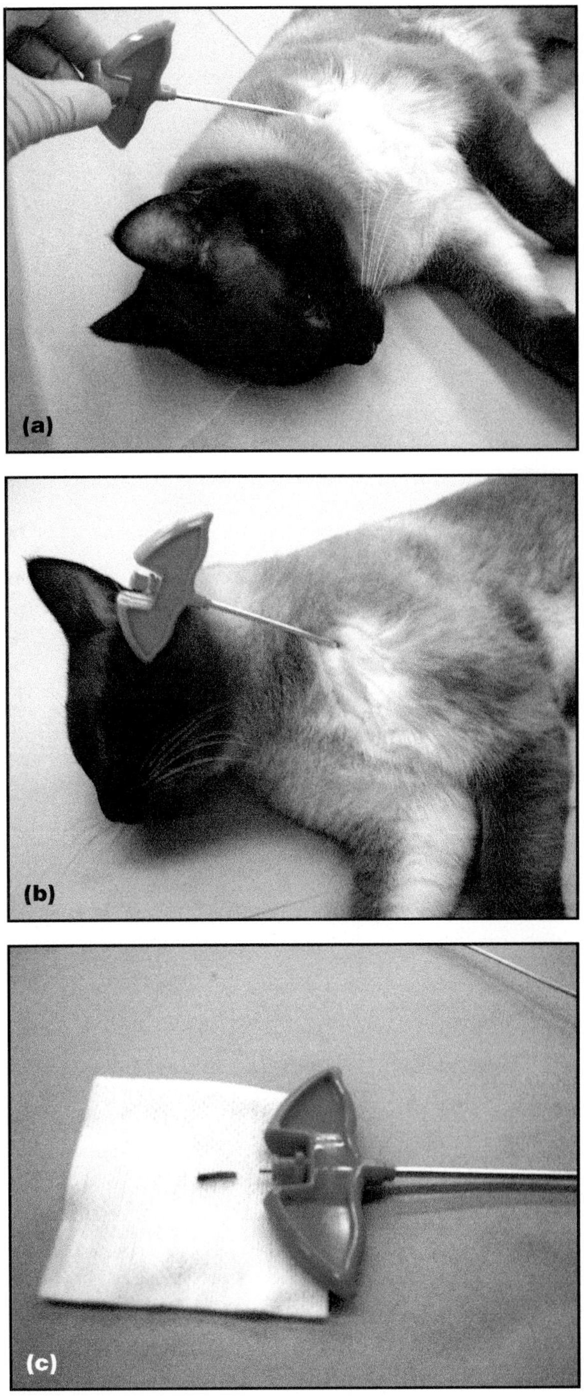

2.10 Placement of core biopsy needle in humerus of anaesthetized cat **(a)**; removal of sharp stylet and advancement of needle **(b)**; retrograde expulsion of the marrow core with the blunt stylet **(c)**.

Interpretation of bone marrow samples

Proficient interpretation of bone marrow samples requires a thorough knowledge of haemopoiesis, and recognition of all stages of cell development and different disease processes. The skill required for accurate interpretation of bone marrow is difficult to acquire with only occasional practice. Practitioners who wish to examine smears themselves are advised to seek confirmation from experienced haematopathologists until they are proficient. A detailed description of the principles of interpretation is beyond the scope of this text; however, basic concepts and deviations from normal findings are reviewed.

To evaluate bone marrow samples accurately, smears must be examined in a systematic and consistent manner. All normal marrow components are assessed sequentially, changes are described,

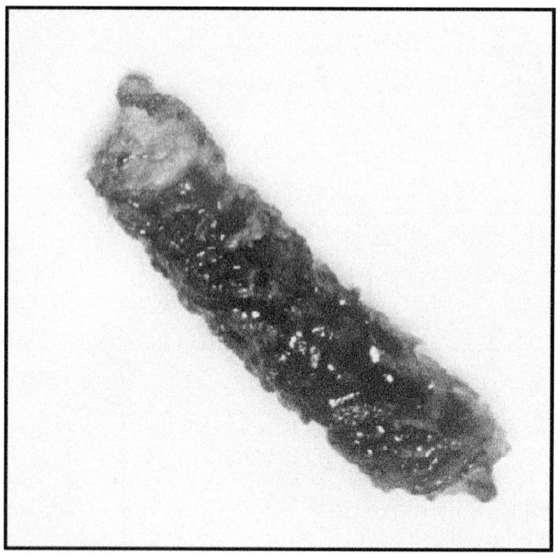

2.11 Normal bone marrow core appears red and should measure at least 1.5 cm.

unusual elements are noted and then a composite interpretation and correlation with the haematological and clinical picture are formulated. Figure 2.12 outlines the approach to interpretation.

Low magnification
• Is the specimen adequate? • How cellular are the marrow granules? • Are there sufficient megakaryocytes of variable maturity? • Are iron stores present? • Which areas are most suitable for closer examination?
High magnification
• What is the proportion of granulocytic vs. erythrocytic cells? • What is the granulocyte:erythrocyte ratio? • Is maturation synchronous in erythrocytes, granulocytes and megakaryocytes? • Are there increased plasma cells, lymphocytes or histiocytes? • Are there infectious agents such as fungal spores or hyphae, or morulae? • Are there necrotic cells or cell debris?
Interpretation
• Summary of the morphological findings • Correlation with results of the CBC and physical and other laboratory findings

2.12 Systematic microscopic evaluation of bone marrow smears.

Low magnification

Adequate marrow smears should have several intact particles on the slide that allow estimation of cellularity ('feathered edge' smear) and slides where particles are spread apart ('squash preparation'), and the cells should be in a single layer to enable assessment of morphology. Marrow particles from young animals are very cellular, but with age there is progressive replacement of the active marrow with fat. Particles comprised of 25–75% cells are considered normal for adult animals, whereas those containing 80–90% fat are typical in healthy elderly animals (Jacobs and Valli, 1988). Particle cellularity corresponds well to overall bone marrow cellularity as assessed on histological preparation of core biopsy specimens. On smears prepared with Wright's stain, megakaryocytes are readily identifiable as giant cells with multilobulated nuclei. Immature megakaryocytes have a moderate amount of dark basophilic cytoplasm, and with progressive maturity, the cytoplasmic volume increases and appears more eosinophilic and granular. On average 5–10 megakaryocytes are associated with a particle, although occasionally megakaryocytes are present only singly at the feathered edge of a smear. Accurate estimates of megakaryocyte numbers are best derived from evaluation of core biopsy samples, because the variable cellularity of aspirates may preclude objective evaluation. Megakaryocyte hyperplasia is common with immune-mediated thrombocytopenia (IMTP), whereas a lack of megakaryocytes has been reported in cases of IMTP where the immune response is thought to be directed against both platelets and their precursors in the marrow (Putsche and Kohn, 2008). Iron stains dark brown to black with Wright's stain and should be evident on marrow smears from adult dogs, but not cats. Lack of stainable iron is a consistent finding in the marrow of animals with advanced iron deficiency. Increased iron stores have been associated with anaemia of chronic disease. Finally, an area of the smear where the cells are spread apart, usually the 'tail' of a particle on a 'squash preparation', should be selected for closer examination.

High magnification

Normal erythropoiesis and granulopoiesis are characterized by a predominance of the maturing stages of cell development. Granulocyte maturation proceeds from undifferentiated round myeloblasts with nucleoli to promyelocytes containing cytoplasmic azurophilic granules to myelocytes with gradually decreasing nuclear size and increasing chromatin condensation. At the metamyelocyte stage nuclei become indented and then progress to band-shaped and eventually mature segmented forms (Figure 2.13). Myeloblasts, promyelocytes and myelocytes undergo mitosis and therefore constitute

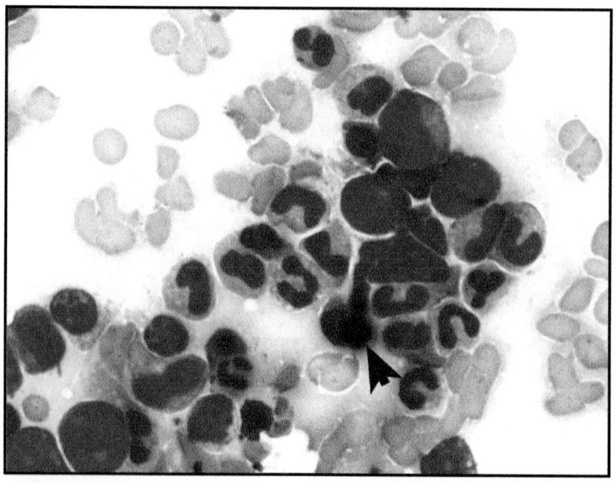

2.13 Bone marrow smear with granulocytic hyperplasia comprised of segmented and band neutrophils, metamyelocytes, promyelocytes, myelocytes and extracellular iron (arrowhead).

the proliferating component of granulocytes. The three maturing stages of metamyelocytes, band and segmented neutrophils, normally comprise 70–80% of all cells in the granulocytic series and are the maturing stages of granulopoiesis.

Development from rubriblast to metarubricyte is distinguished by a progressive decrease in cell size, loss of cytoplasmic basophilia and increased haemoglobin synthesis, imparting the characteristic pink colour of mature red blood cells (Figure 2.14). The nucleus gradually condenses and is extruded from metarubricytes before the polychromatic erythrocyte stage and exit from the marrow. Synchronous erythroid maturation is indicated by about 80% of erythroid cells being at the late rubricyte to metarubricyte stage. The ratio of granulocytic to nucleated erythroid cells (the G:E ratio, also called the myeloid:erythroid (M:E) ratio) ranges from 3:1 to 5:1 in healthy dogs and cats.

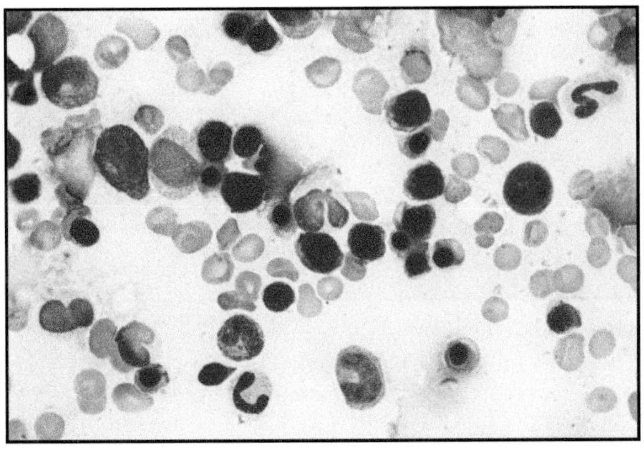

2.14 Bone marrow smear with erythroid maturation stages. Increasing nuclear condensation and acquisition of cytoplasmic haemoglobin indicates progressive maturity.

Benign conditions of the bone marrow

An appropriate marrow response to tissue demand for increased neutrophils or erythrocytes is an overall increase in the proportion of the particular cell line, but with retained orderly maturation and a predominance of maturing stages (hyperplasia). Therefore, the marrow of a dog with a responsive anaemia has a decreased G:E ratio and an absolute increase in erythroid cells, but still with predominance of later stage rubricytes. A chronic inflammatory disease with suppuration, such as pyoderma, increases the G:E ratio by stimulating increased neutrophil production, albeit that most of the granulocytes will be metamyelocytes and band and segmented neutrophils (see Figure 2.13). On the other hand, early recovery from a non-specific cytotoxic insult to the bone marrow (canine or feline parvoviral infection, chemotherapy or radiation) leads to increased proportions of immature forms that are easily mistaken for a neoplastic process. Granulocytic cells will be most affected, because the longer lifespan of red cells entails a slower rate of production. In these cases, re-sampling bone marrow after 1 week should indicate a progressive return to orderly maturation, with accumulation of late erythroid and granulocytic cells.

Pure red cell aplasia is characterized by profound anaemia, a near complete lack of erythroid cells in the bone marrow, normal myelopoiesis and thrombopoiesis and a profoundly increased G:E ratio. Aplastic anaemia manifests as a reduction in all cellular elements, and commonly only reticular cells and plasma cells are observed in the bone marrow (Figure 2.15). In myelofibrosis, proliferation of the stromal cells in the bone marrow, with excessive production of extracellular collagen, leads to gradual destruction of the normal haemopoietic space (Figure 2.16). Myelofibrosis may occur for unknown reasons, may accompany or precede neoplastic diseases of the bone marrow (Weiss, 2006) or may occur subsequent to chronically stimulated erythropoiesis in some cases of severe haemolytic anaemia (Reagan, 1993). Aspiration of marrow in these instances is difficult or impossible, and the diagnosis is based on histopathological findings.

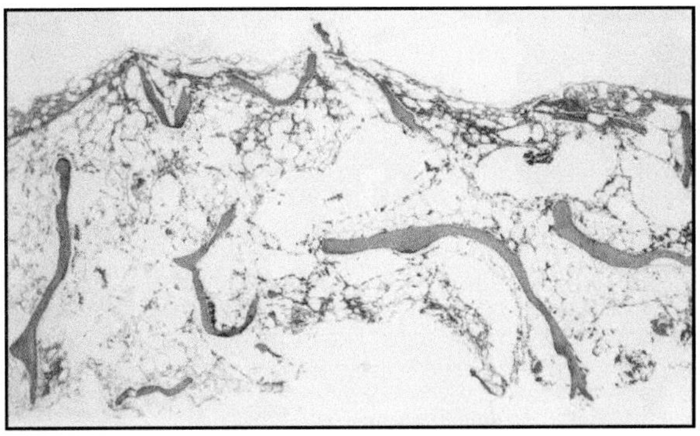

2.15 Histological section of bone marrow from a cat with aplastic anaemia. There are only rare haemopoietic cells apparent among adipocytes.

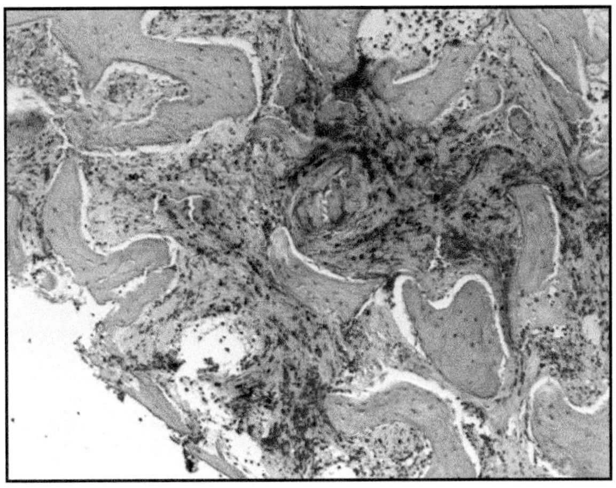

2.16 Histological section of bone marrow from a dog with advanced myelofibrosis. Normal haemopoietic tissue is replaced by fibrocytes and extracellular collagen and there is abundant focal iron deposition.

Diagnosis of leukaemia

Neoplasms of the haemopoietic cells are broadly divided into acute and chronic leukaemias (McManus, 2005), and non-lymphoid (myeloid) and lymphoid leukaemias. Generally, acute leukaemias manifest with marked cytopenias in the peripheral blood, and bone marrow aspirates have a predominance or increased proportion of immature (blast) cells (Figures 2.17 and 2.18). Blast cells are characterized by a moderate amount of cytoplasm, large nuclei, one or several nucleoli and no differentiating morphological features. Some normal haemopoietic cells may be present in the bone marrow, and the G:E ratio may be close to normal, but the synchronicity of maturation in the neoplastic cell line will be severely disturbed. The neoplastic cells may be characterized by cytochemical assays that detect

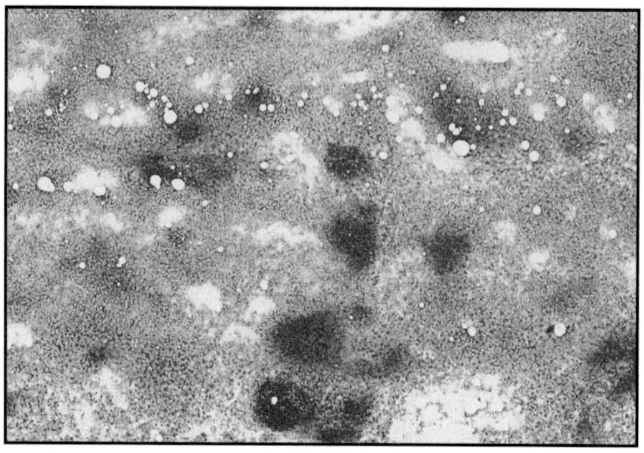

2.17 Bone marrow smear with profound hypercellularity consisting of numerous undifferentiated large cells. The dog had acute leukaemia and pancytopenia on a haemogram.

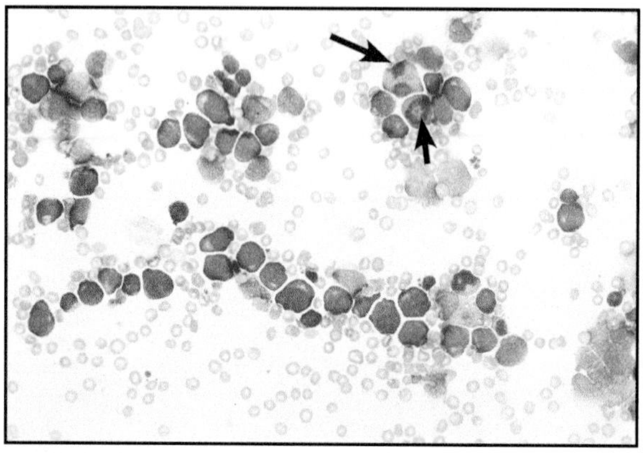

2.18 Higher magnification of Figure 2.17. Most of the cells are blasts with a perinuclear clear area (Golgi zone). Two cells are in mitosis (arrowed) and normal haemopoietic cells are nearly absent.

cytoplasmic enzymes unique for certain cell types, or by immunophenotyping. Immuno-phenotyping involves labelling cells with antibodies to antigens specific for certain cell types, such as cluster of differentiation (CD)3 for T lymphocytes, CD21 for B lymphocytes, or CD41 for megakaryocytes. Binding of fluorescent antibodies to cells in a fluid medium may be detected and quantified with a flow cytometer. Alternatively, bone marrow smears may be labelled by immunohistochemistry with antibodies that yield a colour reaction. Such assays may only be offered by specialized laboratories, but are utilized increasingly to classify leukaemias of animals. Immunophenotypically, most canine acute leukaemias appear to be of granulocytic origin (Figure 2.19), followed by lymphocytic and undifferentiated leukaemias (Vernau and Moore, 1999). Electron microscopy may also allow classification of leukaemic cells by ultrastructural features. The prognosis for acute leukaemias in small animals is poor to grave.

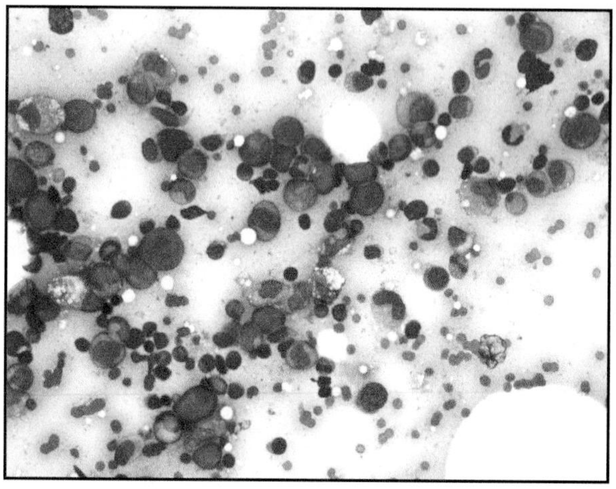

2.19 Bone marrow smear from a dog with acute leukaemia with granulocytic differentiation. The number of blast cells is increased, and differentiation to metamyelocytes and band neutrophils is apparent. There is a marked paucity of erythroid cells and megakaryocytes.

In contrast, chronic leukaemias (now termed myeloproliferative neoplasms (MPNs)) typically consist of an accumulation of cells with relatively normal morphology. Changes in the haemogram consist of an increase in cells of the neoplastic lineage, and possibly mild anaemia, neutropenia or thrombocytopenia. A bone marrow aspirate may sometimes be difficult to obtain, although the core biopsy will show profound hypercellularity. Morphologically, maturation of the affected cell line may be relatively synchronous; however, the G:E ratio may be noticeably increased owing to an absolute increase in cells of the neoplastic lineage. Many chronic leukaemias (Figure 2.20) with gradual progression have been described in small animals. For example, chronic lymphocytic leukaemias in dogs most often have large granular lymphocyte (LGL) morphology and express a T-cell receptor (Vernau and Moore, 1999). These leukaemias originate in the red pulp of the spleen and involve the bone marrow only in advanced disease.

It has been suggested that a blast cell count of more than 20% in the blood or bone marrow indicates an acute leukaemia, whereas a count of less than 20% in the bone marrow suggests

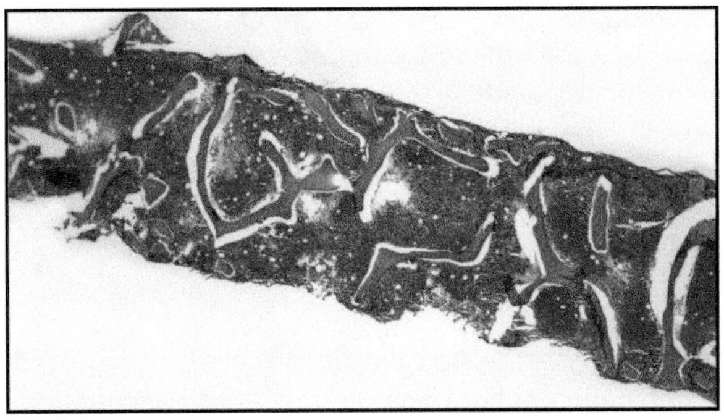

2.20 Histological section of bone marrow from a dog with chronic lymphocytic leukaemia. The cells are packed densely in the bone marrow and there is an absence of megakaryocytes evident at low magnification.

chronic leukaemia, myelodysplastic syndrome or a leukaemoid reaction (Juopperi *et al.*, 2011). Compared to humans, dogs and cats generally present at a later stage of the disease process, and distinction of acute from chronic leukaemia may not be obvious. Survival times exceeding 4 years have been reported in dogs with chronic lymphocytic leukaemia treated with chemotherapy, but studies evaluating the chemoresponsiveness of acute leukaemias in animals are largely missing.

Myeloid leukaemia

Leukaemias are classified in animals as in humans, although many of the molecular and cytogenetic assays employed in human patients are unavailable for animals. Nevertheless, acute myeloid leukaemia (AML) in animals is classified, according to the absence or presence and type of differentiating features, into types M0 to M7. For example, ≥ 90% myeloblasts in the bone marrow indicates M1 AML, while ≥ 30% megakaryoblasts corresponds to M7 AML. Acute erythroleukaemia with erythroid predominance is of M6-Er type, and consists of a proliferation of morphologically abnormal rubricytes, most commonly observed in cats infected with feline leukaemia virus (FeLV). Affected cats typically present with a rubricytosis consisting of immature and mature rubricytes and with variable leucopenia and thrombocytopenia.

Chronic myeloid leukaemia (CML) can usually be readily classified based on morphological features into types such as chronic granulocytic leukaemia. Thrombocythaemia, due to very high platelet counts in blood, is characteristic of chronic megakaryocytic leukaemia. Primary polycythaemia vera is a neoplastic proliferation of multiple differentiated bone marrow cells reflected in an increased haematocrit, granulocytosis and thrombocytosis in the blood (Khanna and Bienzle, 1994). Primary erythrocytosis, on the other hand, is a CML resulting from proliferation of erythrocytes, and manifests with very high haematocrit but usually normal leucocyte and platelet numbers. Conversely, chronic tissue hypoxia or ectopic production of erythropoietin results in physiological or paraneoplastic polycythaemia, respectively, but these are not haemopoietic neoplasms. Marked increases in erythrocytes due to leukaemia or secondary polycythaemia increase blood viscosity, and the animal may present with seizures or blindness secondary to nervous system hypoxia.

The myelodysplastic syndromes (MDS) encompass a variety of abnormal haemopoietic processes characterized by blood cytopenias, abnormal cell maturation and increased blast cells in the bone marrow, and possibly myelofibrosis. The condition is often pre-leukemic, and in cats may be associated with FeLV infection.

Myeloma and lymphoma

Clonal proliferation of immunoglobulin-producing plasma cells in the bone marrow, with a monoclonal gammopathy and lytic bone lesions, characterizes most forms of canine multiple myeloma. The diagnosis of the tumour is based on identifying clusters of plasma cells in aspirates or core biopsy specimens from lytic bone lesions (Figure 2.21), and the presence of monoclonal immunoglobulin in serum or urine. Haematologically normal animals may have 5–10% plasma cells in the marrow, and increased proportions of plasma cells have been observed in myelofibrosis, anaemia of renal failure, and aplastic anaemia (Weiss, 2005). In cases of anaemia of renal failure and aplastic anaemia, however, the plasma cells are morphologically mature and dispersed throughout the marrow, and lytic lesions are not observed. Myeloma in cats manifests less commonly with bone lesions (Mellor *et al.*, 2006).

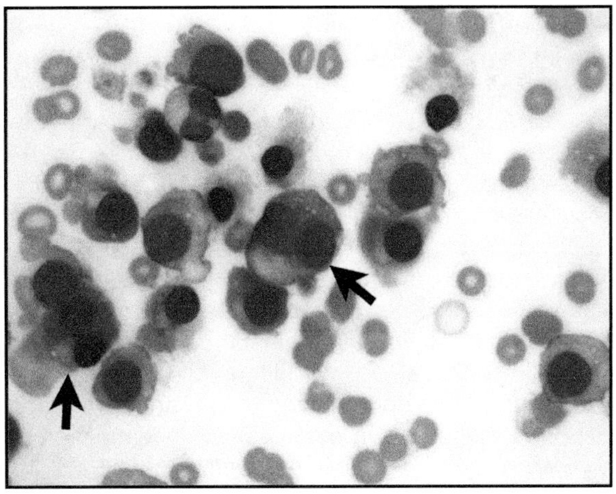

2.21 Bone marrow smear from a dog with multiple myeloma. There are malignant plasma cells, sometimes with two nuclei (arrows), and rare granulocytic or erythroid cells.

Low-grade involvement of the bone marrow is common in dogs with lymphoma, but rarely results in cytopenia and does not adversely affect prognosis. Subtle involvement of the marrow in lymphoma is difficult to detect and quantify, and the clinician should be aware that morphological evaluation of one marrow biopsy specimen is not a sensitive indicator.

Mast cell tumours

Mast cell tumours in the dog may metastasize via the haemolymphatic system to the bone marrow (Welle *et al.*, 2008), and this may be detected by buffy coat smears and bone marrow aspirates. Morphologically indistinguishable benign mastocytosis may, however, occur in a variety of non-neoplastic conditions. Hence, a diagnosis of metastatic mast cell tumour must be based on the detection of clusters of mast cells in bone marrow biopsy specimens or aspirates in the absence of inflammatory diseases such as dermatitis or enteritis, which have been associated with benign mastocytosis (Figure 2.22).

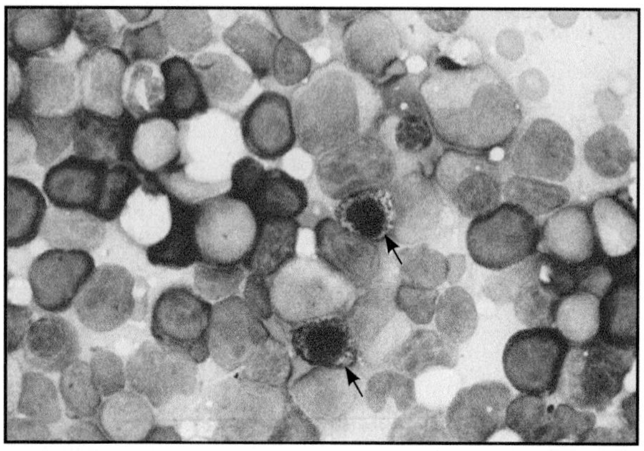

2.22 Bone marrow smear showing two mast cells (arrows) among erythroid and granulocytic cells. The dog had multiple cutaneous mast cell tumours.

Histiocytic tumours

The bone marrow commonly is involved in proliferative diseases of histiocytic cells. Clusters of large vacuolated cells with phagocytosed red cells or haemosiderin in the bone marrow and other tissues are characteristic of the haemophagocytic variant of histiocytic sarcoma (Affolter and Moore, 2002), while multinucleation and anisokaryosis are more prominent features of the dendritic cell variant of histiocytic sarcoma (Moore *et al.*, 2006). Bone marrow histiocytic hyperplasia is observed in mycotic, protozoal or mycobacterial infections that induce granulomatous inflammation, and in storage diseases that result in cytoplasmic accumulation of non-degradable metabolic products.

Metastatic carcinoma

Lastly, neoplasms of epithelial origin may metastasize to the bone marrow, although this seems to be an infrequent or a clinically inapparent occurrence in animals. Clusters of adherent epithelial cells in smears or histological sections of marrow suggest metastatic carcinoma. The prognostic significance of metastatic carcinomas is undetermined for most small animal neoplasms.

Most attempts to diagnose metastasis rely solely on morphological identification of neoplastic cells and thus are limited by the size of the sample, the relative presence of the neoplastic cell population and the expertise of the pathologist. Immunohistochemical staining for epithelial cell markers would probably increase sensitivity.

Summary

Examination of the bone marrow is an essential tool for the diagnosis of most haematological diseases, and aids in the assessment of many other systemic and neoplastic conditions. Providing adequate specimens is paramount for accurate interpretation, and pathological findings must be interpreted in conjunction with physical and laboratory data, and with the peripheral blood picture. Communication between the clinician and the pathologist is an invaluable component in deriving a diagnosis from a bone marrow sample.

References and further reading

Affolter VK and Moore PF (2002) Localized and disseminated histiocytic sarcoma of dendritic cell origin in dogs. *Veterinary Pathology* **39**, 74–83

Jacobs RM and Valli VEO (1988) Bone marrow biopsies, principles and perspectives of interpretation. *Seminars in Veterinary Medicine and Surgery* **3**, 176–182

Juopperi TA, Bienzle D, Bernreuter DC *et al.* (2011) Prognostic markers for myeloid neoplasms: a comparative review of the literature and goals for future investigation. *Veterinary Pathology* **48**(1), 182–197.

Khanna C and Bienzle D (1994) Polycythemia vera in a cat, bone marrow culture in erythropoietin-deficient medium. *Journal of the American Animal Hospital Association* **30**, 45–49

McManus PM (2005) Classification of myeloid neoplasms, a comparative review. *Veterinary Clinical Pathology* **34**, 189–212

Mellor PJ, Haugland S, Murphy S *et al.* (2006) Myeloma-related disorders in cats commonly present as extramedullary neoplasms in contrast to myeloma in human patients, 24 cases with clinical follow-up. *Journal of Veterinary Internal Medicine* **20**, 1376–1383

Moore PF, Affolter VK and Vernau W (2006) Canine hemophagocytic histiocytic sarcoma, a proliferative disorder of $CD11d^+$ macrophages. *Veterinary Pathology* **43**, 632–645

Naresh KN, Lampert I, Hasserjian R *et al.* (2006) Optimal processing of bone marrow trephine biopsy, the Hammersmith Protocol. *Journal of Clinical Pathology* **59**, 903–911

Putsche JC and Kohn B (2008) Primary immune-mediated thrombocytopenia in 30 dogs (1997-2003). *Journal of the American Animal Hospital Association* **44**, 250–257

Reagan WJ (1993) A review of myelofibrosis in dogs. *Toxicological Pathology* **21**, 164–169

Vernau W and Moore PF (1999) An immunophenotypic study of canine leukemias and preliminary assessment of clonality by polymerase chain reaction. *Veterinary Immunology and Immunopathology* **69**, 145–164

Weiss DJ (1987) A review of the techniques for preparation of histopathologic sections of bone marrow. *Veterinary Clinical Pathology* **16**, 90–94

Weiss DJ (2005) Recognition and classification of dysmyelopoiesis in the dog, a review. *Journal of Veterinary Internal Medicine* **19**, 147–154

Weiss DJ (2006) A retrospective study of the incidence and the classification of bone marrow disorders in the dog at a veterinary teaching hospital (1996-2004). *Journal of Veterinary Internal Medicine* **20**, 955–961

Welle MM, Bley CR, Howard J and Rüfenacht S (2008) Canine mast cell tumours, a review of the pathogenesis, clinical features, pathology and treatment. *Veterinary Dermatology* **19**, 321–339

3

Anaemia

Jenny Mills

Introduction

Anaemia is a common clinical and laboratory test finding which in itself does not constitute a diagnosis. The ultimate aim for the veterinary practitioner is to determine the pathogenesis of the anaemia in order to deliver the most appropriate therapy for the patient and to instigate steps to prevent the condition recurring.

This chapter explores the pathophysiological mechanisms of anaemia in dogs and cats, and examines the steps involved in diagnosing the cause of anaemia in a patient. Clinical findings are combined with clues from the haematological report and the blood smear to arrive at a useful pathological diagnosis of the underlying problem. If the initial blood test is not fully revealing, further tests may be required to reach a definitive diagnosis.

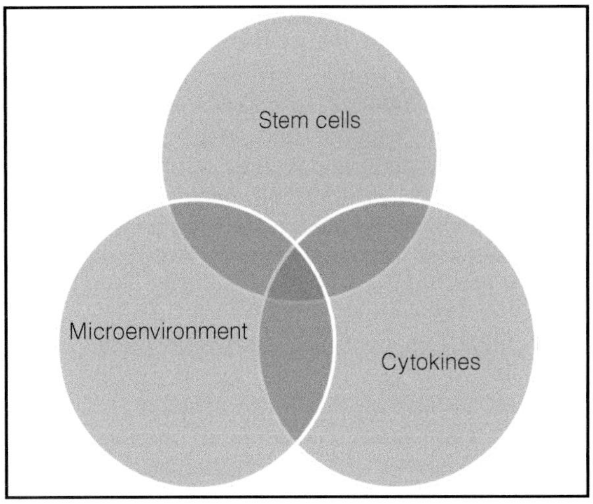

3.1 Three essential components required for haemopoiesis are stem cells, cytokines and an appropriate marrow microenvironment. The microenvironment may consist of an adequate supply of oxygen and nutrients such as iron, amino acids, glycine and vitamins B_{12}, B_6 and folate. The nutrients required for red cell production may be considered in two categories: those needed for nucleotide synthesis; and those for haemoglobin synthesis. The end products, the mature red blood cells, are released into the peripheral circulation by migration through vascular sinusoids.

Red cell production

The process of haemopoiesis and erythropoiesis requires three basic components: stem cells, cytokines and an appropriate microenvironment (Figure 3.1). The microenvironment required for red cell production includes factors such as a supply of oxygen, nutrients, iron and amino acids. In adult mammals, erythropoiesis proceeds within the bone marrow under the influence of specific cytokines, which act directly on surface receptors of the erythroid stem cells: BFU-E (burst-forming unit – erythroid) and CFU-E (colony-forming unit – erythroid). These cytokines include interleukin (IL)-3, 'burst-forming activity' and erythropoietin. Erythropoietin acts on the committed erythroid stem cells, stimulating them into active cell cycle and proliferation. The effect of increased levels of erythropoietin is to increase the number of committed erythroid stem cells, to enhance the survival of developing erythroid cells, to promote the release of maturing red cells, releasing the most mature cells first, and ultimately to increase the number of red cells effectively produced by the bone marrow. Red cell production time is 4 days (range 3–5 days). The effect of erythropoietin on stem cells is modulated and enhanced by other hormones such as androgens, thyroxine, growth hormone, corticosteroids and prostaglandins E_1 and E_2. For this reason, males have a slightly higher red cell count than females; similarly patients with hypothyroidism may have a mild anaemia.

Other factors act to inhibit erythropoiesis by down-regulating the expression of receptors on the surface of the erythroid stem cells. Suppressive factors include the inflammatory cytokines IL-1 and tumour necrosis factor (TNF)-α, both of which are released from macrophages during inflammation. Oestrogen and prostaglandin $F_{2\alpha}$ also suppress erythropoiesis. The dog is particularly sensitive to suppression of erythropoiesis by high levels of oestrogen. In cats, the p15E component of the feline leukaemia virus (FeLV) also acts to inhibit erythropoiesis. These mechanisms result in non-regenerative anaemia.

Definition of anaemia

Anaemia is defined as a situation in which the total erythron mass in peripheral blood is reduced, and the loss or destruction of red cells exceeds the rate of red cell production. The three primary values of the erythron that determine whether an animal is anaemic are haemoglobin (Hb), packed cell volume (PCV) or haematocrit (Hct), and red blood cell (RBC) count. The PCV is measured by centrifugation of a blood sample. The Hct is a value roughly equivalent to PCV and is calculated by a haematological analyser from the direct measurements of red cell count and mean red cell volume in a patient.

When interpreting any laboratory values, an awareness of factors that may influence the results is needed. Of the primary values above, the RBC count is likely to be the least accurate because of the methods of measurement. The Hb concentration will be falsely increased in lipaemic samples. The Hb concentration, PCV and RBC count will be affected by the total plasma volume of the animal. Consequently, dehydrated animals will have a contracted plasma volume and therefore may show haemoconcentration and high erythron values. If the resting erythron values were originally low, a dehydrated animal may have a 'masked anaemia', with the measured primary erythron values possibly falling within reference range. Similarly, if a patient receives intravenous fluids, a tendency to overhydration may occur, resulting in a lowering of the PCV.

Anaemia may be relative or absolute. In relative anaemia, there is a normal total red cell mass but an expanded plasma volume. Examples of relative anaemia are haemodilution after administration of intravenous fluids and sequestration of red cells as a result of splenomegaly. In absolute anaemia the total red cell mass is decreased while the plasma volume is normal. For this reason it is desirable to assess the primary erythron values in conjunction with knowledge of the patient's total protein levels. The remainder of this chapter deals only with absolute anaemia.

Variables that characterize anaemia

Once the presence of anaemia is established from the primary haematological data, the first step in defining the pathophysiology of the problem involves assessment of:

- The regenerative response: reticulocyte count and polychromasia
- Red cell indices: mean corpuscular volume (MCV) and mean corpuscular Hb concentration (MCHC)
- Red cell morphology on a blood smear
- Other qualitative features of the erythron determined by flow cytometric haematology analysers; these features include the red cell distribution width (RDW), which reflects the degree of variation in red cell size (anisocytosis).

The regenerative response

There is a physiological limit to the regenerative response of the bone marrow to anaemia. The greatest regenerative responses are seen with haemolytic anaemia (six- to eightfold increase), and moderate regenerative responses are usually seen with haemorrhagic anaemia (two- to fourfold increase). Exceptions, however, do occur. Anaemias seen within 2–4 days after blood loss or haemolysis may show no signs of regeneration in peripheral blood, because of the production time of red cells. Such conditions are termed pre-regenerative. However some reticulocytes may be seen within 48 hours of red cell loss with a peak at 4–7 days (Cowgill *et al.,* 2003). An absence of reticulocytes in an ongoing anaemia indicates a defect in production and warrants further investigation. The degree of polychromasia (Figure 3.2) and the reticulocyte count are used to assess the extent of the regenerative response of the erythron, subjectively and objectively respectively. The reticulocyte count is determined by using a supravital stain such as new methylene blue or brilliant cresyl blue and by quantifying the proportions of those red cells that contain blue-staining RNA in a reticular network (Figure 3.3). The absolute reticulocyte count is then derived by multiplying the reticulocyte percentage by the patient's total RBC

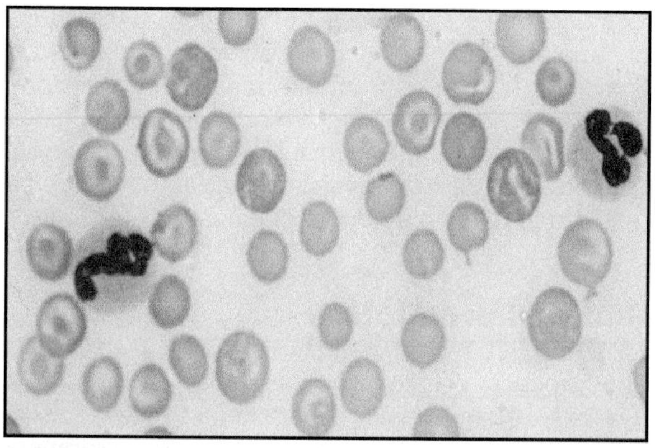

3.2 Blood smear from a dog with moderately severe haemolytic anaemia showing a good regenerative response with many (11) large polychromatic RBCs. Platelets are missing from this field.

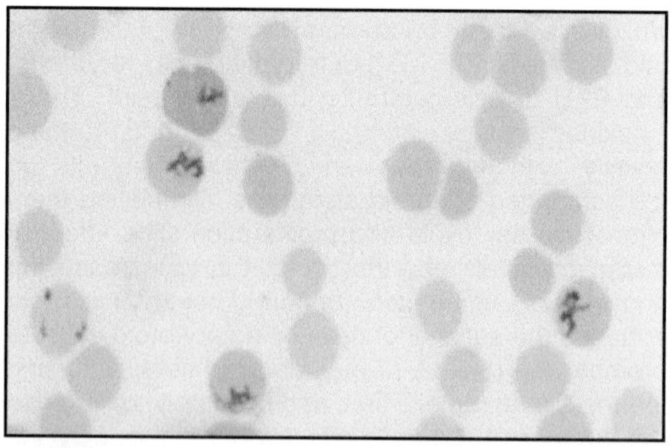

3.3 Reticulocytes stained with the supravital stain new methylene blue to demonstrate RNA. There are four cells showing a classical reticular network and one with a punctate form (this cell is older and is not included in the percentage count). Punctate forms may be quantified separately in cats. Given that reticulocytes continue to mature in the circulation, reticulocyte staining will only be valid on a fresh blood sample.

count. This calculation adjusts for the degree of anaemia and allows conclusions to be drawn on the adequacy of the bone marrow response to the anaemia.

The normal absolute reticulocyte count for a dog ranges from < 60 to 80 × 10^9/l. Using a working value of 60 × 10^9/l, an increase to 360 × 10^9/l will therefore represent a six-fold increase in erythroid production. Cats differ from dogs in that they have punctate reticulocytes as well as normal aggregate forms. The punctate forms represent aged reticulocytes, but only the aggregate forms should be counted when assessing the regenerative response. Absolute reticulocytes in cats range from < 15 to 42 × 10^9/l (Cowgill *et al.,* 2003).

Red cell indices

Red cell indices define the quality of the red cells produced by describing the average red cell size (MCV) and average red cell Hb content (MCHC). In a very strong regenerative response, a macrocytic (high MCV) hypochromic (low MCHC) population of red cells is expected. Microcytic (low MCV), hypochromic (low MCHC) populations, however, are likely to occur in conditions of defective Hb synthesis such as iron deficiency.

Macrocytosis may also be seen in myelodysplasia in cats and dogs, in association with the administration of chemotherapeutic and antiepileptic drugs, and rarely in some Poodles (Toy and Miniature). The condition in Poodles does not require treatment. Microcytosis may be seen normally in the Japanese Akita and Shiba Inu breeds of dog and in some dogs with portosystemic shunts.

Red cell morphology

Red cell morphology is evaluated by examination of a stained blood smear, looking particularly in the monolayer area (Figure 3.4). Any changes in shape from the classic biconcave disc are identified and semiquantified, and may lead to a specific diagnosis or interpretation. Compared with red cells from a dog, those from a cat are smaller (MCV 39–55 fl *versus* 60–77 fl), not as biconcave and show less central pallor on smears.

In very strongly regenerative anaemias, the degree of variation in red cell size is likely to be wider than normal. This feature may be expressed as anisocytosis when examining the blood smear or be reflected in a higher RDW value when using a haematology analyser.

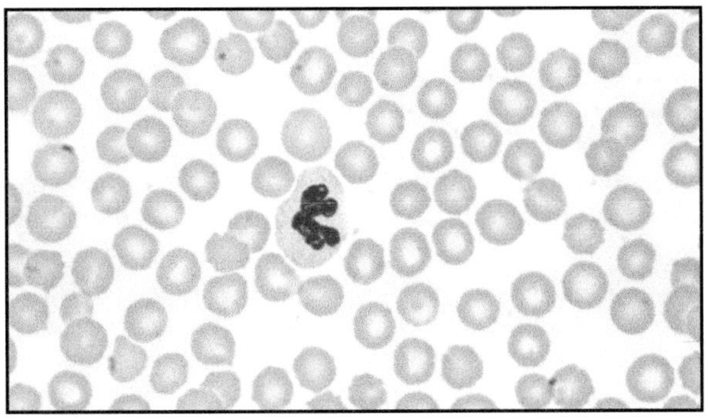

3.4 Blood smear from a non-anaemic dog showing normal distribution of red blood cells in the monolayer area of the slide. Note that there is little space between the cells to insert another red cell. Also note the degree of central pallor of the red cells and the abnormal absence of platelets in this field; the platelets were clumped at the feather end of the slide.

Erythron disorders without anaemia

Anaemia only occurs when the rate of red cell loss or destruction exceeds the rate of red cell production. Changes in red cell production and/or loss may occur without significant reductions in PCV, Hb concentration or RBC count. Compensated anaemia may be seen in some haemolytic states where the rate of production matches the rate of red cell destruction. In these cases, there are obvious signs of erythroid regeneration in the peripheral blood, with high levels of reticulocytes and possibly some morphological change in the red cells. Examples of this have been reported with immune-mediated haemolysis (Mills, 1997) and in a hereditary red cell defect in a young dog (Mills and Marsden, 1999). Another example of canine hereditary elliptocytosis has been described in which the patient was not anaemic and had very few polychromatophilic erythrocytes (Di Terlizzi *et al.,* 2009).

Defects in bone marrow production and disorders that affect the haemoglobinization process, which lead to ineffective erythropoiesis, may be associated temporarily with normal erythron values before anaemia develops. This condition will be described later. Examples of ineffective erythropoiesis include lead poisoning and deficiencies of folic acid, vitamin B_{12} and iron.

The spleen plays a role in the red cell life cycle, in that in most domestic animal species it contains narrow vascular sinusoids through which the red cells traverse. Senescent red cells lose their deformability and consequently are phagocytosed by macrophages in the spleen. In this way the spleen acts as the ‘rubbish sorter’ of blood, removing other particles such as Howell–Jolly bodies and nuclei of immature red cells. Consequently, enlargement of the spleen for any reason can trap or sequester more red cells, contributing to an apparent anaemia caused mainly by redistribution of cells to this organ. However, the effect of adrenaline in causing splenic enlargement is minimal in the dog and cat compared with that in the horse, where up to 30% of the blood volume may be trapped in an enlarged spleen. The spleen of cats does not contain a sinusoidal structure, thereby permitting longer survival of particles such as Heinz bodies within red cells.

If the rate of red cell production exceeds the rate of loss, a state of erythrocytosis (secondary polycythaemia) with high PCV, Hb concentration and RBC count may develop eventually. Increased erythroid production, and consequently reticulocytosis, may occur in response to the high erythropoietin concentrations that follow tissue anoxia. Conditions associated with erythrocytosis include obstructive pulmonary disease, cardiovascular disorders (e.g. ventricular septal defects, patent ductus arteriosus), high altitude states, renal hypoxia or renal abnormalities (e.g. embryonal nephroma, renal cysts). Autonomous production of mature red cells, irrespective of erythropoietin concentrations, represents a neoplastic state of haemopoiesis known as polycythaemia vera (primary polycythaemia).

Classification of anaemia

The classification of anaemia according to basic pathophysiological mechanisms provides a useful approach to the diagnosis of the underlying problem.

Anaemias of bone marrow dysfunction involve reduced red cell production, defects in nucleotide synthesis, defects in haemoglobin synthesis and myelodysplastic syndromes. Anaemias of increased red cell destruction involve haemolysis of normal red cells or haemolysis caused by either genetic defects of red cells or acquired defects of red cells. Anaemias of increased red cell loss involve internal or external haemorrhage. Figure 3.5 shows examples of anaemia, Figure 3.6 shows an outline of causes of anaemia based on diagnostic decisions or observations and Figure 3.7 illustrates a diagnostic algorithm.

Feature	Interpretation
Large number of spherocytes	Immune-mediated haemolysis
Schistocytes (fragmented cells)	Intravascular red cell injury
Keratocytes (horn shapes)	Intravascular red cell injury
Heinz bodies	Heinz body haemolysis, oxidant injury
Dacryocytes (teardrop shapes)	Iron deficiency, myelofibrosis
Echinocytes (burr cells)	Renal azotaemia, chemotherapy
Acanthocytes (spur cells)	Splenic neoplasia, liver disease

3.5 Examples of changes in red cell morphology from the classical biconcave disc and their relevant interpretation.

Anaemias of bone marrow dysfunction

The basic requirements for production of red cells are stem cells, cytokines and an appropriate marrow environment, which includes blood supply, oxygen and nutrients. When any of these components are lacking, erythropoiesis will be affected.

Reduced red cell production

Anaemias in this category will be non-regenerative, normocytic (normal MCV) and normochromic (normal MCHC). A concurrent leucopenia and thrombocytopenia should alert the clinician to the possibility of aplastic anaemia or myelophthisis. In these two conditions, multipotential stem cells may be injured, suppressed (aplasia; no growth) or displaced (myelophthisis; marrow wasting). Some of these effects may be mediated by cytokines or regulatory lymphocytes, which may alter the bone marrow microenvironment. These anaemias can be severe and difficult to treat, but in some instances the administration of cytokines has been found to be helpful in promoting cell development and maturation. Examples of causes of marrow aplasia include the injurious effects of irradiation, toxic plants (e.g. bracken fern in cattle), viruses (e.g. FeLV), hormones (e.g. oestrogen, particularly in dogs and ferrets, not in cats), drugs (e.g. phenylbutazone, chloramphenicol, sulpha drugs), chemicals that accumulate in fat (e.g. DDT, trichlorethylene, cyclic hydrocarbons) and infectious agents such as *Ehrlichia* and *Leishmania*.

Myelophthisis represents a space-occupying lesion in bone marrow that inhibits or displaces normal haemopoietic cells. Examples are marrow neoplasms, leukaemias, metastatic neoplasms (e.g. carcinomas, melanomas), myelofibrosis and granulomatous inflammatory diseases of the marrow, such as systemic fungal infections, histoplasmosis and miliary tuberculosis. The development of myelofibrosis may be idiopathic, representing a clonal proliferation in the marrow, or occur after prolonged marrow stimulation or as a terminal event in myeloproliferative disease. Myelofibrosis is considered to be associated with large numbers of megakaryocytes and with platelet-derived growth factors, and marrow mastocytosis may be seen in these patients.

Pure red cell aplasia refers to reductions in committed (unipotential) erythroid stem cells only. Leucocytes and platelets are unaffected. This condition may be caused by FeLV, by direct suppression of BFU-E stem cells, or may be immune-mediated in dogs, in which antibodies may be specifically directed at epitopes on the immature erythroid cells. In the last case, some spherocytes may be seen in peripheral blood and the Coombs' test may give a positive result. Reductions in the concentrations of erythropoietin or cytokines that affect erythropoiesis have a role in the production of non-regenerative anaemia associated with chronic renal failure or endocrine dysfunction (e.g. hypothyroidism, hyperoestrogenism, hypoadrenocorticism or pituitary hypofunction). The dog is particularly prone to suppression of haemopoiesis by oestrogen, from either hyperoestrogenism in Sertoli cell tumours, interstitial cell tumours, ovarian granulosa cell tumour or after excessive stilboestrol administration (Sontas *et al.*, 2009). The suppression is considered to be mediated by an inhibitor produced by the thymus in response to oestrogen and which suppresses haemopoiesis at the stem cell level (Brockus, 1998).

The anaemia of chronic renal failure is usually mild to moderate and non-regenerative. It is primarily caused by a lack of erythropoietin production by the kidneys. Other factors that contribute to the anaemia of chronic renal failure include:

- Reduced half-life of red cells as a result of uraemic toxins
- Haemorrhagic loss from gastrointestinal ulcers

Category of anaemia	Mechanisms	Examples of causes
Reduced marrow production (stem cell, marrow microenvironment)	Marrow aplasia (results in pancytopenia or bicytopenia)	Irradiation Toxic plants (e.g. bracken fern in cattle) Viruses (e.g. FeLV) Hormones (e.g. oestrogen, particularly in dogs and ferrets, not in cats) Drugs (e.g. phenylbutazone, chloramphenicol, sulpha drugs) Chemicals that accumulate in fat (e.g. DDT, trichlorethylene, cyclic hydrocarbons) Infectious agents (e.g. *Ehrlichia* spp., *Leishmania* spp.)
	Myelophthisis (results in pancytopenia or bicytopenia)	Marrow neoplasms, leukaemias, metastatic neoplasms (e.g. carcinomas, melanomas) Myelofibrosis Granulomatous inflammatory disease of marrow (e.g. systemic fungal infections, histoplasmosis, miliary tuberculosis)
Reduced red blood cell (RBC) production	Pure red cell aplasia (reduced RBCs only)	Immune-mediated (dogs) FeLV-related (cats)
	Reduced erythropoietin and suppression by cytokines	Chronic renal failure Endocrine dysfunction (e.g. hypothyroidism, hypoadrenocorticism or pituitary hypofunction, hyperoestrogenism)
	Cytokine suppression and other complex mechanisms	Anaemia of inflammatory disease Chronic parasitism (e.g. *Trypanosoma congolense*) Chronic liver disease
Ineffective erythropoiesis (lack of specific nutrients)	Defects in nucleotide synthesis	Deficiencies of folic acid, vitamin B_{12}, cobalt and intrinsic factor (e.g. chemotherapy, sulpha drugs, antiepileptic drugs, mysoline, phenobarbital, dilantin)
	Defects in haemoglobin synthesis	Iron deficiency anaemia (e.g. chronic external blood loss, gastrointestinal defects) Deficiencies of copper and vitamin B_6 Lead poisoning Hereditary porphyria (cats)
Myelodysplastic syndromes	Dysplasia in one or more of the haemopoietic cell lines	FeLV Idiopathic, drug-induced
Haemolysis	Genetic defects of red cells	Abnormal RBC shape or membrane (e.g. elliptocytes, stomatocytes) Biochemical RBC defect (e.g. deficiency in pyruvate kinase, phosphofructokinase, methaemoglobin reductase, calcium pump ATPase)
	Acquired defects of RBCs	Biochemical changes (e.g. Heinz bodies, hypophosphataemia) Chemical haemolysins (e.g. heavy metals, lead, zinc, silver; arsenicals; excessive copper and cyclic hydrocarbons) Bacterial, animal or plant haemolysins (e.g. lysins from *Leptospira icterohaemorrhagica*, *Clostridium haemolyticum*; spider and snake venoms; ricin from castor oil beans) Immune-mediated haemolytic anaemia – coating of red cells by antibody and/or complement Mechanical injury of red cells (e.g. vascular pathology, malignancies) Parasites (e.g. *Babesia canis*, *Mycoplasma haemofelis*)
	Lysis of normal RBCs	Hypersplenism (e.g. splenic torsion, malignancy)
Haemorrhage	Loss of blood	Trauma (e.g. ruptured liver, spleen) Surgery Parasitism: internal/external (e.g. fleas, ticks, lice, *Ancylostoma*, *Uncinaria* in dogs) Coagulopathy Platelet defects or deficiency Ruptured aneurysm or neoplasm (e.g. haemangiosarcoma) Pathology of the gastrointestinal or urogenital tract (e.g. GI ulcers, drug-induced ulcers, inflammatory bowel disease, neoplasms)

3.6 Causes of anaemia.

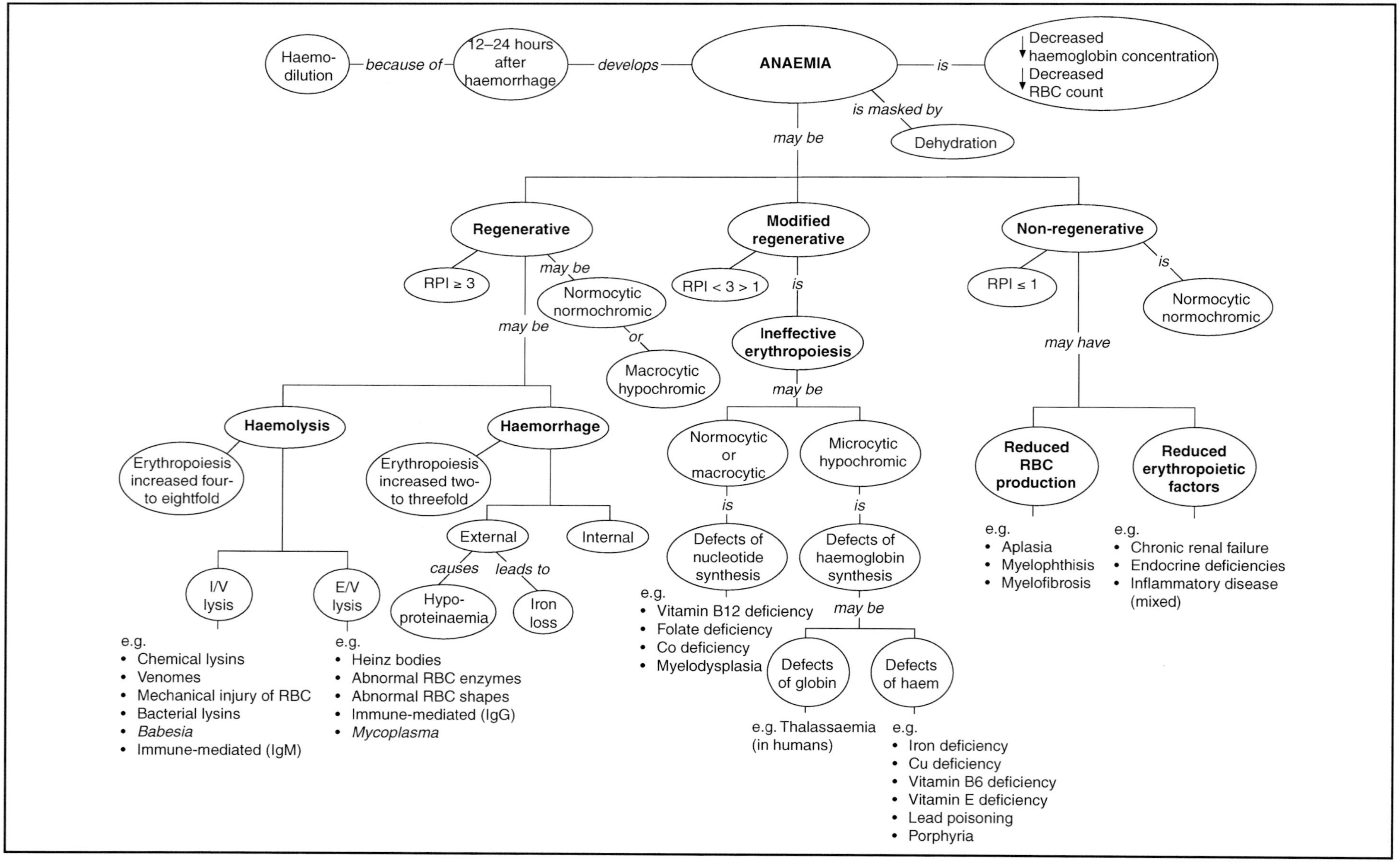

3.7 Concept map of anaemia illustrating a pathway for diagnosing anaemia. Linking words are italicized. RBC, red blood cell; RPI, reticulocyte production index; Cu, copper; Co, cobalt; I/V, intravascular; E/V, extravascular.

- Increased bleeding tendency due to reduced platelet function
- Accumulation of increased levels of hepcidin (a peptide that indirectly inhibits release of iron stores)
- Suppression of erythropoiesis by high concentrations of parathyroid hormone
- Reduced nutrient intake caused by inappetence
- Injury of red cells attributable to glomerular pathology and renal fibrosis.

Consequently echinocytes and some schistocytes and keratocytes can be seen in the anaemia of renal failure.

The anaemia of inflammatory disease – the commonest form of anaemia in domestic animals – is associated with both acute and chronic inflammation. A key mediator of the anaemia of inflammatory and chronic disease is considered to be hepcidin, a peptide produced by hepatocytes that increases in inflammatory conditions (Ganz, 2006). Hepcidin was initially recognized as having antimicrobial properties and is responsible for making iron unavailable; it inhibits the export of iron from cells such as macrophages and enterocytes by binding to the iron export protein, ferroportin. The pathogenesis of the anaemia of inflammatory disease also involves a complex of changes mediated by the cytokines TNF-α and IL-1 released from activated macrophages. The pro-inflammatory cytokines suppress erythropoiesis by down-regulating the surface erythropoietin receptors of committed erythroid stem cells. At the same time, other cytokines stimulate granulocyte production to produce the leucocytes required to combat the infection. Under the influence of IL-1, storage iron is converted from ferritin to the less available form of haemosiderin; iron is tightly bound to haptoglobin and lactoferrin in leucocytes at the site of infection, becoming unavailable for both red cell production and bacterial use. The concentration of circulating serum iron is consequently reduced, but so is its transport protein, transferrin. Rather than measuring transferrin, the functional capacity to transport iron can be measured as the total iron binding capacity. In addition, red cells from affected patients bind increased surface immunoglobulin and consequently have a shortened life span, being phagocytosed more readily than normal.

Other conditions that can cause non-regenerative anaemia include dietary protein deficiency or suppression of erythropoiesis by TNF-α in some parasitic infections. An example of the latter occurs in trypanosomiasis caused by *Trypanosoma congolense*, where expression of erythropoietin receptors is reduced (Suliman *et al.*, 1999).

Chronic liver disease may also be associated with anaemia for a variety of reasons, but usually there is a degree of red cell regeneration, possibly associated with some haemorrhagic loss and red cell injury. In about 60% of dogs with portosystemic shunts, microcytosis may be evident. Disturbances in iron metabolism, copper storage/toxicity and chronic inflammation are likely to contribute to the pathogenesis of the anaemia in chronic liver disorders. Poikilocytosis (abnormal erythrocyte shape) is expected in hepatic disease, with acanthocytosis and ovalocytes (elliptical erythrocytes) seen in many cats with hepatic lipidosis.

Defects in nucleotide synthesis

In conditions of this category, stem cells and cytokines are adequate, but the microenvironment is deficient, lacking a supply of nutrients essential for nucleotide synthesis. Erythropoietin concentrations are increased and cell production proceeds abnormally. Defects in DNA or RNA synthesis cause delays in nuclear synthesis, which result in asynchrony in cell development. Consequently, nuclear development lags behind cytoplasmic development and the cells produced may be large or megaloblastic. Many cells are recognized as abnormal and are destroyed in the bone marrow. This results in ineffective erythropoiesis. The problem extends to all cells attempting to undergo mitosis.

Examples of this form of anaemia occur with deficiencies of folic acid, vitamin B_{12}, cobalt and intrinsic factor. These conditions are rare in animals but may be induced by administration of folate antagonists such as methotrexate or may occur in patients with malignancies, in which the stores of these nutrients may be exhausted. Administration of sulpha drugs and potentiated sulpha drugs can inhibit folate metabolism and thymidine synthesis. Long-term administration of antiepileptic drugs (e.g. mysoline, phenobarbital and dilantin) can also deplete serum folate concentrations. Macrocytosis may be found in human patients with these conditions, but has rarely been described in animals.

A congenital selective malabsorption of vitamin B_{12} in Giant Schnauzers has been reported to cause a non-regenerative anaemia with poikilocytosis and neutropenia with hypersegmentation. The condition was inherited as an autosomal recessive trait. Affected dogs showed a dramatic response to injections of vitamin B_{12}. A similar condition has been reported in a Beagle. The same disorder described in Border Collies resulted in failure to thrive and metabolic acidosis, and was characterized by haematological abnormalities with ketonuria.

Defects in haemoglobin synthesis

In a similar way, defects in the production of components essential for Hb manufacture can lead to ineffective erythropoiesis. In this case, inadequate quantities of Hb are produced and cells appear pale and hypochromic, and cytoplasmic development lags behind nuclear development. These conditions may be considered as defects of either haem or globin synthesis. Examples of defects of globin synthesis are seen in the genetic abnormalities that affect the production of the α or β amino acid chains of Hb in humans, for example thalassaemia and sickle cell anaemia, none of which has been recorded to date in animals. There are many variants of thalassaemia in humans, and these may result in red cells being more fragile than normal, having a shortened lifespan, being abnormal in shape and showing microcytosis and hypochromasia. Similarly, red cells of patients with sickle cell anaemia have abnormal crescent shapes and a shortened lifespan.

Iron deficiency anaemia is a classic example of a defect in haem synthesis (Figure 3.8). In this condition erythropoietin concentrations are high and stem cells are adequate, but the lack of available iron leads to delayed and defective cytoplasmic maturation of red cells. The developing cells may undergo an additional mitosis at the basophilic rubricyte stage while awaiting the haemoglobinization process, consequently becoming smaller (microcytic) and hypochromic. The resulting cells are more fragile than normal, some show tear-drop shapes (dacryocytes) and many are destroyed prematurely. A marked decrease in the expression of the hepcidin gene has been found in dogs with nutritional iron deficiency, with an increase in the expression of the transferrin receptor gene, thereby potentially enhancing the utilization of iron when it becomes available (Fry *et al.*, 2009).

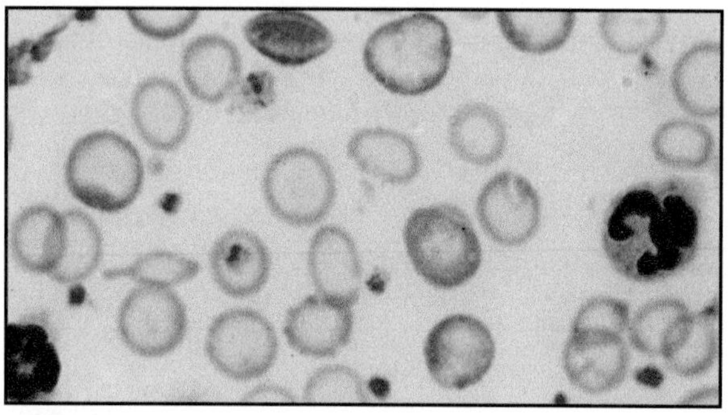

3.8 Blood smear from a dog with iron deficiency anaemia showing severely hypochromic red cells with a wide area of central pallor. One dacryocyte (tear drop-shaped cell) is present on the left side; some cells are smaller than normal. Note the plentiful platelets.

About 50% of patients with iron deficiency anaemia may have concurrent thrombocytosis, with large numbers of small platelets and consequently a tendency to form microthrombi. Thrombocytosis may occur in patients that have concurrent chronic external blood loss that has led to the development of the iron-deficient state. Chronic external haemorrhage is the commonest cause of iron deficiency anaemia (caused by internal or external blood-sucking parasites, gastrointestinal ulcers or neoplasms, etc.). Reduced intake of iron may be seen in young animals around the time of weaning. In older animals, blood loss through the gastrointestinal tract is the most common cause of iron deficiency anaemia.

Deficiencies of copper and vitamin B_6 may show similar haematological signs to iron deficiency in humans, with microcytosis and hypochromasia, but rarely cause anaemia in animals. Copper in the enzyme ferroxidase (caeruloplasmin) is essential for the utilization of iron, converting ferrous to ferric iron, in which form it is transported by transferrin to the bone marrow. Within the marrow it is converted back to the ferrous form to be incorporated in red cell production at the haem synthetase step.

Other conditions that lead to defects in haem synthesis in small animals are lead poisoning and erythropoietic porphyria. Lead blocks sulphydral groups within enzymes involved in haem synthesis. Characteristically, large numbers of metarubricytes are found in the peripheral blood of animals with acute lead poisoning, but there is no concurrent anaemia or polychromasia. Basophilic stippling may be seen in about 30% of affected dogs, but is not a specific finding.

Hereditary porphyria has been reported as a dominant trait in anaemic Siamese cats and in some non-anaemic Domestic Shorthaired cats. Affected animals will have ineffective erythropoiesis in which large quantities of the isomer I of protoporphyrin are produced instead of isomer III. Isomer I is unable to combine normally with iron to form haem. There may be some haemolysis of red cells with 'port wine'-coloured urine, photosensitization, and fluorescence of teeth and urine in ultraviolet light caused by oxidized porphyrins in these tissues. It is interesting to note that hereditary porphyria in humans is thought to have given rise to the legends of werewolves.

Myelodysplastic syndromes (MDS)

These conditions are characterized by dysplasia (abnormal development) in one or more haemopoietic cell lines in a hypercellular bone marrow as a result of ineffective haemopoiesis, with concurrent refractory cytopenias and non-regenerative anaemia in the peripheral blood; the cells produced may be dysfunctional. Although myelodysplasia is rare in dogs, myelodysplasia in cats is often associated with FeLV infection and may manifest with macrocytosis. Bone marrow examination is essential to characterize the pathology.

By definition, there will be fewer than 20% blastic cells in the bone marrow in MDS. Six types of MDS are described in humans, which have implications in management strategies, although all may not be directly applicable to animals (Valli, 2007). These categories are:

- Refractory anaemia with an excess of blasts (RAEB subtypes 1 and 2)
- Refractory anaemia with/or without ringed sideroblasts
- Refractory cytopenia with multilineage dysplasia
- MDS unclassified (most frequently identified in dogs).

Myelodysplastic syndromes may be primary, resulting from a genetic transformation in a multipotential stem cell, or secondary and associated with administration of a chemotherapeutic drug or irradiation therapy. The secondary conditions may resolve on withdrawal of the offending drug. In most myelodysplastic syndromes the haemopoietic cells have increased apoptosis, reduced capacity of cells to differentiate and the microenvironment may have overproduction of IL-1 and TNF-α. The primary conditions are variable in their response to haemopoietic cytokines that act as maturation factors. Cases of MDS with higher percentages of blastic cells in the marrow have a shorted survival time and poorer prognosis, whereas MDS with refractory anaemia, cytopenia or erythroid predominance appear to respond to recombinant haemopoietic cytokines or erythropoietin and such patients have a longer survival (Weiss, 2003). Patients with refractory cytopenias with multilineage dysplasia and with a higher percentage of blasts may progress into overt acute myelogenous leukaemia at a later date, but may respond temporarily to topotecan and cytarabine (Valli, 2007).

These conditions must be distinguished from ineffective erythropoiesis caused by nutrient deficiencies (e.g. vitamin B_{12}, folic acid, iron), lead or arsenic toxicity or drug reaction by bone marrow examination, biochemical assays and clinical history.

Chronic idiopathic myelofibrosis is a rare condition that was previously known as myeloid metaplasia with myelofibrosis and represents a clonal proliferation in bone marrow (Valli, 2007). It involves hyperplasia of the myeloid and megakaryocytic series with variable asynchrony in the early developmental cells but maturation through to the end-stage cells. The erythroid cells are reduced and many dacryocytes appear in the peripheral blood along with a mild leucoerythroblastic reaction and splenomegaly. Ineffective granulopoiesis may occur, leading to leucopenia. In due course, fibrosis of the marrow develops and is closely associated with megakaryocyte hyperplasia. Core biopsies of marrow will be more diagnostic than marrow aspirates once myelofibrosis develops.

Anaemias of increased red cell destruction

Haemolysis may be considered the result of an intrinsic or extrinsic defect of the red cell, which causes the cells to be destroyed at a higher rate than normal. Consequently these cells have a short half-life and may show some morphological change. Specific changes in red cell shape may provide clues to the cause of the haemolysis. Examples include immune-mediated haemolytic anaemia (IMHA; with marked spherocytosis; Figure 3.9), signs of mechanical intravascular injury (e.g. schistocytes, keratocytes; Figures 3.10, 3.11 and 3.12), biochemical change (e.g. Heinz bodies, eccentrocytes, ovalocytes, sphero-echinocytes) or cellular parasites (e.g. *Mycoplasma* (formerly *Haemobartonella*), *Babesia* spp.). Changes to the red cell membrane are also seen in echinocytes (burr cells) and acanthocytes (spur cells; Figure 3.13). The mechanism of destruction of the red cells may be by direct lysis within the bloodstream (intravascular haemolysis) or by erythrophagia by macrophages in the spleen, liver, marrow or lymph nodes (extravascular haemolysis), or both.

Clinically, intravascular haemolysis may have a more deleterious effect on the patient than extravascular haemolysis, because, in addition to the effects of low tissue oxygenation, there are also fragments of free red cell membrane in circulation, which may trigger disseminated intravascular coagulation (DIC). The presence of free Hb released from red cells is injurious to tissues and some may appear in urine when concentrations exceed renal thresholds. In addition, the rate of destruction of red cells may also exceed the capacity of the liver to process

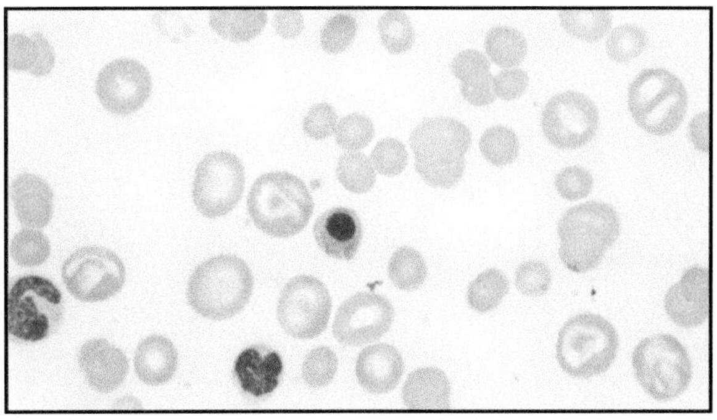

3.9 Blood smear from a dog with immune-mediated haemolytic anaemia showing many large polychromatic erythrocytes and smaller spherocytes; this represents a classical biphasic red cell population. Platelets are also missing from this field. They may be consumed in concurrent anti-platelet destruction or coagulopathy (disseminated intravascular coagulation and thromboemboli).

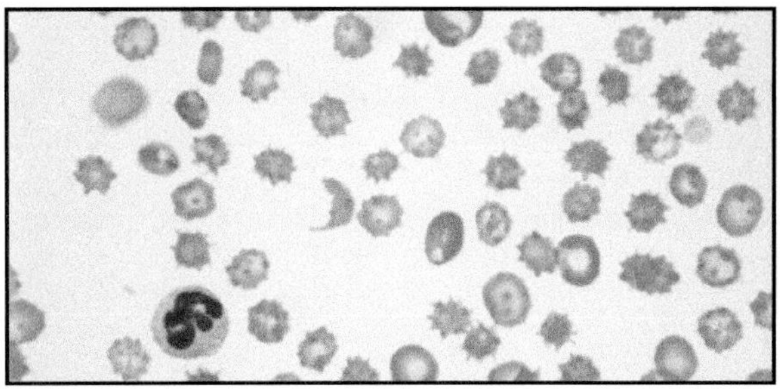

3.10 Blood smear from a dog with a schizocyte in the centre of the field indicating mechanical red cell injury. There is a moderate regenerative anaemia associated with a vascular neoplasm, haemangiosarcoma, and there is marked poikilocytosis with many echinocytes (burr cells). Only one platelet is present in this field.

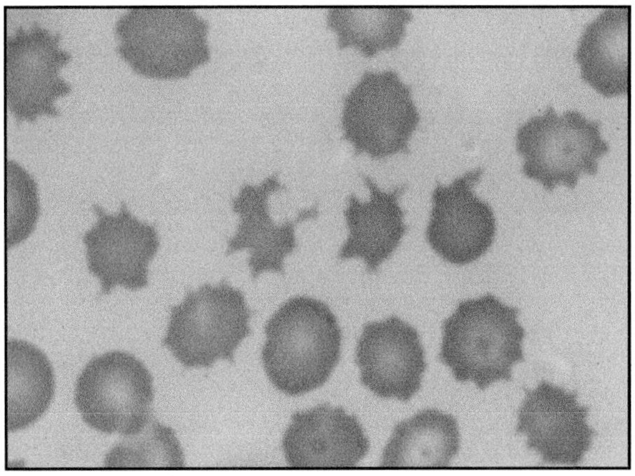

3.11 Blood smear from a dog with severe schizocytosis associated with a malignancy, causing mechanical red cell injury and moderate anaemia.

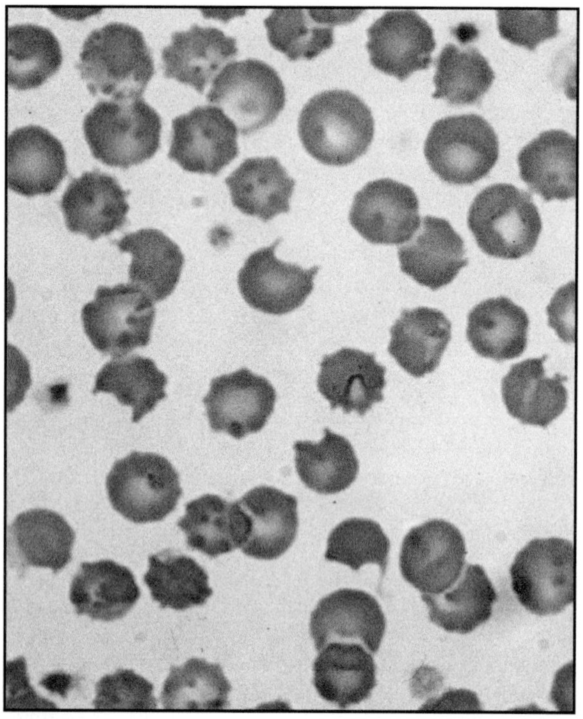

3.12 Blood smear from a dog with mechanical red cell injury and moderate regenerative anaemia associated with disseminated intravascular coagulation. Three horn-shaped cells, keratocytes, are present in the centre of the field. There is also moderate echinocytosis (burr cells).

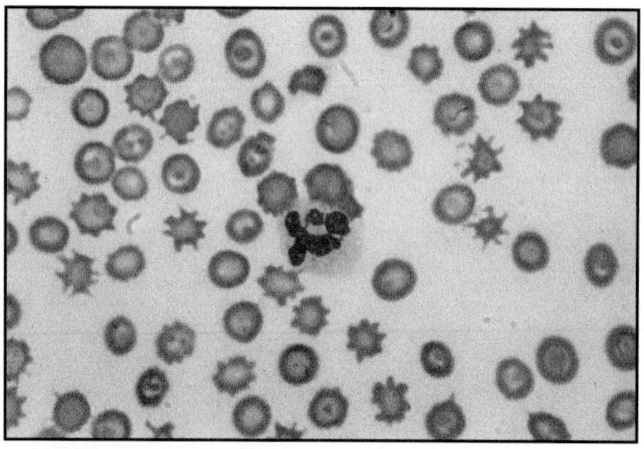

3.13 Blood smear from a dog with many acanthocytes (spur cells – star-shaped appearance with long cytoplasmic projections) with a moderate regenerative anaemia associated with splenic haemangiosarcoma.

bilirubin, and, combined with poor oxygenation, reduced liver function contributes to the appearance of clinical jaundice in many patients with intravascular haemolysis.

Extravascular haemolysis may proceed within macrophages in the spleen, liver or marrow and consequently mild splenic enlargement associated with extravascular haemolysis may be detected on abdominal palpation. Although affected patients show all the signs of anaemia, there are no signs of the haemoglobinaemia, haemoglobinuria or tissue injury usually associated with intravascular haemolysis. In addition, jaundice is rare in extravascular haemolysis.

The anaemia in haemolytic conditions will usually be strongly regenerative. The maximum marrow response may be an eightfold increase in red cell production, as detected by the absolute reticulocyte count. In the long term, however, continued haemolysis and marrow stimulation, particularly with hereditary haemolytic disorders, can lead eventually to myelofibrosis and in some cases osteosclerosis.

Haemolysis due to genetic defects of red cells

In these rare conditions, red cells may have an abnormal shape or membrane (e.g. elliptocytes, stomatocytes) or a biochemical defect (e.g. deficiency in pyruvate kinase (PK), phosphofructokinase (PFK), methaemoglobin reductase, calcium pump ATPase), which acts to shorten their lifespan. Other inherited haemolytic conditions may be associated with copper storage defects, malabsorption of vitamin B_{12} and hepatic disorders.

Hereditary stomatocytosis has been described in some dwarf Alaskan Malamutes, Pomeranians and Miniature and Standard Schnauzers. Hereditary elliptocytosis (Figure 3.14) has been reported in a crossbred line of dogs, a mixed breed dog (Di Terlizzi *et al.,* 2009) and a Silky Terrier (Mills and Marsden, 1999). These conditions were associated with either minimal anaemia or compensated anaemia and were discovered incidentally.

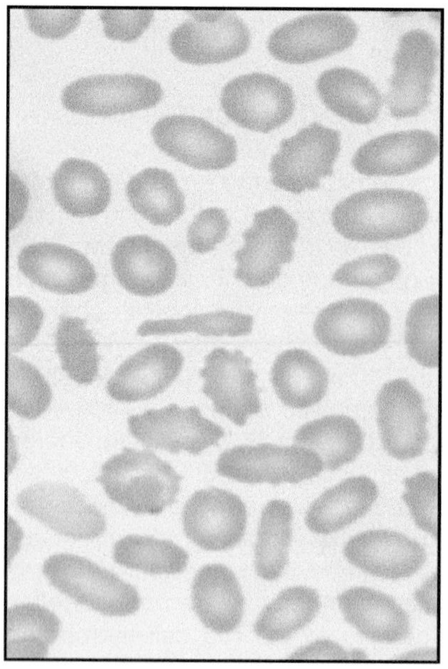

3.14 Blood smear from a young dog with poikilocytosis caused by hereditary elliptocytosis and a compensated anaemia.

Increased RBC osmotic fragility due to a spectrin deficiency of RBC membranes has been reported in Golden Retrievers from the Netherlands (Slappendel *et al.,* 2005), and increased osmotic fragility is also recognized in Abyssinian and Somali cats.

PK deficiency of red cells is an autosomal recessive trait described in Basenjis, Beagles, West Highland White Terriers, Cairn Terriers, Abyssinian and Somali cats and several other breeds of dog. PK is required in the anaerobic glycolytic pathway of RBCs. Affected cells are unable to maintain normal shape, lose potassium and have reduced oxygen affinity. Red cells become sphero-echinocytic and have a lifespan reduced to about 20 days. Erythrocytes from affected dogs lack the normal R-type PK isoenzyme, and instead have an abnormal M-2 type PK isoenzyme (Giger *et al.*, 1991). Specific laboratory tests are required to diagnose a PK deficient dog, rather than simply measuring total PK activity. Carrier dogs, with half normal activity, can also be identified. Genetic tests are available to detect affected and carrier dogs.

A non-spherocytic haemolytic anaemia of Beagles is associated with a defect in the ATPase calcium pump system. The defect affects older red cells more than young cells. Other non-spherocytic anaemias have been recorded in Miniature Poodles and Beagles. In these cases, chronic haemolysis leads to myelofibrosis and osteosclerosis.

A compensated intravascular haemolysis with bilirubinuria associated with PFK deficiency of red cells is an autosomal recessive condition that has been described in English Springer Spaniels, American Cocker Spaniels, mixed breed dogs and Whippets (Harvey and Smith, 1994; Gerber *et al.*, 2009). PFK is a rate-controlling enzyme in glycolysis in RBCs. The affected red cells showed increased fragility in alkaline conditions; this is a result of decreased intracellular concentrations of 2,3-diphosphoglycerate, the major organic acid within red cells. PFK may also be decreased in muscle cells, causing clinical signs of cramp and muscle weakness. Genetic tests are available to detect this condition in affected and carrier dogs.

A separate polysystemic disorder involving dyserythropoiesis, polymyopathy, megaoesophagus and cardiomegaly has been described in English Springer Spaniels; the exact mechanism causing these defects has not been defined (Holland *et al.*, 1991).

Methaemoglobin reductase deficiency has been described in a cat and in three dogs (a Miniature Poodle, Toy Alaskan Eskimo bitch and Pomeranian puppy). The affected animals showed persistent cyanosis of mucous membranes and occasional seizures. Methaemoglobin concentrations were increased to 19–25% of the total Hb concentration. In contrast to the condition in humans, these dogs did not respond to oral riboflavine therapy.

Macrocytosis may be seen in some Toy and Miniature Poodles, with MCVs of 85–95 fl (normal range 60–77 fl). Although marrow examination will reveal abnormal nucleated erythrocytes and incomplete mitosis with some dyserythropoiesis, no therapy is indicated. Similarly, Japanese Akita and Shiba Inu dogs have smaller red cells than other breeds, with MCVs as low as 55–64 fl. Their red cells contain a higher level of intracellular potassium than those of other dogs, thereby causing spurious hyperkalaemia in haemolysed blood samples.

Haemolysis caused by acquired defects of red cells

Acquired defects of red cells are the most common cause of haemolysis. The ultimate mechanism of lysis is usually either direct membrane injury or osmotic lysis. Morphological changes to red cells are usually seen in haemolytic anaemia. The causes are listed in Figure 3.6 and include:

- Biochemical changes (e.g. Heinz bodies, hypophosphataemia)
- Exposure to chemical haemolysins (e.g. heavy metals such as lead, zinc, silver; arsenicals; excessive copper and cyclic hydrocarbons)
- Bacterial, animal or plant haemolysins (e.g. lysins from *Leptospira icterohaemorrhagica*, *Clostridium haemolyticum*; some spider and snake venoms, particularly black snake; and the ricin from castor oil beans, which causes direct lysis)
- Coating of red cells by antibody and/or complement (this will shorten their lifespan and lead to IMHA, with the appearance of marked spherocytosis and anisocytosis)
- Mechanical injury of red cells (cell injury that occurs while in the circulation may result in intravascular haemolysis; examples are conditions associated with vascular and valvular lesions or some malignancies)
- Parasites: infection with intracellular or extracellular parasites such as *Babesia canis* or *Mycoplasma haemofelis* will cause haemolytic anaemia, which may be compounded by immune-mediated haemolysis.

Biochemical changes: Prolonged exposure to oxidant drugs or chemicals may lead to exhaustion of reduced glutathione and the rate-limiting enzyme, glutathione 6-phosphate dehydrogenase, within red cells, causing denaturation of Hb. As a result, Heinz bodies form in the older red cells first, making them more rigid than normal, and these cells are either phagocytosed as they pass through the splenic sinuses or lysed directly within the circulation. Heinz bodies are 0.5–1 μm in diameter and their presence may be shown by a supravital stain such as new methylene blue. The methaemoglobin reductase (diaphorase) system is also vulnerable to oxidant injury, resulting in the formation of methaemoglobin. In this state, iron within red cells is oxidized to the ferric form, which cannot transport oxygen. As a result, affected animals may not only have severe anaemia but also hypoxaemia. Ingestion of onions is a common cause of Heinz body formation in dogs, and toxicity is dose dependent, i.e. the larger the animal the more onion is needed to cause toxicity. Garlic also contains the same toxic agents; however, the toxic dose is unknown. The toxic agents in onions and garlic are *n*-propyl disulphide, *s*-methylcysteine sulphoxide, methyl disulphide and allyl disulphide. High doses of vitamins K_1 and K_3 have also resulted in Heinz body formation.

Cats are more prone to Heinz body formation because their Hb molecules contain eight to ten sulphydryl groups, compared with only two or three groups in other species. However, the spleen in cats is non-sinusoidal, allowing longer survival of red cells containing Heinz bodies. Cats with diabetes mellitus, lymphoma or hyperthyroidism have a higher incidence of Heinz bodies than normal cats. Cats fed a semi-solid diet of tinned food containing the preservative propylene glycol may develop Heinz bodies, and many other oxidizing substances can also lead to Heinz body formation.

Cats are particularly prone to haemolysis associated with severe hypophosphataemia; this may occur in cats with diabetes mellitus or hepatic lipidosis (Adams *et al.*, 1993). For this reason, phosphate supplementation is recommended for cats with serum phosphate concentrations of < 0.5 mmol/l (Di Bartola, 2006).

Immune-mediated haemolysis: Anaemias in this category are mediated by antibody and/or complement on the surface of red cells. Erythrolysis may occur either within the bloodstream or extravascularly. Intravascular lysis is more likely to be associated with IgM antibody or with high concentrations of IgG antibody, and with more severe clinical signs. The distinguishing features of immune-mediated haemolysis include a biphasic population of red cells (many spherocytes and large polychromatic cells), a positive result with a direct Coombs' test and, in some cases, gross agglutination. Spherocytes form as a result of loss by phagocytosis of red cell membrane and attached immune complexes. The injured cell is able to reseal its membrane without loss of internal contents but loses surface area in the process.

In some cases, the antibody is directed against immature developing red cells within the bone marrow, rather than against mature erythrocytes. Patients with this phenomenon will have little polychromasia, but some spherocytes should be observed within the peripheral blood. This condition is equivalent to pure red cell aplasia.

Anti-red cell antibody may be actively produced by the patient or acquired passively by transfusion or colostral ingestion. The appearance of antibody may be genetically modulated and occur spontaneously, or may follow cell injury or adsorption of foreign proteins or haptens on the red cell surface. Examples of the latter are virus particles, drugs (e.g. antibiotics, tranquillizers), chemicals or red cell parasites. In conditions in which a specific causative agent or underlying disease process cannot be identified, the term autoimmune haemolytic anaemia (AIHA) may be applied. Conditions in which a causative agent or underlying disease can be identified are termed immune-mediated haemolytic anaemia (IMHA).

Some animals with IMHA may also have antibody specific for platelet epitopes, and in these cases destruction of red cells and platelets (immune-mediated thrombocytopenia, IMTP) results in severe thrombocytopenia and both haemolytic and haemorrhagic anaemia. However, although one third of dogs with IMHA have been reported to also have IMTP, clinical signs of surface bleeding seem to be rare. Concurrent coagulopathy may also contribute to the thrombocytopenia noted in some patients with IMHA.

IMHA in the dog may be classified into one of five categories on the basis of the type of antibody present. Classes I and II are associated with gross agglutination and intravascular haemolysis respectively, and require aggressive therapy. Class III is the most common, does not involve spontaneous agglutination and requires a Coombs' test for verification of the diagnosis. Classes IV and V involve cold-reacting antibodies, which cause agglutination and lysis, respectively, at 4°C.

Mechanical injury: Mechanical injury of red cells was recognized in human patients receiving the early heart valve transplants that consisted of a mechanical ball valve prosthesis. Cells were damaged as they collided at high velocity with the obstacle in their path. Injured cells were recognized on the blood smear as fragmented schistocytes and keratocytes. Similar cells may be found in animals with DIC, severe heartworm infection, vasculitis, (splenic) haemangiosarcoma, patent ductus arteriosus, myelofibrosis, malignancies, haemolytic–uraemic syndrome and, to some extent, glomerulonephritis. Many of these conditions are associated with microangiopathy.

Haemolysis of normal red cells

Any condition that results in hypersplenism (e.g. splenic torsion, malignancy) may be associated with increased phagocytosis of red cells by splenic macrophages. The microenvironment within an enlarged spleen will expose cells to high pH and low glucose concentrations, resulting in premature ageing of the cells. Patients with this condition will have a regenerative anaemia with increased metarubricytes, Howell–Jolly bodies, poikilocytes and usually a mild thrombocytopenia. Patients with splenic haemangiosarcoma are likely to show severe poikilocytosis with acanthocytes, schizocytes, echinocytes and evidence of red cell regeneration.

Anaemias of increased red cell loss

Haemorrhage is a passive loss of whole blood and may involve internal or external blood loss, or both. Both forms can be severe and life-threatening, depending on the extent of the blood loss. Loss of 30–40% of total blood volume leads to hypovolaemic shock; death is likely after loss of more than 40% of total blood volume. The total blood volume in dogs is about 84 ml/kg (range 78–88 ml/kg) and that in cats is 64 ml/kg (range 62–66 ml/kg).

In internal haemorrhage, most red cells are reabsorbed via the lymphatics within a few days and re-enter the circulation in a slightly damaged form. Other cells are phagocytosed and their iron is recycled via haemosiderin deposition in the macrophages. External haemorrhage involves loss of both iron and plasma protein from the body, thereby depleting body stores of iron and diminishing the potential for the erythron to regenerate successfully in the long term. The availability of iron is a rate-limiting step in red cell production. Consequently, in managing animals with external haemorrhage, the administration of iron should be considered.

Compared with those with haemolysis, patients with haemorrhage show noticeable changes in haemodynamics. After a peracute haemorrhagic episode there may be hypotension with a normal PCV. Anaemia and hypoproteinaemia may not develop until 4–24 hours after the haemorrhagic episode, following haemodilution from fluid shifts. Interstitial fluid shifts occur within a few hours, causing mild reductions in erythron values after 4 hours. Significant reductions in plasma protein, PCV and Hb concentration occur after 12–24 hours, when plasma volume has expanded to approximately normal levels.

Haemorrhagic anaemia is classically regenerative, but this response is seen only after 3–4 days. In the interim period, the anaemia may be considered pre-regenerative.

The degree of response depends on the availability of iron. Iron is less readily available in the ferric form in haemorrhagic anaemia than in haemolytic anaemia. This accounts for the lower average increase in red cell production of two- to fourfold normal that is seen in haemorrhagic anaemia, as assessed by absolute reticulocyte counts. Exceptions to these general guidelines will occur. Peak reticulocyte counts may be seen a week after the haemorrhagic episode.

The plasma protein concentration will be reduced in haemorrhagic patients, particularly those with external haemorrhage. A decrease in plasma protein concentration may occur as early as 4 hours after haemorrhage. A persistently low plasma protein concentration should lead to a suspicion of ongoing external haemorrhage. After a single episode of severe haemorrhage, plasma protein should return to normal levels by 5–7 days.

Platelet counts in patients with haemorrhage may or may not decrease initially, but any decrease may be followed by an increase. A thrombocytosis is usually expected in haemorrhagic anaemia of several days' duration. Thrombocytosis is initially caused by movement of platelets from the spleen as a result of the adrenaline response, but general marrow stimulation or stimulation of both the erythroid and megakaryocytic cell lines may occur.

Leucocyte numbers are not decreased in haemorrhage, and in fact they are likely to be increased in acute haemorrhage due to the effects of adrenaline. Mild neutro-philia may occur in the dog concurrently with a marked regenerative erythron response.

Some strongly regenerative anaemias may be macrocytic and hypochromic in the early stages. With continuing external haemorrhage, the anaemia is classically normocytic and normochromic and protein concentration remains low. If iron deficiency develops as a result of continued external haemorrhage, the anaemia may become microcytic and hypochromic.

The causes of haemorrhagic anaemia are listed in Figure 3.6. Clinical signs and further tests will provide diagnostic clues. For example, coagulation profiles will be helpful in patients with signs such as haematomas, haemarthroses and haemorrhage into body cavities; fluid cytology diagnosis may be an aid in the diagnosis of haemorrhagic neoplasms.

When to collect bone marrow samples and do further tests

Bone marrow aspirates or core biopsies are advocated in the following situations:

- Pancytopenia or bicytopenia
- Non-regenerative or poorly regenerative anaemia where the cause is not obvious
- Neutropenia or thrombocytopenia where the cause is not obvious
- Suspected haematopoietic neoplasia, myelodysplasia or marrow dysfunction as indicated by ineffective haemopoiesis, dacryocytes or leucoerythroblastosis (the presence of some immature cells of both myeloid and erythroid series in the peripheral blood)
- Leukaemia.

Marrow biopsy can also be used to assess the amount of storage iron and to evaluate the regenerative erythroid response. In short, marrow biopsies are recommended if any defect of the production of cells is suspected, with either excessive or insufficient numbers of mature cells. Core biopsies are particularly recommended in patients suspected of having myelofibrosis, because aspiration biopsies may be unrewarding.

Haemopoietic neoplasia

Neoplasia of the haemopoietic system involves haemopoietic cell lines in bone marrow that have undergone a genetic neoplastic transformation and are proliferating autonomously. The end result is leukaemia. The cells produced may accumulate in bone marrow before appearing in the circulation. Some leukaemic cells such as neoplastic neutrophils may have a longer lifespan in circulation than normal and may have functional defects such as altered adhesive properties, reduced phagocytic and bactericidal capabilities and altered chemotaxis. Neoplastic platelets may have reduced adhesive and functional properties, paradoxically resulting in bleeding.

From a haematological perspective, neoplasms of the haemopoietic system may be suspected when either blastic haemopoietic cells appear in the circulation, or an unexplained pancytopenia or bicytopenia or a marked leucocytosis is present in peripheral blood. The presence of haemopoietic neoplasia will cause variable degrees of myelophthisis, and consequently the peripheral blood will show some degree of cytopenia and mild to moderate poorly regenerative anaemia. Myelophthisis may be due to the physical presence of the neoplasm as well as the effects of marrow suppressive factors associated with the tumour. Thrombocytopenia may also occur as a result of reduced platelet production and some splenic sequestration, resulting in haemorrhage.

Bone marrow samples are required in the diagnosis of leukaemia, and characterization of the cell line involved will involve immunophenotyping and assessment of clonality by molecular genetic analysis.

Causes of anaemia in perspective

The commonest cause of anaemia in all domestic animal species is the anaemia of inflammatory disease. This usually causes only a mild to moderate anaemia and is normocytic, normochromic and non-regenerative. Some published surveys have shown that dogs are likely to have non-regenerative and haemorrhagic anaemias in about equal proportions, whereas about 70% of reported anaemias in cats are non-regenerative. It is possible that this may be associated with factors unique to the cat such as the prevalence of viral infections, shorter lifespan of the red cells and reduced amounts of iron stored in the bone marrow.

References and further reading

Adams LG, Hardy RM, Weiss DJ and Bartges JW (1993) Hypophosphatemia and hemolytic anemia associated with diabetes mellitus and hepatic lipidosis in cats. *Journal of Veterinary Internal Medicine* **7**, 226–271

Boone L, Moriano J and Knauer K (1996) Treatment of dyserythropoiesis with refractory anaemia and excess of blasts in a dog using human recombinant erythropoietin (abstract). *Veterinary Pathology* **33**, 573

Brockus CW (1998) Endogenous estrogen myelotoxicosis associated with functional cystic ovaries in a dog. *Veterinary Clinical Pathology* **27**, 55–56

Cowgill ES, Neelm JA and Grindem CB (2003) Clinical application of reticulocyte counts in dogs and cats. *The Veterinary Clinics of North America, Small Animal Practice* **33**, 1223–1244

Di Bartola SP (2006) *Fluid, Electrolyte and Acid–Base Disorders in Small Animal Practice, 3rd edn*, p.200. Saunders Elsevier, St. Louis, MO

Di Terlizzi R, Gallagher PG, Mohandas N *et al.* (2009) Canine elliptocytosis due to a mutant β-spectrin. *Veterinary Clinical Pathology* **38**, 52–58

Fry MM, Kirk CA, Liggett JL *et al.* (2009) Changes in hepatic gene expression in dogs with experimentally induced nutritional iron deficiency. *Veterinary Clinical Pathology* **38**, 13–19

Ganz T (2006) Molecular pathogenesis of anemia of chronic disease. *Pediatric Blood Cancer* **46**, 554–557

Gerber K, Harvey JW, D-Agorne S, Wood J and Giger U (2009) Hemolysis, myopathy, and cardiac disease associated with hereditary phosphofructokinase deficiency in two Whippets. *Veterinary Clinical Pathology* **38**, 46–51

Giger U, Mason GD and Wang P (1991) Inherited erythrocyte pyruvate kinase deficiency in a Beagle dog. *Veterinary Clinical Pathology* **20**, 83–87

Harvey JW and Smith JE (1994) Haematology and clinical chemistry of English springer spaniel dogs with phosphofructokinase deficiency. *Comparative Haematology International* **4**, 70–75

Holland CT, Canfield PJ, Watson ADJ and Allan GS (1991) Dyserythropoiesis, polymyopathy, and cardiac disease in three related English springer spaniels. *Journal of Veterinary Internal Medicine* **5**, 151–159

Jain NC, Blue JT, Grindem CB *et al.* (1991) Proposed criteria for classification of acute myeloid leukaemia in dogs and cats. *Veterinary Clinical Pathology* **20**, 63–82

Mills JN (1997) Compensated haemolytic anaemia in a dog. *Australian Veterinary Journal* **75**, 24–26

Mills JN and Marsden CA (1999) Presumed hereditary elliptocytosis in a dog. *Australian Veterinary Journal* **77**, 15–16

Slappendel RJ, Van Zweiten R, Van Leeuwen M and Schneijdenberg CTWM (2005) Hereditary spectrin deficiency in Golden Retriever dogs. *Journal of Veterinary Internal Medicine* **19**,187–192

Sontas HB, Dokuzeylu B, Turna O and Ekici H (2009) Estrogen-induced myelotoxicity in dogs: a review. *Canadian Veterinary Journal* **50**, 1054–1058

Suliman H, Logan-Henfrey L, Majiwa P, Ole-Moiyoi O and Feldman B (1999) Analysis of erythropoietin and erythropoietin receptor genes expression in cattle during acute infection with *Trypanosoma congolense* (abstract). *Veterinary Clinical Pathology* **28**, 118–119

Valli VE (2007) *Veterinary Comparative Hematopathology*, Blackwell Publishing, Ames, Iowa

Weiss DJ (2003) New insights into the physiology and treatment of acquired myelodysplastic syndromes and aplastic pancytopenia. *The Veterinary Clinics of North America: Small Animal Practice* **33**, 1317–1334

Weiss DJ and Lulich J (1999) Myelodysplastic syndrome with sideroblastic differentiation in a dog. *Veterinary Clinical Pathology* **28**, 59–63

4

Polycythaemia

Elizabeth Villiers and Simon Tappin

Introduction

Polycythaemia is characterized by an increase in the packed cell volume (PCV), red blood cell (RBC) count and haemoglobin (Hb) concentration. It may be relative (owing to diminished plasma volume) or absolute. Absolute polycythaemia may result from increased concentrations of erythropoietin (secondary polycythaemia) or from the myeloproliferative disease polycythaemia vera (primary polycythaemia). The term polycythaemia implies an increased number of several haemopoietic cell lines, and human patients with polycythaemia vera have erythrocytosis accompanied by neutrophilia and thrombocytosis. However, dogs and cats with polycythaemia vera usually have normal neutrophil and platelet counts and so the term primary erythrocytosis may be more appropriate.

Erythropoiesis

In the bone marrow the pluripotent stem cell gives rise to the committed erythrocyte progenitor cell known as a burst-forming unit (BFU), which divides and differentiates into colony-forming units (CFUs). These in turn divide and differentiate into erythroblasts, which continue to divide into early, intermediate and then late normoblasts. Reticulocytes are formed when the nucleus is extruded from late normoblasts and the red cells reach full maturation in the bloodstream. The key regulator of erythropoiesis is erythropoietin (EPO). This hormone is produced in the kidneys and acts by stimulating the CFUs and, to a lesser extent, the BFUs. EPO also hastens the release of reticulocytes into the bloodstream. The synthesis of EPO is not regulated by the number of circulating red cells but by the degree of renal hypoxia. Hypoxia triggers an increased rate of production of EPO, whereas high tissue oxygenation results in a reduced rate. Other hormones, such as cortisol and thyroxine, stimulate EPO production but have no intrinsic EPO activity.

Relative polycythaemia

Relative polycythaemia arises when the plasma volume is decreased, usually as a result of fluid loss. Thus the PCV is increased, but the total mass of circulating red blood cells is normal. Relative polycythaemia may arise in animals with acute diarrhoea, extensive burns, heat stroke or water deprivation, and clinical signs of dehydration are usually obvious. The PCV is mildly increased and there is an accompanying increase in plasma proteins (unless plasma protein has been lost, as in burn injuries). Occasionally, relative polycythaemia may result from splenic contraction after stress (e.g. severe pain) or excitement. Splenic contraction leads to the release of large numbers of red cells into the circulation. Relative polycythaemia resolves after rehydration or removal of the cause of splenic contraction.

Secondary polycythaemia

Secondary polycythaemia results from increased EPO production. This may be a physiologically appropriate response to systemic hypoxia or may occur in the absence of systemic hypoxia, known as physiologically inappropriate polycythaemia. This condition occurs most commonly in association with renal neoplasia. In animals with secondary polycythaemia, serum EPO concentrations are usually increased.

Physiologically appropriate secondary polycythaemia

Two of the most common causes of tissue hypoxia are chronic pulmonary disease (e.g. feline allergic bronchitis) and right-to-left shunting cardiovascular disease. Right-to-left shunting may occur with a patent ductus arteriosus. Initially there is a left-to-right shunt leading to increased blood flow in the pulmonary artery. Pulmonary hypertension and compensatory right ventricular hypertrophy result in increased pulmonary artery pressure, and when this exceeds the aortic pressure the direction of blood flow in the patent ductus reverses. Thus deoxygenated blood is delivered into the descending aorta, resulting in hypoxia in the caudal half of the body and a subsequent increase in EPO production. Right-to-left shunting may also occur in animals with a coexisting atrial septal defect and pulmonic stenosis, and in those with tetralogy of Fallot in which there is a large ventricular septal defect and pulmonic stenosis.

Physiologically appropriate polycythaemia may also occur in animals living at high altitude. In humans, polycythaemia may be caused by massive obesity and haemoglobinopathies. Obesity has not been recognized as a cause of polycythaemia in dogs and cats. Haemoglobinopathies such as methaemoglobin reductase deficiency may cause polycythaemia (Hasler and Giger, 1996), but these disorders are rare in dogs and cats.

Physiologically inappropriate secondary polycythaemia

The most common cause of physiologically inappropriate secondary polycythaemia is renal neoplasia. Polycythaemia has been most often reported in association with renal adenocarcinoma (also known as renal cell carcinoma) (Klainbart *et al.*, 2008), but also in association with renal lymphoma (Snead, 2005) and renal fibrosarcoma (Nitsche, 2004).

The mechanism of inappropriate EPO production is not fully understood. It may be due to increased production/secretion of EPO or an EPO-like substance from the tumour, or it may result from local tissue hypoxia in the kidney, which is caused by a disruption of the renal microvasculature by the tumour.

In humans, several extrarenal tumours have been associated with secondary polycythaemia, including hepatoma, uterine leiomyoma, ovarian carcinoma and phaeochromocytoma. Polycythaemia secondary to extrarenal neoplasia is uncommon in the dog and cat, but has been reported in a dog with a nasal fibrosarcoma (Couto *et al.*, 1989), a dog with a schwannoma (Yamauchi *et al.*, 2004) and a dog with a caecal leiomyosarcoma (Sato *et al.*, 2002). In all three cases the tumours were found to have high EPO activity, suggesting that the tumour cells produced EPO. The polycythaemia resolved in all cases after surgical resection of the tumours.

Non-neoplastic renal diseases such as renal cysts and hydronephrosis are well recognized causes of secondary polycythaemia in humans. However, in dogs and cats only small numbers of such cases have been documented. Hasler and Giger (1996) reported secondary polycythaemia in one cat with a renal capsular effusion and in a second cat with fatty infiltration of the kidney. EPO concentrations were noticeably increased in these two cats, confirming secondary polycythaemia. Secondary polycythaemia caused by pyelonephritis has been reported in two dogs in association with *Cryptococcus neoformans* infection (Waters and Prueter, 1986), and necrotizing pyelonephritis associated with suspected *Klebsiella* infection has also been reported (Kessler, 2008). Secondary polycythaemia in the dog with necrotizing pyelonephritis resolved fully after nephrectomy.

Mild polycythaemia may result from hyperadrenocorticism in dogs and hyperthyroidism in cats, given that both cortisol and thyroid hormones stimulate increased production of EPO.

Primary polycythaemia

Primary polycythaemia (polycythaemia vera, primary erythrocytosis) is a chronic myeloproliferative disease characterized by a clonal expansion of haematopoietic progenitor cells that leads to the accumulation of morphologically and functionally normal red cells. Red cell proliferation occurs independently of EPO and does not respond to normal feedback mechanisms. In human patients an acquired mutation in the tyrosine kinase JAK2 leads to its constitutive activation and is present in more than 80% of cases of polycythaemia vera. This mutation also occurs in some cases of idiopathic myelofibrosis and essential thrombocythemia (Vainchenker and Constantinescu, 2005). Detection of a JAK2 mutation is an important diagnostic test in human patients as clinical trials using JAK2 inhibitors are showing great promise in the treatment of these disorders (Verstovsek, 2009). Recently, identical mutations in JAK2 kinase have been discovered in dogs with primary polycythaemia (Beurlet *et al.*, 2011), although as yet there is no research using JAK2 inhibitors in animals with primary polycythaemia.

In the dog, secondary polycythaemia is more common than primary polycythaemia. In the cat, primary polycythaemia is the more common form, and although infiltrative renal diseases such as lymphoma and feline infectious peritonitis are common in the cat, these diseases rarely result in polycythaemia.

Consequences of polycythaemia

An excessive number of RBCs results in increased blood volume and increased blood viscosity. The blood viscosity increases disproportionately with increases in the PCV above 50%. Capillaries and veins are distended to accommodate the increased blood volume, which results in erythema (Figure 4.1).

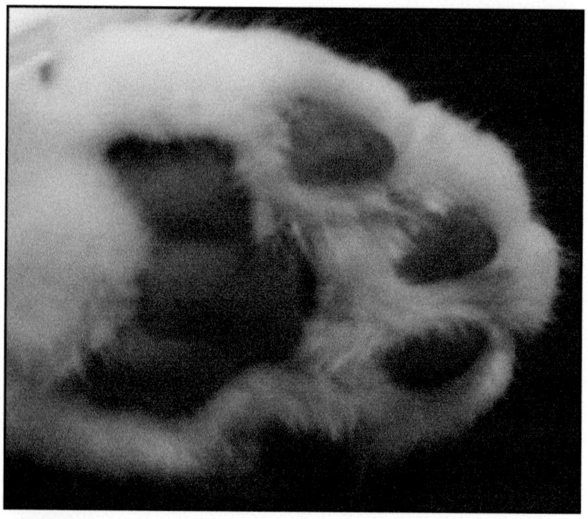

4.1 Erythematous foot pads of a cat with primary polycythaemia, prior to phlebotomy.

Bleeding episodes such as epistaxis, haematuria and haematemesis may occur, and result from mechanical rupture of capillaries caused by overdistension. Hyperviscosity leads to sludging of blood in small vessels, which leads to tissue hypoxia. The three organs most affected by increased blood viscosity are the central nervous system (CNS; in particular the cerebral cortex), the kidneys and the heart. Disorders of the CNS such as seizures, lethargy, weakness, ataxia, dementia, depression and coma may be seen. Glomerulonephropathy may result from glomerular and interstitial capillary hypoxia and lead to proteinuria and clinical signs of polydipsia and polyuria. Hyperviscosity and increased vascular resistance result in increased cardiac effort, and there may be an associated myocardial hypertrophy, which may progress to mild hypertrophic cardiomyopathy. Ocular abnormalities including distended tortuous blood vessels (Figure 4.2), uveitis (Snead, 2005) and occasionally retinal haemorrhage may be present. The sluggish blood flow that results from hyperviscosity may predispose to thrombus formation. Figure 4.3 summarizes the clinical signs that may be seen in polycythaemic animals.

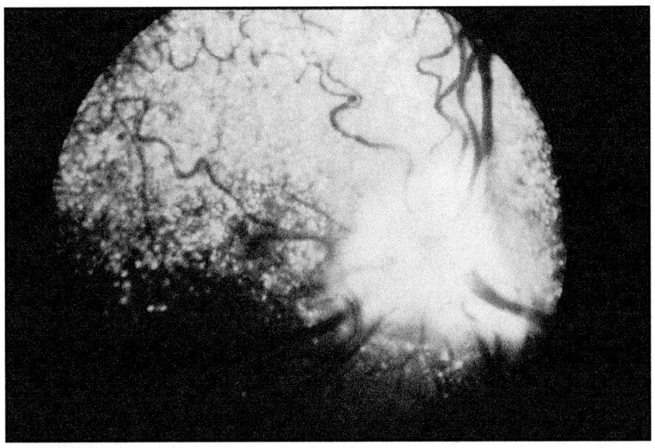

4.2 Distended and tortuous retinal vessels resulting from hyperviscosity. (Image courtesy of Neil Gorman)

Hyperaemic mucous membranes
• Not always seen
Neurological signs
• Disorientation • Depression, stupor, coma • Seizures • Weakness • Blindness • Ataxia
Renal signs
• Polydipsia/polyuria
Bleeding episodes
• Epistaxis • Haematemesis • Haematuria • Haemorrhagic diarrhoea
Ocular signs
• Tortuous distended retinal vessels • Retinal haemorrhage • Distended scleral vessels
Other
• Splenomegaly occasionally seen in cats with primary erythrocytosis • Paroxysmal sneezing quite common in dogs (increased blood viscosity in nasal mucosa)

4.3 Clinical signs of polycythaemia.

Laboratory findings and diagnosis

An increase in PCV (> 55% in dogs and > 45% in cats) indicates polycythaemia. In dogs and cats with absolute polycythaemia the PCV is often as high as 70–90%, whereas in relative polycythaemia the PCV is usually mildly increased (e.g. 60%). In absolute polycythaemia there may be a mild reticulocytosis, and microcytosis is sometimes seen in dogs; this occurs because of a relative iron deficiency in an active bone marrow. Primary polycythaemia is sometimes accompanied by a mild thrombocytosis.

Once polycythaemia is recognized, subsequent evaluation is aimed at determining whether the polycythaemia is relative, primary or secondary. Relative polycythaemia is identified when the PCV is increased but the red cell mass is normal. The red cell mass can be measured using an isotope dilution technique, but in practice this is rarely necessary, because animals with relative polycythaemia usually have obvious clinical signs of dehydration, and the PCV returns to normal when the patient is rehydrated. In addition, increased plasma protein concentration and a mild degree of polycythaemia both suggest relative polycythaemia.

Once relative polycythaemia has been excluded, investigations should aim to distinguish primary from secondary polycythaemia. This is achieved by searching for possible causes of secondary polycythaemia (e.g. cardiopulmonary disease or renal disease) and by evaluation of EPO concentrations.

Clinical signs of respiratory disease (e.g. coughing, dyspnoea) or cardiac disease (e.g. cardiac murmur, arrhythmia, cyanosis) point towards secondary appropriate polycythaemia. Thoracic radiography, echocardiography and electrocardiography are useful in diagnosing pulmonary or cardiac disease. Ideally, arterial blood gas evaluation should be performed to measure the partial pressure of oxygen in arterial blood (P_aO_2). The dorsal metatarsal artery is the most suitable sampling site. Samples must be stored aerobically and on ice if they are not analysed immediately. The normal P_aO_2 in a dog or cat breathing room air is 80–100 mmHg. In cases of physiologically appropriate polycythaemia the P_aO_2 is usually noticeably reduced (e.g. < 60 mmHg). A pulse oximeter may be used to measure the arterial haemoglobin saturation (S_aO_2). The normal S_aO_2 is > 97%. As with the P_aO_2, the S_aO_2 is noticeably reduced in appropriate secondary polycythaemia. Animals with primary polycythaemia may have mildly reduced S_aO_2 and P_aO_2, which may be due to blood hyperviscosity resulting in poor tissue perfusion.

If systemic hypoxia has been ruled out, the investigation aims to search for potential causes of inappropriate polycythaemia. This is most commonly caused by renal neoplasia, although non-neoplastic renal disease should also be considered. A cranial abdominal mass or renomegaly may be obvious on clinical examination or may be detected on plain radiographs. Ultrasound examination of the kidneys is used to identify neoplasia or other renal disease (Figure 4.4). When renal abnormalities are detected, a fine needle aspirate or Trucut biopsy sample may be obtained. Other tests such as biochemical screening and urine analysis are helpful. Serum urea and creatinine concentrations are usually normal in cases of renal neoplasia unless both kidneys are involved. In cases of renal neoplasia, urine analysis may reveal proteinuria, haematuria and an active sediment. Proteinuria may also be caused by glomerulonephropathy, which may be secondary to polycythaemia. Non-specific changes such as splenomegaly and hyperechoic renal parenchyma may be seen in primary polycythaemia and are thought to be secondary to increased viscosity.

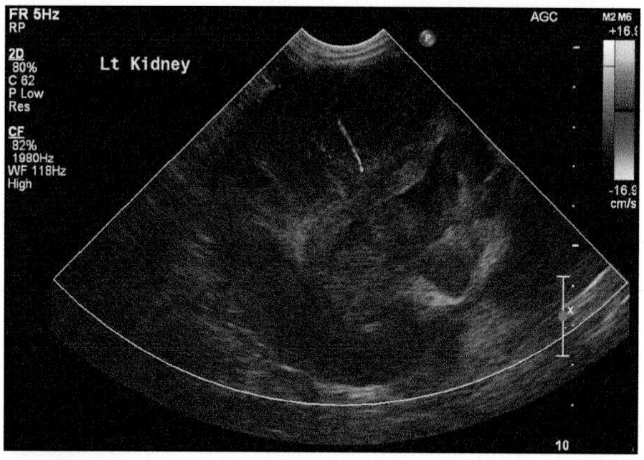

4.4 Ultrasound examination of the left kidney, revealing disruption of the cortex and medulla. Biopsy later revealed this to be due to lymphoma. (Image courtesy of Samuel Jakovljevic)

Glomerulonephropathy may be caused by polycythaemia as a result of renal hypoxia caused by hyperviscosity (Page *et al.*, 1990). Renal diseases such as pyelonephritis may cause secondary polycythaemia. Thus it may be difficult to determine whether non-neoplastic renal disease is a consequence of primary polycythaemia or whether it is the underlying cause of the polycythaemia, and in this situation the serum EPO concentration should always be evaluated.

A diagnosis of primary polycythaemia is made if causes of secondary polycythaemia have been excluded and if serum EPO concentrations are low or normal. As primary polycythaemia is largely a diagnosis of exclusion, the accuracy of this diagnosis depends on the extent of the clinicopathological investigation. Figure 4.5 summarizes the diagnostic approach to polycythaemia.

Serum EPO concentrations

Assessment of serum EPO concentrations is helpful in distinguishing primary from secondary polycythaemia, because high values point towards secondary polycythaemia and low or normal values are consistent with primary polycythaemia. EPO can be measured by radioimmunoassay or enzyme-linked immunosorbent assay (ELISA), although these assays are currently not widely available. In the United Kingdom, EPO concentrations in the dog and cat may be assayed at Cambridge Specialist Laboratory Services Ltd (PO Box 967, Stapleford, Cambridge CB2 5XY). A serum sample or a plasma sample collected in ethylenediamine tetra-acetic acid (EDTA) may be used.

Dogs and cats with primary polycythaemia have low or low–normal concentrations of EPO; and a low or normal serum EPO value in an animal with no signs of secondary polycythaemia supports a diagnosis of primary polycythaemia. High concentrations of serum EPO are only seen in secondary polycythaemia. A study using a radioimmunoassay in polycythaemic dogs found that serum EPO concentrations were slightly to moderately increased in dogs with congenital heart disease and pulmonary disorders and moderately to noticeably increased in dogs with renal tumours (Cook and Lothrop, 1994). However, not all cases of secondary polycythaemia are associated with high serum EPO concentrations, because cats with renal tumours have been reported to have normal serum EPO concentrations (Cook and Lothrop, 1994; Hasler and Giger, 1996). Possible explanations for this are that the renal tumours may have produced an EPO-like substance that was not recognized by the assay or that EPO production was cyclic. EPO concentrations may also be normal in animals with polycythaemia secondary to chronic hypoxia (Cook and Lothrop, 1994; Hasler and Giger, 1996). The animal may in time adapt to hypoxia, resulting in a gradual decrease in EPO production. Hence EPO concentrations should always be interpreted in conjunction with the clinical findings and their measurement should never replace a thorough clinicopathological evaluation.

Evaluation of bone marrow

In people with primary polycythaemia, the features of bone marrow include hypercellularity, erythroid hyperplasia, mild granulocytic hyperplasia and increased numbers of megakaryocytes, often in clusters and with atypical morphology (Lakey *et al.*, 2010). It is stated commonly that bone marrow evaluation is not helpful in distinguishing primary and secondary polycythaemia in dogs and cats, since both conditions lead to increased cellularity with erythroid hyperplasia. However, megakaryocytic and granulocytic hyperplasia may be seen in primary polycythaemia, sometimes with abnormal megakaryocyte morphology and clustering. These features are not expected in secondary polycythaemia. Hence, bone marrow evaluation may aid in the identification of primary polycythaemia. More detailed studies of bone marrow findings in this disease are warranted.

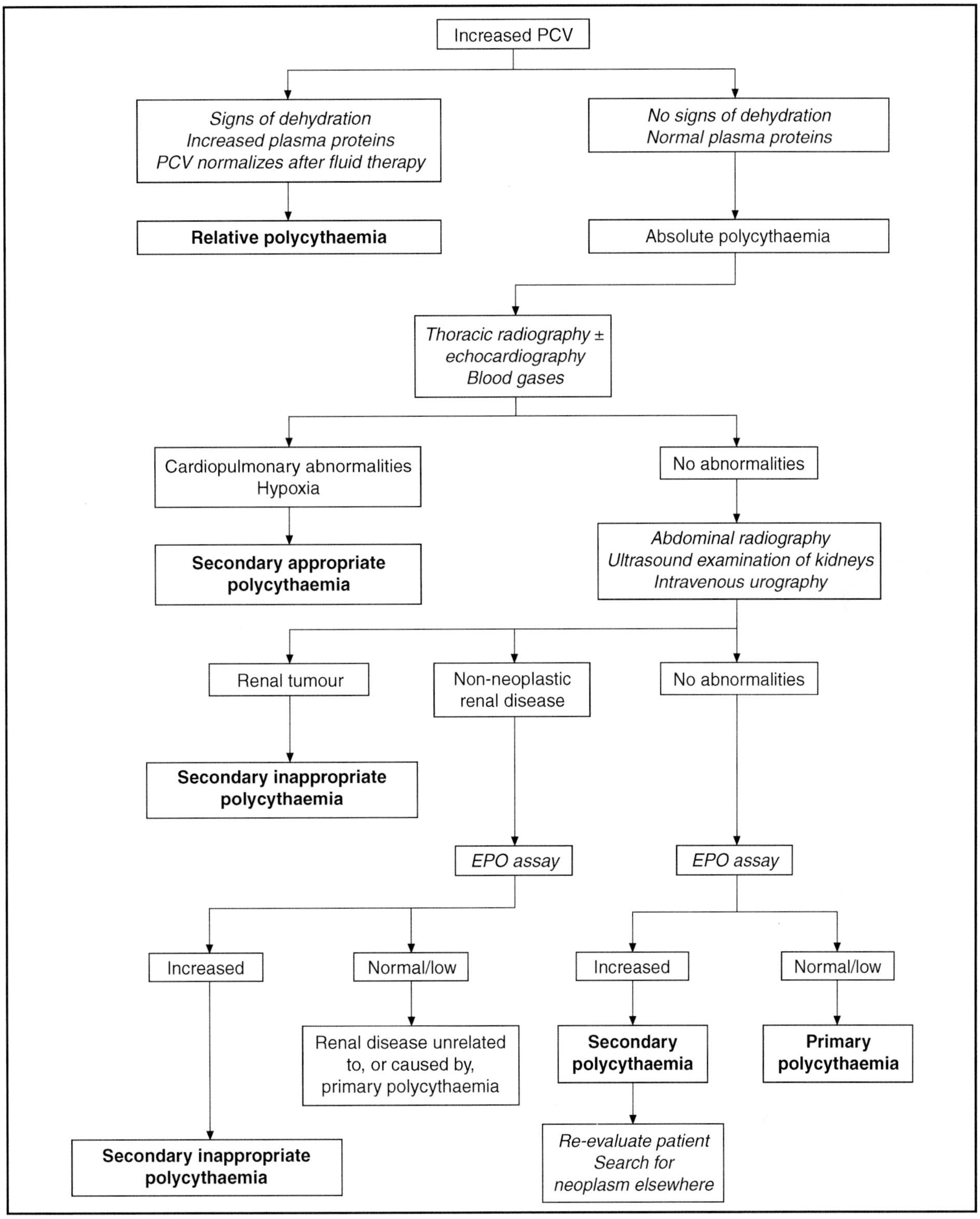

4.5 Approach to the polycythaemic patient. EPO, erythropoietin; PCV, packed cell volume.

Treatment

The treatment of polycythaemia depends on the underlying cause of the disease. Animals with relative polycythaemia should be treated with fluid therapy to correct dehydration. Initial treatment of absolute polycythaemia, irrespective of the cause, is aimed at reducing the blood viscosity by reducing the number of circulating red cells. This is achieved by performing serial phlebotomies, removing aliquots of 10–20 ml/kg of blood and replacing the removed volume with crystalloid solution until the target PCV is reached or the clinical signs resolve. In primary polycythaemia the target PCV is < 55% for dogs and < 50% for cats. Removing 20 ml/kg of blood decreases the PCV by about 15%. The jugular vein is generally used, and blood is collected in a similar manner to the collection of blood for transfusion. In dogs, blood may be collected using a blood transfusion collection set, whereas in cats a 60 ml syringe and a 19 gauge butterfly needle are useful. If collected with the appropriate anticoagulant and stored correctly, this blood could be used for auto-transfusion if needed; it should not be transfused into other patients. Blood should be stored at this stage for later EPO measurement, because phlebotomy can increase EPO concentrations. The use of leeches has been suggested as an alternative to phlebotomy and is useful in patients where phlebotomy is difficult owing to increased blood viscosity (Figure 4.6). The medical leech *Hirudo medicinalis* can suck 5–10 ml of blood over a 2–4 hour period, and the procedure is usually well tolerated by patients because local anaesthetic agents are present in leech saliva. As a result of the anti-thrombotic and vasodilatory substances contained within the leech saliva a similar amount of blood to that removed during phlebotomy is usually lost over the following 24 hours (Nett *et al.*, 2001).

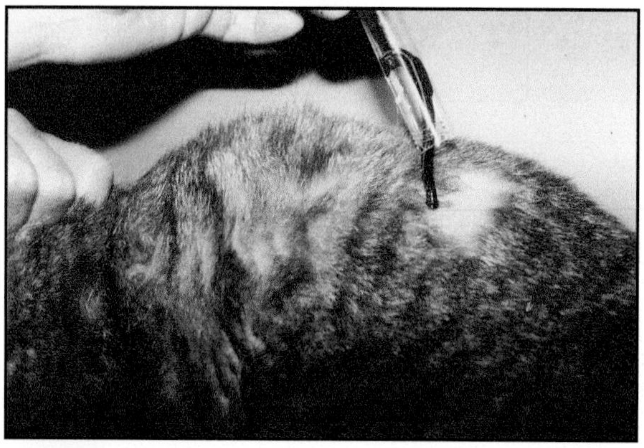

4.6 Application of a medical leech (*Hirudo medicinalis*) to treat primary polycythaemia in a cat. (Image courtesy of Claudia Nett and Tony Glaus)

In animals with polycythaemia secondary to chronic hypoxia, a more cautious approach is recommended because sudden removal of a large amount of blood may exacerbate the hypoxia and may result in hypotension. Therefore aliquots of 5 ml/kg of blood are removed at one time, and this is repeated as needed until the PCV has decreased to 55–60%. Dogs with polycythaemia secondary to a right-to-left shunting patent ductus arteriosus can have a reasonable short term prognosis (6–22 months) with myelosuppressive chemotherapy using hydroxycarbamide (40–50 mg/kg every other day) (Moore and Stepien, 2001). Hydroxycarbamide therapy is discussed further below.

In animals with polycythaemia secondary to surgically resectable renal tumours, it is important to carry out phlebotomy before surgery because hyperviscosity is associated with an increased risk of thrombosis and/or excessive haemorrhage. Renal adenocarcinomas may be contained within the renal capsule or may invade surrounding structures such as the vena cava and may not be amenable to surgical excision. Occasionally, both kidneys may be affected. In dogs with renal adenocarcinoma, metastases to regional lymph nodes, liver, lungs and bone are seen, with a reported incidence of between 16% (Bryan *et al.*, 2006) and 48% of cases (Klein *et al.*, 1988). In cases where surgical excision is possible, the median survival time after surgery is reported as 16 months, range 0–59 months (Bryan *et al.*, 2006). In animals with polycythaemia secondary to undergoing nephrectomy for renal adenocarcinoma, the presence of polycythaemia does not appear to affect the prognosis adversely (Bryan *et al.*, 2006; Klainbart *et al.*, 2008).

Primary polycythaemia

Three treatment modalities have been used in the treatment of primary polycythaemia: repeated phlebotomy, myelosuppressive therapy (most often with hydroxycarbamide) and radioactive phosphorus, although the latter is no longer used. Combinations of phlebotomy and hydroxycarbamide, or phlebotomy and radioactive phosphorus, have also been used.

Phlebotomy

In humans, phlebotomy alone is usually used as the first line of treatment, because this is safe and immediately effective. It may lead to iron deficiency, but this is not undesirable because it will slow down erythropoiesis. Severe iron deficiency leading to anaemia is treated with judicious iron replacement. Therapy with aspirin or anagrelise (which inhibits platelet maturation) is often used concurrently to combat thrombosis (Spivak, 2002). Treatment with chemotherapy, usually hydroxycarbamide, is thought to reduce the risk of thrombotic complications but carries an increased risk of transformation to acute leukaemia and so is usually only used in patients at high risk of thrombosis (older people and those with a prior history of thrombosis (Finazzi and Barbui, 2008)).

In dogs and cats there are few reported cases of primary polycythaemia treated by phlebotomy alone. In one report a cat survived for more than 20 months (Foster and Lothrop, 1988), and in another report a dog survived for a year and was generally free of clinical signs (Meyer *et al.*, 1993). Providing that the procedure is well tolerated, this method of treatment is safe and effective, although the risk of thrombosis may be increased, as it is in human patients. In the report by Meyer *et al.* (1993) the dog died suddenly, and the authors postulated that this may have been due to thrombosis. The frequency of phlebotomies is determined by the PCV, which, together with the clinical response, should be monitored frequently (e.g. monthly). If phlebotomy is required more frequently than every 4–6 weeks, myelosuppressive therapy is recommended, and this is usually in the form of chemotherapy.

Hydroxycarbamide

Hydroxycarbamide is the myelosuppressive drug of choice for the medical management of erythrocytosis, although alkylating agents, such as chlorambucil and busulfan, have also been suggested.

Hydroxycarbamide causes reversible bone marrow suppression by inhibiting DNA synthesis without affecting RNA or protein synthesis. After an initial phlebotomy, a loading dose of 30 mg/kg/day is given for 7–10 days, followed by a maintenance dose of 15 mg/kg/day. Haematology is monitored at intervals of 7–14 days until the PCV is stable and within the normal range, and then every 6–8 weeks. If the PCV increases while the animal is on maintenance therapy, phlebotomy may be repeated and/or the dose of hydroxycarbamide may be increased for 7–10 days, after which time the dose is reduced to the maintenance dose again. Given that the drug causes bone marrow suppression it has the potential to cause thrombocytopenia, which may result in spontaneous bleeding, and neutropenia, which may result in life-threatening sepsis. It is therefore mandatory to monitor the patient's haematology parameters regularly while on maintenance treatment. If thrombocytopenia or neutropenia occurs, hydroxycarbamide treatment should be suspended temporarily until the counts return to normal and then reintroduced at a lower dose. Antibiotics should be given while the patient is neutropenic. Other potential side effects in the dog include anorexia, vomiting and sloughing of the claws (Marconato *et al.*, 2007). In practice, such side effects are rarely seen.

Hydroxycarbamide is most commonly supplied in 500 mg capsules, which should not be opened because this exposes the cytotoxic contents. Capsules can either be reformulated using a compounding pharmacist (Nova Laboratories Ltd within the UK) or the total number of milligrams required for a set period can be calculated and the 500 mg capsules spread evenly over that period. For example, a cat weighing 3.5 kg would require a daily maintenance dose of 52.5 mg, so 50 mg capsules could be compounded for daily administration, or if a bolus approach is used 50 mg equates to one tenth of a 500 mg capsule, thus one tablet should be given every 10 days. This bolus-type dosing may occasionally result in an adverse reaction in cats, leading to methaemoglobinaemia and haemolytic anaemia with Heinz bodies (Watson *et al.*, 1994). If such a reaction is encountered, daily dosing of compounded hydroxycarbamide should be given. An alternative bolus protocol has also been suggested for cats (125 mg every other day for 2 weeks, then 250 mg twice a week for 2 weeks, then 500 mg once a week); however, the risk of causing methaemoglobinaemia is higher and hospitalization prior to each dose increase is suggested (Watson *et al.*, 1994). Treatment for life-threatening methaemoglobinaemia includes oxygen therapy, red cell transfusion, methylene blue and *N*-acetylcysteine.

Radioactive phosphorus

Radioactive phosphorus (^{32}P) has been used in a small number of dogs with polycythaemia. After administration, ^{32}P is taken up by bone where it decays, thereby irradiating the adjacent haemopoietic cells in the bone marrow. It is well tolerated and associated with minimal short-term side effects, although the potential carcinogenic effects seen in human patients presumably also affect the dog. In a report by Smith and Turrel (1989), a single treatment resulted in long-term control in about 40% of cases, although 25% of cases showed no response. The main disadvantage of this treatment is the requirement for isolation of the animal in purpose-built premises.

Prognosis

The prognosis for polycythaemic animals depends on the underlying cause. Primary polycythaemia has a guarded prognosis, although successful long term management has been reported. Animals with secondary polycythaemia have a variable prognosis, which depends on the underlying cause.

References and further reading

Bryan JN, Henry CJ, Turnquist SE *et al.* (2006) Primary renal neoplasia of dogs. *Journal of Veterinary Internal Medicine* **20**, 1155–1160

Beurlet S, Krief P, Sansonetti A *et al.* (2011) Identification of JAK2 mutations in canine primary polycythemia. *Experimental Hematology* **39**, 542–543

Cook SM and Lothrop CD (1994) Serum erythropoietin concentrations measured by radioimmunoassay in normal, polycythaemia and anaemic dogs and cats. *Journal of Veterinary Internal Medicine* **8**, 18–25

Couto CG, Boudrieau RJ and Zanjani ED (1989) Tumour-associated erythrocytosis in a dog with nasal fibrosarcoma. *Journal of Veterinary Internal Medicine* **3**, 183–185

Finazzi G and Barbui T (2008) Evidence and expertise in the management of polycythemia vera and essential thrombocythemia. *Leukemia* **8**, 494–502

Foster ES and Lothrop CD (1988) Polycythaemia in a cat with cardiac hypertrophy. *Journal of the American Veterinary Medical Association* **192**, 1736–1738

Hasler AH and Giger U (1996) Serum erythropoietin values in polycythaemic cats. *Journal of the American Animal Hospital Association* **32**, 294–301

Kessler M (2008) Secondary polycythaemia associated with high plasma erythropoietin concentrations in a dog with a necrotising pyelonephritis. *Journal of Small Animal Practice* **49**, 363–366

Klainbart S, Segev G, Loeb E, Melamed D and Aroch I (2008) Resolution of renal adenocarcinoma-induced secondary inappropriate polycythaemia after nephrectomy in two cats. *Journal of Feline Medicine and Surgery* **3**, 264–268

Klein MK, Cockrell GL and Withrow SJ (1988) Canine primary renal neoplasms: a retrospective review of 54 cases. *Journal of the American Animal Hospital Association* **24**, 443–452

Lakey MA, Pardanani A, Hoyer JD *et al.* (2010) Bone marrow morphologic features in polycythemia vera with *JAK2* exon 12 mutations. *American Journal of Clinical Pathology* **133**, 942–948

Marconato L, Bonfanti U and Fileccia I (2007) Unusual dermatological toxicity of hydroxyurea in two dogs with spontaneously occurring tumours. *Journal of Small Animal Practice* **48**, 514–517

Meyer HP, Slappendel RJ and Greydanaus-van de Putten SWM (1993) Polycythaemia vera in a dog treated by repeated phlebotomies. *Veterinary Quarterly* **14**, 108–111

Moore KW and Stepien RL (2001) Hydroxyurea for treatment of polycythemia secondary to right-to-left shunting patent ductus arteriosus in 4 dogs. *Journal of Veterinary Internal Medicine* **15**(4), 418–421

Nett CS, Arnold P and Glaus TM (2001) Leeching as initial treatment in a cat with polycythemia vera. *Journal of Small Animal Practice* **42**, 554–556

Nitsche EK (2004) Erythrocytosis in dogs and cats. Diagnosis and management. *Compendium of Continuing Education for the Practicing Veterinarian* **26**, 104–119

Page RL, Stiff ME, McEntee MC and Walter LG (1990) Transient glomerulonephropathy associated with primary erythrocytosis in a dog. *Journal of the American Veterinary Medical Association* **196**, 620–622

Sato K, Hikasa Y, Morita T *et al.* (2002) Secondary erythrocytosis associated with high plasma erythropoietin concentrations in a dog with cecal leiomyosarcoma. *Journal of the American Veterinary Medical Association* **220**, 486–490

Smith M and Turrel JM (1989) Radiophosphorus treatment of bone marrow disorders in dogs: 11 cases (1970–1987). *Journal of the American Veterinary Medical Association* **194**, 98–102

Snead EC (2005) A case of bilateral renal lymphosarcoma with secondary polycythemia and paraneoplastic syndromes of hypoglycaemia and uveitis in an English Springer Spaniel. *Veterinary and Comparative Oncology* **3**, 139–144

Spivak JL (2002) Polycythemia vera: myths, mechanisms and management. *Blood* **100,** 4272–4290

Vainchecker W and Constantinescu S (2005) A unique activating mutation in JAK2 (V617F) is at the origin of polycythemia vera and allows a new classification of myeloproliferative disease. *Haematology* **14**, 195–200

Verstovsek S (2009) Therapeutic potential of JAK2 inhibitors. *Hematology* **1**, 636–642

Waters DJ and Prueter JC (1986) Secondary polycythemia associated with renal disease in the dog: two case reports and review of the literature. *Journal of the American Animal Hospital Association* **31**, 29–33

Watson ADJ, Moore AS and Helfand SC (1994) Primary erythrocytosis in the cat: treatment with hydroxyurea. *Journal of Small Animal Practice* **35**, 320–325

Yamauchi A, Ohta T, Okada T *et al.* (2004) Secondary erythrocytosis associated with schwannoma in a dog. *Journal of Veterinary Medical Science* **66**, 1605–1608

5

Iron deficiency anaemia

Mary C. Lewis and Mike Stone

Introduction

Iron deficiency anaemia develops as a result of a lack of iron during red blood cell (RBC) production. In small animal medicine, two causes of iron deficiency anaemia are commonly recognized: insufficient dietary iron and chronic blood loss. Iron deficiency anaemia is typically not a disease itself, but a manifestation of disease. The clinical presentation may include features of the underlying disease process as well as those of anaemia. However, some patients may require medical attention because of signs of anaemia alone.

Iron metabolism and pathophysiology

Iron exists in three main compartments: transport iron (transferrin); storage iron (ferritin and haemosiderin); and a functional compartment (haemoglobin (Hb), myoglobin and various enzymes). Iron moves throughout the body between these different compartments to maintain iron homeostasis (Figure 5.1). Most iron in the body is located inside erythrocytes in the form of Hb. With iron deficiency, Hb and erythrocyte production takes priority and the other compartments will become depleted before the development of anaemia. Conversely, when treating iron deficiency the haematocrit (Hct) will rise before the storage pools are replenished. Therefore, therapy for iron deficiency must be continued beyond the time it takes to return the Hct to normal in order to replace storage pools.

Iron absorption occurs in the small intestine, predominantly the duodenum and jejunum. Intestinal absorption and release of iron from enterocytes into the plasma is regulated by a small peptide hormone called hepcidin. Hepcidin is produced in the liver and its production is influenced by hypoxia, plasma iron levels and inflammation (Vokurka *et al.*, 2006). Iron is carried in the plasma bound to the transport protein transferrin. Transferrin is produced in the liver, and liver iron stores regulate its production.

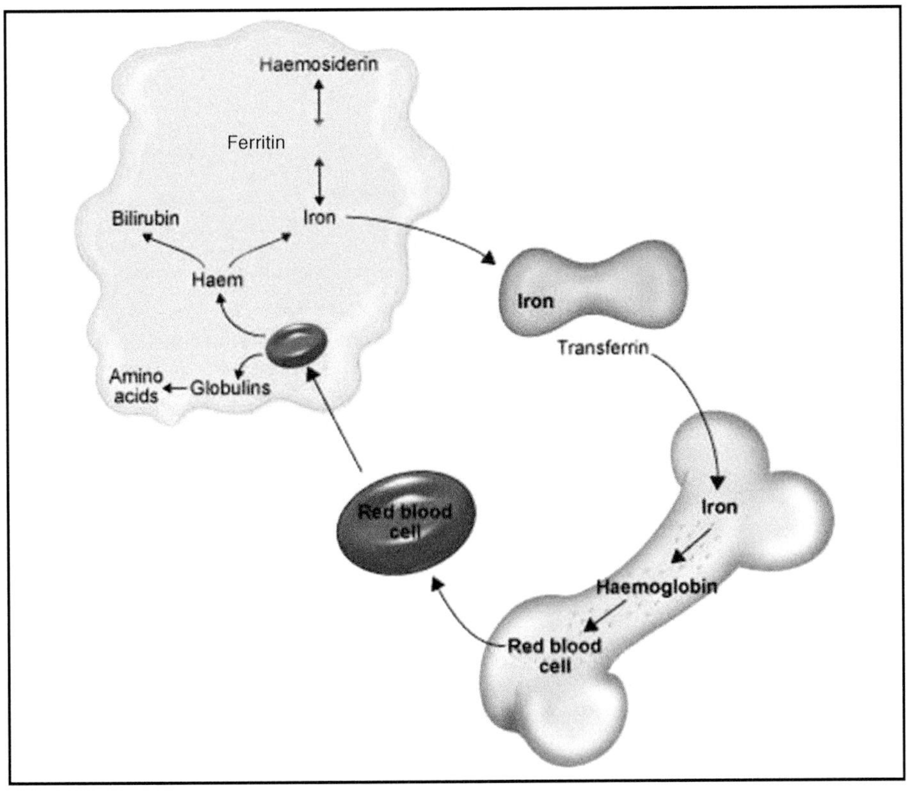

5.1 The body is able to reutilize iron from the breakdown of haemoglobin within mononuclear phagocytic cells. The iron binds to transferrin and is returned to the bone marrow and used to produce more haemoglobin.

Transferrin concentrations increase with iron deficiency in some species, although not in dogs (Weeks *et al.*, 1990).

Transferrin receptors are most numerous in tissues with high iron requirements, such as erythroid progenitor cells in the bone marrow. In developing erythrocytes, iron is added to protoporphyrin IX to form haem. Haem is then incorporated into Hb after several more steps. The maturation and division rate of erythrocyte precursors is affected by their Hb concentration. If Hb synthesis is incomplete or impaired (as with iron deficiency), erythroid cells continue to divide. As a result, erythrocytes released into circulation are smaller in size (microcytes) and have a lower Hb concentration (hypochromasia).

Normal erythrocyte degradation occurs in macrophages. Senescent erythrocytes are phagocytosed in the spleen, liver or bone marrow and Hb is broken down into haem and globulins. Globulins are degraded to amino acids, while haem is broken down into bilirubin and unbound iron. Most iron is immediately returned to the plasma and bound to transferrin, while a smaller portion is stored in macrophages, as either haemosiderin or ferritin. Although ferritin is primarily intracellular, a small amount circulates in serum in proportion to total iron stores, and this is useful diagnostically. Unlike ferritin, which is soluble and lost during tissue processing, haemosiderin may be visualized in tissues by light microscopy.

Causes of iron deficiency

The major causes of iron deficiency anaemia in animals are summarized in Figure 5.2.

Insufficient intake
• Nursing kittens and puppies
Chronic, external blood loss
• Internal parasitism • External parasitism • Bleeding ulcers in gastrointestinal tract • Bleeding gastrointestinal tract tumours • Inflammatory bowel disease • Inherited haemostatic defects • Thrombocytopenia • Inflammatory bowel disease • Repeated phlebotomy • Chronic epistaxis • Urogenital haemorrhage
Rapid erythropoiesis
• Erythropoietin therapy for anaemia

5.2 Causes of iron deficiency.

Nursing animals

Iron deficiency anaemia is common in young and nursing animals and is accepted as a normal phenomenon. The packed cell volume (PCV) of puppies and kittens is normal at birth, decreases until weaning, and then returns to normal. The development of anaemia in kittens can be lessened by giving iron, suggesting iron deficiency as its cause (Weiser and Kociba, 1983).

Iron deficiency anaemia is common in nursing animals because milk is a poor source of iron and requirements for iron are usually higher than intake at this age. From birth until weaning, animals fed exclusively a diet of milk must rely upon their own iron stores to create Hb. Piglets raised without access to soil are commonly supplemented with iron at birth to prevent iron deficiency, iron deficiency anaemia, and poor growth. This practice has not seemed to be necessary in other domestic species, even though iron deficiency anaemia is recognized. In humans, iron deficiency (even when not severe enough to cause anaemia) in childhood may lead to behavioural disturbances and developmental delay, which may not be fully reversible (Lozoff *et al.*, 1991).

Adult animals

Blood loss

Iron deficiency anaemia in older animals is most commonly caused by chronic external blood loss. Parasites, bleeding gastrointestinal (GI) tumours or ulcers, inherited haemostatic defects, thrombocytopenia, inflammatory bowel disease and repeated phlebotomies are potential causes of iron deficiency anaemia. Early in these conditions, body iron stores are used for erythropoiesis, so anaemia, if present, is mild and moderately to markedly regenerative. However, after weeks to months of bleeding (and iron loss), body iron stores become progressively depleted, insufficient iron is available for normal erythrocyte production and the bone marrow becomes increasingly unable to replace the red blood cells that are being lost. Moreover, those erythrocytes that are produced contain less iron and are therefore more fragile, decreasing their lifespan. At this time, the anaemia is usually more severe, microcytic and hypochromic. Patients may have few clinical signs despite a very low Hct because the body has had time to adjust to the anaemia. GI lesions or parasites may cause occult bleeding that remains unnoticed until signs of anaemia supervene.

Blood donation

Each 450 ml blood collection removes approximately 200 mg of iron from the body (each ml of blood contains approximately 0.5 mg iron). Frequent blood donations may lead to iron deficiency and replacement should be considered.

Copper deficiency

Copper deficiency results in a functional iron deficiency. Decreased activity of the copper-dependent enzymes caeruloplasmin and hephaestin prevents the release of iron from body iron stores and the intestines, respectively. Decreased iron availability leads to defective Hb synthesis and ultimately a microcytic, hypochromic anaemia. Copper deficiency is uncommon in small animals but has been reported in dogs (Seguin and Bunch, 2001).

Erythropoietin therapy

Administration of erythropoietin (EPO) may result in a 'functional iron deficiency' even when body iron stores are replete. The intense erythropoietic stimulus may require more iron than can be released quickly from body stores. Patients who have chronic renal failure and poor response to EPO therapy may benefit from iron supplementation.

Tests for evaluating iron status

The diagnostic approach to the anaemic patient should include a complete blood count with evaluation of erythrocyte morphology, reticulocyte and platelet count, biochemical profile, urinalysis and faecal flotation. If the cause of blood loss is not readily apparent (e.g. fleas, intestinal parasites, haematuria) careful examination of the GI tract as a source of bleeding should be performed. Abdominal ultrasonography or radiography may be useful in identifying a mass, while a faecal occult blood test may be useful when overt melaena is not appreciated. Concurrent mild to moderate hypoproteinaemia is expected, depending on the severity of blood loss. A variety of tests are available for evaluating iron status in small animals. These tests are discussed in detail below and include: haematology and red cell indices (mean corpuscular volume (MCV), mean corpuscular haemoglobin concentration (MCHC), red cell distribution width (RDW)); serum iron; transferrin or serum total iron-binding capacity (TIBC); serum ferritin; and bone marrow iron.

Haematology

Iron deficiency secondary to blood loss is typically associated with a regenerative response, characterized by reticulocytosis. However, over time the regenerative response may be less than expected for the degree of anaemia. Classically, microcytic and hypochromic anaemia is present. However, the red cell indices will vary depending on the severity of iron deficiency. For example, the presence of microcytic cells may not be reflected in the MCV when the regenerative response of the bone marrow to blood loss causes the release of large reticulocytes into circulation. These cells have a higher MCV than mature erythrocytes and, when combined with the low MCV of microcytes, the reported MCV may remain within the normal reference range. The presence of both large reticulocytes and microcytes will cause the RDW to increase. A histogram depicts the varying sizes of red cells graphically (Figure 5.3). These graphs help to highlight a microcytic population that is not sufficient to cause the MCV to decrease below the reference interval.

Although the presence of microcytic anaemia is a common indicator of iron deficiency, microcytosis may be seen in other conditions as well as in some specific dog breeds. These circumstances, detailed in Figure 5.4, should be taken into consideration when assessing a patient with a microcytic anaemia. For example, an Akita with a microcytic anaemia may have developed anaemia secondary to a disease other than iron deficiency and the administration of iron is unlikely to be helpful.

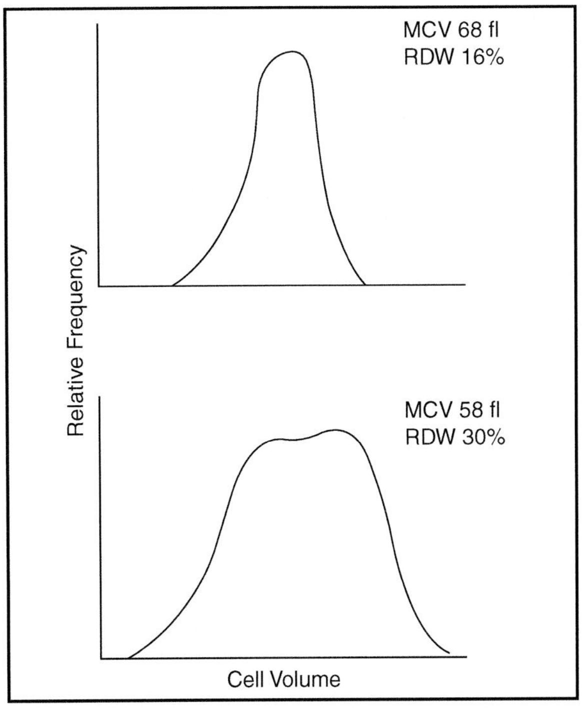

5.3 Idealized histograms of normal (above) and iron deficient (below) canine erythrocytes. The widening of the curve in iron deficient erythrocytes represents a population of erythrocytes of varied size (microcytic, normocytic and, if the anaemia is regenerative, macrocytic erythrocytes). MCV, mean corpuscular volume; RDW, red cell distribution width.

- Iron deficiency
- Portosystemic shunt
- Chronic liver disease
- Breed variation (Akita, Shiba Inu)
- Young animals (< 3–4 months of age)
- Anaemia of inflammatory disease
- Copper deficiency
- Artefact[a]
- Aluminium toxicity[b]
- Dyserythropoiesis (English Springer Spaniel)

5.4 Causes of microcytosis. Decreased mean corpuscular volume (MCV) is a normal finding in certain breeds. (Sources: [a] Boisvert *et al.*, 1999; [b] Segev *et al.*, 2009).

Iron deficiency anaemia is often associated with a concurrent thrombocytosis (Schloess *et al.*, 1965). The cause of the thrombocytosis associated with iron deficiency is unknown.

Examination of a blood smear may reveal hypochromic erythrocytes with a pale centre and only a narrow red-staining rim (Figure 5.5). Iron deficient erythrocytes are more fragile and less deformable, which decreases their lifespan and can result in erythrocyte morphological abnormalities, including schistocytes, keratocytes and target cells (Figures 5.5 to 5.7).

Reticulocyte Hb content and size (rMCV) may be useful markers of early (before the development of anaemia) iron deficiency (Fry and Kirk, 2006).

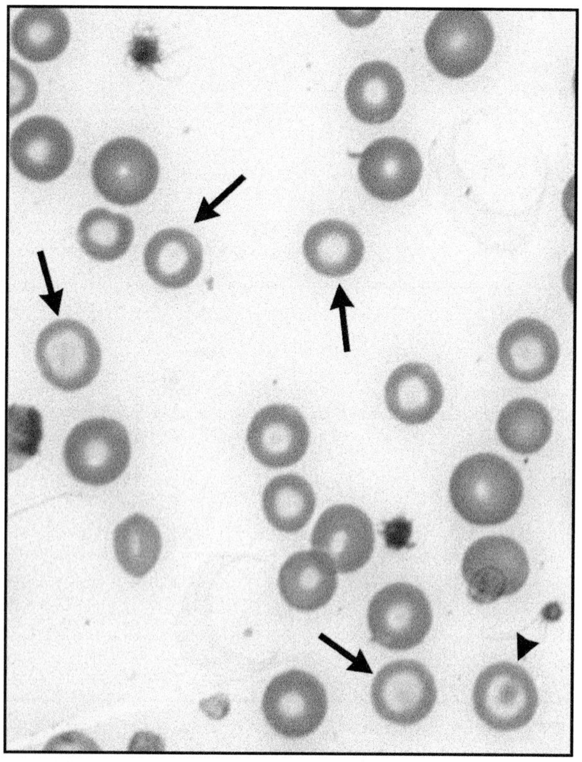

5.5 Hypochromic erythrocytes (arrows) and a codocyte (target cell, arrowhead).

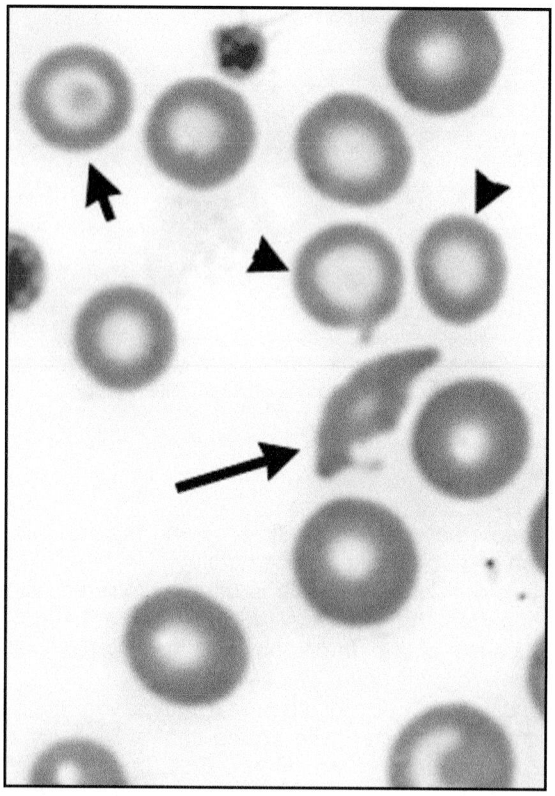

5.6 Schistocyte (arrow), hypochromic erythrocytes (arrowheads), codocyte (target cell; short arrow) and two platelets.

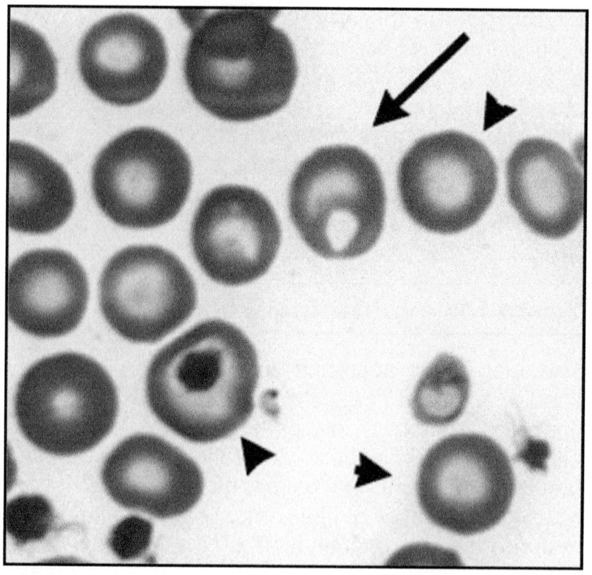

5.7 A keratocyte, sometimes referred to as a 'blister cell' or 'helmet cell', is indicated by the arrow and is surrounded by several hypochromatic erythrocytes (arrowheads).

Canine and feline erythrocytes have a lifespan of 60–90 days, but they circulate as reticulocytes for only a few days. As a result, their Hb content and MCV provide a more real-time assessment of iron availability. If iron stores are low, reticulocytes will have lower Hb content and reduced rMCV.

Serum iron concentration

Serum iron concentrations are expected to be low with iron deficiency anaemia. Unfortunately decreased serum iron lacks specificity for the diagnosis of iron deficiency, because decreased iron may be seen with other conditions, such as acute or chronic inflammatory reactions and congenital portosystemic shunts. Conversely, normal to elevated serum iron concentrations in an anaemic patient should exclude iron deficiency as the cause of anaemia, as long as causes of false increases in serum iron concentration can be excluded. Serum iron levels can be falsely increased with haemoglobinaemia (haemolysis) and high serum ferritin concentrations in some iron assays.

Serum total iron-binding capacity (TIBC) and percentage saturation of transferrin

The TIBC represents an indirect measure of the amount of transferrin present in the serum. Although transferrin can be measured directly via immunological methods, transferrin is usually measured indirectly, as TIBC, by re-measuring serum iron concentrations after the serum has been saturated with iron. Given that transferrin can bind more iron than is normally present in the blood, the TIBC is greater than the serum iron concentration. The percentage saturation of transferrin represents serum iron divided by the transferrin concentration (Figure 5.8). Because transferrin concentrations do not increase in dogs with iron deficiency, the measurement of TIBC and percentage saturation appears to add little diagnostic value to the measurement of serum iron alone (Weeks *et al.*, 1990).

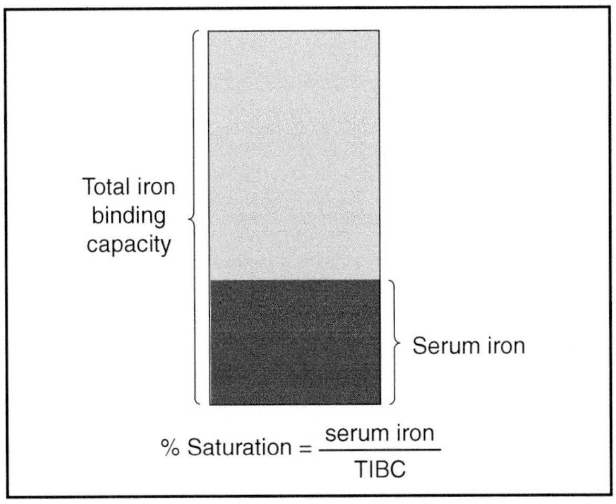

5.8 Relationship between serum iron, total iron binding capacity (TIBC) and percentage saturation of transferrin.

Serum ferritin

In the absence of confounding factors, discussed below, serum ferritin is the single best measure of total body iron stores. Serum ferritin levels are expected to be low in iron deficiency and normal with adequate iron stores. However, a normal value does not exclude iron deficiency completely, because levels may be elevated by inflammatory diseases, histiocytic neoplasia, hepatitis and haemolysis. Species-specific immunoassays must be used for measurement.

Bone marrow iron

Evaluation of the bone marrow can provide a subjective assessment of the amount of storage iron (haemosiderin). In this method, a bone marrow aspirate (or biopsy specimen) is either examined with routine stains or stained with Perl's Prussian blue, which highlights the presence of iron. This test is subjective and although the presence of stainable iron excludes the diagnosis of iron deficiency, the converse may not be true. For example, healthy cats have little to no haemosiderin in their marrow. Evidence from study of human patients also suggests that negative iron staining is not predictive of iron deficiency (Ganti *et al.*, 2003).

Summary

Iron deficiency anaemia is classically a microcytic, hypochromic anaemia with a variable regenerative response. If iron deficiency is a suspected cause of anaemia, measurements of serum iron concentration and ferritin levels are recommended. A decrease of both would confirm the diagnosis of iron deficiency. Additional testing may reveal normal to increased TIBC, low transferrin saturation, decreased Hb content and rMCV, and lack of stainable iron in the marrow.

Anaemia secondary to inflammatory disease (anaemia of chronic disease) is typically normocytic and normochromic, although in some cases may appear microcytic and hypochromic. The serum iron concentration is also low in this condition; however, the increased stores of body iron may be demonstrated by examination of a marrow aspirate or inferred from an elevated concentration of ferritin. With the anaemia of inflammatory disease, the stores of iron are actually increased, but the release of iron to the erythroid marrow is inadequate (Andrews, 1999).

Treatment of iron deficiency

Management is focused on repletion of iron stores as well as correcting the cause of iron deficiency. A blood transfusion may be needed if severe anaemia is present. A transfusion will help to assure adequate oxygen transport and is a good source of iron. Iron is effective in treating anaemia caused by iron deficiency, but is not beneficial for anaemias that are not associated with iron deficiency, such as the anaemia of inflammatory disease. Iron should not be administered indiscriminately to patients with undiagnosed anaemia.

The oral administration of ferrous sulphate at 2–5 mg/kg/day is the safest treatment for iron deficiency. Ferrous fumarate or ferrous gluconate are also effective. Side effects of oral administration may include abdominal pain, nausea, vomiting, diarrhoea or constipation. Food reduces absorption of iron and it may be preferable to give iron in the fasting state, even if the dose must be reduced (Hillman, 1990).

Injectable iron dextran may be indicated in patients with malabsorptive disease or when intolerance prevents effective oral therapy. In humans, intramuscular injections can cause prolonged pain at the injection site, anaphylaxis, skin discoloration, sterile abscesses and local sarcomas, and they are therefore discouraged (Hillman, 1990). Iron dextran has been administered at 50 mg by intramuscular injection to 18-day-old kittens (Weiser and Kociba, 1983). Intravenous administration has replaced intramuscular administration in human patients, although the authors do not know whether this route is safe in small animals.

The response to therapy can be evaluated by increases in PCV and may be evident as early as 4–7 days after beginning iron therapy. The PCV should be normal or nearly so within 4 weeks of therapy. If the response is inadequate by this time, the diagnosis should be reconsidered.

The duration of therapy is governed by the need to replace iron stores. If iron therapy is stopped after the Hct has returned to normal, but before replenishment of iron stores, the animal is at risk of recurrence of iron deficiency should further bleeding occur. Iron supplementation is therefore recommended for several months to replace body stores adequately (Hillman, 1990).

References and further reading

Andrews NC (1999) Disorders of iron metabolism. *New England Journal of Medicine* **341**(26), 1986–1995

Boisvert AM, Tvedten HW and Scott MA (1999) Artifactual effects of hypernatremia and hyponatremia on red cell analytes measured by the Bayer H*1 analyzer. *Veterinary Clinical Pathology* **28**(3), 91–96

Fry MM and Kirk CA (2006) Reticulocyte indices in a canine model of nutritional iron deficiency. *Veterinary Clinical Pathology* **35**(2), 172–181

Ganti AK, Moazzam N, Laroia S *et al.* (2003) Predictive value of absent bone marrow iron stores in the clinical diagnosis of iron deficiency anemia. *In Vivo* **17**(5), 389–392

Hillman R (1990) Drugs effective in iron deficiency and other hypochromic anemias. In: *The Pharmacological Basis of Therapeutics*, ed. AG Gilman, pp.1282–1292. Pergamon Press, New York

Lozoff B, Jimenez E and Wolf AW (1991) Long-term developmental outcome of infants with iron deficiency. *New England Journal of Medicine* **325**(10), 687–694

Ottenjan M, Weingart C, Arndt G *et al.* (2006) Characterization of the anemia of inflammatory disease in cats with abscesses, pyothorax, or fat necrosis. *Journal of Veterinary Internal Medicine* **20**(5), 1143–1150

Schloess LL, Kipp MA and Wenzel FJ (1965) Thrombocytosis in iron-deficiency anemia. *Journal of Laboratory and Clinical Medicine* **66**(1), 107–114

Segev G, Bandt C, Francey T *et al.* (2008) Aluminum toxicity following administration of aluminum-based phosphate binders in 2 dogs with renal failure. *Journal of Veterinary Internal Medicine* **22**(6), 1432–1435

Seguin MA and Bunch SE (2001) Iatrogenic copper deficiency associated with long-term copper chelation for treatment of copper storage disease in a Bedlington Terrier. *Journal of the American Veterinary Medical Association* **218**(10), 1593–1597, 1580

Vokurka M, Krijt J, Sulc K *et al.* (2006) Hepcidin mRNA levels in mouse liver respond to inhibition of erythropoiesis. *Physiologic Research* **55**(6), 667–674

Weeks BR, Smith JE and Stadler CK (1990) Effect of dietary iron content on hematologic and other measures of iron adequacy in dogs. *Journal of the American Veterinary Medical Association* **196**(5), 749–753

Weiser MG and Kociba GJ (1983) Sequential changes in erythrocyte volume distribution and microcytosis associated with iron deficiency in kittens. *Veterinary Pathology* **20**(1), 1–12

6

Immune-mediated haemolytic anaemia

Michael J. Day†

Introduction

Antibody and/or complement-mediated destruction of circulating red blood cells (RBCs) is known as immune-mediated haemolytic anaemia (IMHA). The immunological destruction of the RBCs occurs by a classical type II hypersensitivity reaction (Day and Mackin, 2008). This involves extravascular phagocytosis of opsonized RBCs in the spleen or liver, or intravascular osmotic lysis following the generation of terminal membrane attack complexes of the complement pathway (Figure 6.1). The former mechanism is most likely to involve IgG antibody, and the latter is more closely associated with the binding of IgM to the surface of the RBCs. Although either intra- or extravascular haemolysis may be dominant in any one patient, it is possible for combinations of these two mechanisms to occur. In some cases, the bone marrow erythroid precursors (instead of, or in addition to the circulating erythrocytes) are targeted, giving rise to more severe diseases termed non-regenerative IMHA (NRIMHA) and pure red cell aplasia (PRCA) (Stokol *et al.*, 2000; Weiss, 2002).

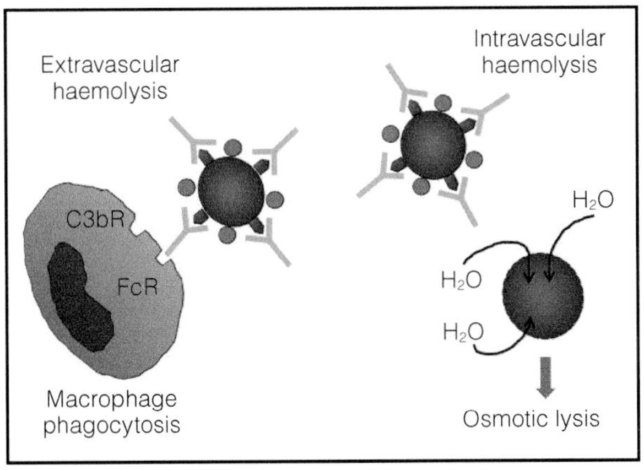

6.1 Mechanisms of RBC destruction in IMHA. In extravascular haemolysis, antibody and complement-coated RBCs are removed from the circulation by macrophages in the spleen and liver. Macrophages carry surface Fc receptors (FcR) for antibody and complement C3b receptors (C3bR) that enhance this interaction. In intravascular haemolysis, the binding of antibody and complement proceeds to formation of the membrane attack complex of the terminal pathway of the complement system. Multiple transmembrane pores form in the RBC membrane; these permit a net influx of ions and water. The swollen RBC ruptures (osmotic lysis), releasing haemoglobin into the circulation. This generally occurs on a massive scale and is associated with the onset of icterus and haemoglobinuria.

The diagnostic label IMHA covers a spectrum of clinical disease. The basic distinction is between primary and secondary disease. In primary IMHA no underlying cause for the presence of RBC-associated antibody can be identified on thorough clinical and laboratory investigation. Primary IMHA may therefore be considered to be a true idiopathic, autoimmune disease and the diagnostic label autoimmune haemolytic anaemia (AIHA) can be applied. AIHA and autoimmune thrombocytopenia (AITP) may occur concurrently (Evans' syndrome) or AIHA may be part of a multisystemic autoimmune syndrome (e.g. systemic lupus erythematosus). AIHA may also occur in combination with autoimmune neutropenia (AINP), and sometimes all three immune-mediated cytopenias may be concurrent. By contrast, in secondary IMHA, the presence of erythrocyte-associated antibody is secondary to an underlying cause or trigger factor that is identified historically or on clinical or laboratory examination.

Autoimmune disease

In primary idiopathic AIHA the specificity of the autoantibodies is for an autoantigen – in this context a protein or glycoprotein that is a normal component of the erythrocyte membrane. The target membrane antigens in canine AIHA have been defined, and they include the anion exchange molecule (band 3), the cytoskeletal molecule spectrin, and a series of membrane glycoproteins (glycophorins) (Day, 1999). The same range of membrane antigens is targeted in AIHA in human patients and in rodent models of the disease.

The production of autoantibodies involves the same series of stages that characterize the synthesis of any immunoglobulin. The key event in the initiation of the autoimmune response is the activation of the autoreactive T lymphocyte. Although the majority of self-reactive T cells are deleted during development in the thymus, a proportion escapes this control point and is released into the circulation. Normal humans and animals (including dogs) have circulating T lymphocytes with specificity for erythrocyte or platelet autoantigenic peptides; however, these cells are normally kept in check so that autoimmunity does not develop. Failure of the control of self-reactive T lymphocytes may lie largely with reduced activity of regulatory (suppressor) T cells.

A high proportion of dogs with IMHA are believed to have true primary, idiopathic AIHA, and a recent UK study reported 43 of 77 dogs with IMHA to have primary disease (Warman *et al.*, 2008). Further evidence for the existence of primary AIHA in the dog comes from the strong breed and familial associations that are documented. Pedigrees of Cocker Spaniels and Old English Sheepdogs have been studied extensively, and English Springer Spaniels in the UK are predisposed. A predisposition amongst Clumber Spaniels is widely recognized in North America and the Maltese Terrier is over-represented in Australia (McAlees, 2010). Recent research has defined associations between primary IMHA and combinations of alleles (haplotypes) of genes of the major histocompatibility complex (MHC) in some of these breeds (Kennedy *et al.*, 2006), and genome-wide association studies (GWAS) are currently searching for genetic associations in English Cocker and Springer Spaniels. Autoimmunity is multifactorial in nature, and may require a combination of predisposing and trigger factors (e.g. stress, oestrus, whelping, infection), acting on an appropriate genetic background, to upset the normal homeostatic regulation of autoreactive T cells and induce clinical autoimmune disease.

Primary IMHA is thought to be relatively less common than secondary disease in the cat (Day, 1996a; Kohn *et al.*, 2006; Tasker *et al.*, 2010). There is little evidence for breed-associated or familial feline AIHA (Gunn-Moore *et al.*, 1999). PRCA is rarely recognized in the cat (Zini *et al.*, 2007).

Secondary immune-mediated disease

By current clinical definitions, many animals with IMHA have primary, idiopathic autoimmune disease that responds to immunosuppressive therapy. By contrast, there is a proportion of cases in which the immune-mediated blood dyscrasia is clearly secondary to an underlying cause.

Neoplasia

Canine IMHA is recognized to occur secondary to a range of neoplastic diseases (e.g. lymphoma, leukaemia, myeloproliferative disease in dogs and cats or haemangiosarcoma in the dog). The mechanisms underlying these associations are at present only speculation. A recent investigation of the well described association between human chronic lymphocytic leukaemia and IMHA has shown that the neoplastic B cells are able to present erythrocyte autoantigen and stimulate autoreactive T cells (Galletti *et al.*, 2008). In human $CD5^+$ B-cell lymphoma, the neoplastic B cells are the source of autoantibody.

Chronic inflammation

Chronic inflammatory disease has been associated with secondary IMHA. Examples include dogs with inflammatory bowel disease and cats with abscesses, feline infectious peritonitis virus infection, pancreatitis or chronic interstitial nephritis. The mechanisms of such associations are unknown, but probably relate to non-specific stimulation of the immune system with activation of autoreactive T and B cells.

Infection

An increasing range of infectious agents is known to trigger secondary IMHA in the dog and cat. Many of these are arthropod-borne microparasites (e.g. *Babesia*, *Ehrlichia*, *Leishmania*, *Rickettsia*, *Cytauxzoon*) (Shaw *et al.*, 2001a, b) but other agents (feline leukaemia virus (FeLV) and *Leptospira*) have also been implicated. These are clearly major differentials in geographical areas in which these diseases are endemic, and the travel history of all animals with IMHA should be evaluated carefully (Shaw *et al.*, 2003). Dogs with babesiosis may be Coombs' test positive, but recent studies have suggested that this may more commonly occur with *Babesia gibsoni* (small form *Babesia*) or *Babesia canis vogeli* infections (Carli *et al.*, 2009). All cats with presumptive IMHA should have retroviral screening (FeLV and feline immunodeficiency virus (FIV)) and be tested for *Mycoplasma* infection. FeLV infection may trigger IMHA through a variety of mechanisms, and although now less common than historically, may still induce lymphoma. Wherever possible, quantitative real-time polymerase chain reaction (PCR) should be used to test for infection with the three feline haemoplasma species (*Mycoplasma haemofelis, 'Candidatus* Mycoplasma haemominutum' and *'Candidatus* Mycoplasma turicensis') and to determine the infectious load. There is a strong association between feline haemoplasma infection (*M. haemofelis*), haemolytic anaemia and Coombs' positivity. Recent experimental studies have shown that erythrocyte antibody develops just after anaemia – which suggests that the antibody does not initiate the anaemia, but may contribute to it once developed (Tasker *et al.*, 2009). Recently, interest has focused on canine haemoplasmas (*Mycoplasma haemocanis, 'Candidatus* Mycoplasma haematoparvum') as a potential trigger for IMHA. An unpublished abstract from Germany has suggested that up to 18% of dogs with IMHA may carry this infection, but a large survey of UK dogs with IMHA and other forms of anaemia has shown no association, although *M. haemocanis* has been identified in splenectomized UK dogs (Warman *et al.*, 2010).

Vaccination

Recent administration (within 4 weeks preceding the onset of disease) of a vaccine (polyvalent, modified-live vaccines are generally incriminated) has been recognized as a trigger factor for canine IMHA (Duval and Giger, 1996). Since the initial description of this phenomenon, numerous other retrospective studies have suggested that vaccination is not a common risk factor for development of IMHA, although in individual patients there is a clear temporal association between these events. UK data give an incidence of 0.001 cases of canine IMHA per 10,000 doses of vaccine sold (Veterinary Products Committee, 2002).

Drug therapy

IMHA may be triggered by administration of drugs, and the best example of this phenomenon involves administration of trimethoprim/sulphonamide antimicrobials to Dobermanns and dogs of a range of other breeds (Trepanier *et al.*, 2003). In the cat, medical management of hyperthyroidism with carbimazole/methimazole is well recognized to be associated with possible induction of a range of immune-mediated side effects including IMHA, IMTP and serum antinuclear antibody positivity (Petersen *et al.*, 1988).

Mechanisms

The precise immunological mechanisms by which these secondary causes give rise to IMHA are largely a matter of speculation. Drugs may act as immunological haptens, and by attaching to the red cell membrane they may induce an immune response to the drug or drug/protein combination that causes 'bystander destruction' of the red cell. A similar mechanism has been proposed for some infectious agents (e.g. haemoplasmas) but some microbes are also thought to trigger the production of true autoantibodies reactive solely with red cell membrane antigens (e.g. canine small babesiosis). Other infectious agents (e.g. *Leishmania*) cause massive (inappropriate) activation of humoral immunity, including the production of antibodies that may cause the secondary immune-mediated components of clinical infection. Vaccine antigens might act as 'molecular mimics' of red cell membrane proteins, or the induction of autoantibody may reflect incorporation of extraneous proteins into the vaccine or be attributed to the effects of adjuvant within these products (Day, 2006). Neoplastic lymphocytes might be a source of erythrocyte autoantibody, or cytokines produced by these cells may upset immunological regulation and activate other autoreactive lymphoid populations. In the case of haemangiosarcoma, traumatized erythrocytes (schistocytes) may have abnormal membrane antigen conformation, making these cells targets for immune-mediated destruction.

Clinical signs

In general terms, two clinical presentations of canine IMHA are recognized. The most common involves a relatively slow onset (days to weeks) of clinical signs, including anorexia and increasing lethargy and exercise intolerance. Physical examination reveals pale mucous membranes, and in cases of concurrent thrombocytopenia, petechiae can be seen. Tachypnoea and tachycardia are present to compensate for anaemia. A systolic cardiac murmur can develop as a result of chronic anaemia. There may be evidence of hepatosplenomegaly and mild lymphadenomegaly as a reflection of erythrocyte destruction, extramedullary haemopoiesis and immune activation in these tissues.

The alternative clinical presentation is an acute or peracute onset of a haemolytic crisis. These patients may be relatively normal one day, and collapsed the next. Such patients will more frequently have haemoglobinuria and icterus caused by sudden and severe intravascular haemolysis that overwhelms the capacity of the liver to conjugate bilirubin and allows loss of haemoglobin through the renal glomerulus (Figure 6.2).

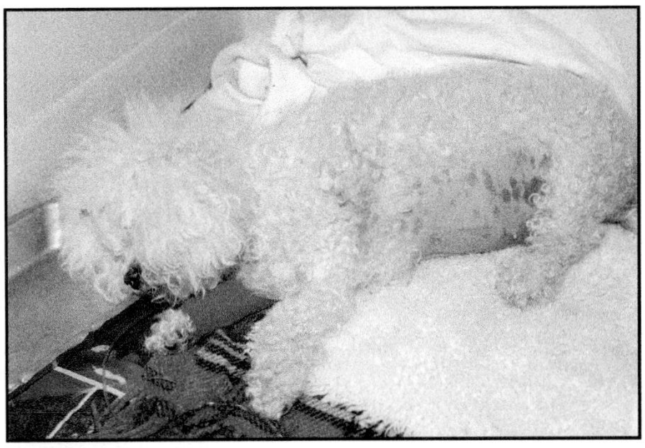

6.2 This dog has severe acute onset immune-mediated haemolytic anaemia (IMHA) with marked tissue jaundice. Sudden intravascular haemolysis has overwhelmed the capacity of the liver to conjugate bilirubin, leading to hyperbilirubinaemia. The dog also probably has haemoglobinuria.

Pulmonary (and other organ) thromboembolism associated with disseminated intravascular coagulation (DIC) is a recognized complication of canine IMHA and considered an important risk factor for mortality. The pathogenesis of this effect is poorly understood, although hypercoagulability and increased aggregability of platelets are widely recognized. A recent study has shown no evidence for autoantibodies against vascular endothelium, as are often observed in human thromboembolic processes (Wells *et al.*, 2009), and the 'lupus anticoagulant' (an anti-phospholipid autoantibody that enhances platelet aggregation and decreases regulation of the coagulation pathways) is also rarely identified in dogs with IMHA.

The same spectrum of clinical disease may occur in the cat, but because cats appear better able to compensate for chronic anaemia, the anaemia may be more severe at the time of presentation.

Diagnosis

The diagnostic approach to cases of IMHA proceeds through stages of increasing complexity. Initial clinical and historical assessments are supported by haematological analysis and bone marrow assessment in non-regenerative forms of disease.

Haematology

Haematological analysis is the most important diagnostic procedure, and key features of the haemogram that are consistent with IMHA are listed below.

- **Strongly regenerative, severe haemolytic anaemia.** The exceptions to this will be cases of

NRIMHA/PRCA, or in disease of peracute onset in which there has not been sufficient time for the bone marrow to compensate. Approximately one third of cases of IMHA will be non-regenerative at the time of admission. The reticulocyte count should be determined. In cats, the distinction between aggregate and punctate reticulocytes should be made, with release of aggregate reticulocytes indicative of active regeneration.

- **Autoagglutination of erythrocytes** macro- or microscopically. Macroscopic agglutination should be further investigated by the 'in-saline agglutination test' which will distinguish true agglutinates from rouleaux. This simple diagnostic procedure can be performed readily in practice. A tube of ethylene diamine tetraacetic acid (EDTA)-anticoagulated blood from the patient should be placed in the refrigerator (4°C) for 30 minutes. After this time, the tube should be examined for the presence of agglutinates of red blood cells. If these are seen, a drop of the blood should be placed on a microscope slide and diluted with an equal volume (drop) of saline. The slide should be rocked gently. If this procedure leads to dispersal of the aggregated RBCs then the clumping effect was a result of rouleaux formation rather than true agglutination. Persistence of the effect is a positive 'in-saline agglutination test' and is indicative of the presence of haemagglutinating antibody (generally of the IgM class) (Figure 6.3). Such antibodies often have preferential reactivity at colder temperature and may elute from the surface of the erythrocytes at body temperature. The in-saline agglutination test should always be performed where cold-reactive agglutination is present, but in reality this effect is relatively uncommon. A positive test provides useful diagnostic information, but a negative test does not rule out IMHA. In cats, additional saline dilution may be required compared with dogs because feline RBCs are often naturally more aggregable than those of the dog.
- **Spherocytosis** is major indicator of IMHA in the dog. A spherocyte is a partially phagocytosed RBC that has lost a portion of its membrane after encountering a phagocyte on transit through the spleen or liver (Figures 6.4 and 6.5). Spherocytosis is highly indicative of IMHA in dogs, but spherocytes are not distinguished in the cat because these animals normally have smaller and denser erythrocytes.
- **Left shift neutrophilia.** This may sometimes be

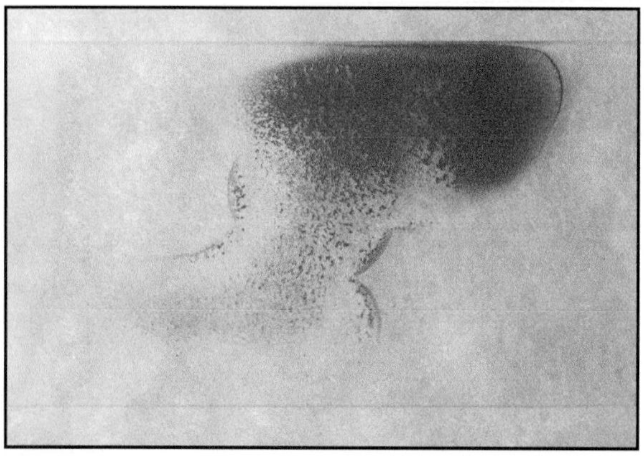

6.3 The in-saline agglutination test. A drop of EDTA blood from a dog with suspected IMHA is placed on a microscope slide. Small flecks within the sample indicate the presence of probable agglutinates of RBCs. An equal volume of saline is added to the drop of blood. The slide is rocked gently and after a few seconds the aggregated RBCs remain present. This indicates agglutination rather than rouleaux formation and indicates a positive in-saline agglutination test.

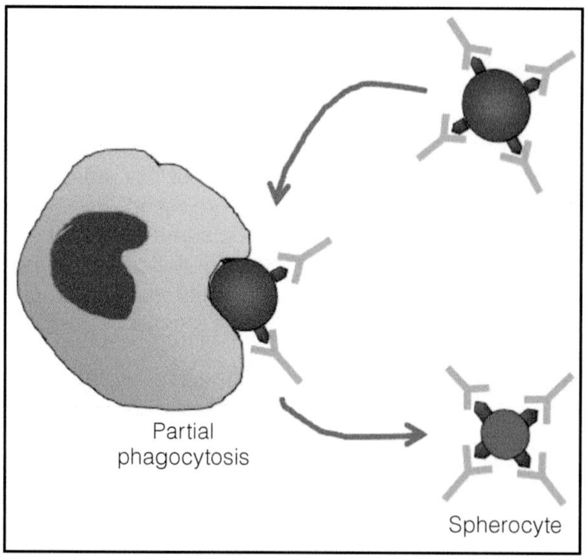

6.4 Formation of spherocytes. An antibody-coated red blood cell (RBC) passes through the spleen and encounters a macrophage. Following interaction with the Fc receptor, the macrophage is unable to engulf (phagocytose) the RBC entirely, but instead removes a portion of the cell membrane. The damaged RBC 'repairs' itself by closing over the defect, leading to formation of a smaller cell that lacks the classical zone of central pallor typical of a canine RBC. This cell passes back into the circulation where it appears as a spherocyte.

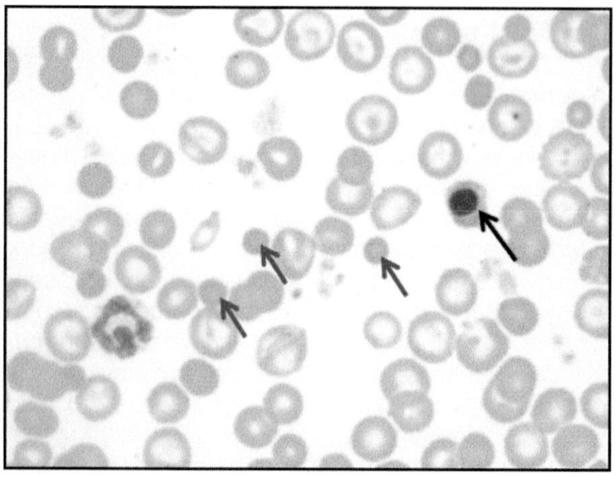

6.5 Blood smear from a dog with IMHA. The anisocytosis, polychromasia, spherocytosis (blue arrows) and nucleated erythrocytes (black arrow) are all highly indicative of IMHA.

profound and require differentiation from myeloproliferative disease. The reasons for this change are suggested to include centrilobular hepatocyte degeneration and necrosis as a consequence of anaemia, production of proinflammatory cytokines by activated macrophages, and non-specific bone marrow stimulation.
- **Concurrent thrombocytopenia** in Evans' syndrome or neutropenia in concurrent IMNP.

The blood smear should always be evaluated to assess for potential underlying causes of disease (e.g. leukaemic cells, erythrocyte parasites).

Recent studies have shown a high prevalence of haemostatic abnormalities in dogs with IMHA and have suggested that these may underlie the predisposition to development of pulmonary thromboembolism (Scott-Moncrieff *et al.*, 2001; Sinnott and Otto, 2009). The acute phase proteins (APPs) C-reactive protein (CRP) and $\alpha 1$ acid glycoprotein (AAG) are elevated at the time of presentation with IMHA but normalize as dogs stabilize with treatment. There is a correlation between APP concentration and the packed cell volume (PCV) and white blood cell (WBC) count, which suggests that APPs may be a useful means of monitoring response to treatment (Griebsch *et al.*, 2009; Mitchell *et al.*, 2009).

Laboratory tests

The identification of erythrocyte-bound antibody and/or complement is based on the Coombs' or direct antiglobulin test, which remains the mainstay for definitive diagnosis and is widely available in a commercial setting, although not all laboratories offer complete testing using multiple antisera that are fully titrated at different incubation temperatures. The Coombs' test involves the demonstration of antibody and/or complement on the surface of RBCs from the patient, and uses incubation of a washed red cell suspension with antisera that will cause gross agglutination (Figure 6.6). The polyvalent Coombs' reagent detects all immunoreactants, while specific antisera (to IgG, IgM and complement C3) may be used in parallel to define the nature of the immune reaction further (Figure 6.7). Recent studies have reported that testing with a panel of reagents is more likely to give a positive diagnosis than testing with polyvalent reagent alone (Overmann *et al.*, 2007; Warman *et al.*, 2008). Moreover, there are distinct differences in the pattern of test reactivity between dogs with primary and secondary disease. Dogs with primary disease are more likely to have IgG antibody and less likely to have IgM antibody compared with dogs that have secondary IMHA.

Although ELISA-based tests for IMHA have been developed, they are more complicated than is required for routine clinical diagnosis. In some countries the osmotic fragility test is favoured as an adjunct diagnostic test. More recently, a flow cytometric method for detection of erythrocyte-bound antibody has been applied to canine samples (Wilkerson et al., 2000). This test may have greater sensitivity, but lower specificity, than the Coombs' test and depends on the availability of a flow cytometer. A recent study of 147 anaemic and 145 non-anaemic dogs tested by flow cytometry for the presence of erythrocyte-bound IgG and IgM revealed a strong association with IMHA and thrombocytopenia, but dogs with infectious disease were often also positive (Moreley et al., 2008).

The latest innovation is the development of rapid,

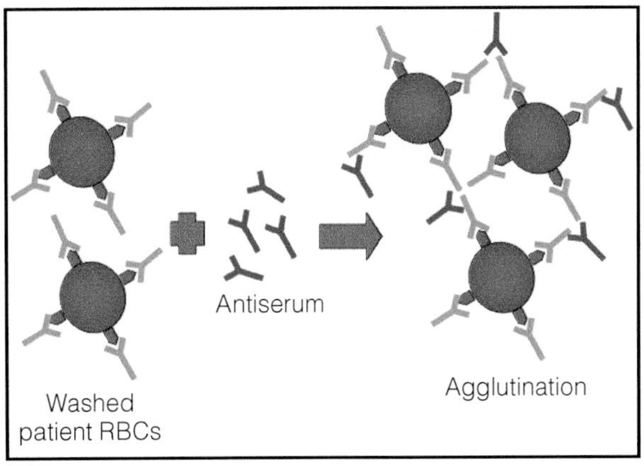

6.6 Principle of the Coombs' test. A suspension of washed antibody- and/or complement-coated red blood cells (RBCs) from the patient is incubated with an antiserum specific for one or more of the immunological molecules that coat the surface of the RBCs (i.e. IgG, IgM or complement C3). In this example, rabbit antiserum specific for canine IgG binds the canine IgG molecules coating the patient RBCs, leading to formation of a lattice-like arrangement that appears grossly as agglutination.

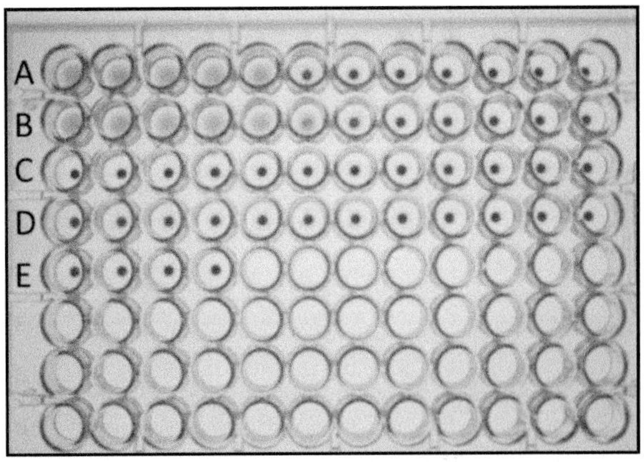

6.7 The Coombs' test is performed in a microtitration system. In this plate, four different antisera are titrated across the plate from left to right. Row A contains polyvalent canine Coombs' reagent, row B contains anti-dog IgG, row C contains anti-dog IgM and row D contains anti-dog complement C3. The antisera are most concentrated on the left side, and with each doubling dilution made towards the right side of the plate they become more dilute. Row E contains saline as a negative control. An equal volume of a suspension of washed patient RBCs is added to each well and the plate is incubated (duplicate plates at both 4 and 37°C). A positive reaction (agglutination) appears as a diffuse mat of RBCs and a negative reaction as a button of RBCs at the base of the well. The titre of the reaction is the inverse of the dilution of antiserum present in the last well of the series that gives a positive result. This dog is Coombs' positive and the RBCs are coated with IgG (titre 160).

in-house, tube-based tests for both dog and cat. These simply determine a positive/negative result using polyvalent antiserum but appear to work well in validation studies (Piek *et al.*, 2011). However, in order to use these tests it is necessary to purchase a specific centrifuge from the manufacturer.

It is often stated that the Coombs' test is invalid in cats. This suggestion is based on the results of a single, rather old and poorly validated study in which it was reported that a proportion of clinically normal cats had a low-titred positive Coombs' test using IgM antiserum (Dunn *et al.*, 1984). In fact, the Coombs' test may be performed for cats in exactly the same way as for dogs (although anti-complement reagents are not available for this species) and it provides the same useful diagnostic information (Day 1996a; Kohn *et al.*, 2006). A recent large validation study showed good correlation between the feline Coombs' test and haemolytic anaemia (Tasker *et al.*, 2010).

The increasing availability of sophisticated laboratory diagnostic tests will mean that animals with secondary IMHA will be identified more readily. For example, animals with Coombs' positive anaemia may be readily screened for microparasitic diseases by PCR using a peripheral blood sample, and these methods are far more sensitive than attempts to detect circulating parasitaemia by examination of a blood smear. Advances in molecular diagnosis may mean that further underlying causes of immune-mediated blood dyscrasias (e.g. subclinical lymphoma identified by clonality testing) may be identified more readily in the future.

Treatment

For those cases in which IMHA is secondary to a defined underlying cause, appropriate therapy for the primary disease must be administered. Any drugs that the animal has been receiving should be withdrawn unless their administration is absolutely necessary.

Transfusion

Adjunct therapy for the anaemic state may also be considered, particularly transfusion of whole blood or packed erythrocytes in severely anaemic patients. Blood products should be as fresh as possible because with prolonged storage there is erythrocyte damage, leading to release of phospholipid that enhances the risk of DIC. It is often considered that transfusion is contraindicated in IMHA as it may 'add fuel to the fire', but even though transfused erythrocytes may have a shorter lifespan than normal, transfusion may still mean the difference between death and survival in the acute stages of disease and transfusion should never be withheld. Recent studies have suggested that use of a purified bovine haemoglobin product (Oxyglobin) may worsen the outcome in canine IMHA, but again this product should not be withheld if it may make a difference with respect to survival. Oxyglobin has also been used to effect in cats with IMHA (Weingart and Kohn, 2008).

Heparin and aspirin

Adjunct administration of heparin or ultra-low-dose aspirin is now routinely practised as a means of preventing the potential secondary thromboembolic complications of IMHA. A recent study compared three such modalities (in conjunction with standard immunosuppression) (Helmond *et al.*, 2009; Orcutt *et al.*, 2009). The three protocols tested were:

1. Ultra-low dose aspirin (0.5 mg/kg/day orally) in 25 cases
2. Constant low-dose unfractionated heparin (150 IU/kg s.c. q6h) in 7 cases
3. Individually adjusted dose of unfractionated heparin (attempting to maintain a therapeutic plasma level of 0.3–0.7 IU/ml using an anti-Factor Xa assay; this required administration of 180–712 IU/kg q6–8 h) in 8 cases.

The success of these protocols was judged by 6-month survival and the incidence of thromboembolic events (TEE).

- Protocol 1: 10 of 25 dogs treated were alive at 6 months; 6 of these 15 died from TEE.
- Protocol 2: 1 of 7 dogs treated was alive at 6 months; 5 dogs had a TEE, which was fatal in 3 cases.
- Protocol 3: 7/8 dogs treated were alive at 6 months; only 2 dogs had a TEE, which was fatal in 1 case.

These results support the use of individually adjusted dosing with unfractionated heparin, although in practical terms this procedure is unlikely to be widely available.

Splenectomy

Splenectomy was once widely practised as an adjunct treatment in canine IMHA. The rationale for this procedure was the removal of a major site of erythrocyte destruction, but given that extravascular haemolysis may also occur elsewhere (e.g. the liver) and that the spleen is also important for extramedullary haemopoiesis, there is little to recommend this practice.

Immunosuppressive drug therapy

The specific medical therapy for these disorders involves administration of immunosuppressive drugs. The choice of agents depends upon the clinical presentation of the patient and the severity of disease, and relies largely on clinical acumen.

Dogs with compensated regenerative anaemia of chronic onset should respond to simple glucocorticotherapy. In such patients, the major beneficial effect of glucocorticoids is in down-regulating Fc receptor expression by phagocytic cells, thereby slowing the extravascular haemolysis that is the primary mechanism in this form of disease. The glucocorticoid of choice is oral prednisolone administered at the immunosuppressive dose (2 mg/kg/day for dogs or 4 mg/kg/day for cats, given once or split twice daily) and slowly tapered. An H2 receptor antagonist and sucralfate may be administered in order to prevent gastrointestinal ulceration. Although dogs may show a rapid clinical and haematological response to glucocorticotherapy, the drug should not be withdrawn early because relapse is common. There are a number of tapering protocols, but a simple regime involves step reduction of the dose by one quarter every 2 weeks, ending with administration of 0.5 mg/kg every other day. This assumes that there is no relapse of disease. In most cases it will be possible to withdraw therapy completely after the stage of dosing every other day with 0.5 mg/kg, but in some patients this leads to relapse and lifelong maintenance therapy is required.

For dogs with severe disease of more acute onset, or in relapse, clinical judgement would suggest that adjunct immunosuppressive agents might be incorporated into the treatment regime. A range of other drugs (e.g. danazol, azathioprine, cyclophosphamide, ciclosporin, leflunomide, mycophenolic acid and liposomal-encapsulated clodronate) has been co-administered with glucocorticoids in various regimes to reduce the likelihood of glucocorticoid side effects ('steroid sparing') or to have additional immunomodulatory effects. Despite the widespread use of such protocols, there is no clear consensus as to which (if any) combination is most efficacious, and which individual cases are the most likely candidates for combined therapy (Burgess *et al.*, 2000; Grundy and Barton, 2001; Weinkle *et al.*, 2005). In fact, some studies suggest that the use of some adjunct drugs has no added value (ciclosporin), or even results in a less successful clinical outcome than the use of glucocorticoid alone (cyclophosphamide) (Mason *et al.*, 2003). These studies are difficult to interpret because those dogs receiving combination therapy (as opposed to glucocorticoid monotherapy) most likely had more severe clinical disease with a greater likelihood of fatal outcome. At present, the majority of authors favour azathioprine (2 mg/kg/day orally) when an adjunct to glucocorticoid is required. It should be remembered that this drug has a delayed onset of action (10–14 days) and the decision to use it should be made at the time of initial assessment. Azathioprine is a much cheaper drug than either ciclosporin or mycophenolic acid, but both of the latter agents are being assessed currently for their benefit in the management of canine IMHA (Husbands *et al.*, 2004). These adjunct drugs all have specific side effects for which patients must be monitored during therapy.

Immunoglobulin therapy

Administration of high dose intravenous human immunoglobulin (IVIG) has proven useful, but the expense and availability of this product generally precludes its widespread application (Kellerman and Bruyette, 1997). The large quantity of human immunoglobulins in such an injection bind to macrophage Fc receptors and block access of the canine antibody attached to the RBCs. Repeated doses of human immunoglobulin should be avoided because there is the potential for immunological sensitization to the foreign protein and development of subsequent hypersensitivity responses. Moreover, it is now suggested that administration of IVIG may promote coagulability and this would be undesirable in the management of a disease in which a hypercoagulable state already exists (Tsuchiya *et al.*, 2009).

Considerations for cats

The management of feline IMHA also involves immunosuppressive glucocorticoids (as above) or chlorambucil (0.1–0.2 mg/kg tapering dose), remembering that the use of azathioprine in cats is generally to be avoided. All cats should be tested for haemoplasma infection and if positive an appropriate course of antimicrobial therapy (e.g. doxycycline) is required.

Prognosis

IMHA is a severe disease and in a referral setting several studies have now shown that approximately 50% of dogs will die during initial hospitalization (Weinkle *et al.*, 2005). This may in part reflect the fact that only more severe cases are referred rather than being managed in first opinion practice. The outcome is even worse for dogs with secondary IMHA where the underlying disease may be the cause of death. IMHA with evidence of intravascular haemolysis (hyperbilirubinaemia, icterus, haemoglobinaemia, haemoglobinuria), autoagglutination, cold-reactive IgM antibodies identified in the Coombs' test, targeting of bone marrow precursors, thrombocytopenia or development of pulmonary thromboembolism or DIC carries a more guarded prognosis. Risk factors for thromboembolic complications include thrombocytopenia and hyperbilirubinaemia (Carr *et al.*, 2002). Those animals that recover from the initial disease episode are at risk for relapse, often months or years later. Careful monitoring should be performed, most simply by haematological analysis (e.g. packed cell volume), for at least 6 months after an episode of disease and at intervals for the lifetime of the animal. Monitoring Coombs' test positivity is not helpful because many dogs that have recovered from IMHA may remain Coombs' positive for long periods of time after recovery, despite being clinically and haematologically normal (Day, 1996b).

In one recent study, the estimated 6-month survival rate in dogs with primary IMHA that were treated with a standard protocol of prednisolone, azathioprine and a blood transfusion if necessary, was 72.6%. The highest mortality occurred in the first 14 days after diagnosis, and multivariate analysis identified uraemia, band neutrophilia, thrombocytopenia and petechiae as the major independent variables that were negative prognostic indicators during the first 2 weeks after diagnosis. Those animals that survived the first 2 weeks after diagnosis had a 6-month survival rate of 92% (Piek *et al.*, 2008). In the study with the poorest outcome figures, there was an overall mortality rate of 70% in a series of 70 cases of IMHA, with 41% of dogs dying whilst hospitalized and 36% of the remaining dogs that were discharged from hospital dying within a 3-month period (Reimer *et al.*, 1999).

References and further reading

Burgess KA, Moore A, Rand W *et al.* (2000) Treatment of immune-mediated hemolytic anemia in dogs with cyclophosphamide. *Journal of Veterinary Internal Medicine* **14**, 456–462

Carli E, Tasca S, Trotta M *et al.* (2009) Detection of erythrocyte binding IgM and IgG by flow cytometry in sick dogs with *Babesia canis canis* or *Babesia canis vogeli* infection. *Veterinary Parasitology* **162**, 51–57

Carr AP, Panciera DL and Kidd L (2002) Prognostic factors for mortality and thromboembolism in canine immune-mediated hemolytic anemia: a retrospective study of 72 dogs. *Journal of Veterinary Internal Medicine* **16**, 504–509

Day MJ (1996a) Diagnostic assessment of the feline immune system, part II. *Feline Practice* **24**, 14–25

Day MJ (1996b) Serial monitoring of clinical, haematological and immunological parameters in canine autoimmune haemolytic anaemia. *Journal of Small Animal Practice* **37**, 523–534

Day MJ (1999) Antigen specificity in canine autoimmune haemolytic anaemia. *Veterinary Immunology and Immunopathology* **69**, 215–224

Day MJ (2006) Vaccine side-effects: fact and fiction. *Veterinary Microbiology* **117**, 51–58

Day MJ and Mackin AJ (2008) Immune-mediated haematological disease. In: *Clinical Immunology of the Dog and Cat, 2nd edn*, ed. MJ Day, pp.94–121. Manson Publishing, London

Dunn JK, Searcy GP and Hirsch VM (1984) The diagnostic significance of a positive direct antiglobulin test in anemic cats. *Canadian Journal of Comparative Medicine* **48**, 349–353

Duval D and Giger U (1996) Vaccine-associated immune-mediated hemolytic anemia in the dog. *Journal of Veterinary Internal Medicine* **10**, 290–295

Galletti J, Canones C, Morande P *et al.* (2008) Chronic lymphocytic leukemia cells bind and present the erythrocyte protein band 3: possible role as initiators of autoimmune hemolytic anemia. *Journal of Immunology* **181**, 3674–3683

Griebsch C, Arndt G, Raila J *et al.* (2009) C-reactive protein concentration in dogs with primary immune-mediated hemolytic anemia. *Veterinary Clinical Pathology* **38**, 421–425

Grundy SA and Barton C (2001) Influence of drug treatment on survival of dogs with immune-mediated hemolytic anemia: 88 cases (1989-1999). *Journal of the American Veterinary Medical Association* **218**, 543–546

Gunn-Moore DA, Day MJ, Graham MEA *et al.* (1999) Immune-mediated haemolytic anaemia in two sibling cats associated with multicentric lymphoblastic infiltration. *Journal of Feline Medicine and Surgery* **1**, 209–214

Helmond SE, Polzin DJ, Armstrong PJ *et al.* (2009) Treatment of canine immune-mediated haemolytic anaemia with individually adjusted heparin dosing: a pilot study. *Journal of Veterinary Internal Medicine* **23**, 693

Husbands B, Polzin D, Armstrong PJ *et al.* (2004) Prednisone and cyclosporine vs. prednisone alone for treatment of canine immune-mediated hemolytic anemia. *Journal of Veterinary Internal Medicine* **18**, 389

Kellerman DL and Bruyette DS (1997) Intravenous human immunoglobulin for the treatment of immune-mediated hemolytic anemia in 13 dogs. *Journal of Veterinary Internal Medicine* **11**, 327–332

Kennedy LJ, Barnes A, Ollier WER *et al.* (2006) Association of a common DLA class II haplotype with canine primary immune-mediated haemolytic anaemia. *Tissue Antigens* **68**, 502–506

Kohn B, Weingart C, Eckmann V *et al.* (2006) Primary immune-mediated haemolytic anemia in 19 cats: diagnosis, therapy and outcome (1998-2004). *Journal of Veterinary Internal Medicine* **20**, 159–166

Mason N, Duval D, Shofer FS *et al.* (2003) Cyclophosphamide exerts no beneficial effect over prednisone alone in the initial treatment of acute immune-mediated hemolytic anemia in dogs: a randomized controlled clinical trial. *Journal of Veterinary Internal Medicine* **17**, 206–212

McAlees TJ (2010) Immune-mediated haemolytic anaemia in 110 dogs in Victoria, Australia. *Australian Veterinary Journal* **88**, 25–28

Mitchell KD, Kruth SA, Wood RD *et al.* (2009) Serum acute phase protein concentrations in dogs with autoimmune hemolytic anemia. *Journal of Veterinary Internal Medicine* **23**, 585–591

Moreley P, Mathes M, Guth A *et al.* (2008) Anti-erythrocyte antibodies and disease associations in anemic and non-anemic dogs. *Journal of Veterinary Internal Medicine* **22**, 886–892

Orcutt ES, Polzin DJ, Armstrong PJ *et al.* (2009) Comparison of individually monitored unfractionated heparin versus low-dose aspirin on survival of dogs with immune-mediated hemolytic anemia. *Journal of Veterinary Internal Medicine* **23**, 693

Overmann JA, Sharkey LC, Weiss DJ *et al.* (2007) Performance of 2 microtiter canine Coombs" tests. *Veterinary Clinical Pathology* **36**, 179–183

Peterson ME, Kintzer PP and Hurvitz AI (1988) Methimazole treatment of 262 cats with hyperthyroidism. *Journal of Veterinary Internal Medicine* **2**, 150–157

Piek CJ, Junius G, Dekker A *et al.* (2008) Idiopathic immune-mediated hemolytic anemia: treatment outcome and prognostic factors in 149 dogs. *Journal of Veterinary Internal Medicine* **22**, 366–373

Piek CJ, Teske E, van Leeuwen MW *et al.* (2011) Good agreement and high specificity of the Diamed gel test in comparison with direct Coombs" testing in the dog and cat. Manuscript submitted.

Reimer ME, Troy GC and Warnick LD (1999) Immune-mediated hemolytic anemia: 70 cases (1988-1996). *Journal of the American Animal Hospital Association* **35**, 384–391

Scott-Moncrieff JC, Treadwell NG, McCullough SM *et al.* (2001) Hemostatic abnormalities in dogs with primary immune-mediated hemolytic anemia. *Journal of the American Animal Hospital Association* **37**, 220–227

Shaw SE, Birtles RJ and Day MJ (2001a) Arthropod-transmitted infectious diseases of cats. *Journal of Feline Medicine and Surgery* **3**, 193–209

Shaw SE, Day MJ, Birtles RJ *et al.* (2001b) Tick-borne infectious diseases of dogs. *Trends in Parasitology* **17**, 74–80

Shaw SE, Lerga AI, Williams S *et al.* (2003) Review of exotic infectious diseases in small animals entering the United Kingdom from abroad diagnosed by PCR. *Veterinary Record* **152**, 176–177

Sinnott VB and Otto CM (2009) Use of thromboelastography in dogs with immune-mediated haemolytic anemia: 39 cases (2000-2008). *Journal of Veterinary Emergency Critical Care* **19**, 484–488

Stokol T, Blue JT and French TW (2000) Idiopathic pure red cell aplasia and nonregenerative immune-mediated anemia in dogs: 43 cases (1988-1999). *Journal of the American Veterinary Medical Association* **216**, 1429–1436

Tasker S, Murray JK, Knowles TG *et al.* (2010) Coombs", haemoplasma and retrovirus testing in feline anaemia. *Journal of Small Animal Practice* **51**, 192–199

Tasker S, Peters IR, Papasouliotis K *et al.* (2009) Description of outcomes of experimental infection with feline haemoplasmas: copy numbers, haematology, Coombs" testing and blood glucose concentrations. *Veterinary Microbiology* **139**, 323–332

Trepanier LA, Danhof R, Toll J *et al.* (2003) Clinical findings in 40 dogs with hypersensitivity associated with administration of potentiated sulfonamides. *Journal of Veterinary Internal Medicine* **17**, 647–652

Tsuchiya R, Akutsu Y, Ikegami A *et al.* (2009) Prothrombotic and inflammatory effects of intravenous administration of human immunoglobulin G in dogs. *Journal of Veterinary Internal Medicine* **23**, 1164–1169

Veterinary Products Committee (VPC) Working Group on Feline and Canine Vaccination (2002) *Final Report to the VPC*. Defra, London

Warman SM, Helps CR, Barker EN *et al.* (2010) Haemoplasma infection is not a common cause of canine immune-mediated haemolytic anaemia in the UK. Manuscript submitted.

Warman SM, Murray JK, Ridyard A *et al.* (2008) Pattern of Coombs" test reactivity has diagnostic significance in dogs with immune-mediated haemolytic anaemia. *Journal of Small Animal Practice* **49**, 525–530

Weingart C and Kohn B (2008) Clinical use of a haemoglobin-based oxygen carrying solution (Oxyglobin®) in 48 cats (2002-2006). *Journal of Feline Medicine and Surgery* **10**, 431–438

Weinkle TK, Center SA, Randolph JF *et al.* (2005) Evaluation of prognostic factors, survival rates, and treatment protocols for immune-mediated hemolytic anemia in dogs: 151 cases (1993-2002). *Journal of the American Veterinary Medical Association* **226**, 1869–1880

Weiss DJ (2002) Primary pure red cell aplasia in dogs: 13 cases (1996-2000). *Journal of the American Veterinary Medical Association* **221**, 93–95

Wells R, Guth A, Lappin M *et al.* (2009) Anti-endothelial cell antibodies in dogs with immune-mediated hemolytic anemia and other diseases associated with high risk of thromboembolism. *Journal of Veterinary Internal Medicine* **23**, 295–300

Wilkerson MJ, Davis E, Shuman W *et al.* (2000) Isotype-specific antibodies in horses and dogs with immune-mediated hemolytic anemia. *Journal of Veterinary Internal Medicine* **14**, 190–196

Zini E, Hauser B, Meli ML *et al.* (2007) Immune-mediated erythroid and megakaryocytic aplasia in a cat. *Journal of the American Veterinary Medical Association* **230**, 1024–1027

7

Haemoplasmosis

Séverine Tasker

Introduction

Feline and canine haemoplasmas are small bacteria that live on the surface of red blood cells (RBCs; Figure 7.1). Infection can result in a haemolytic anaemia. Haemoplasmas are also known as 'haemotropic mycoplasmas'. *Haemobartonella felis* has now been renamed *Mycoplasma haemofelis*, whilst *Haemobartonella canis* is now called *Mycoplasma haemocanis*. Additional feline and canine haemoplasmas also exist such as '*Candidatus* Mycoplasma haemominutum' and '*Candidatus* Mycoplasma haematoparvum'. These different species differ in pathogenicity.

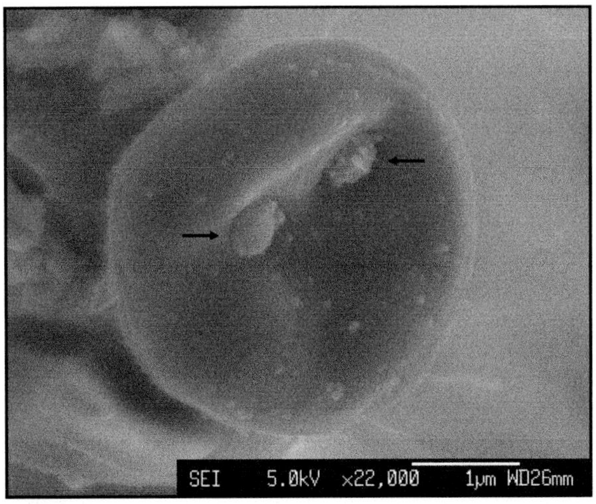

7.1 Scanning electron micrograph of a feline erythrocyte infected with *Mycoplasma haemofelis*. Two *M. haemofelis* organisms attached to the surface of the erythrocyte are highlighted by arrows. (Reproduced with permission from Tasker S (2010))

Feline haemoplasma species and geographical distribution

At least three feline haemoplasma species exist worldwide (Figure 7.2). One study from the United States suggested that cats could also be infected with an organism similar to the canine haemoplasma species '*Candidatus* M. haematoparvum' (Sykes *et al.*, 2007), but other studies have failed to find evidence of this infection. '*Candidatus* M. haemominutum' is generally the most common species, while fewer cats are infected with '*Candidatus* M. turicensis' and *M. haemofelis* (Figure 7.2). Some countries (e.g. South Africa and Canada) may have a higher prevalence of '*Candidatus* M. turicensis' and *M. haemofelis*. Of 1585 feline samples submitted to a United Kingdom diagnostic service for

Species name	Host species	Summary of pathogenicity	Prevalence
Mycoplasma haemofelis	Cat	Usually induces haemolytic anaemia during acute infection	10–32.1%
'*Candidatus* Mycoplasma haemominutum'	Cat	Can result in a decrease in red blood cell parameters, but not severe enough to induce anaemia unless cat has concurrent disease or is immunocompromised	0.4–46.6%
'*Candidatus* Mycoplasma turicensis'	Cat	Can result in a decrease in red blood cell parameters, but not severe enough to induce anaemia unless cat has concurrent disease or is immunocompromised	0.4–26%
'*Candidatus* Mycoplasma haematoparvum-like'	Cat	No data on pathogenesis currently available	0–0.7%
Mycoplasma haemocanis	Dog	Only induces haemolytic anaemia in splenectomized or immunocompromised dogs	0.5–45%
'*Candidatus* Mycoplasma haematoparvum'	Dog	Only induces haemolytic anaemia in splenectomized or immunocompromised dogs	0–33%

7.2 Summary of the pathogenicity and prevalence of feline and canine haemoplasma species. Several haemoplasma species have been assigned the *Candidatus* status to reflect the fact that they represent newly described species that have not yet been fully characterized owing to our inability to culture them *in vitro*.

haemoplasma polymerase chain reaction (PCR) testing, 11.2% were positive for '*Candidatus* M. haemominutum', 2.8% for *M. haemofelis* and 1.7% for '*Candidatus* M. turicensis' (Peters *et al.*, 2008).

Published studies usually include asymptomatic carrier cats in their prevalence figures because cats that recover from acute haemoplasma infection can remain chronically infected. Long-term carrier status is especially common following '*Candidatus* M. haemominutum' infection, although suspected clearance of this infection has also been reported both with and without antibiotic treatment. Cats infected with *M. haemofelis* and '*Candidatus* M. turicensis' may spontaneously clear infection from the peripheral blood after infection, without antibiotic treatment. In any carrier cat the potential for reactivation of infection exists, which can result in clinical disease, but this seems to be uncommon once the haemoplasma infection becomes chronic, after a couple of months.

Transmission of feline haemoplasmas

The cat flea, *Ctenocephalides felis*, is implicated in transmission of haemoplasmas between cats, with transient *M. haemofelis* transmission (detected by PCR) documented between cats via haemophagous activity (Woods *et al.*, 2005), although clinical and haematological signs of *M. haemofelis* infection were not induced in the recipient cat. Haemoplasma DNA has been found in fleas collected from pet cats and stray cats, as well as in ticks. The clustered geographical distribution of infection in some studies supports the role of an arthropod vector in transmission of haemoplasmas, but real evidence confirming their role in natural transmission is still lacking.

Haemoplasma DNA is found in the saliva of infected cats. Cat bite abscesses, outdoor roaming and male gender are risk factors for infection, so it may be that horizontal transmission of haemoplasma occurs via fighting. However, recent attempts to transmit '*Candidatus* M. turicensis' with saliva were not very successful (Museux *et al.*, 2009). It may be that transmission of haemoplasma via social contact is unlikely, but aggressive interaction (e.g. cat bites) may allow transmission of infection if the recipient cat is exposed to infectious blood rather than just saliva.

Vertical transmission of haemoplasmas, from queen to kittens, may occur during pregnancy, at birth or via lactation. Transmission via contaminated blood transfusions can also occur. Although not reported, transmission may also be possible via the use of the same equipment (e.g. surgical instruments) in different cats without appropriate cleaning/sterilization, particularly if blood contamination is significant and recent.

Pathogenesis of feline haemoplasma infection

Feline haemoplasma species vary in pathogenicity, with some isolates inducing anaemia consistently whilst others result in few noticeable clinical signs (Figure 7.3). Concurrent disease or retrovirus

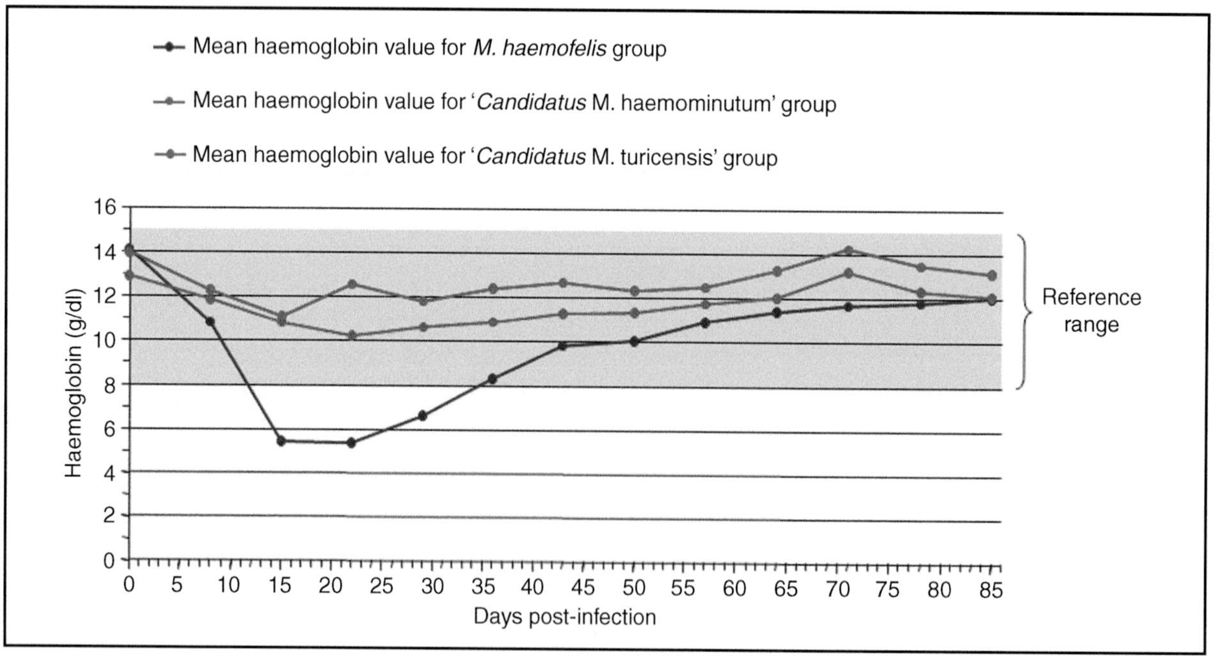

7.3 Representative mean haemoglobin (Hb) values for three groups of cats infected with either *M. haemofelis*, '*Candidatus* M. haemominutum' or '*Candidatus* M. turicensis'. The reference range for Hb is represented by the grey shaded area (8–15 g/dl). Only the cats infected with *M. haemofelis* became anaemic, with the lowest Hb values recorded 2–3 weeks following infection. Cats infected with '*Candidatus* M. haemominutum' and '*Candidatus* M. turicensis' did not become anaemic, although a slight fall in Hb was apparent during the first 2–3 weeks of infection. (Reproduced with permission from Tasker S (2010))

infection can also influence the outcome of infection, and younger cats may be more susceptible to clinical disease. The number of haemoplasma organisms inducing infection, the particular isolate of the haemoplasma species involved and the route of infection may also play a role. In contrast to non-feline haemoplasma species, splenectomy is not required for feline haemoplasmas to induce disease in their hosts, although immunocompromise may increase the pathogenicity of '*Candidatus* M. haemominutum' and '*Candidatus* M. turicensis'.

The primary pathogenic outcome of infection recognized with haemoplasma infection is haemolysis, although other clinical effects are also seen. Most of the haemolysis is extravascular in nature, occurring in the spleen and liver, but intravascular haemolysis has also been reported.

M. haemofelis

M. haemofelis is the most pathogenic feline haemoplasma species. Acute infection often results in haemolytic anaemia (see Figure 7.3), but studies in naturally infected cats have not always demonstrated an association between the presence of anaemia and *M. haemofelis* infection. This is probably because different studies have sampled different populations of cats, different isolates of *M. haemofelis* are involved and/or because cats chronically infected with *M. haemofelis* are less likely to be anaemic than acutely infected cats.

Both persistent autoagglutination and positive Coombs' tests, indicating the presence of erythrocyte-bound antibodies, have been demonstrated in anaemic *M. haemofelis*-infected cats (Tasker *et al.*, 2009). These antibodies could mediate immune-mediated destruction of red blood cells, although they have been shown to appear after the onset of anaemia. Although this could reflect a low sensitivity of detection of antibody early in infection, it could also suggest that the antibodies appear as a result of haemoplasma-induced haemolysis rather than that they initiate the haemolysis. These antibodies can disappear following antibiotic and supportive treatment alone, without specific glucocorticoid treatment, an observation that further questions their role in haemoplasma-induced anaemia.

'*Candidatus* M. haemominutum'

'*Candidatus* M. haemominutum' infection rarely results in significant clinical signs. A fall in red cell indices can occur following infection (see Figure 7.3), but these changes are not usually severe enough to result in anaemia. However, significant anaemia has been reported in retrovirus-infected cats, especially those infected with feline leukaemia virus (FeLV), following '*Candidatus* M. haemominutum' infection, as well as in cats with other concurrent diseases. Therefore, the underlying health status of the cat is likely to play an important role in the outcome of infection, but 'primary' (i.e. not associated with any other underlying diseases or conditions) '*Candidatus* M. haemominutum'-associated anaemia has also been described. '*Candidatus* M. haemominutum' infection has been associated with a blunted erythrocyte regenerative response.

'*Candidatus* M. turicensis'

'*Candidatus* M. turicensis' infection was initially reported in association with haemolytic anaemia, although others have found no evidence of anaemia following infection. As for '*Candidatus* M. haemominutum' infection, a fall in red blood cell indices occurs following infection with '*Candidatus* M. turicensis' (see Figure 7.3), but these changes are not usually severe enough to result in anaemia. Co-infection with other haemoplasma species is often seen with '*Candidatus* M. turicensis'-infection. Concurrent diseases or infections are believed to be important in the pathogenesis of infection with '*Candidatus* M. turicensis'.

Clinical signs of feline haemoplasmosis

Clinical signs of feline haemoplasmosis depend upon the haemoplasma species involved, the stage of infection, whether the haemoplasma infection is primary or secondary to another disease process, stress or infection, and the degree and speed of onset of anaemia. Common clinical signs (Figure 7.4) include pallor, lethargy, anorexia, weight loss, depression and dehydration. Intermittent pyrexia is often seen, particularly in the acute stages of disease, as well as splenomegaly, which may reflect extramedullary haemopoiesis. Icterus is uncommon, but is occasionally seen with severe acute haemolysis.

- Pale mucous membranes
- Lethargy
- Anorexia
- Weight loss
- Depression
- Dehydration
- Pyrexia (can be intermittent)
- Splenomegaly
- Jaundice

7.4 Summary of clinical signs that may occur with feline haemoplasma infection.

Diagnosis of feline haemoplasmosis

Haematology

Clinical haemoplasmosis typically results in a regenerative anaemia (Figure 7.5), although reticulocyte counts can be problematic to obtain in parasitaemic cats because the organisms interfere with the identification of reticulocytes. Significant reticulocytosis is not always seen as a result of cats being in the early stages of anaemia (i.e. before regeneration has occurred), concurrent retroviral infections or other disease processes, or a blunting effect of the haemoplasma infection on the bone marrow. Release of sequestered erythrocytes from the spleen may also result in a marked rise in red blood cell count without accompanying reticulocytosis. Normoblastaemia may be present and positive

- Macrocytic normo- or hypochromic anaemia
- Reticulocytosis[a]
- Normoblastaemia
- Autoagglutination that is persistent following washing of red blood cells in saline
- Positive Coombs' test
- Hyperproteinaemia
- Raised liver enzyme levels
- Hyperbilirubinaemia

7.5 Summary of laboratory changes that may occur with feline haemoplasma infection. [a]May be absent owing to concurrent retroviral infection or other diseases, or a blunting effect of the haemoplasma infection on the bone marrow, or if the cat was sampled in the pre-regenerative phase of the anaemia.

Coombs' tests and persistent autoagglutination can occur with *M. haemofelis.*

Biochemistry

Serum biochemistry (Figure 7.5) may reveal hyperproteinaemia due to an acute phase response or dehydration, and increased liver enzyme levels may arise from hepatic hypoxic damage. Hyperbilirubinaemia has occasionally been reported with severe haemolysis.

Cytology

Previously, the most commonly used method for diagnosis of haemoplasma infection was demonstration of organisms on a Romanowsky-stained (e.g. Wright's, Giemsa or Diff-Quik™) blood smear. Round haemoplasmas are visible on the surface of the erythrocyte singly, in pairs or in chains (Figure 7.6). Although it has been suggested that '*Candidatus* M. haemominutum' is smaller than *M. haemofelis*, differentiation cannot be performed reliably by blood smear examination alone. '*Candidatus* M. turicensis' organisms have not yet been demonstrated cytologically.

Cytology is known to be associated with both false negative and false positive diagnoses. Sensitivity is a particular issue owing to fluctuating parasitaemia, so a negative result on cytology cannot be taken to reflect an absence of haemoplasmosis. A sensitivity of 0–37.5% has been reported in various studies. Given that the organisms detach from red blood cells quite rapidly once blood has been collected into EDTA or heparin anticoagulant, smears for cytological examination should be made soon after blood collection. The specificity of cytology can also be poor, as a result of stain precipitate or Howell–Jolly bodies being mistaken for organisms. The specificity of cytology for the diagnosis of haemoplasmosis is better (84–98%) than the sensitivity, but these figures are based upon board-certified clinical pathologists performing the cytological examination, which is not always the case in practice.

Polymerase chain reaction (PCR)

PCR amplifies specific lengths of DNA so that the small amounts present in, for example, a blood sample become detectable. PCR is now considered to be the diagnostic test of choice for haemoplasma infection. The sensitivity and specificity of PCR assays should always be made available by laboratories that offer the tests commercially, so that their reliability can be evaluated objectively. In addition, laboratories offering PCR must always use appropriate negative and positive controls to monitor for contamination or problems with the PCR assay. Internal controls for PCR amplification are being increasingly used in veterinary PCR assays (see below). PCR is much more sensitive than cytology for diagnosis of haemoplasmosis. All PCR assays described so far for feline haemoplasmas are based on amplification of segments of the 16S rRNA gene, using primers specific for this gene in the haemoplasmas. Only a small volume of blood (usually 0.5 ml EDTA-anticoagulated blood) is required for analysis, and because the DNA in blood samples is quite stable, there are no special transport requirements. Blood samples for PCR should not be collected while a cat is undergoing antibiotic treatment, although a positive result with high organism numbers during antibiotic treatment would indicate that the therapy is not being optimally effective.

Conventional non-quantitative PCR (cPCR) assays have been developed that detect and

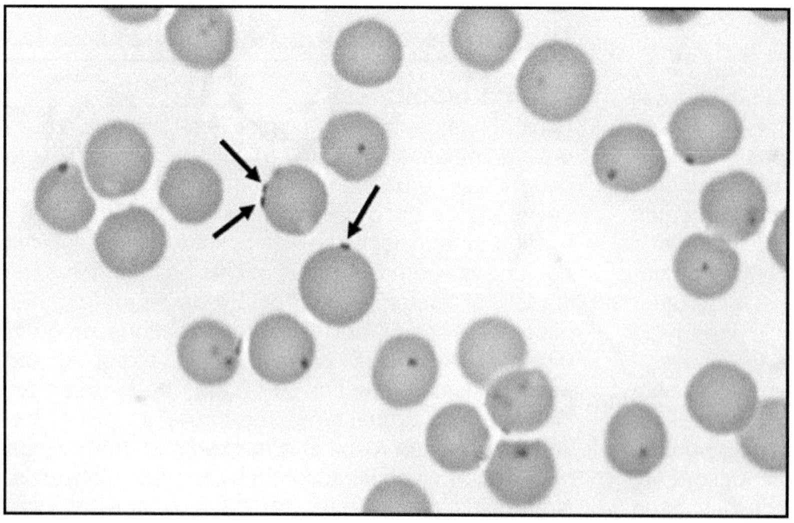

7.6 Blood smear (Wright's stain) from a cat with asymptomatic infection with '*Candidatus* M. haemominutum'. Arrows indicate individual organisms.

distinguish both *M. haemofelis* and '*Candidatus* M. haemominutum' infections. However '*Candidatus* M. turicensis' is usually not amplified or cannot be differentiated from *M. haemofelis* using these cPCR assays, necessitating sequencing or an additional PCR to detect '*Candidatus* M. turicensis'. The diagnostic laboratory being used for PCR should be consulted to determine which haemoplasma species its assays are able to detect. Real-time quantitative PCR (qPCR) assays for feline haemoplasmas offer an additional level of specificity over cPCR because they include fluorogenic probes specific to a particular haemoplasma species as well as primers. Several qPCR assays have been described that amplify and differentiate all three feline haemoplasma species. In addition, some assays are duplexed to amplify concurrently, by PCR, an internal control such as feline 28S rDNA to ensure that negative PCR results do not arise as a result of problems with DNA extraction, quality or PCR inhibition. Importantly, qPCR also allows quantification of the amount of haemoplasma DNA present in the patient's blood, which may help to determine the significance of infection and/or allow monitoring of the response to treatment (see below). qPCR offers other advantages over cPCR, such as a reduced risk of contamination, because the tubes containing the PCR product are never opened during analysis, and a quicker throughput time.

Given that asymptomatic carrier cats exist, a positive PCR result does not necessarily mean that haemoplasma infection is the cause of the cat's clinical signs. PCR only detects infection, rather than confirming the cause of the cat's disease. PCR results should therefore always be interpreted alongside clinical signs and haematological findings.

Treatment and prognosis of feline haemoplasmosis

Antibiotics

Tetracyclines (e.g. doxycycline) and fluoroquinolones (e.g. marbofloxacin and pradofloxacin) are effective in the treatment of feline haemoplasma infection. These antibiotics improve clinical signs and haematological abnormalities, and reduce the number of haemoplasma organisms in the blood. However, consistent predictable elimination of haemoplasma infection has not yet been shown with any antibiotic treatment protocol. Different haemoplasma isolates, as well as different haemoplasma species, are believed to respond to antibiotic treatments differently.

Doxycycline (10 mg/kg/day orally) is the antibiotic of choice to treat feline haemoplasmosis, with longer treatment courses (up to 8 weeks) recommended by some to increase the chance of eliminating infection. Doxycycline appears to be effective against *M. haemofelis*, '*Candidatus* M. haemominutum' and '*Candidatus* M. turicensis', although controlled studies have only been published for *M. haemofelis*. Some doxycycline formulations (particularly the doxycycline hydrate form, which has high acidity) have been associated with oesophagitis and oesophageal strictures in cats, so the doxycycline dose should be followed by a small amount of food or syringing of water to encourage complete passage of tablets into the stomach.

Enrofloxacin (5 mg/kg orally q24h) has been used successfully to treat *M. haemofelis* infection in controlled studies, but diffuse retinal degeneration and acute blindness have been reported in some cats given enrofloxacin. Although this side effect is said to be rare, extreme caution must be taken with use of this drug in cats. Marbofloxacin was effective in the treatment of *M. haemofelis* and '*Candidatus* M. haemominutum' infection in controlled studies, using the recommended UK dose of 2 mg/kg orally q24h, although the fall in the number of '*Candidatus* M. haemominutum' organisms in the blood was less pronounced than that in *M. haemofelis* numbers. Marbofloxacin treatment has not been associated with ocular abnormalities in cats (Ishak *et al*., 2008). Pradofloxacin (5 mg/kg orally q24h) has also been shown to be effective for the treatment of *M. haemofelis* infection.

Supportive care

Cats with clinical haemoplasmosis are often dehydrated, so fluid therapy is an important component of treatment. Encouraging food intake and nutritional support is important in inappetent cats. Although cats often tolerate anaemia remarkably well, if the anaemia has developed acutely and/or is severe and accompanied by clinical signs, a blood transfusion or treatment with an oxygen-carrying haemoglobin compound such as Oxyglobin may be required (see Chapter 36).

Corticosteroids

Corticosteroids have been recommended as adjunctive therapy for the proposed immune-mediated haemolysis that may accompany haemoplasma infection. However, their value in treatment remains unproven. Clinically ill cats that are Coombs' positive usually respond to antibiotic treatment alone. It has also been shown that a cat that received methylprednisolone acetate prior to '*Candidatus* M. turicensis' infection developed a more severe anaemia than a cat that was not pretreated, so corticosteroids also have the potential to exacerbate haemoplasmosis. Prednisolone treatment (2–4 mg/kg/day orally) should therefore be reserved for use in cases in which immune-mediated haemolysis is believed to be a major component of the anaemia and/or in cases in which there is clinical deterioration despite appropriate antibiotic treatment for haemoplasmosis.

Monitoring response to treatment

In addition to seeing an improvement in clinical signs and haematological parameters, qPCR is a means of assessing the response to antibiotic therapy (Tasker, 2010). Cats can become PCR negative during effective antibiotic treatment (but it may take a number of days or even weeks for the haemoplasma levels to fall to below PCR detection limits) and may become PCR positive again when antibiotic treatment is stopped. Ideally repeat blood samples for qPCR should be collected a week or two after starting antibiotics to ensure that therapy is effective at lowering haemoplasma copy numbers. If efficacy is seen, therapy should be continued for up to 8 weeks, ideally with documentation of negative PCR results at the completion of treatment. A goal of any treatment protocol for haemoplasmosis should be to eliminate infection, although proving that infection has been eliminated is difficult. Repeated (monthly is suggested, two to three times) negative results on blood samples tested with a sensitive PCR assay are probably the most reliable means of demonstrating elimination. If negative results do not result from treatment, control of clinical signs and a reduction of copy numbers in the blood still indicate that treatment has been helpful. However recrudescence of disease remains possible in these cases as long as they remain haemoplasma positive.

Prognosis

The long-term prognosis of cats after recovery from uncomplicated haemoplasmosis appears to be good if a definitive diagnosis is made and effective therapy instigated quickly. Concurrent illness or disease may worsen the disease and/or slow recovery from infection. Chronic asymptomatic haemoplasma carrier cats remain at risk of recrudescence of disease although this is not believed to be common.

Canine haemoplasma species

Two haemoplasma species, *M. haemocanis* and '*Candidatus* Mycoplasma haematoparvum', have been described in dogs. Both species tend to induce haemolytic anaemia only in splenectomized dogs or those that are immunocompromised (e.g. by chemotherapy or immunosuppressive corticosteroid treatment). Immune-mediated haemolytic anaemia (IMHA) in association with *M. haemocanis* infection has been described recently in a splenectomized dog in the UK (Hulme-Moir *et al.*, 2010), but a survey of 37 UK dogs with primary IMHA did not reveal any underlying haemoplasma infection in any case (Warman *et al.*, 2010).

Recent work has evaluated the prevalence of canine haemoplasma infection in dog populations worldwide by PCR with prevalences of 0.5–45% and 0–33% reported for *M. haemocanis* and '*Candidatus* M. haematoparvum', respectively. Risk factors associated with canine haemoplasma infection include living in kennels, young age, being crossbred and mange infection (Novacco *et al.*, 2010). The proposed vector for transmission of the infection is the brown dog tick *Rhipicephalus sanguineus*. Little work has been done regarding canine haemoplasma carrier status but asymptomatic carrier dogs infected with '*Candidatus* M. haematoparvum' and *M. haemocanis* do exist.

The cytological appearance of canine haemoplasmas is similar to that of the feline organisms, although chains of organisms are more commonly seen with *M. haemocanis* (Figure 7.7). However, cytological examination is still insensitive for the diagnosis of canine haemoplasmosis, and diagnostic qPCR assays for the detection and quantification of both *M. haemocanis* and '*Candidatus* M. haematoparvum' in canine blood samples are now available.

Controlled studies of treatments for canine haemoplasmosis have not been published, but tetracyclines and fluoroquinolones have been reported to be effective in individual cases, although elimination of infection does not always result (Hulme-Moir *et al.*, 2010).

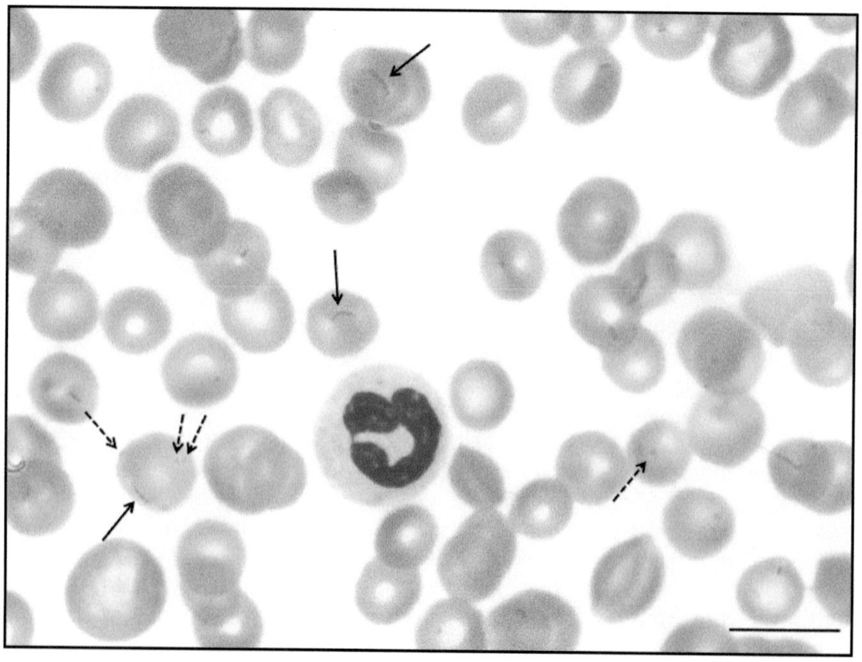

7.7 Blood smear (May–Grünwald's Giemsa stain) from a splenectomized dog with haemolytic anaemia associated with *M. haemocanis* infection. Bar = 10 µm. Dashed arrows indicate individual *M. haemocanis* organisms. Solid arrows indicate chains of *M. haemocanis* organisms on the surface of the red blood cells. (With kind permission of Lisa Hulme-Moir)

References and further reading

Hulme-Moir KL, Barker EN, Stonelake A *et al.* (2010) Use of real-time polymerase chain reaction to monitor antibiotic therapy in a dog with naturally acquired *Mycoplasma haemocanis* infection. *Journal of Veterinary Diagnostic Investigation* **22**, 582–587

Ishak AM, Dowers KL, Cavanaugh MT *et al.* (2008) Marbofloxacin for the treatment of experimentally induced *Mycoplasma haemofelis* infection in cats. *Journal of Veterinary Internal Medicine* **22**, 288–292

Museux K, Boretti FS, Willi B *et al.* (2009) *In vivo* transmission studies of '*Candidatus* Mycoplasma turicensis' in the domestic cat. *Veterinary Research* **40**, 45–59

Novacco M, Meli ML, Gentilini F *et al.* (2010) Prevalence and geographical distribution of canine hemotropic mycoplasma infections in Mediterranean countries and analysis of risk factors for infection. *Veterinary Microbiology* **142**, 276–284.

Peters IR, Helps CR, Willi B *et al.* (2008) The prevalence of three species of feline haemoplasmas in samples submitted to a diagnostic service as determined by three novel real-time duplex PCR assays. *Veterinary Microbiology* **126**, 142–150

Sykes JE, Drazenovich NL, Ball LM *et al.* (2007) Use of conventional and real-time polymerase chain reaction to determine the epidemiology of hemoplasma infections in anemic and nonanemic cats. *Journal of Veterinary Internal Medicine* **21**, 685–693

Tasker S (2010) Haemotropic mycoplasmas: what's the real significance in cats? *Journal of Feline Medicine and Surgery* **12**, 369–381

Tasker S, Peters IR, Papasouliotis K *et al.* (2009) Description of outcomes of experimental infection with feline haemoplasmas: copy numbers, haematology, Coombs' testing and blood glucose concentrations. *Veterinary Microbiology* **139**, 323–332

Warman SM, Helps CR, Barker EN *et al.* (2010) Haemoplasma infection is not a common cause of canine immune-mediated haemolytic anaemia in the UK. *Journal of Small Animal Practice* **51**, 534–539

Woods JE, Brewer MM, Hawley JR *et al.* (2005) Evaluation of experimental transmission of '*Candidatus* Mycoplasma haemominutum' and *Mycoplasma haemofelis* by *Ctenocephalides felis* to cats. *American Journal of Veterinary Research* **66**, 1008–1012

8

Babesiosis and cytauxzoonosis

Peter Irwin

Babesiosis

Introduction

Until recently most veterinary practitioners in the United Kingdom and other northern European countries would have considered the risk of transmitting haemoparasites by a blood transfusion to be remote. Unfortunately this risk is now very real; vector-borne diseases in general are on the rise as a consequence of expanding vector ranges and relaxed travel restrictions, and subclinical infection with these organisms is much more common than was previously recognized. Recent reviews of tick distribution in the UK indicate that potential tick vector species are present in focal geographical areas (http://data.nbn.org.uk) and a recent description of fatal babesiosis in an untravelled dog in the UK (Holm *et al.*, 2006) serves to remind us about the reality of vector-borne disease. Furthermore, widespread application of molecular tools for research and diagnosis has not only identified new species of *Babesia* and other related haemoprotozoans; there is now evidence that at least one species is transmitted from dog to dog by blood exchanged during fighting, without the need for a tick vector. When selecting a potential blood donor, therefore, it is imperative that the veterinary surgeon determines whether there is any history of travel or fighting, and screens the donor's blood carefully with a variety of diagnostic tests to ensure that they are free of infection.

Canine and feline piroplasm species, life cycle and transmission

The name 'piroplasm' is a collective term that describes large and small intra-erythrocytic protozoan parasites of the genera *Babesia*, *Theileria* and *Cytauxzoon*. Since the last edition of this book was published a number of new species have been described and the geographical ranges of these haemoparasites are continually revised, so any list is anticipated to become outdated in a relatively short time. Currently there are 11 piroplasm species reported in dogs and seven species in domestic cats worldwide (Figures 8.1 and 8.2). Some of these have been detected by molecular techniques (polymerase chain reaction; PCR) only and little is known about their clinical significance and natural biology in companion animals.

In Europe the predominant piroplasm species in dogs are *Babesia canis* and *Babesia vogeli*, with *Babesia gibsoni* and a *Babesia microti*-like organism (also referred to as *Theileria annae*) considered to be important emerging infections. Although molecular evidence for piroplasm infection in cats exists, to date there have been few clinical descriptions of babesiosis in cats living in Europe. Indeed, our understanding of feline piroplasms in general is more limited compared with those of dogs; *Cytauxzoon felis* in North America and *Babesia felis* in South Africa are the best described piroplasms in this species. The known geographical distributions of the piroplasms of dogs and cats are given in Figures 8.1 and 8.2.

Piroplasms (Figures 8.3 to 8.5) are tick-borne parasites; their life cycle in mammalian hosts and vectors is well understood for many species of *Babesia* and *Theileria*. Infective sporozoites are injected into the dog or cat in the tick's saliva as it feeds; they enter the host's bloodstream where, in the case of *Babesia* spp., they invade and multiply within erythrocytes during repeated phases of asexual reproduction, releasing merozoites that find and invade other erythrocytes. *Theileria* spp. have an exoerythrocytic stage in leucocytes where they undergo schizogony before infecting erythrocytes, as described previously for *Babesia*. Transmission back to a tick may occur at any time that a parasitaemia exists. After ingestion by the tick the piroplasms develop by sexual reproduction and maturation, eventually migrating to the cells of the tick's salivary glands in readiness for the next feeding or to its ovaries (in the case of *Babesia* only) for transovarial transmission to the next generation of ticks. As would be expected from this close biological relationship between piroplasm and haematophagous arthropod, the geographical distributions of canine and feline piroplasms generally reflect the ecological habitats of the vector tick species around the world (refer to occurrence maps at http://www.cvbd.org), and veterinary practitioners working in these areas are usually familiar with the clinical disease that they cause. Unfortunately, piroplasm infections may also develop in dogs and cats when least expected, in regions far from recognized tick habitats. Such infections arise for a variety of reasons; they may occur in pets that have travelled to or originated in endemic regions, or may be true autochthonous cases, reflecting the worrisome spread of the parasite into the local arthropod population where none existed previously. Wildlife reservoirs may also provide insight into the mode of

Size	Species	Synonyms	Vectors	Main geographical distribution	Comments
Small	*Babesia gibsoni*	*Babesia gibsoni* Asia strain	*Haemaphysalis longicornis*, *H. bispinosa*	Asia and sporadic occurrence worldwide	Outside Asia mainly associated with Pit Bull Terriers and other fighting dogs
	Babesia conradae	*B. gibsoni* (in original reports), Western piroplasm	Unknown	Western USA (California)	Genetic similarity with piroplasms isolated in humans and wildlife in western USA
	Babesia microti-like Spanish isolate/agent	*Theileria annae*	*Ixodes hexagonus* (putative)	Iberian peninsular (Spain and Portugal), Europe, USA	Red foxes are a wildlife reservoir and potentially the natural host
	Theileria spp.	Un-named *Theileria* spp., South African *Theileria* spp.	Unknown	South Africa	Molecular detection only
	Theileria annulata		Unknown	Africa, Europe, Asia	Molecular detection only
	Theileria equi	*Babesia equi*	Unknown	Africa, Europe, Asia	Molecular detection only
Large	*Babesia vogeli*	*Babesia canis vogeli*	*Rhipicephalus sanguineus*	Wide range: tropical, subtropical and Mediterranean regions	
	Babesia canis	*Babesia canis canis*	*Dermacentor* spp.	Europe	
	Babesia rossi	*Babesia canis rossi*	*Haemaphysalis elliptica* (formerly *H. leachi*)	Sub-Saharan Africa, South Africa	
	Babesia sp.	Un-named large *Babesia* sp., North Carolina isolate	Unknown	Eastern and southeastern USA	Genetic similarity with piroplasms isolated from cattle and horses
	Babesia sp.		Unknown	UK	Single report. Genetic similarity with *B. vogeli*

8.1 Piroplasm species of domestic dogs.

Size	Species	Synonyms	Vectors	Main geographical distribution	Comments
Small	*Cytauxzoon felis*		*Dermacentor variabilis*, *Amblyomma americanum*	Southern and eastern USA	Emerging disease
	Cytauxzoon spp.		Unknown	Reports from Europe, Asia and Africa	Molecular detection only
	Babesia felis		Unknown	Southern Africa	
	Babesia microti-like spp.	*Theileria annae*			Molecular detection only
Large	*Babesia presentii*		Unknown	Israel	
	Babesia cati		Unknown	India	
	Babesia canis canis			Spain and Portugal	Molecular detection only

8.2 Piroplasm species of domestic cats.

autochthonous infections in companion animals, and the recognition recently that the *Babesia microti*-like piroplasm (*T. annae*) is endemic in foxes in certain regions of the USA and Europe is a good example. It is these cases that pose a significant diagnostic challenge for the veterinary surgeon, when the all-important 'clinical suspicion' may be absent. This is a concern not only for dogs and cats with clinical illness, but is also a consideration for the selection of blood donors. Issues pertaining to the diagnosis of piroplasmosis are discussed in a later section.

While vector-borne transmission is the natural means by which most pets develop babesiosis, other routes of infection are theoretically possible and have been well documented. As noted above, piroplasms are readily transferred between mammalian hosts in blood products, whether deliberately as a means of initiating an experimental infection, or inadvertently by therapeutic blood transfusion (Stegeman *et al.*, 2003). Canine babesiosis has been reported in neonates, presumably as a result of transplacental transmission, but this seems to be a relatively unusual occurrence and is rarely of clinical significance.

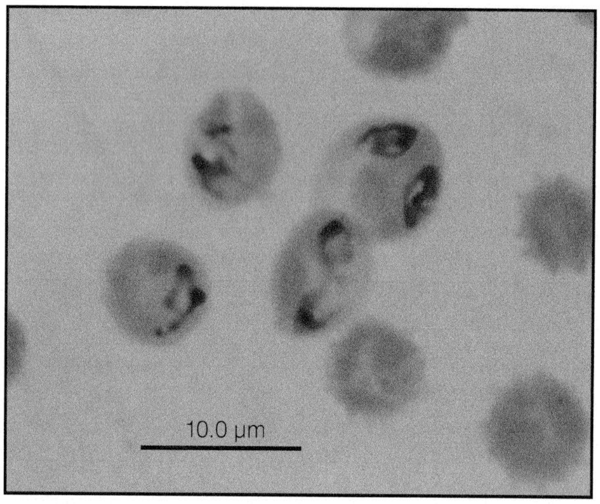

8.3 Large intra-erythrocytic piroplasms from a dog in northern Australia: *Babesia vogeli* (Giemsa stain).

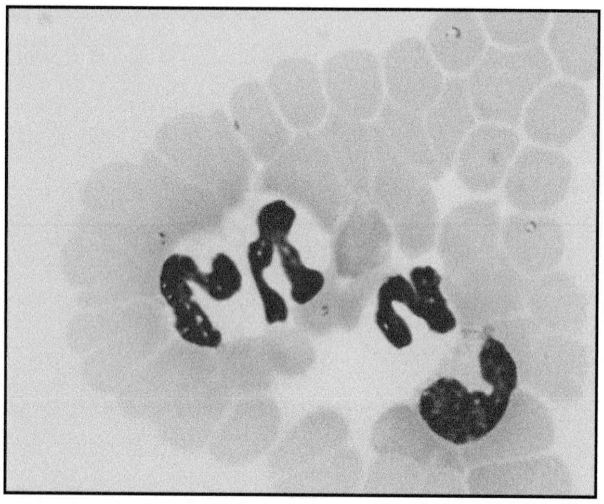

8.4 Small intra-erythrocytic piroplasms from a dog in Malaysia: *Babesia gibsoni* (Giemsa stain).

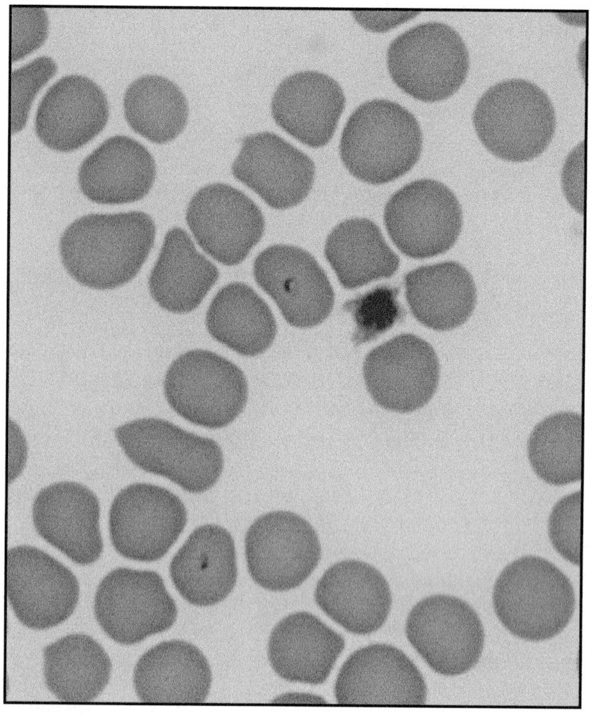

8.5 Small intra-erythrocytic piroplasms from a cat imported into Australia: *Babesia felis* (Giemsa stain).

Of epidemiological and clinical significance is the recognition that transmission of *Babesia gibsoni* during aggressive interactions by dogs fighting is the major route of infection for this species of piroplasm and is the reason for its expanding global distribution. It is best documented among breeds of dogs that are used for fighting, such as the American Pit Bull and Staffordshire Bull Terriers, and the Tosa Inu in Japan, yet transmission to other dog breeds after they have been bitten by members of these 'fighting breeds' has also been documented. It is presumed that the introduction of parasites occurs when blood from an infected dog enters the bite wound(s) of the recipient; there is no evidence that transmission occurs via the saliva from the infected dog.

Pathogenesis

The pathophysiological effects of piroplasmosis vary widely, yet some degree of haemolytic anaemia and thrombocytopenia is generally noted in all affected individuals at some stage after infection. The main determinant of pathogenesis seems to be the species of piroplasm responsible; it is generally accepted that the most pathogenic of the well recognized species in dogs is *Babesia rossi* in Africa, and *Cytauxzoon* infection in cats is also associated with a high mortality (see later). Small piroplasms such as *B. gibsoni*, *B. conradae*, the *Babesia microti*-like agent (*Theileria annae*) and *B. canis* (sensu strictu) show moderate to severe virulence in dogs, while *Babesia vogeli* and the recently described large *Babesia* in North America are the least pathogenic in terms of their ability to cause haemolysis. Such generalizations should be viewed with caution however, because other factors such as the age and immune status of the host, and the presence of concurrent infections, will influence pathogenicity in an individual. As an example, *Babesia vogeli* infection in adult dogs is frequently asymptomatic and results in only mild to moderate thrombocytopenia, yet natural infection of puppies less than 12 weeks old with this species is often fatal (Irwin and Hutchinson, 1991). To date, the un-named *Babesia* sp. from North America has been reported predominantly in splenectomized dogs, which suggests that immunocompromise is required to permit patent infection and illness with this species (Sikorski *et al.*, 2010).

Babesiosis is often referred to as being 'complicated' or 'uncomplicated' in terms of its pathogenesis. Uncomplicated babesiosis is generally associated with mild to moderate anaemia, causing pallor, weakness, icterus and fever, and varying degrees of pigmenturia (haemoglobinuria and bilirubinuria). Complicated babesiosis refers to pathological manifestations that cannot be readily explained as a consequence of haemolysis alone and is characterized by dysfunction of one or more organs and a high mortality. This type of babesiosis has been studied extensively in South Africa in association with *Babesia rossi* infection, but has also been reported in association with serious *Babesia canis* infections in Europe (Matijatko *et al.*, 2009).

Primary parasite-induced intravascular and extravascular haemolysis occurs as a result of increased osmotic fragility and oxidative injury of infected cells, but secondary immune-mediated mechanisms are thought to be responsible for the majority of clinical manifestations within the haematological system and more widespread changes in other organs such as the kidney, liver and central nervous system (CNS). Hypoxaemia, haemoglobinuric nephropathy and glomerulonephritis caused by piroplasmosis may result in renal failure, and azotaemia has been identified as a risk factor and predictor of mortality in dogs infected with a *Babesia microti*-like agent in northern Spain (Camacho *et al.*, 2004).

Clinical and laboratory manifestations

In addition to the complicated and uncomplicated presentations referred to in the previous section, babesiosis is recognized clinically as acute or chronic. New infections lead to an acute (or sometimes 'per acute') phase with clinical signs that range in severity from mild anaemia and/or thrombocytopenia through to severe haemolysis, widespread organ failure and death. However, depending upon the species of piroplasm and various host factors, it is possible that some infections may go unnoticed by the owner, or are so mild or non-specific as to avoid presentation for veterinary examination.

Typical laboratory abnormalities in acute babesiosis include a regenerative anaemia and normal serum total protein, consistent with haemolysis, and thrombocytopenia. In some cases a normochromic, normocytic anaemia is observed and may reflect preregenerative disease or chronic infection with less pathogenic piroplasms. Serum biochemistry findings are non-specific but may include mild to moderate elevations in alanine transaminase (ALT), aspartate transaminase (AST) and alkaline phosphatase (ALP) activities, and hyperbilirubinaemia. Azotaemia is common but may be prerenal in origin; urine analysis, specifically urine specific gravity (USG), is required to determine whether there is renal insufficiency.

A chronic phase of infection develops in most cases regardless of whether or not treatment is given. It is important to stress again that such infections may be asymptomatic; the dog or cat may act as a carrier of the organism, and the infection may or may not recrudesce at times of stress or immunosuppression (such as chemotherapy or splenectomy). This is pertinent to the selection of blood donors, because these individuals will be healthy in all outward respects (see later). Furthermore, splenectomy of dogs (or cats) that live in endemic regions poses a risk for the development of more severe babesiosis due to parasite recrudescence or a new infection. Complicated babesiosis has been associated with severe neurological dysfunction (e.g. stupor, coma and seizures), bleeding diatheses (petechial and ecchymotic haemorrhages), respiratory failure (pulmonary oedema) and weakness (hypotension, acid–base disturbances and acute renal failure).

Diagnosis of babesiosis

The approach to a diagnosis of babesiosis, or piroplasmosis, is governed largely by the clinical situation and the resources available. On the one hand babesiosis may be considered as a differential diagnosis in a dog or cat with one or more of the clinical signs or laboratory abnormalities described above. Alternatively the diagnostic question might arise when the veterinary surgeon needs to select a blood donor that is free of infection. In both situations it is worth reflecting on the fact that animals infected with *Babesia* spp. (or other piroplasms) are quite likely to be co-infected with other tick-borne pathogens such as *Ehrlichia* spp., *Anaplasma* spp. (Chapters 18, 19) or *Bartonella* spp. A history of tick exposure (living in or previous travel to a tick-endemic area) or recent injury from a dog fight should all prompt a specific investigation for babesiosis.

Dogs and cats with clinical signs consistent with babesiosis, and those with anaemia and/or thrombocytopenia, should receive a haematological evaluation that must include a careful microscopic search for intra-erythrocytic inclusions. When acute babesiosis is suspected, a microscopic examination of a blood smear remains the simplest and most accessible diagnostic test. In acute disease microscopy is reasonably sensitive for detecting intra-erythrocytic piroplasms, providing that the blood smears are well prepared and the veterinary surgeon is practised at performing a haematological examination. Parasites must be differentiated from artefact and cell or stain debris, and reference to images of piroplasms is useful in order to avoid over-diagnosis (see Figures 8.3 to 8.5). Visualization of one or more piroplasms is sufficient to warrant specific treatment in most cases (see later) but the true identity (or genotype) of the organism cannot be determined by morphology alone; this requires molecular tools such as PCR and sequence analysis. Failure to visualize red cell parasites, however, does not exclude a diagnosis of piroplasmosis and if no other cause for the haematological changes is found then samples (EDTA and serum) should be submitted to a commercial laboratory for piroplasm PCR and serological testing respectively.

Molecular testing is useful to confirm the diagnosis in acute babesiosis, but a combination of serology and PCR is absolutely mandatory for the detection of chronic infections in (carrier) dogs and cats, because in these cases the parasitaemia will be too low for a reliable microscopic diagnosis. When selecting blood donors, the current recommendation is to screen suspected cases or blood donors initially by serology and subsequently to test seronegative dogs with an appropriate piroplasm PCR (Wardrop *et al.*, 2005; Wang *et al.*, 2010).

Serological testing

The immunofluorescent antibody test (IFAT) is the

principal serological test that is available on a commercial basis; most dogs develop antibodies within 7–10 days of infection. However cross-reactions between different piroplasm species have resulted in reduced specificity, and antibodies to some of the more recently described piroplasms may not be detected by conventional IFAT assays, resulting in reduced sensitivity and the potential to overlook infection if only serology is used. In addition, validated IFAT testing for canine babesiosis is offered by only relatively few laboratories around the world.

To date, bench-top enzyme-linked immunosorbent assay (ELISA)-based colorimetric tests for in-clinic diagnosis of babesiosis are not available commercially, as they are for some of the other vector-borne diseases (e.g. canine monocytic ehrlichiosis or anaplasmosis). The development of such assays is currently of research interest, and suitable tests, based on the production of recombinant immunodominant proteins, may become available in the future.

Molecular diagnosis

The PCR has revolutionized the diagnosis of infectious and parasitic organisms, especially those that are either too small to visualize readily or are present in such low numbers as to be beyond the detection limits of conventional methods. Veterinary surgeons should be aware, however, that PCR testing has its limitations and should ensure that their diagnostic laboratory uses validated methodology and appropriate controls with every reaction. Amplicon sequencing is also recommended in order to be certain of identity of a positive isolate. In chronic infections the parasitaemia is generally very low; in fact piroplasms may be present in such low numbers in the blood (or at times, not at all) that their DNA is beyond the detection limits of the PCR. In this situation it may be possible to get a false negative result. The second major limitation of molecular testing pertains to the design of the primers used in the PCR. Primers designed to amplify the DNA of specific piroplasm species may fail to amplify others. Primer design is therefore critical and the veterinary surgeon should enquire whether the laboratory they send samples to for testing uses a PCR that is likely to detect all known species, not only those that have been reported previously in the local region or country.

Therapy and prevention

Both specific and supportive treatment protocols have been developed for the management of dogs and cats with piroplasmosis (Figure 8.6). Although many drugs have been developed over the years, there is little scientifically robust evidence regarding the efficacy of any of them. Babesiosis is a frustrating disease to manage because most, if not all, dogs and cats treated with specific anti-piroplasm drugs are unlikely to be cured of their infection, and

Host	Morphology or *Babesia sp.*	Drug	Recommended dose and frequency	Notes/comments
Dog	Large (*B. canis*)	Imidocarb (dipropionate and dihydrochloride)	5–7 mg/kg s.c. or i.m., repeat in 14 days	Pain at site of injection; nodule may develop at site of injection. Cholinergic signs (vomiting, diarrhoea) controlled with atropine (0.05 mg/kg s.c.)
		Trypan blue	10 mg/kg i.v. once	Tissue irritant, use as 1% solution. Reversible staining of body tissues occurs
	Large and small	Phenamidine (isethionate)	15 mg/kg s.c., once or repeat q24h	Nausea, vomiting and CNS signs are common side effects
		Pentamidine (isethionate)	16.5 mg/kg i.m., repeat q24h	Nausea, vomiting and CNS signs are common side effects
		Diminazine aceturate	3.5 mg/kg i.m., once	Unpredictable and idiosyncratic toxicity; CNS signs may be severe. Some preparations contain antipyrone
	Small (*B. gibsoni*)	Parvaquone	20 mg/kg s.c., once	
		Atovaquone + azithromycin	13.3 mg/kg orally q8h for 10 days atovaquone + 10 mg/kg orally q24h for 10 days azithromycin	Absorption of atovaquone is improved if given with food. Safe, with rapid removal of piroplasms from blood. Resistance reported
		Clindamycin	25 mg/kg q12h orally	Causes morphological changes to piroplasms, efficacy uncertain
		Clindamycin + metronidazole + doxycycline	25 mg/kg q12h orally clindamycin + 15 mg/kg orally q12h metronidazole + 5 mg/kg orally q12h doxycycline	Uncertain efficacy
Cat	*B. felis*	Primaquine (phosphate)	0.5 mg/kg orally, once	
	C. felis	Imidocarb dipropionate	6 mg/kg i.m., repeat in 14 days	Uncertain efficacy

8.6 Management of piroplasmosis. CNS, central nervous system; i.m., intramuscular; i.v., intravenous; s.c., subcutaneous.

it would be most unwise to assume that treatment of an intended blood donor, for example, would clear a *Babesia* infection. A dog or cat in which infection has been confirmed should be regarded as potentially infected for life, despite specific treatment and remission of clinical signs.

Dogs and cats with tick burdens should be treated immediately upon entry to the clinic with a rapid 'knock-down' acaricide (e.g. fipronil) and individual ticks should be removed and destroyed whenever possible. These precautions reduce the risk of ticks contaminating the ward environment; this can become a significant hygiene issue that increases the risk of nosocomial vector-borne infection and that requires proactive cleaning and disinfection (with acaricidal agents) of all areas where patients are hospitalized.

Supportive treatment for piroplasmosis

Supportive treatment is aimed at restoring adequate tissue oxygenation by correction of the anaemia, especially if this is severe, and managing dehydration and any electrolyte disturbances. One or more blood transfusions are indicated to restore and maintain the packed cell volume (PCV) at a normal value; details of how much blood to give and other considerations regarding transfusion protocols can be found elsewhere in this book. As with all anaemic animals, fluid therapy should be used judiciously and is indicated primarily if the patient is also dehydrated or anorexic. Oxygen therapy in anaemic patients is of questionable benefit unless concurrent lung pathology is affecting respiratory function and oxygen exchange. Good nursing support (e.g. warmth, nutrition) should also be provided.

Anti-piroplasm treatment

Specific treatments for piroplasmosis and their dose regimes are listed in Figure 8.6. At the very least, the general morphology of the piroplasm infection should be determined to provide a guide to appropriate drug choice (Figure 8.6). In dogs the large *Babesia* spp. are treated with imidocarb dipropionate or diminazine aceturate. Diminazine or the atovaquone and azithromycin combination therapy is used to treat small piroplasm infections and *Babesia gibsoni* in particular. There is even less reliable information pertaining to the treatment of feline babesiosis; in South Africa where this disease is most prevalent (caused by *B. felis*), affected cats are treated primarily with primaquine. Many of the drugs listed in Figure 8.6 result in a reduction of parasitaemia and amelioration of clinical signs, but recrudescence, relapse and/or re-infection are frequently reported by practitioners in endemic regions, leading to speculation about drug resistance and raising questions about efficacy. To date, only atovaquone has been confirmed experimentally to induce drug resistance by causing a mutation of the *cytochrome b* gene in isolates of *Babesia gibsoni*.

Prevention of babesiosis

It used to be thought that if a dog (or cat) could be simply kept free of tick exposure then there would be no risk of developing babesiosis. However, the recognition that *B. gibsoni* is transmitted through bite wounds has changed this thinking, and although dog fighting is banned in most countries, for some breeds this activity is clearly a significant risk factor for babesiosis and illegal dog fighting still occurs in many locations. Nevertheless, in tick-endemic regions especially, regular and systematic application of acaricidal agents, together with daily tick searches, is recommended to reduce the risk of a dog contracting babesiosis. Ectoparasiticides that contain repellent compounds, such as permethrin, are recommended because they prevent the ticks from attaching.

Vaccines are available in some countries to protect dogs against certain types of piroplasm (*B. canis* and *B. rossi* for example). While these show reasonable efficacy and may ameliorate the disease, complete protection is not achieved.

Cytauxzoonosis

Introduction

Cytauxzoon felis is a tick-borne protozoan parasite of domestic and wild felids that is reported predominantly throughout the south-central and southeastern United States, but with recent reports extending its range further in a north-easterly direction (see Figure 8.2). Its natural host is the North American bobcat (*Lynx rufus*), but domestic cats become infected when they are bitten by *Dermacentor variabilis* or (as recently demonstrated by experimental transmission studies) by *Amblyomma americanum* ticks, typically in the summer months. Clinical signs in cats include fever, anorexia, listlessness, icterus, dyspnoea and collapse. Cytauxzoonosis is considered to be a serious disease in the USA and most affected individuals are presented to the veterinary surgeon in a moribund state. However, although cytauxzoonosis is generally associated with a high mortality and guarded prognosis there have been recent reports of subclinical cases, suggesting that asymptomatic parasitaemic carriers exist and that the infection is not always fatal (Brown *et al.*, 2008). This suggests that a carrier cat could pose a risk of transmission if selected as a blood donor.

Life cycle and pathogenesis

Cytauxzoon felis is the only piroplasm of companion animals to have a confirmed exoerythrocytic life cycle stage. Sporozoites injected into the feline host during tick feeding quickly invade mononuclear phagocytes throughout the body and undergo schizogeny, a process that results in the development of large, morphologically distinct schizonts that may be observed in fine needle aspirates of organs such as the spleen, liver or lung. Merozoites are released from these schizonts in large numbers and invade erythrocytes, resulting in high parasitaemias in acute disease in some individuals (Figure 8.7).

The pathogenesis of cytauxzoonosis is attributed to the schizogenous phase that causes mechanical obstruction to the blood flow through various organs, notably the lungs, and results in a shock-like state.

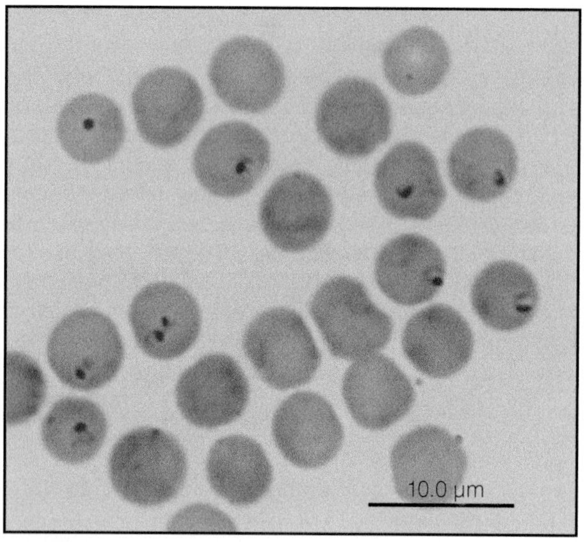

8.7 *Cytauxzoon felis* piroplasms in a peripheral blood film (Giemsa stain). (Specimen kindly provided by Dr J Meinkoth)

Vascular occlusion and damage is associated further with the release of inflammatory mediators and the development of disseminated intravascular coagulation (DIC). Intravascular and extravascular haemolysis both occur as a result of invasion of erythrocytes by merozoites.

Diagnosis of cytauxzoonosis

Similar to the other piroplasm infections described previously, the diagnosis of cytauxzoonosis is made during acute infections by examination of a blood smear. The parasitaemia is variable but in most cases the intraerythrocytic piroplasms are readily observed in Giemsa-stained blood smears (Figure 8.7). *Cytauxzoon felis* appears in a number of morphological varieties including the signet-ring form, bipolar oval forms, tetrads and dark-staining 'dots', the latter of which may be mistaken for feline haemotropic *Mycoplasma* spp. ('haemobartonellosis'; see Chapter 7). Stain precipitate is also easily mistaken for *C. felis* organisms by less experienced microscopists. A unique, yet uncommon, finding in cytauxzoonosis is the appearance of tissue phase schizonts in blood smears and buffy coat preparations. As noted above, however, these forms are best demonstrated in impression smears from bone marrow, spleen or lymph nodes, where they are typically numerous.

Haematology and serum biochemistry abnormalities are typical of haemolytic anaemia. Initially the anaemia is pre-regenerative (normochromic and normocytic), but it progresses to a strong regenerative response, characterized by the presence of nucleated red cells by the time of death. Moderate to severe leucopenia is typical and thrombocytopenia, sometimes profound, is commonly reported with or without DIC. Prolongation of clotting times (prothrombin time (PT) and activated partial thromboplastin time (aPTT)) has been recorded and has been used to support a diagnosis of DIC. Icteric plasma is noted several days after infection, and other non-specific clinicopathological changes that have been recorded include hyperglycaemia, hypokalaemia, hypocholesterolaemia and elevations in serum ALT and ALP.

Currently there is no serological test available commercially for cytauxzoonosis, however highly sensitive and specific PCR tests are available at certain diagnostic and research laboratories in the USA.

Treatment of cytauxzoonosis

The management of seriously ill cats with cytauxzoonosis poses significant challenges for the veterinary surgeon. Currently there is no widely accepted treatment regime, apart from the provision of proactive supportive care aimed at minimizing the systemic haemolytic, inflammatory and coagulation disturbances; isotonic fluid therapy, blood transfusions, and heparinization are widely used. However, there is little scientifically robust evidence that any of the antimicrobial drugs that have been described to treat cytauxzoonosis are specifically efficacious. Enrofloxacin and tetracyclines (doxycycline) appear to be widely used, often in conjunction with imidocarb dipropionate (see Figure 8.6), yet the use of clindamycin, penicillin and diminazine has also been reported.

References and further reading

Brown HM, Latimer KS, Erikson LE *et al.* (2008) Detection of persistent *Cytauxzoon felis* infection by polymerase chain reaction in three asymptomatic domestic cats. *Journal of Veterinary Diagnostic Investigation* **20**, 485–488

Camacho AT, Guitian FJ, Pallas E *et al.* (2004) Azotaemia and mortality among *Babesia microti*-like infected dogs. *Journal of Veterinary Internal Medicine* **18**, 141–146

Holm LP, Kerr MG, Trees AJ *et al.* (2006) Fatal babesiosis in an untravelled British dog. *Veterinary Record* **159**, 179–180

Irwin PJ and Hutchinson GW (1991) Clinical and pathological findings of *Babesia* infection in dogs. *Australian Veterinary Journal* **68**, 204–209

Matijatko V, Kiš I, Torti M *et al.* (2009) Septic shock in canine babesiosis. *Veterinary Parasitology* **162**, 263–70

Sikorski LE, Birkenheuer AJ, Holowaychuk MK *et al.* (2010) Babesiosis caused by a large *Babesia* species in 7 immunocompromised dogs. *Journal of Veterinary Internal Medicine* **24**, 127–131

Stegeman JR, Birkenheuer AJ, Kruger JM and Breitschwerdt EB (2003) Transfusion-associated *Babesia gibsoni* infection in a dog. *Journal of the American Veterinary Medical Association* **222**, 959–963

Wang C, Ahluwalia SK, Li Y *et al.* (2010) Frequency and therapy monitoring of canine *Babesia* spp. infection by high-resolution melting curve quantitative FRET-PCR. *Veterinary Parasitology* **168**, 11–18

Wardrop KJ, Reine N, Birkenheuer A *et al.* (2005) Canine and feline blood donor screening for infectious disease. *Journal of Veterinary Internal Medicine* **19**, 135–42

9

Non-regenerative anaemia

Jed A. Overmann and Douglas J. Weiss

Introduction

Non-regenerative anaemias lack peripheral indicators of a bone marrow response. As discussed in Chapter 3, the non-regenerative nature of an anaemia is recognized by evaluation of the absolute reticulocyte count and/or the degree of polychromasia present in peripheral blood. In cases of non-regenerative anaemia, these two measures remain persistently low or within reference intervals and do not increase as would be expected if the bone marrow was responding to the anaemia. In general, non-regenerative anaemias result from reduced or ineffective erythropoiesis; however, identification of a specific underlying cause is important, because the prognosis and treatment will depend on the underlying pathogenesis. Non-regenerative anaemias are a common laboratory finding in ill animals, and being aware of the causes and their diagnostic features is important for quality patient care.

Anaemia of inflammation and neoplasia

This is the most frequent cause of a mild to moderate non-regenerative anaemia in dogs and cats (see Chapter 11).

Anaemia of chronic renal disease

Non-regenerative anaemia is a frequent finding in dogs and cats with chronic renal disease, often correlating with the severity of renal failure (see Chapter 10).

Aplastic anaemia

Aplastic anaemia (also called aplastic pancytopenia) is characterized by marked depletion of haemopoietic cells in the bone marrow and replacement of these cells by adipose tissue. This condition results primarily from damage to early haemopoietic precursors or haemopoietic stem cells in bone marrow. Other factors that may contribute are damage to the bone marrow microenvironment and altered cytokine production. Causes of aplastic anaemia include infectious agents (e.g. *Ehrlichia canis* and parvovirus), drugs, toxins, immune-mediated mechanisms, and exposure to radiation. Many cases, however, are classified as idiopathic, with no clear underlying cause. Animals present with bi- or pancytopenia, which in many cases reflects the time course of the condition. In more acute cases, neutrophil and platelet numbers will decline first, while the haematocrit (Hct) remains within reference intervals, a result of the relatively long circulating lifespan of erythrocytes. Chronic cases of aplastic anaemia present with pancytopenia. Typical cases have a moderate to severe, normocytic, normochromic, non-regenerative anaemia, neutropenia and thrombocytopenia. Patients present with clinical signs and physical examination findings consistent with anaemia (e.g. lethargy, exercise intolerance and pale mucous membranes), and in some cases additional clinical signs associated with decreased leucocytes (e.g. fever) and platelets (e.g. petechiae and epistaxis).

Idiopathic aplastic anaemia

Idiopathic aplastic anaemia is a common cause of aplastic anaemia in the dog and is also seen relatively frequently in the cat (Weiss, 2006a,b). The onset of disease is usually chronic in nature. Animals tend to be young to middle aged with no clear sex or breed predilection. The diagnosis is based on the complete blood count (CBC) and the results of bone marrow aspirate and biopsy, in addition to ruling out other causes of aplastic anaemia. As described previously, bone marrow biopsy reveals a severe generalized hypoplasia to aplasia of haemopoietic precursors, along with replacement of the cells by adipocytes (Figure 9.1). An immune-mediated basis for this condition has not been established, but neither has it been excluded. Treatment generally consists of supportive care such as transfusions of blood and platelets, along with broad-spectrum antibiotic therapy. Immunosuppressive therapy (e.g. steroidal, non-steroidal and combinations thereof) has been used, but a response to immunosuppressive therapy has not been clearly established. The prognosis for these patients is generally considered guarded to poor, but some animals experience full haematological recovery.

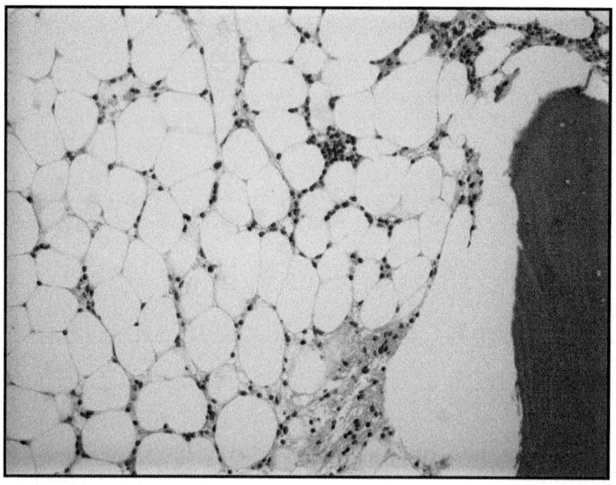

9.1 Histological section of bone marrow from a dog with aplastic anaemia. The few cells remaining are primarily small lymphocytes.

Infectious causes of aplastic anaemia

Infectious organisms cause non-regenerative anaemia through various mechanisms. Most have the potential to induce the anaemia of inflammatory disease (Chapter 11); however, some can also have direct pathological effects on the bone marrow that contribute to a non-regenerative anaemia and potentially other cytopenias. Some organisms (e.g. parvovirus, *Histoplasma* spp., *Leishmania* spp.) invade bone marrow directly and suppress or destroy haemopoietic precursors. Others (e.g. bacteria) can induce an inflammatory response indirectly through the release of toxins.

Viral infection

Parvoviral infections are known to cause bone marrow injury and hypoplasia. Both feline panleucopenia virus and canine parvovirus infect rapidly dividing haemopoietic precursors. In cats, there is an association between feline leukaemia virus (FeLV) infection and non-regenerative anaemia/ aplastic anaemia (Chapter 17).

Rickettsial infection

Some dogs with chronic *Ehrlichia canis* infection develop aplastic anaemia (Chapter 18).

Bacterial infection

Bacterial infection and sepsis can lead to pathological changes in the bone marrow as a result of acute inflammation. Given that various pathological changes are present in the bone marrow, these conditions are not classified as aplastic anaemia. However, if the condition persists, the marrow may appear aplastic after resolution of the acute lesions. Bacteria can invade bone marrow directly, resulting in microabscesses. More frequently these changes consist of bacterial toxin-induced microvascular injury, which results in haemorrhage, oedema, fibrin deposition and variable infiltrates of neutrophils. Localized or diffuse bone marrow ischaemia can follow, leading to areas of myelonecrosis.

Fungal infection

Systemic fungal diseases (e.g. histoplasmosis, blastomycosis, cryptococcocis and coccidioidomycosis) can infiltrate bone and/or marrow. *Histoplasma capsulatum*, in particular, is known to infect bone marrow (Figure 9.2). Organisms can be identified on smears made from bone marrow aspirates and are frequently accompanied by various degrees of granulomatous inflammation.

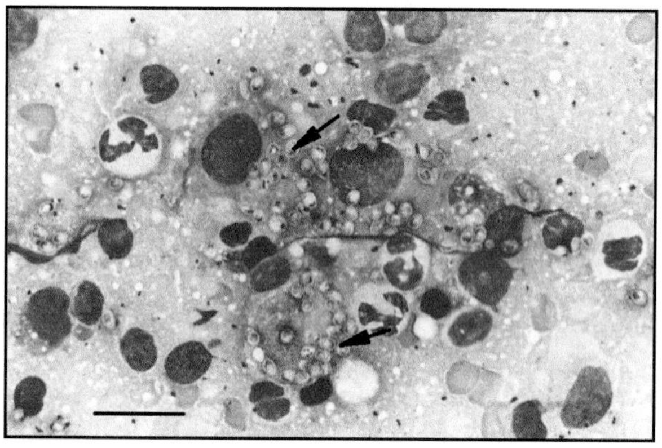

9.2 Bone marrow aspirate from a dog showing macrophages containing *Histoplasma capsulatum* organisms (arrows). Bar, 20 μm.

Protozoal infection

Non-regenerative anaemia and thrombocytopenia are common findings in dogs infected with *Leishmania* spp. Aspirates of bone marrow or lymph nodes can be diagnostic of infection because they often reveal the presence of *Leishmania* spp. amastigotes (Chapter 20). Bone marrow aspirates also typically contain large numbers of macrophages.

Drug-related causes of aplastic anaemia

A variety of drugs have been implicated as a cause of aplastic anaemia and generalized bone marrow toxicity in the dog and cat (Figure 9.3). Primary mechanisms causing bone marrow pathology include direct damage to mitotically active cells and immune-mediated damage to early haemopoietic precursors. Drugs listed here have been associated with either chronic aplastic anaemia or bone marrow toxicity/necrosis. While the latter may not necessarily represent a true aplastic anaemia as defined by characteristic bone marrow alterations, drugs that cause bone marrow toxicity or necrosis are considered here as a potential cause of multiple cytopenias, including a non-regenerative anaemia. The therapy for these patients consists of discontinuation of the drug along with supportive care.

Chemotherapeutics

Chemotherapeutic drugs are known to suppress haemopoiesis, often in a dose-dependent fashion, as a result of targeting rapidly dividing haemopoietic precursors in the bone marrow. Because this is an acute insult to the bone marrow, cytopenias develop in a sequential fashion after initiation of treatment, with neutropenia appearing within 5 days

Drug class	Drugs	Species	Suspected mechanism
Antineoplastics	Class effect	Dog, cat	MS, D, N
Endocrine drugs	Oestrogen	Dog	MS
Anti-inflammatory agents	Phenylbutazone	Dog, cat	MS, IM
	Azathioprine	Dog, cat	MS
	Carprofen	Dog	N
Antimicrobials	Cephalosporins	Dog	IM, MS, D
	Sulphonamides	Dog	IM, MS
	Metronidazole	Dog	MS, N
Anticonvulsants	Phenobarbital	Dog	MS, N
Anti-parasitics	Levamisole	Dog	MS
	Albendazole	Dog, cat	MS
	Fenbendazole	Dog	MS, N

9.3 Drugs suspected of causing or confirmed to cause non-regenerative anaemia, bi- or pancytopenia. D, dysmyelopoiesis; IM, immune-mediated blood cell destruction; MS, bone marrow suppression; N, bone marrow necrosis.

to a week, followed by thrombocytopenia within 2 weeks. Anaemia caused by bone marrow suppression is not evident, owing to the relatively long lifespan of erythrocytes; however, some patients may be anaemic for other reasons such as a concurrent anaemia of inflammation or blood loss. Neutropenia and thrombocytopenia frequently resolve within 3–4 days after cessation of therapy.

Oestrogen

Oestrogen-induced bone marrow suppression in the dog can be seen secondary to administration of therapeutic doses of oestradiol or diethylstilboestrol, or as the result of increased endogenous levels of oestrogen (e.g. Sertoli cell tumour or ovarian granulosa cell tumour) (Sontas *et al.*, 2009). The mechanism probably involves haemopoietic stem cell destruction, but is poorly characterized. Bone marrow suppression secondary to oestrogen therapy occurs in a dose-dependent manner and is typically reversible, however some dogs exhibit an idiosyncratic reaction characterized by extreme sensitivity to oestrogens. Dogs with increased sensitivity to oestrogens, those receiving repeated therapeutic doses, or those with increased endogenous sources may develop severe aplastic anaemia. The prognosis for these dogs is poor, but recovery has been documented in some patients after prolonged symptomatic therapy. Treatment includes removal of the oestrogen source along with supportive care such as blood and platelet transfusions, and broad-spectrum antibiotic therapy.

Anti-inflammatory drugs

Phenylbutazone (dog) and azathioprine (dog, cat) therapy have both been associated with aplastic anaemia in some animals. Phenylbutazone therapy has been associated with transient agranulocytosis (presumably immune mediated), aplastic anaemia, and bone marrow necrosis and myelofibrosis. Cats may be especially susceptible to azathioprine-induced bone marrow aplasia (Beale *et al.,* 1992). Severe myelonecrosis leading to cytopenias has been described in some dogs treated with carprofen (Weiss, 2006b). Reported cases have recovered after discontinuation of the treatment.

Antimicrobials

Multiple cytopenias or aplastic anaemia have been associated with the use of antimicrobial sulphonamides (e.g. trimethoprim/sulfadiazine) and cephalosporins (e.g. cefonicid, cefazedone) in the dog, and may be due to an immune-mediated mechanism (Bloom *et al.*, 1988; Trepanier, 2004). Sulphonamides induce both an idiosyncratic syndrome (neutropenia, thrombocytopenia, haemolytic anaemia, fever, polyarthropathy or hepatopathy) and aplastic anaemia. Dobermanns may be at increased risk of sulphonamide hypersensitivity. The mechanism for the idiosyncratic syndrome appears to be immune mediated and does not appear to be related to folate deficiency. Evidence of an immune-mediated aetiology includes demonstration of drug-dependent anti-platelet antibodies and a positive direct Coombs' test (Giger *et al.* 1985). In dogs with sulfadiazine-induced aplastic anaemia, pancytopenia usually occurs 10–14 days after initiation of treatment. The bone marrow is typically aplastic with the haemopoietic space replaced by adipose tissue. The haematological dyscrasia usually resolves within 2 weeks of discontinuing treatment. Bone marrow necrosis leading to pancytopenia has been reported in dogs receiving metronidazole (Weiss, 2006b).

Anticonvulsants

Phenobarbital therapy has been associated with several types of haematological dyscrasia in dogs. The mildest haematological disorder is neutropenia and thrombocytopenia. The presence of granulocyte hyperplasia in the bone marrow indicates that the neutropenia is due to destruction of mature granulocytes. A more frequent adverse drug reaction is bone marrow necrosis or myelofibrosis. Dogs with bone marrow necrosis are frequently bicytopenic or pancytopenic. The bone marrow is characterized by multifocal areas of coagulation-type necrosis with variable degrees of myelofibrosis (Weiss and Smith, 2002). Bone marrow necrosis leading to pancytopenia has been reported in dogs receiving metronidazole (Weiss, 2006b). Dogs with myelofibrosis, without concurrent necrosis, frequently have a severe non-regenerative anaemia. The myelofibrosis may represent the chronic stage of bone marrow necrosis.

Antiparasitic drugs

Albendazole (dog and cat) and fenbendazole (dog) appear to cause idiosyncratic reactions in some animals, resulting in either aplastic anaemia or bone marrow toxicity leading to pancytopenia (Stokol *et al.*, 1997; Weiss, 2006b).

Non-regenerative immune-mediated haemolytic anaemia

Immune-mediated haemolytic anaemia (IMHA) is frequently associated with a regenerative bone marrow erythroid response; however, a significant percentage of dogs and cats with IMHA will present with non-regenerative anaemia (Stokol *et al.*, 2000; Kohn *et al.*, 2006; Weiss, 2008). It is possible that some of these animals are experiencing a peracute immune-mediated haemolytic process, in which the 3–4 days necessary to develop a regenerative response (i.e. reticulocytosis) has not elapsed. However, in many animals, the non-regenerative nature of the anaemia persists (i.e. > 5 days), indicating a failed bone marrow response. Interestingly, bone marrow evaluation in these animals often reveals erythroid hyperplasia. Failure to develop reticulocytosis is attributed to immune-mediated destruction of erythrocyte precursors, as well as pathological events in the bone marrow resulting in ineffective erythropoiesis. In some patients this immune-mediated destruction of erythroid precursors is clearly evident in bone marrow aspirates and biopsy specimens as a maturation arrest. In a maturation arrest, erythrocyte precursors develop normally up to a certain stage and are then targeted by antibodies and destroyed. A maturation arrest is not always evident, which suggests that additional factors may contribute to the non-regenerative nature of the anaemia in some patients with non-regenerative IMHA. Bone marrow pathology in dogs and cats with non-regenerative IMHA has been described recently, and a significant percentage of these animals had one or more pathological changes, including dysmyelopoiesis, bone marrow necrosis, myelofibrosis, haemorrhage, oedema or acute inflammation (Figure 9.4; Weiss, 2008). These pathological changes are thought to inhibit normal function of the bone marrow, resulting in ineffective erythropoiesis.

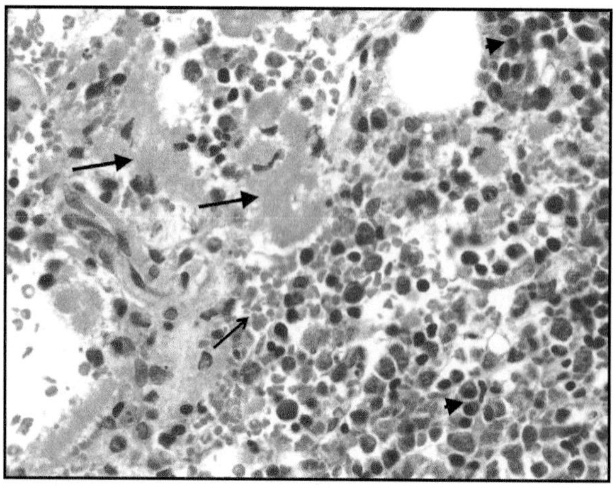

9.4 Histological section of bone marrow from a dog showing haemorrhage (small arrow), oedema and fibrin deposition (large arrows), and an increase in plasma cells (arrowheads).

Presentation and diagnosis

In dogs, the predilection is similar to regenerative IMHA with middle-aged, neutered females being overrepresented. Affected cats tend to be relatively young. A study of IMHA in cats, the majority of which showed non-regenerative anaemia, reported a mean age of 3.2 years for affected animals (Kohn *et al.*, 2006). Patients present with moderate to severe anaemia that is typically normocytic and normochromic. The leucocyte count tends to be within the reference interval or mildly increased, which is in contrast to regenerative IMHA in which relatively high leucocyte counts and moderate to severe left shifts are frequently present (Stokol *et al.*, 2000). Platelet counts also tend to be within reference intervals or increased. It is important to note that neutropenia and thrombocytopenia can be present in some cases. The diagnosis in some patients relies on traditional indicators of IMHA such as a positive direct Coombs' test, spherocytosis (dog) and autoagglutination of erythrocytes (Chapter 6). Bone marrow aspiration and biopsy are important for supporting the diagnosis of non-regenerative IMHA, and are critical in those patients that lack or have mild indicators of IMHA in the peripheral blood. In addition, bone marrow evaluation is important in differentiating non-regenerative IMHA from other conditions such as pure red cell aplasia (PRCA) because these two processes can have similar findings in the peripheral blood. Bone marrow aspiration and biopsy samples reveal variable degrees of erythroid hyperplasia and in some cases a maturation arrest in the erythroid line. Other frequent findings are dysmyelopoiesis, bone marrow necrosis, myelofibrosis, haemorrhage, oedema, lymphocytosis (cats) and plasmacytosis (dogs).

Treatment and prognosis

Treatment of IMHA is described in Chapter 6, and is similar whether the anaemia is regenerative or non-regenerative. The time frame for the response to treatment is somewhat variable, but typically takes weeks. The risk of complications associated with thromboembolic disease appears to be somewhat lower in patients with non-regenerative IMHA (especially those with a subacute to chronic course) when compared with patients with acute regenerative IMHA. The prognosis is guarded, and a recent study of dogs and cats with non-regenerative IMHA reported the 60-day survival rate to be 61% for dogs and 63% for cats (Weiss, 2008).

Pure red cell aplasia

PRCA is typified by a selective absence of erythroid precursors within the bone marrow. Granulopoiesis and thrombopoiesis are relatively unaffected. The selective erythroid aplasia is most frequently the result of immune-mediated destruction of early erythroid precursors (i.e. immune-mediated PRCA), but has been described with other conditions such as parvoviral infection/vaccination, treatment with recombinant human erythropoietin, and infection with FeLV (subgroup C). The remainder of the discussion will focus on immune-mediated PRCA, because this is the most common type. Immune-mediated PRCA is considered to be a type of non-regenerative IMHA, with the immune-mediated destruction targeting very early erythroid precursors. PRCA, however, has distinct and characteristic bone marrow alterations that contrast to those seen with other types of non-regenerative IMHA.

Presentation and diagnosis

In dogs there is a predilection for the disease in middle-aged neutered females, as with IMHA. A sex predilection has not been observed in cats but animals tend to be relatively young, with one study reporting an age range of 8 months to 3 years (Stokol and Blue, 1999). Both dogs and cats present with severe, normocytic, normochromic, non-regenerative anaemia. The mean PCV is 10% for dogs and 7% for cats. Leucocyte and platelet counts tend to be within or occasionally above reference intervals. Traditional indicators of IMHA are not reliably present. The direct Coombs' test is frequently negative and spherocytes are observed only occasionally in dogs. Bone marrow aspiration and biopsy are critical for the diagnosis of PRCA, and reveal a normal to hypercellular marrow with normal granulopoiesis and thrombopoiesis, but severe hypoplasia to aplasia of the erythroid lineage. Additional findings in bone marrow include an increase in plasma cells in dogs and an increase in small lymphocytes in cats. When diagnosing immune-mediated PRCA it is important to differentiate PRCA from non-regenerative IMHA, anaemia of chronic renal disease (Chapter 10), myelofibrosis, myelodysplastic syndromes and other causes of PRCA such as parvoviral infection/vaccination.

Treatment and prognosis

Immunosuppressive therapy is the cornerstone of treatment, along with blood transfusion in many cases. Prednisolone is routinely used (dogs 1–3 mg/kg orally q12h, cats 3.5–5.5 mg/kg orally daily in divided doses), sometimes in combination therapy with cyclophosphamide or azathioprine (for dogs). In dogs, the response to therapy is frequently delayed, with one study reporting a median of 38 days for the initial response (i.e. the time to an increase in Hct of ≥ 5%) and 118 days for complete resolution (i.e. Hct within the reference interval; Weiss, 2002). Resolution of the anaemia in cats occurs within 3–5 weeks; however, in contrast to dogs, most cats required long-term immunosuppressive therapy after resolution (Stokol and Blue, 1999). The 60-day survival rate for dogs and cats with PRCA has been reported as 79% and 88%, respectively (Weiss, 2008).

Myelofibrosis

Myelofibrosis is characterized by proliferation of fibroblasts and deposition of variable amounts of collagen and/or reticulin fibres in the bone marrow space. Myelofibrosis can be either primary or secondary in nature. In humans primary myelofibrosis (also termed idiopathic myelofibrosis) is a condition associated with a distinct myeloproliferative disorder. Small numbers of dogs with myelofibrosis have had findings that appear to fit human criteria for the diagnosis of primary myelofibrosis (Breuer *et al.*, 1999). However, most cases of myelofibrosis in dogs and cats appear to be secondary (Weiss and Smith, 2002; Weiss, 2007). The causes of secondary myelofibrosis include: IMHA; bone marrow necrosis; leukaemia; myelodysplastic syndromes; non-haematological neoplasia; treatment with certain drugs (e.g. phenobarbital, phenylbutazone); congenital pyruvate kinase deficiency; and irradiation. Of these causes, IMHA, neoplasia/leukaemia and myelodysplastic syndrome account for a relatively large percentage of all cases. The aetiology of myelofibrosis is not well understood. There is some evidence that increased stimulation of fibroblasts by fibrogenic cytokines released from megakaryocytes and macrophages may play a role. In addition, an association of myelofibrosis with bone marrow necrosis may suggest that fibrosis is a chronic response to marrow necrosis or inflammation, similar to scar tissue formation.

Presentation and diagnosis

Dogs and cats with myelofibrosis almost invariably present with a moderate to severe, normocytic, normochromic, non-regenerative anaemia. Platelet counts are generally within reference intervals or decreased, and most animals have a normal leucocyte count. As a result of the anaemia, fatigue, weakness, weight loss and pale mucous membranes are frequent clinical signs/physical examination findings. A diagnosis of myelofibrosis is based on evaluation of bone marrow core biopsy samples. Bone marrow aspirates from these patients are often of low yield ('dry tap'), lacking bone marrow spicules and significant numbers of haemopoietic precursors for evaluation. The degree of marrow fibrosis and overall cellularity are highly variable from patient to patient. Some samples are hypercellular, while others are hypocellular, and fibrosis can range from mild to severe. Special stains can be used to highlight reticulin fibrosis (Gomori's reticulin stain) and collagen fibrosis (Masson's trichrome stain). Additional findings may include areas of necrosis or inflammation, and in many cases increased amounts of haemosiderin (Figure 9.5). The latter has been suggested as a potential cause of fibrosis, but its presence does not appear to correlate with the severity of fibrosis.

The diagnostic work-up should include a search for the underlying cause of the myelofibrosis. The patient's history should be explored to determine whether any drugs or toxin exposure may have caused bone marrow injury. A search for infectious agents and neoplasia should be conducted. In addition, because of the frequency of IMHA as a cause of myelofibrosis, it is prudent to screen all patients for immune-mediated diseases.

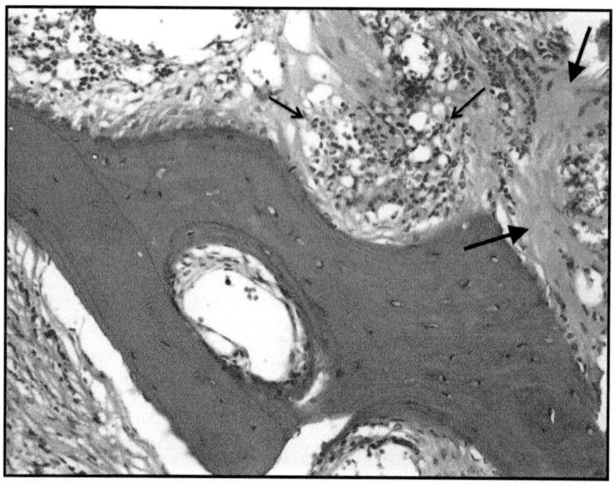

9.5 Histological section of bone marrow from a dog showing an area of fibrosis (large arrows) and an acute inflammatory infiltrate (small arrows).

Treatment and prognosis

The management of secondary myelofibrosis has traditionally consisted of treatment of the underlying condition (if identified) along with immunosuppressive doses of corticosteroids and blood transfusions. Approximately half of all dogs with secondary myelofibrosis exhibit haematological recovery. Those animals with malignant neoplasia as an underlying cause have a worse prognosis. In addition, the degree of fibrosis does not appear to correlate with long-term survival in dogs, and other potential markers of survival such as the degree of marrow cellularity and severity of anaemia have been inconsistent in their prognostic value (Villiers and Dunn, 1999; Weiss and Smith, 2002).

Myelodysplastic syndromes (MDS)

Myelodysplastic syndromes are a heterogeneous group of clonal disorders of the bone marrow and blood. Characteristic features are peripheral cytopenias, along with dysplastic changes seen in one or more cell lines in blood or bone marrow. Bone marrow samples are usually normo- to hypercellular in these patients. Myeloblasts are increased (5–20%) in some patients. The presence of an increased percentage of myeloblasts is a negative prognostic indicator and is a major factor in classification of the various types of MDS. Presently, animals with > 20% myeloblasts are considered to have acute leukaemia. Increased apoptosis of haemopoietic precursors and abnormal growth and differentiation of these cells is thought to result in ineffective haemopoiesis (i.e. death of haemopoietic precursor cells in the marrow) with resultant peripheral cytopenias. Acquired genetic abnormalities underlying the clonal nature of these disorders can be spontaneous (i.e. primary), or secondary to exposure to radiation, drugs or toxins. Most cases of MDS in dogs are assumed to be spontaneous in their origin; however, in cats there is an association with FeLV infection. Although MDS has been categorized by several classification systems, the World Health Organization Classification System is currently recommended and that terminology will be used here (Figures 9.6 and 9.7). In dogs, refractory anaemia (RA) and refractory anaemia with excess blasts (RAEB) are the major types of MDS. In cats, refractory cytopenias with multilineage dysplasia (RCMD) and RAEB are the major types of MDS. These will be described below. Other types of MDS occur infrequently and the reader is referred elsewhere for a complete discussion of MDS types (Valli, 2007; Weiss, 2010). In diagnosing MDS it is important to differentiate this condition from secondary dysmyelopoiesis. Secondary dysmyelopoiesis is a non-clonal condition in which dysplastic features are also evident in the bone marrow. Secondary dysmyelopoiesis has been associated with certain disease processes (e.g. IMHA, immune-mediated thrombocytopenia, lymphoma), administration of drugs (e.g. phenobarbital, oestrogen, cephalosporins, chloramphenicol), iron deficiency, lead poisoning, and sepsis. Differentiating MDS from secondary dysmyelopoiesis can be difficult in some cases.

Refractory anaemia in dogs

Dogs affected with RA have an insidious onset of clinical signs consisting of lethargy and exercise intolerance. Pale mucous membranes, increased heart and respiratory rates, and anaemia-related heart murmurs are frequent findings on physical examination. Haematological alterations consist of non-regenerative, normocytic, normochromic

Condition	Clinical signs	Peripheral blood findings	Bone marrow findings	Prognosis
Refractory anaemia [a]	Lethargy, exercise intolerance	Normocytic, normochromic, non-regenerative anaemia	Dyserythropoiesis, variable increase in rubriblasts, < 5% myeloblasts	Guarded
Refractory anaemia with ringed sideroblasts (RARS)	Lethargy, exercise intolerance	Hypochromic non-regenerative anaemia with siderocytes	Dyserythropoiesis, variable increase in rubriblasts, sideroblasts	Guarded
Refractory cytopenias with multilineage dysplasia (RCMD)	Uncertain	Variable	Ringed sideroblasts, dysplasia in multiple cell lineages, < 5% myeloblasts	Guarded
Refractory anaemia with excess blasts (RAEB) [a]	Lethargy, anorexia, fever, petechiae	Bicytopenia or pancytopenia	Dyserythropoiesis, dysgranulopoiesis, dysmegakaryopoiesis, 5–20% myeloblasts	Poor

9.6 Classification and characteristics of myelodysplastic syndromes in dogs. [a] MDS types most frequently reported in the dog.

Condition	Clinical signs	Peripheral blood findings	Bone marrow findings	Prognosis
Refractory anaemia	Not reported			
Refractory anaemia with ringed sideroblasts (RARS)	Few cases reported			
Refractory cytopenias with multilineage dysplasia (RCMD) [a]	Anorexia, depression, weight loss, weakness	Macrocytic normochromic non-regenerative anaemia, bicytopenia or pancytopenia, metarubricytosis	Dysplasia in multiple cell lineages, < 5% myeloblasts	Guarded
Refractory anaemia with excess blasts (RAEB) [a]	Lethargy, anorexia, fever, petechial haemorrhage	Normocytic or macrocytic non-regenerative anaemia, bicytopenia or pancytopenia	Dyserythropoiesis, dysgranulopoiesis, dysmegakaryopoiesis, 5–20% myeloblasts	Poor

9.7 Classification and characteristics of myelodysplastic syndromes in cats. [a] MDS types most frequently reported in the cat.

anaemia with leucocyte and platelet counts within reference intervals. The bone marrow is normocellular or hypercellular. Rubriblasts are frequently increased in number, ranging between 5 and 30% of all nucleated bone marrow cells, and myeloblasts are consistently < 5%. Dysplastic features are usually limited to the erythroid series.

The treatment of dogs with RA has included cyclophosphamide, cytarabine and erythropoietin. Most dogs for which follow-up was available survived for months to years with no reports of progression to acute leukaemia. In the limited number of cases reported, response to treatment or survival did not appear to be dependent on the percentage of rubriblasts in the bone marrow.

RAEB in dogs

RAEB is the most frequently occurring type of MDS in dogs. RAEB is a disease of middle-aged to old dogs with no apparent breed or sex predilection. Affected dogs are usually more ill than those with RA. Signs of illness include lethargy, depression, anorexia, diarrhoea and fever. Haematological alterations include normocytic, normochromic, non-regenerative anaemia, neutropenia and thrombocytopenia. The bone marrow is usually hypercellular. A defining feature of RAEB is the presence of 6–20% myeloblasts in the bone marrow. Dysplastic features are typically present in all bone marrow cell lineages.

Treatment of RAEB in dogs has been mostly supportive. Broad-spectrum antibiotics are indicated when severe neutropenia is present and to treat fever or sepsis. Red blood cell (RBC) or whole blood transfusions are indicated to treat severe anaemia. Erythropoietin and other haemopoietic growth factors have been given. Although these treatments may improve the cytopenias, they do not appear to prolong survival significantly. Administration of chemotherapeutic agents, including hydroxycarbamide (hydroxyurea), low-dose cytarabine and low-dose aclarubicin has been tried in individual cases. Hydroxycarbamide has been used most frequently. Some individual animals appear to respond to chemotherapy. At present, the survival of dogs with RAEB is short, with survival times ranging from days to months. Progression to acute myeloid leukaemia has been documented in approximately 25% of reported cases.

RCMD in cats

Clinical signs frequently encountered in cats with RCMD include anorexia, depression, weakness and weight loss. Affected cats have a moderate to severe, macrocytic, normochromic, non-regenerative anaemia and frequently have metarubricytosis and autoagglutination (note that the presence of autoagglutination can lead to confusion with IMHA). Most cats have thrombocytopenia and some have leucopenia. The bone marrow is normocellular or hypercellular, myeloblasts are not increased, and rubriblasts are typically increased. Dysplastic features are present in the erythroid lineage of all affected cats and are frequently present in granulocyte and megakaryocyte lineages.

Although the prognosis is guarded, some cats with RCMD respond partially or completely to symptomatic therapy and show prolonged survival. Therapy has consisted of prednisolone, prednisolone and cytarabine, ciclosporin, or combination chemotherapy consisting of daunorubicin, cytarabine, vincristine and prednisolone. Cats with RCMD are less likely to progress to acute myeloid leukaemia and have longer survival compared with those with RAEB.

RAEB in cats

Cats with RAEB are characterized by multiple cytopenias, dysplasia in all cell lineages and increased myeloblasts in the bone marrow. In studies in which most affected cats were FeLV-positive, the median age was approximately 3 years, whereas in studies in which the majority of affected cats were FeLV-negative, the median age was approximately 9 years. Cats with RAEB tend to be severely ill with clinical signs including anorexia, weakness, depression, weight loss, fever, vomiting, diarrhoea and platelet-related bleeding. Cats with RAEB have a moderate to severe, non-regenerative anaemia and some have metarubricytosis and autoagglutination. Most cats are thrombocytopenic and some are leucopenic. The bone marrow is usually normocellular or hypercellular, but may be hypocellular. Cats that are FeLV-positive frequently have erythroid hypoplasia. By definition, all affected cats have 6–20% myeloblasts in the bone marrow, with variable increases in rubriblasts. Dysplastic features are present in all cell lines. Presently, survival for cats with RAEB varies from days to a few months, with frequent progression to acute myeloid leukaemia.

Neoplasia/leukaemia

Non-regenerative anaemia can be present in patients with leukaemia and neoplasia metastatic to the bone marrow. Myelophthisis, defined as crowding out or displacement of normal haemopoietic cells by neoplastic cells, occurs in these conditions. A reduction in the number of haemopoietic precursors along with disruption of the bone marrow microenvironment leads to decreased erythrocyte production. In addition, mechanisms described in Chapter 11 contribute further to anaemia in animals with neoplasia/leukaemia.

References and further reading

Beale KM, Altman D, Clemmons RR *et al.* (1992) Systemic toxicosis associated with azathioprine administration in domestic cats. *American Journal of Veterinary Research* **53**, 1236–1240

Bloom JC, Theim PA, Sellers TS *et al.* (1988) Cephalosporin-induced immune cytopenias in the dog: demonstration of erythrocyte-, neutrophil-, and platelet-associated IgG following treatment with cefazedone. *American Journal of Hematology* **28**, 71–78

Brazzell JL and Weiss DJ (2006) A retrospective study of aplastic pancytopenia in the dog: 9 cases (1996–2003). *Veterinary Clinical Pathology* **35**, 413–417

Breuer W, Darbes J, Hemanns W *et al.* (1999) Idiopathic myelofibrosis in a cat and in three dogs. *Comparative Haematology International* **9**, 17–24

Giger U, Werner LL, Millichamp NJ *et al.* (1985) Sulfadiazine-induced allergy in six Doberman Pinschers. *Journal of the American Veterinary Medical Association* **186**, 479–484

Kohn B, Weingart C, Eckmann V *et al.* (2006) Primary immune-mediated hemolytic anemia in 19 cats: diagnosis, therapy, and outcome (1998–2004). *Journal of Veterinary Internal Medicine* **20**, 159–166

Sontas HB, Dokuzeylu B, Turna O *et al.* (2009) Estrogen-induced myelotoxicity in dogs: a review. *The Canadian Veterinary Journal* **50**, 1054–1058

Stokol T and Blue JT (1999) Pure red cell aplasia in cats: 9 cases (1989–1997). *Journal of the American Veterinary Medical Association* **214**, 75–79

Stokol T, Blue JT and French TW (2000) Idiopathic pure red cell aplasia and nonregenerative immune-mediated anemia in dogs: 43 cases (1988–1999). *Journal of the American Veterinary Medical Association* **216**, 1429–1436

Stokol T, Randolph JF, Nachbar S *et al.* (1997) Development of bone marrow toxicosis after albendazole administration in a dog and cat. *Journal of the American Veterinary Medical Association* **210**, 1753–1756

Trepanier LA (2004) Idiosyncratic toxicity associated with potentiated sulfonamides in the dog. *Journal of Veterinary Pharmacology and Therapeutics* **27**, 129–138

Valli VE (2007) Myelodysplastic syndromes. In: *Veterinary Comparative Hematopathology,* pp. 473–489. Blackwell, Ames, IA

Villiers EJ and Dunn JK (1999) Clinicopathological features of seven cases of canine myelofibrosis and the possible relationship between the histological findings and prognosis. *Veterinary Record* **145**, 222–228

Weiss DJ (2002) Primary pure red cell aplasia in dogs: 13 cases (1996–2000). *Journal of the American Veterinary Medical Association* **221**, 93–95

Weiss DJ (2006a) Short communication: Aplastic anemia in cats – clinicopathological features and associated disease conditions 1996–2004. *Journal of Feline Medicine and Surgery* **8**, 203–206

Weiss DJ (2006b) A retrospective study of the incidence and classification of bone marrow disorders in the dog at a veterinary teaching hospital (1996–2004). *Journal of Veterinary Internal Medicine* **20**, 955–961

Weiss DJ (2007) Feline myelonecrosis and myelofibrosis: 22 cases 1996–2006. *Comparative Clinical Pathology* **16**, 181–185

Weiss DJ (2008) Bone marrow pathology in dogs and cats with non-regenerative immune-mediated haemolytic anaemia and pure red cell aplasia. *Journal of Comparative Pathology* **138**, 46–53

Weiss DJ (2010) Myelodysplastic syndromes. In: *Schalm's Veterinary Hematology, 6th edn,* ed. DJ Weiss and J Wardrop, pp. 467–474. Wiley-Blackwell, Ames, Iowa

Weiss DJ and Smith SA (2002) A retrospective study of 19 cases of canine myelofibrosis. *Journal of Veterinary Internal Medicine* **16**, 174–178

10

Anaemia of chronic renal disease

Andreas H. Hasler

Introduction

Anaemia is a common problem in cats and dogs with chronic renal disease (CRD). The severity of the anaemia correlates with the degree of renal disease as expressed by the creatinine and/or the urea concentration (King *et al.*, 1992). Hence, in stages I and II of the International Renal Interest Society (IRIS) classification, anaemia is often absent or mild, whereas in stages III and IV anaemia is present to severe. The signs and symptoms of anaemia in patients with CRD do not differ from those seen in other patients with chronic anaemia, and include pallor of the mucous membranes and skin, tachycardia, tachypnoea, lethargy, weakness and anorexia. These problems increase the morbidity and mortality of CRD. Compensatory mechanisms such as increased cardiac output, lowered peripheral vascular resistance and an increase in 2,3-diphosphoglycerate (2,3-DPG) may improve oxygenation and alleviate the clinical signs.

Pathophysiology

The pathophysiology of anaemia in animals with CRD is multifactorial and may involve bone marrow failure, blood loss or haemolysis. Bone marrow failure (i.e. failure of erythropoiesis) caused by reduced production of erythropoietin (EPO) by diseased kidneys is the major contributing factor in both human and veterinary patients (Cowgill, 1992).

Erythropoietin deficiency

A classic endocrine feedback system tightly regulates the red cell mass under normal circumstances (Erslev, 1990). EPO is the key factor in the regulation of red cell mass and erythrocyte production (Figure 10.1). EPO is a polypeptide hormone that belongs to the group of haemopoietic growth factors. It has a high degree of amino acid sequence homology among mammals, which explains the interspecies cross-reactivity of hormone assays and the use of heterologous recombinant human EPO (rHuEPO) or its newer derivatives in replacement therapy. Reduced oxygenation of blood reaching the kidney is the key physiological signal for increasing erythropoiesis through increased expression of the *EPO* gene by the fibroblasts of the renal cortex and outer medulla. In hypoxia, the intracellular transcription factor hypoxia-inducible factor (HIF) binds to a hypoxia-response element (HRE) to stimulate transcription of the *EPO* gene and consequently EPO production (Foley, 2008). Cells that produce EPO may be active or inactive, and the number of active cells parallels the degree of hypoxia. In non-uraemic patients, serum EPO concentrations are inversely correlated with the haematocrit (Hct), which means that EPO concentrations increase in proportion to the severity of anaemia (Figure 10.2). EPO is the primary regulator

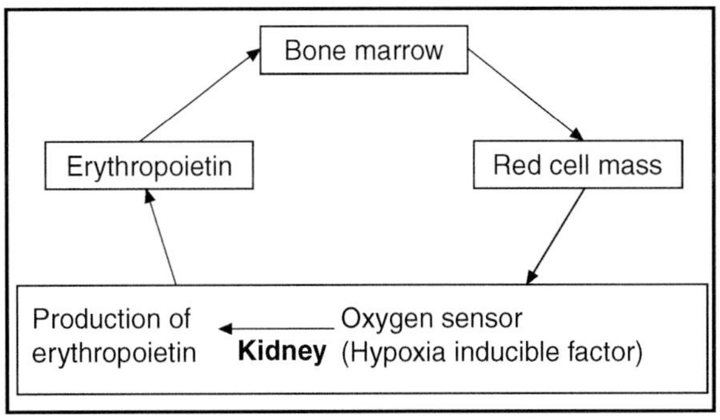

10.1 Synthesis and regulation of erythropoietin.

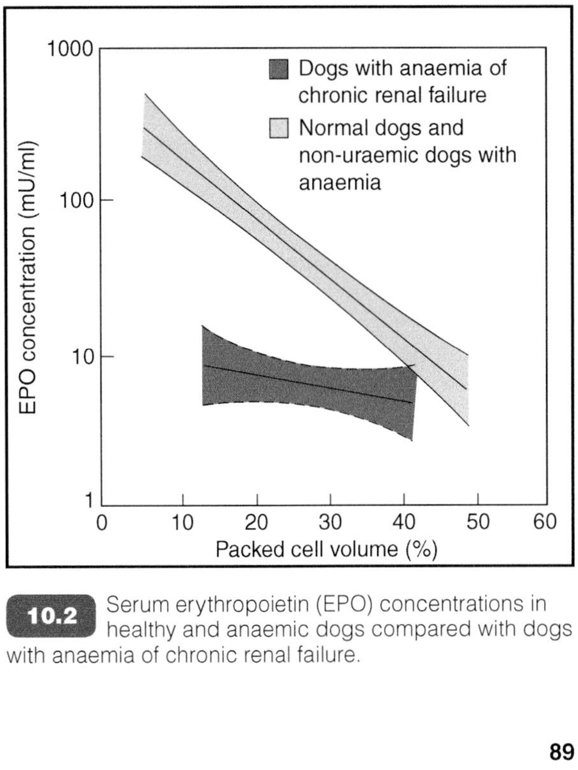

10.2 Serum erythropoietin (EPO) concentrations in healthy and anaemic dogs compared with dogs with anaemia of chronic renal failure.

of the growth and survival of erythroid progenitors. The stimulation of erythropoiesis results in an increase in circulating red cells, and, as a consequence, oxygen-carrying capacity is enhanced.

By contrast, uraemic patients have an impaired regulatory loop, and their ability to produce EPO in response to tissue hypoxia is abolished or decreased. Numerous studies in humans and other species have shown that serum EPO concentrations in uraemic patients are inappropriately low when compared with normal reference values (see Figure 10.2). Anaemic dogs with CRD generally have low or normal plasma EPO concentrations. Mildly increased EPO concentrations may be found occasionally, but they are often inadequately increased in view of the degree of the anaemia (King *et al.*, 1992). In an experimental model of decreased renal mass, the EPO response paralleled the remaining functional renal mass (Oishi *et al.*, 1993). The potential EPO regulation capacity in mild CRF is as conserved as that in normal animals, whereas that in advanced CRF is impaired, which suggests that the underlying mechanisms of low EPO production alter according to the stage of CRF. It has yet to be established whether the decrease in plasma EPO concentration is caused by an impaired oxygen-sensing mechanism, a decreased synthesis of EPO or both.

Myelofibrosis and hyperparathyroidism

Secondary hyperparathyroidism is a common sequel to CRD. An increase in parathyroid hormone (PTH) concentration may lead to myelofibrosis (Rao *et al.*, 1993), and the fibrotic bone marrow has a decreased erythropoietic potential. Furthermore, a direct inhibitory effect of PTH on erythropoiesis has been proposed to act via down-regulation of erythropoietin receptors on erythroid progenitor cells in the bone marrow. One study showed that anaemic dogs with CRD had significantly higher PTH values when compared with non-anaemic dogs with CRD (King *et al.*, 1992). PTH appears to influence erythrocyte survival time, because decreased erythrocyte survival time has been shown in dogs with surgically induced renal failure, and this normalized after parathyroidectomy (King *et al.*, 1992). In addition to the role of PTH and myelofibrosis in the pathogenesis of the anaemia of CRD, there is much interest in the relationship between PTH, myelofibrosis and the response to replacement therapy with exogenous EPO. Hyperparathyroidism and myelofibrosis are thought to be one reason for EPO resistance, and correction of hyperparathyroidism has been shown to improve the response to exogenous EPO (Rao *et al.*, 1993).

Increased osmotic fragility

Osmotic fragility of erythrocytes is increased in human patients with CRD, however a single study of osmotic fragility in dogs with CRD did not find changes in this parameter (King *et al.*, 1992). These results suggest that altered osmotic fragility is not a major contributor to the anaemia of CRD in dogs.

Gastrointestinal and other bleeding

Bleeding into the gastrointestinal (GI) tract may be the most common cause of blood loss anaemia in uraemic patients, and may be manifest clinically as haematemesis, haematochezia or melaena. Gastrin has been implicated in the development of gastric ulcers. The gastrin concentration is increased because its metabolism is reduced in the diseased kidney. The resulting hypergastrinaemia increases acid production, leading to mucosal irritation, ulcers and consequently haemorrhage. GI bleeding may go undetected for a long time and, if persistent, can cause iron deficiency. Uraemia also has a direct effect on platelet function and hence may lead to haemorrhage.

Iron deficiency anaemia

Many dogs and cats with CRD have subnormal serum iron concentration and transferrin saturation below 15% (Cowgill, 1992). It is not clear whether this is related to decreased iron intake, diminished iron absorption or excessive iron loss. In humans and mice the acute phase protein hepcidin is increased in end-stage CRD. Hepcidin is a major player in iron homeostasis and down-regulates iron absorption and release. Recent studies suggest that the dog has hepcidin metabolism comparable to that of mice and humans (Frye, 2008).

Clinical evaluation

The minimal database for anaemia of CRD consists of the history, physical examination, complete blood count (CBC; including red cell indices and reticulocyte count) and a complete serum biochemistry panel including albumin, phosphate, blood urea nitrogen (BUN), creatinine, calcium and a complete urinalysis. Stool analysis for parasites and occult blood may be helpful to exclude GI bleeding. The diagnosis of CRD should be based on findings consistent with the disease. It must be remembered that other diseases (e.g. hypoadrenocorticism) may cause concurrent azotaemia, isosthenuria and anaemia.

Complete blood count

The packed cell volume (PCV) is commonly used to assess anaemia in veterinary medicine. The red blood cell (RBC) count or the haemoglobin (Hb) concentration can also be used to document anaemia, but for simplicity only the PCV is mentioned in the following discussion. Furthermore, a very small amount of blood is necessary for PCV determination, compared with that required for a CBC. The degree of anaemia should be re-evaluated once the animal has been rehydrated. Patients with CRD are often dehydrated, and the haemo-concentration may mask the full extent of the anaemia. Red cell indices characterize the anaemia according to the size and Hb content of the erythrocytes. A normocytic–normochromic pattern occurs in the anaemia of erythropoietin deficiency.

Any other pattern suggests a different form of anaemia (e.g. microcytic–hypochromic anaemia due to iron deficiency).

Reticulocyte count

The presence of a regenerative anaemia rules out lack of EPO, and other causes of anaemia must be evaluated (e.g. haemolysis, GI bleeding). Bone marrow examination is generally not indicated for primary evaluation of the anaemia of CRD. The exception may be to document myelofibrosis or the presence of serum antibodies specific for rHuEPO.

Blood loss

Any blood loss should be investigated. Concurrent hypoalbuminaemia may suggest blood loss, or a high BUN:creatinine ratio may suggest GI bleeding. Although parasites (e.g. fleas, hookworms) in otherwise healthy animals rarely cause significant anaemia, they may contribute to anaemia in the patient with CRD.

Serum EPO concentration

It is not necessary to determine serum EPO concentrations to diagnose EPO-deficient anaemia of CRD. To the author's knowledge there is no study that suggests that EPO concentration is a useful prognostic indicator of the progress of the anaemia of CRD or the response to treatment. The finding of an appropriately increased EPO concentration in an anaemic animal may, however, direct the clinician to search for other causes of anaemia (e.g. blood loss).

PTH concentration

Determination of the plasma PTH concentration may sometimes be helpful in cases of CRD, for example in those animals that may be treated with calcitriol.

Hypertension

Arterial hypertension is a common complication of CRD (Syme *et al.*, 2002). Hypertension has been related to survival in cats with CRD (Elliott *et al.*, 2001) and hence blood pressure measurements are indicated. Further, pre-existing hypertension is a relative contraindication for the administration of EPO and should be controlled before such therapy.

Treatment

The anaemia of CRD is multifactorial, and treatment must therefore be tailored to the underlying disease. The approach should be practical and cost effective. The initial management should aim to minimize blood loss, whereas subsequent therapy should be directed towards increasing red cell mass.

Gastrointestinal and other blood loss

Patients with CRD require close monitoring, and hence frequent blood sampling is needed for laboratory tests. Repeated blood collection may quickly render cats and small dogs anaemic. Testing should therefore be optimized and restricted where possible. Intestinal parasites (e.g. hookworms) and flea infestation should be addressed with proper therapy. Gastric ulceration may be alleviated with the use of antacids and sucralfate.

Iron deficiency is treated with oral or injectable iron preparations. Starting doses of 100–300 mg/day for dogs and 50–100 mg/day for cats have been recommended. Side effects of oral iron supplementation include vomiting and diarrhoea. Therapy should be evaluated by monitoring plasma iron concentrations and transferrin saturation.

Blood transfusions

Prior to the availability of rHuEPO, the anaemia of CRD was treated by transfusion of whole blood or packed red blood cells. This approach remains the modality of choice in an acute situation where rapid improvement is a necessity. Transfusion in cats with CRD accounts for about 10–20% of all transfusions (Castellanos *et al.*, 2004). However, there are several inherent problems associated with such transfusions, which make this procedure unsuitable for long-term management:

- Even with careful cross-matching, incompatibilities may develop with repeated transfusions, and prohibit further use
- Few veterinary clinics have reliable access to blood products
- It is nearly impossible to restore the PCV to the normal range in animals with anaemia of CRD, thus the patient remains anaemic.

Recombinant human EPO

Following the discovery that the major determinant of uraemic anaemia is a relative or absolute deficiency of EPO, treatment has focused on replacement with exogenous EPO. Since the first trial of rHuEPO in human medicine in 1985, a large body of literature has shown the efficacy and benefits of treatment with EPO in humans and domestic animals, and rHuEPO has emerged as the mainstay for correction of uraemic anaemia in human patients (Erslev and Besarab, 1997). Newer formulations have emerged (e.g. darbepoetin) and have partially replaced the original EPO medications. In line with the development of different strategies (e.g. HIF stabilization) the umbrella term 'erythropoiesis stimulating agents' (ESAs) has emerged.

Benefits

Treatment with rHuEPO produces a dose-dependent increase in PCV in virtually every human patient (Erslev and Besarab, 1997). Similarly, in dogs it can be expected that the PCV will increase by 0.5–1% per day, and usually the red cell mass can be restored within a month (Cowgill *et al.*, 1998). Thrombocytosis, but not leucocytosis, may accompany the increase in PCV. Thrombocytosis appears to be a direct effect of administration of rHuEPO (Vaziri, 2009).

In addition to improvements in PCV, the most

impressive benefits of effective ESA therapy are significant subjective improvements in wellbeing, increased appetite and increased physical activity, documented in both humans and other species (Cowgill *et al.*, 1998). The gain in appetite improves nutritional status, and resolution of hypokalaemia has been reported in cats.

Indications

Treatment with ESA is indicated in patients with moderate to severe anaemia caused by EPO deficiency and where clinical judgement suggests a possible benefit.

Contraindications

There are relative, but no absolute, contraindications to the use of rHuEPO in dogs and cats, one such case being animals with mild anaemia. Although these animals might benefit from an increased PCV and exhibit the same increase in wellbeing and quality of life, the potential for development of the major side effect (see section below on safety and side effects) and the cost of therapy should be considered and discussed with the owner.

EPO preparations

Commonly used ESAs are available as epoetin alfa, epoetin beta and darbepoetin; the last has a longer activity. All preparations must be stored in a refrigerator. In the past, most treatments in animals have been with epoetin alfa but the advantage of darbepoetin has led to transition. No commercial EPO preparations are authorized for use in domestic animals, and it is necessary to receive written consent from the client.

Injection

The subcutaneous route is used most often because the drug can be administered by owners at home with suitable instruction (similar to insulin injections).

Starting treatment

Replacement therapy can be divided into an initiation and a maintenance phase. The initiation phase is characterized by an increase in PCV, and the dose is higher during this phase (Figure 10.3). An empirical dose for darbepoetin (in micrograms) is about 1:200 of a rHuEPO (in IU) dosage, which translates for a dog to about 1.5 μg/kg once weekly and for an average cat to about 6.25 μg/cat s.c. once weekly. The dose for rHuEPO is 100 IU/kg three times a week. This has been shown to promote an erythropoietic response in most animals. This dose is continued until the PCV has reached the lower end of the target value (25–30% for cats and 35–45% for dogs), which signals the end of the initiating phase (usually within 4–8 weeks). At this point, the dose and interval is reduced and then titrated to effect (Figure 10.4). In the maintenance phase, darbepoetin may be given every 2–4 weeks, or rHuEPO may be given weekly. The reaction to changes in

Product	Initiation		Maintenance	
	Dose	*Frequency*	*Dose*	*Frequency*
Darbepoetin	Cats: 6.25 μg/cat Dogs: 1.5 μg/kg	Once weekly	Cats: 6.25 μg/cat Dogs: 1.5 μg/kg	Once every 2–4 weeks
Recombinant human erythropoietin (rHuEPO)	100 IU/kg	Three times a week	100 IU/kg	Once weekly

10.3 Recommended dosage of erythropoiesis stimulating agents (ESA).

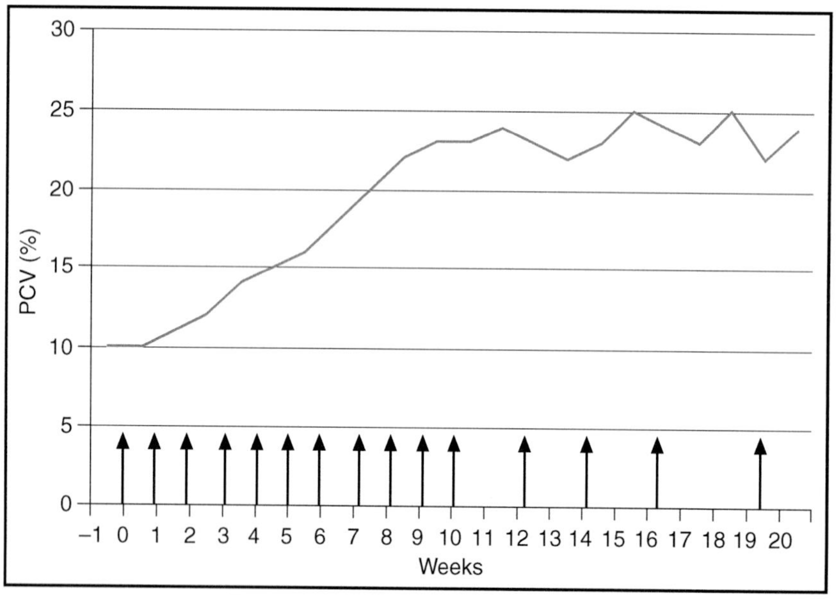

10.4 Response to treatment with darbepoetin in a 13-year-old cat with anaemia of chronic renal failure. The PCV increased to about 25% in response to weekly injections. The frequency of treatment with darbepoetin (arrows) was lowered at that time so that it was given every 2–4 weeks.

dose or interval is slow, and therefore it takes about 3 weeks to assess the impact of a different regime. Hence, changes in ESA dose or interval should not be made more than once every 3 weeks.

The stimulated erythropoiesis puts a high demand on iron stores, which makes concurrent supplementation a necessity. Dosages of oral iron sulphate of 100–300 mg/day for dogs and 50–100 mg/day for cats have been recommended.

Safety and side effects

There is no evidence that treatment with ESA accelerates the progression of renal disease in human patients (Jacobs, 1995). The most detrimental side effect of treatment in animals is the development of antibodies against the human ESA molecule. Such antibodies may bind to both exogenous and endogenous EPO owing to the similarity in their antigenic structure. Consequently, the body becomes resistant to ESA with time, and a progressive decline of PCV will occur. Antibodies do not commonly appear until the fourth week of treatment, but may occur at any time thereafter. Whereas the overall incidence of anti-rHuEPO antibodies may be only 30%, such antibodies developed (along with refractory anaemia) in two of three dogs that were treated for more than 90 days and in five of seven cats that were treated for more than 180 days (Cowgill *et al.*, 1998). These results show that long-term treatment with rHuEPO is associated with a high degree of antibody stimulation. There is an anecdotal impression that darbepoetin is less immunogenic and hence antibodies develop to a much lesser degree. This makes darbepoetin the ESA of choice for dogs and cats with CRD. Although most authors claim that the antibodies disappear upon withdrawal, the memory immune response prohibits a second trial with rHuEPO. A switch from rHuEPO to darbepoetin does not seem to help. These patients will become dependent on blood transfusion. The major sign of antibodies is resistance to treatment after a preliminary response. Unfortunately, there is no commercial test for detection of anti-rHuEPO antibody. A bone marrow sample with a myeloid:erythroid ratio of > 8 is suggestive of resistance to EPO. It is unclear whether concomitant treatment with immunomodulating drugs (e.g. ciclosporin) may postpone or alleviate antibody formation.

Systemic hypertension can develop in patients with no prior record of blood pressure problems. The mechanisms by which ESA therapy may increase blood pressure include increased blood viscosity, loss of hypoxic vasodilatation and a direct vascular effect via increased synthesis of endothelin and other vasoactive substances (Mashio, 1995).

Future directions

Replacement therapy with the present ESAs in small animals has limitations owing to the heterologous origin of the molecules used. Development of antibodies against ESA is rarely a feature of replacement treatment in human patients, and hence it is conceivable that use of a homologous product for dogs (recombinant canine ESA) and cats (recombinant feline ESA) would prevent the induction of antibodies against ESA. The *EPO* gene in dogs and cats has been cloned, and its activity *in vitro* and *in vivo* has been examined and proven (Randolph *et al.*, 2004a, b). At present no information about commercial release is available but the gene was patented in 2009. Gene transfer of an *EPO* gene construct into the musculature of feline patients showed some promise (Walker *et al.*, 2005). Again, a widespread use of this modality has not been established.

The correction of anaemia might improve quality of life and alleviate some of the problems associated with uraemia, but it does not stop the progression of renal disease, and other aspects of the uraemic syndrome may dictate euthanasia. Haemodialysis remains a treatment modality for acute kidney failure, but is not generally available for the management of chronic renal disease in dogs and cats. Renal transplantation in cats (and dogs) is restricted to only a few places in the United States and Australia. The problems to overcome are initially of an ethical nature. Successful renal transplantation will, however, be a major advancement and will resolve the anaemia of CRD along with other uraemic problems.

References and further reading

Castellanos I, Couto CG and Gray TL (2004) Clinical use of blood products in cats: a retrospective study (1997--2000). *Journal of Veterinary Internal Medicine* **18** (4), 529–532

Cowgill LD (1992) Pathophysiology and management of anemia in chronic progressive renal failure. *Seminars in Veterinary Medicine & Surgery (Small Animal)* **7**(3), 175–182

Cowgill LD, James KM, Levy JK *et al.* (1998) Use of recombinant human erythropoietin for management of anemia in dogs and cats with renal failure. *Journal of the American Veterinary Medical Association* **212**(4), 521–528

Elliott J, Barber PJ, Syme HM, Rawlings JM and Markwell PJ (2001) Feline hypertension: clinical findings and response to antihypertensive treatment in 30 cases. *Journal of Small Animal Practice* **42**(3), 122–129

Erslev AJ (1990) Erythropoietin. *Leukemia Research* **14**(8), 683–688

Erslev AJ and Besarab A (1997) Erythropoietin in the pathogenesis and treatment of the anemia of chronic renal failure. *Kidney International* **51**(3), 622–630

Foley RN (2008) Erythropoietin: physiology and molecular mechanisms. *Heart Failure Reviews* **13**(4), 405–414

Frye C (2008) Anemia in chronic renal failure. 1973. *CANNT Journal* **18**(3), 17–18

Jacobs C (1995) Starting rHuEPO in chronic renal failure: when, why, and how? *Nephrology, Dialysis and Transplantation* **10**(Suppl 2), 43–47

King LG, Giger U, Diserens D and Nagode LA (1992) Anemia of chronic renal failure in dogs. *Journal of Veterinary Internal Medicine* **6**(5), 264–270

Maschio G (1995) Erythropoeitin and systemic hypertension. *Nephrology, Dialysis and Transplantation* **10**(Suppl 2), 74–79

Oishi A, Sakamoto H, Shimizu R, Ohashi F and Takeuchi A (1993) Evaluation of erythropoietin production in dogs with reduced functional renal tissue. *The Journal Veterinary Medical Science* **55**(4), 543–548

Randolph JE, Scarlett J, Stokol T and MacLeod JN (2004a) Clinical officacy and safety of recombinant canine erythropoietin in dogs with anemia of chronic renal failure and dogs with recombinant human erythropoietin-induced red cell aplasia. *Journal of Veterinary Internal Medicine* **18**(1), 81–91

Randolph JE, Scarlett J, Stokol T, Saunders KM and MacLeod JN (2004b) Expression, bioactivity, and clinical assessment of recombinant feline erythropoietin. *American Journal of Veterinary*

Research **65**(10), 1355–1366

Rao DS, Shih MS and Mohini R (1993) Effect of serum parathyroid hormone and bone marrow fibrosis on the response to erythropoietin in uremia. *New England Journal of Medicine* **328**(3), 171–175

Syme HM, Barber PJ, Markwell PJ and Elliott J (2002) Prevalence of systolic hypertension in cats with chronic renal failure at initial evaluation. *Journal of the American Veterinary Medical Association* **220**(12), 1799–1804

Vaziri ND (2009) Thrombocytosis in EPO-treated dialysis patients may be mediated by EPO rather than iron deficiency. *American Journal of Kidney Diseases* **53**(5), 733–736

Walker MC, Mandell TC, Crawford PC *et al.* (2005) Expression of erythropoietin in cats treated with a recombinant adeno-associated viral vector. *American Journal of Veterinary Research* **66**(3), 450–456

11

Anaemia of inflammation and neoplasia

Trevor Waner and Shimon Harrus

Introduction

Anaemia of inflammation and neoplasia (AIN), also known as the 'anaemia of chronic disease', is an anaemia that accompanies and complicates infectious, non-infectious and neoplastic disorders. It is the most common type of anaemia in small animal and human medicine, and is one of the most prevalent anaemias in hospitalized patients. The classical features of AIN are mild to moderate non-regenerative, normocytic normochromic anaemia with hypoferraemia accompanying a chronic inflammatory condition such as infection, neoplastic disease or trauma (Rivera and Ganz, 2009). The degree of the anaemia is positively associated with the degree of inflammation, with more advanced diseases displaying a more severe anaemia (Weiss, 2009).

Pathophysiology

Multiple mechanisms contribute to the development of AIN but the condition is considered to be a result of immune activation by an underlying process, mediated by immune and inflammatory cytokines. Several pathophysiological mechanisms have been proposed:

- Iron-limited erythropoiesis mediated by increased levels of hepcidin
- Retention of iron within macrophages (mediated by interferon (IFN)-γ and interleukin (IL)-10) and enterocytes (mediated by IFN-γ and IL-6) leading to hypoferraemia and subnormal saturation of transferrin, which results in a limited availability of iron for erythropoiesis
- An inadequate erythropoietin response in proportion to the degree of the anaemia
- An inhibition of proliferation and differentiation of progenitor erythroid cells in response to erythropoietin, accompanied by apoptosis in the bone marrow caused by IFN-γ, IL-1, tumour necrosis factor (TNF)-α and α-antitrypsin
- A reduction in erythrocyte half-life caused by dyserythropoiesis, erythrocyte damage and increased erythrophagocytosis under the influence of TNF-α.

Of these mechanisms, iron-limited erythropoiesis mediated by increased levels of hepcidin during inflammatory conditions is considered to be the key mechanism (Fry *et al.*, 2004). The disruptive effects of chronic inflammation on iron homeostasis largely explain the mechanism for the onset of AIN. Hepcidin, a liver-derived 25-amino acid cysteine-rich peptide, plays an important role as a regulator of hypoferraemia in inflammation (Park *et al.*, 2001). Hepcidin has antimicrobial properties in human blood and urine (Fry *et al.*, 2004) and is a type II acute phase protein (Nemeth *et al.*, 2003). Essentially, hepcidin acts as a negative regulator of intestinal iron absorption and macrophage iron release. Mice that lack hepcidin mRNA develop iron overload, whereas transgenic mice over-expressing hepcidin die at birth as a result of severe iron deficiency. Hepcidin has been sequenced in humans, mice, rats, pigs, fish and dogs (Fry *et al.*, 2004). A high homology between human and canine hepcidin has been found. In dogs, hepcidin is found mainly in the liver and to a lesser extent in the lung and kidney. This differs from mice and humans, in which hepcidin is not expressed in the kidney.

Absorption of the majority of dietary iron takes place in the duodenum. Steps involved in absorption include reduction of the iron to a ferrous state, uptake by enterocytes, intracellular storage and finally release. Once in the enterocyte, iron may either remain in the cell for use or storage, after which it is lost into the gut lumen as the enterocyte is sloughed, or it can be exported across the membrane into the circulation by an iron transporter, ferroportin-1 (Munoz *et al.*, 2009). The regulation of the rate of iron absorption is controlled by the expression of ferroportin-1, which is localized on the enterocyte membrane. During inflammation, IL-6 acts directly on hepatocytes to release excess hepcidin into the blood. Hepcidin binds to ferroportin-1 in the villous enterocytes of the duodenum, resulting in the internalization of ferroportin-1 and loss of its function, contributing to a state of hypoferraemia (Munoz *et al.*, 2009).

While the major source of iron for the body is dietary, the major cellular system responsible for the adequate supply of iron for erythropoiesis is the monocyte–macrophage system (Weiss, 2009). The majority of iron in the monocytes and macrophages is acquired from recycling of senescent erythrocytes after erythrophagocytosis. Mammalian monocytes and macrophages produce small amounts of hepcidin in response to stimulation by lipopolysaccharide (LPS) or IL-6. The hepcidin released by monocytes and macrophages targets ferroportin in a similar mechanism to that occurring in the enterocytes, resulting in an accumulation of iron in these cells and thus further promoting a state of iron restriction anaemia. The formation of hepcidin by activated macrophages and monocytes has been proposed to be part of a rapid innate immune response aimed to prevent iron export from macrophages, thus reducing the circulating iron concentration and the availability of this nutrient for pathogens (Sow *et al.*, 2007).

Although the mechanism of iron restriction through induction of hepcidin is important in AIN, it cannot fully explain all the aspects of this type of anaemia. A baffling aspect of AIN is the speed with which the condition can develop in severe acute inflammatory conditions. In fact, studies have shown that anaemia can develop at a rapid rate in non-bleeding patients in intensive care (Nguyen *et al.*, 2003). The rapidity with which anaemia can develop has prompted some to propose relinquishing the term 'anaemia of chronic disease'. The rapid progression to anaemia suggests that additional pathophysiological mechanisms take place and require further investigation.

A link between inflammatory conditions and cancer, both of which result in anaemia, has been proposed to be effected through TNF-α (Buck *et al.*, 2009). Abnormally high levels of TNF-α have been detected in a wide range of tumour types in humans, such as kidney, breast, lung and prostate cancers. Correspondingly, TNF-α overproduction has also been found to be involved in numerous chronic inflammatory diseases. TNF-α has proinflammatory, proliferative and apoptotic properties, but it has also been described as an inhibitor of erythroid differentiation and is associated with a number of haematological diseases. Several *in vitro* studies have shown that TNF-α has an inhibitory effect on haemopoietic progenitor cell growth. TNF-α has also been shown to have a direct inhibitory effect on erythropoietin. The negative erythropoietic properties of TNF-α have been proposed to contribute to the state of anaemia in some inflammatory and neoplastic conditions.

Clinical presentation

The history and a thorough physical examination are crucial to the diagnosis of AIN, taking into account that the identification of the underlying condition is an essential element in the diagnosis and treatment of the condition. Typical clinical findings in AIN include pale mucous membranes accompanying a wide variety of inflammatory and neoplastic conditions.

Diagnosis

The physical examination should be supported by a complete blood count (CBC, including evaluation of a blood smear), iron profile and bone marrow examination. Haematological findings indicative of AIN are a mild to moderate, non-regenerative, normocytic normochromic anaemia. The packed cell volume (PCV) usually does not drop below 20% in dogs, and not lower than 15% in cats with AIN. The haemoglobin (Hb) concentration and total erythrocyte count are mildly to moderately reduced, and there is an absence of reticulocytosis, which indicates a lack of bone marrow response to the anaemia. The erythrocyte indices mean corpuscular volume (MCV) and mean corpuscular haemoglobin concentration (MCHC) remain within the normal range.

Anaemia is a common haematological abnormality in patients with cancer, and affects more than 30% of dogs with neoplastic diseases. Tumours in dogs that have been associated with AIN include haemangiosarcoma, leukaemia, lymphoma and multiple myeloma. In canine lymphoma, the anaemia is more likely to occur in dogs older than 10 years of age. In the case of canine osteosarcoma, no correlation was found between age and the presence of anaemia (Miller *et al.*, 2009).

Anaemia has been documented in a high percentage of dogs with acute lymphoblastic leukaemia (98%), acute myeloid leukaemia (97%), chronic lymphocytic leukaemia (75%) and in leukaemic high-grade lymphoma (77%). In all of these forms of neoplasia, the degree of anaemia was mostly mild to moderate. Chronic inflammation associated with chronic lymphocytic leukaemia and leukaemic high-grade lymphoma may be responsible for the mild to moderate anaemia seen in these conditions (Tasca *et al.*, 2009).

Iron parameters are central to the diagnosis of AIN: serum iron concentration and total iron binding capacity (TIBC) are reduced and there is low transferrin saturation (TSAT), whereas serum ferritin may be increased or remain at normal levels. The metals copper and zinc may be modestly increased in AIN, possibly as a result of the increased activity of the copper–zinc metalloenzyme superoxide dismutase, which has been shown to be directly correlated with levels of stored iron. Diagnostic aids that are being clinically evaluated and show promise for the future include tests to measure hepcidin and the expression of the transferrin receptor gene (Fry *et al.*, 2009; Theurl *et al.*, 2009).

The diagnosis of AIN requires differentiation of AIN, iron deficiency anaemia (IDA), and a combined AIN and IDA (AIN/IDA), taking into account that AIN may be accompanied by a concurrent blood loss. The findings of erythrocyte microcytosis and hypochromasia accompanied by thrombocytosis may reflect an IDA rather than AIN. Differentiation of AIN alone from a combined AIN/IDA is clinically important because iron supplementation in patients with AIN alone may have detrimental effects, resulting in promotion of the growth of tumour cells and microorganisms, and may instigate negative effects on innate immune mechanisms. On the other hand, patients with concurrent AIN and IDA may benefit from iron supplementation because the iron is an essential element for basic metabolism and erythropoiesis. Using a rat model, researchers have been able to differentiate between AIN and AIN/IDA by determination of serum hepcidin levels (Theurl *et al.*, 2009). It has been shown that rats with concurrent AIN/IDA had significantly lower blood hepcidin levels than rats with AIN alone. It was suggested that the serum hepcidin level may serve as a valuable tool in distinguishing AIN alone from a combined AIN/IDA. Other methods (e.g. analysis of serum ferritin to distinguish between AIN and AIN/IDA) have not gained widespread acceptance. Staining of bone marrow aspirates with Perl's Prussian blue, although regarded as an accurate means of assessing bone marrow iron stores, represents an invasive method and therefore is not routinely used.

Treatment

AIN can be effectively overcome by correcting the underlying disease. Taking into account the multiple pathways and multiple factors that influence iron homeostasis during inflammation and neoplasia, it is questionable whether a single therapeutic intervention will resolve the anaemia. The only feasible approach appears to be identification of the primary underlying disorder and initiation of specific therapy before any particular treatment for the anaemia is undertaken. As a rule, iron should not be given to patients with AIN unless iron deficiency is proven. In human patients, resolution of AIN occurs within 3 months after alleviation of the primary causative condition.

In a study assessing the impact of anaemia on the outcome and survival time of dogs with lymphoma undergoing chemotherapy, anaemia was found to be a risk factor for poor prognosis and short survival time (Abbo and Lucroy, 2007). Dogs with moderate anaemia were found to have a 2.37-fold greater likelihood of dying than dogs with mild anaemia or no anaemia. This is not the case in patients with osteosarcoma, in which no correlation was found between the survival time and the presence of anaemia (Miller *et al.*, 2009).

Conclusions

AIN, the outcome of iron-limited erythropoiesis, is considered to be the result of immune activation by an underlying process. The role of hepcidin during inflammatory conditions is considered to be the key mechanism of AIN. The diagnosis of AIN is based on the presence of mild to moderate non-regenerative anaemia accompanied by inflammation and/or neoplasia. This type of anaemia can be effectively overcome by correcting the underlying disease. Supplementation of iron may not be appropriate and may even be detrimental. In cases of neoplasia, anaemia may be a risk factor for poor prognosis.

References and further reading

Abbo AH and Lucroy MD (2007) Assessment of anemia as an independent predictor of response to chemotherapy and survival in dogs with lymphoma: 96 cases (1993–2006). *Journal of the American Veterinary Medical Association* **231**, 1836–1842

Buck I, Morceau F, Grigorakaki C *et al.* (2009) Linking anemia to inflammation and cancer: the crucial role of TNF alpha. *Biochemical Pharmacology* **77**, 1572–1579

Fry MM, Kirk CA, Liggett JL *et al.* (2009) Changes in hepatic gene expression in dogs with experimentally induced nutritional iron deficiency. *Veterinary Clinical Pathology* **38**, 13–19

Fry MM, Liggett JL and Baek SJ (2004) Molecular cloning and expression of canine hepcidin. *Veterinary Clinical Pathology* **33**, 223–227

Miller AG, Morley PS, Rao S *et al.* (2009) Anemia is associated with decreased survival time in dogs with lymphoma. *Journal of Veterinary Internal Medicine* **23**, 116–122

Munoz M, Villar I and Garcia-Erce JA (2009) An update on iron physiology. *World Journal of Gastroenterology* **15**, 4617–4626

Nemeth E, Valore EV, Territo M *et al.* (2003) Hepcidin, a putative mediator of anemia of inflammation, is a type II acute-phase protein. *Blood* **101**, 2461–2463

Nguyen BV, Bota DP, Melot C *et al.* (2003) Time course of hemoglobin concentrations in nonbleeding intensive care unit patients. *Critical Care Medicine* **31**, 406–410

Park CH, Valore EV, Waring AJ *et al.* (2001) Hepcidin, a urinary antimicrobial peptide synthesized in the liver. *Journal of Biological Chemistry* **276**, 7806–7810

Rivera S and Ganz T (2009) Animal models of anemia of inflammation. *Seminars in Hematology* **46**, 351–357

Sow FB, Florence WC, Satoskar AR *et al.* (2007) Expression and localization of hepcidin in macrophages: a role in host defense against tuberculosis. *Journal of Leukocyte Biology* **82**, 934–945

Tasca S, Carli E, Caldin M *et al.* (2009) Hematologic abnormalities and flow cytometric immunophenotyping results in dogs with hematopoietic neoplasia: 210 cases (2002–2006). *Veterinary Clinical Pathology* **38**, 2–12

Theurl I, Aigner E, Theurl M *et al.* (2009) Regulation of iron homeostasis in anemia of chronic disease and iron deficiency anemia: diagnostic and therapeutic implications. *Blood* **113**, 5277–5286

Weiss G (2009) Iron metabolism in the anemia of chronic disease. *International Journal of Biochemistry, Biophysics and Molecular Biology* **1790**, 682–693

12

Disorders of leucocyte number

Harold Tvedten

Introduction

Leucocytes are inflammatory cells, and the main reason to measure the total white blood cell (WBC) count and differential WBC count, and to evaluate leucocyte morphology, is to determine whether the animal is showing an inflammatory process and, if so, to characterize the severity and other characteristics of that inflammatory response. Important features to consider include:

- Which types of inflammatory cells are involved
- The severity of any left shift
- Whether lymphopenia is present to suggest stress-related inflammatory disease
- Whether lymphocytosis is present to suggest a chronic immune stimulus
- Whether there are toxic changes in neutrophils that may suggest more severe disease.

The neutrophil is the most common white cell and therefore leucocytosis and neutrophilia are closely associated. Leucocytosis is less commonly due to eosinophilia or monocytosis.

The lymphocyte is the second most common WBC in blood. Lymphopenia is common with stress alone or stress of inflammatory or other diseases, and therefore leucopenia is commonly associated with neutropenia, lymphopenia or often both. Lymphocytosis may be seen in adrenaline-related fear responses in healthy young cats, as part of strong and chronic immune responses or in leukaemia.

Monocytes, eosinophils and basophils are few in number in normal blood. Thus eosinopenia, monocytopenia or basopenia does not cause leucopenia. Specific leucocyte disorders (e.g. leukaemia, neutropenia and eosinophilia) and leucocyte changes related to specific infections are discussed in subsequent chapters.

Neutrophil responses are the most commonly observed changes, signalling inflammation characterized by exudation, suppuration or purulence. Eosinophilic inflammation, granulomatous (i.e. macrophage-dominated inflammation) and even basophilic inflammation also occur. Other processes that alter leucocyte number and morphology include glucocorticoid-related stress effects, adrenaline-related effects of fear, leukaemia and myeloproliferative disorders, drug treatment and the effects of toxins.

The absolute number of each type of leucocyte (i.e. segmented neutrophils, non-segmented neutrophils, lymphocytes, eosinophils, monocytes and basophils) should be interpreted both independently of other cell types and then together as a leucogram. Relative numbers (i.e. percentages and ratios) are affected by total WBC counts and can be misleading if leucopenia or excessive leucocytosis is present. Morphological changes in leucocytes also contribute to the major laboratory conclusions and interpretation of the clinical disease state in the patient. This chapter discusses physiological and pathological processes that affect leucocyte numbers, but discussion of specific diseases and morphology is found in other chapters. Interpretation of numbers and words in the leucogram section of a laboratory report should begin with an understanding of methods used and sources of error and imprecision.

Technical aspects

Total WBC count

Automated counts

The total WBC count as determined by automated instruments is a precise and reliable measurement. The coefficient of variation (CV) for total WBCs is usually very low (< 2%) for most haematology instruments. There are occasionally other blood particles (e.g. fat droplets in lipaemia) that can be counted as WBCs, but laboratory personnel should recognize these by the appearance of graphical displays (e.g. cytograms, dot plots), other instrument flags or by the gross appearance of the sample. Many instruments perform total WBC counts by two methods, so variation between the methods can also indicate an error. Usually the automated total WBC count can be assumed to be accurate.

Manual counts

A manual total WBC count may be performed in a glass counting chamber (haemocytometer) in situations where an automated haematology instrument is not available. This method is cheaper, although time consuming, and has much more imprecision. Variation in the manual total WBC count may be ± 15%, while that of an automated total WBC count may be only ± 1.5%. The manual method may be used to double check cell counts for which the automated cell count is in question. Approximate agreement between automated and manual counts will help to assure clinical accuracy.

Differential counts

The differential leucocyte count is more subject to error than is the total WBC count. Therefore, the absolute count of individual leucocyte types, especially when present in low numbers, can be associated with moderate to large errors. The absolute number of a particular type of leucocyte is usually determined by multiplying the percentage of that type (relative count from the manual differential count) by the total WBC count. Automated instruments may enumerate absolute numbers of each cell type directly.

Manual counting

The manual differential count requires a well trained person to identify the cells. Cells such as canine and feline basophils and 'grey' eosinophils may be difficult to recognize. Differentiation of segmented and non-segmented 'band' neutrophils is subjective and may vary when different people perform a manual differential count.

Differentiation of segmented from non-segmented cells may not be possible when neutrophils are very toxic and many reactive monocytes and reactive lymphocytes are present. In that situation the actual number of different cell types should not be released, but only a verbal description should be reported by the laboratory.

Because only 100–200 WBCs are counted, there is moderate to high imprecision. Imprecision is greater with cells found in low number (i.e. basophils, eosinophils, monocytes and non-segmented neutrophils).

Automated counting

The automated differential count is more precise than the manual differential count, especially for neutrophils and lymphocytes (Figure 12.1). Imprecision is measured by the coefficient of variation (CV). The CV values for the different methods will change with different blood samples, based on the number of different types of leucocyte in the blood. Precision is best with neutrophils, which are normally present in the greatest numbers. Cells found in low numbers (< 5–10%) are associated with the most imprecision in enumeration. Subjectivity in differentiating immature neutrophils from segmented neutrophils and the usually low numbers of non-segmented neutrophils cause great imprecision when counting non-segmented neutrophils. When there are also toxic changes in neutrophils and reactive changes in lymphocytes and monocytes, imprecision can be so great that a specific number (% or absolute number) should not be released from a laboratory. In this situation a verbal description of the cells can allow a reasonable diagnosis, or the conclusion of severe inflammation, to be drawn. Guidelines for acceptable imprecision based on background intra-individual variation for human leucocytes help in interpretation

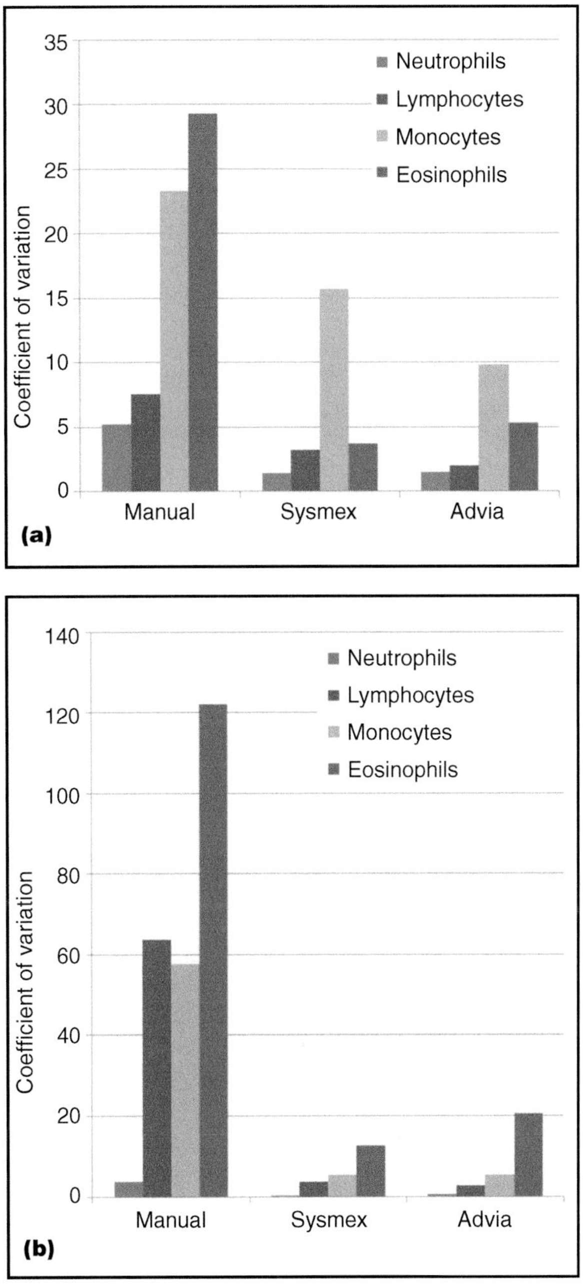

12.1 Imprecision in differential leucocyte counts for three commonly employed methods. Two canine blood samples (a and b) were analysed consecutively 10 times by each method. The manual differential count included 100 WBCs. The Sysmex XT 2000iV and Advia 2120 are automated haematology instruments with veterinary software that perform an automated differential count on thousands of WBCs using a laser-based, flow cytometric system. The automated counts were more precise than the manual count, but still had moderate imprecision for monocytes **(a)** and eosinophils **(b)**. Automated differential monocyte counts had a CV of 10–16% (a), which indicates greater imprecision than achieved by manual differential counts for neutrophils and lymphocytes for that sample. Note that the blood in (b) gave greater imprecision for manual differential counts of lymphocytes (CV 64%), monocytes (CV 58%) and especially eosinophils (CV 122%). The Advia machine also had greater imprecision for eosinophils (CV 21%), as did the Sysmex machine (CV 12%) for sample (b). The greater imprecision in (b) was caused by lymphopenia and severe eosinopenia.

of the CV values in Figure 12.1. Kjelgaard-Hansen and Jensen (2006) suggested that the maximal acceptable imprecision should be 8.1% for neutrophils, 5.2% for lymphocytes, 8.9% for monocytes, 10.5% for eosinophils and 14% for basophils.

Application to diagnosis

Diagnosis and interpretation of disease changes require both total WBC and absolute counts of each leucocyte type. Because of imprecision and sporadic errors in the manual and automated differential counts, veterinary surgeons must use prominent changes in numbers of leucocyte types in diagnosis and when monitoring patient progress.

Two examples from Rumke (1978), a statistician who calculated 95% confidence intervals for variation around a true percentage of a leucocyte type in a differential count based on the number of cells counted, are as follows:

- If there were 2% of a cell type (e.g. eosinophils) in a blood sample, then the 95% confidence limits would be 0.2–7.0, 1.2–3.1 or 1.7–2.3 if 100, 1000 or 10,000 cells were identified, respectively. Most manual differential counts are based on 100 WBCs, so with a sample containing 2% eosinophils, the reported results would be 0 to 7%
- If there were 20% of a cell type (e.g. lymphocytes) in a blood sample, the 95% confidence limits would be 12.7–29.2, 17.6–22.6 or 19.2–20.8 if 100, 1000 or 10,000 cells were identified, respectively. Similarly, a manual 100-cell differential count on a blood sample containing 20% lymphocytes could report 13–29% lymphocytes. Thus a difference of more than twofold is attributable just to sampling (statistical) error.

Although more precise, the automated differential count is also susceptible to errors and omissions. No current instrument can detect basophils in the dog or cat. No automated instrument enumerates non-segmented neutrophils, and there may be sporadic errors in identifying eosinophils or monocytes. Some instruments provide only a three-part differential count, which often means only an estimate of neutrophil and lymphocyte numbers. Enumeration of non-segmented neutrophils is a major criterion for identification of a left shift and therefore inflammation in the patient, so should be included in at least the first haematological evaluation of a sick patient.

Given that the automated differential count is more precise, it is the preferred method for following changes in numbers of a leucocyte type with treatment and time, if the instrument used can identify the cell type in question effectively. Because the manual differential performed by a competent haematologist should detect all cell types in a blood sample, it should be used to evaluate ill patients during the initial diagnosis.

Leucocyte pools

Interpretation of leucocyte numbers requires consideration of rates of production, cell death within the bone marrow or lymphoid organ, emigration from blood into tissues and the distribution of cells in conceptual areas called 'pools'.

Neutrophils are the main cell type in the blood of dogs and cats and the pool concept refers mainly to changes in neutrophil numbers. Neutrophil labelling studies by Prasse *et al.* (1973) in the dog and cat showed the cat to be quite different from the dog (and other species; Figure 12.2). The total blood neutrophil pool (TBNP) is the number of neutrophils in the vascular system. The TBNP is divided into the circulating (CBNP) and marginating (MBNP) pools. The CBNP includes those neutrophils that are circulating freely in the blood and are therefore collected in a blood sample at the time of venepuncture. In the dog and in most other species there is a similar number of neutrophils that are in the vascular system, but that are not collected during venepuncture. These are loosely associated with endothelial cells and are called marginated cells, in the MBNP. Prasse (1973) showed that the cat has a much greater number of neutrophils in the MBNP and thus has much greater potential to shift neutrophils from the MBNP to the CBNP. This observation is used to explain why cats have a much more prominent physiological leucocytosis (adrenaline-associated fear response) than dogs.

Pool	Dog	Cat
Total blood neutrophil pool (TBNP)	10.2 (100%)	28.9 (100%)
Circulating neutrophil pool (CNP)	5.4 (53%)	7.8 (27%)
Marginal neutrophil pool (MNP)	4.8 (47%)	21.0 (73%)

12.2 Neutrophil pools in the dog and cat. The number of neutrophils is given as cells x 10^8/kg body weight, with percentage of the total blood neutrophil pool in parentheses.

Shifts of leucocytes into tissues affect the balance of input and removal of neutrophils. The greatest removal of neutrophils occurs with inflammation of large surfaces such as the gut (e.g. in parvovirus enteritis) or peritoneum (e.g. with a ruptured gut) and not with local inflammation such as in an abscess.

The bone marrow may be divided into production, maturation and storage pools. The dog and cat have a large storage pool of neutrophils (about a 5 days' supply) and can release neutrophils quickly into the blood. Therefore neutropenia is unexpected in acute inflammation and suggests a poor prognosis. Neutropenia can be observed experimentally in dogs by the use of leucophoresis (a method used to remove neutrophils from the blood), but this neutropenia is so short lived that it is not seen in clinical patients. Canine parvovirus enteritis commonly causes neutropenia early in the infection owing to a combination of a tremendous loss of neutrophils through the damaged gut mucosa and viral damage to the bone marrow cells.

Leucocyte responses in inflammation

Left shift

The interpretation that a dog or cat has an inflammatory disease is most specifically and definitely indicated by a left shift, defined as an increase in more immature, non-segmented neutrophils (Cowell and Decker, 2000; Schultze, 2000). However, the differentiation of non-segmented (bands) from mature segmented neutrophils is highly subjective and one of the most imprecise tests in haematology. Imprecision in the classification of non-segmented neutrophils is reflected by a CV that is often 50% or more.

The reference value for canine non-segmented neutrophils is < 0.3–0.5 × 10^9/l in most laboratories, but using 1.0 × 10^9/l is a better threshold for identifying a left shift, owing to imprecision and subjectivity in the test.

Many people are hesitant to identify non-segmented neutrophils, which can make some laboratories appear to have less sensitivity in identifying patients with inflammation. Some laboratories report 'hyposegmentation' when they see more immature neutrophils, but hesitate in reporting them as non-segmented cells. Clinicians may complement a haematology test with measurement of acute phase protein concentrations (e.g. C-reactive protein (CRP) in dogs or serum amyloid A (SAA) in cats) to improve sensitivity in detecting inflammatory processes. Acute phase protein changes in inflammation will also increase the amount of rouleaux in canine blood and the erythrocyte sedimentation rate.

The severity of the left shift reflects severity of the inflammation. Greater increases in non-segmented cells indicate more severe inflammation and a greater demand for neutrophils from the bone marrow. As the storage pool is depleted, younger neutrophils are released from the marrow. If the number of non-segmented cells exceeds that of segmented cells, this is termed a 'degenerative left shift' and is one indicator of a poor prognosis. Increasing numbers of the more immature neutrophil stages also indicate more severe inflammation. Neutrophil stages, in reverse order of maturity, are: segmented; band; metamyelocyte; myelocyte; progranulocyte; and myeloblast. Left shifts usually involve increases in bands only. Increasing numbers of metamyelocytes and even myelocytes indicate that the animal is reaching deeper into the bone marrow to supply adequate neutrophils to match the need for the inflammatory response, and therefore a more severe problem is present. If progranulocytes and myeloblasts are seen, there is reason to consider myeloid leukaemia or myelodysplasia.

A left shift in itself does not indicate a worse prognosis, but the magnitude of increased non-segmented cells is compared with the magnitude of the neutrophilia and leucocytosis. A mild to moderate left shift of 1–4 × 10^9/l is expected and if there are clearly more segmented neutrophils than non-segmented cells, the bone marrow is responding well. Left shifts are most likely early in an inflammatory response, before the bone marrow has had a chance to develop myeloid hyperplasia and increase neutrophil production sufficient to match the demand for neutrophils in the tissues. With time (a few days), myeloid hyperplasia allows the degree of left shift and leucocytosis to return towards normal. Chronic or mild inflammation may not be associated with leucocytosis or a left shift.

Lymphopenia

Lymphopenia is expected as a result of the stress of inflammation, especially during the acute stages of inflammation. Persistent or recurrent lymphopenia during the course of subacute to chronic inflammation indicates persistent or recurrent occurrence of the stress of active inflammation. The return of lymphocyte counts to normal is a positive prognostic sign. Lymphopenia is the most common change in leucocyte number in patient blood and is seen in a wide variety of acute and chronic diseases with inflammatory or non-inflammatory causes.

Lymphocytosis

Differentiation of acute *versus* chronic inflammation on the basis only of haematological results is difficult.

Monocytosis may be seen in more chronic inflammation involving macrophages, but monocytosis in dogs is as often caused by glucocorticoid treatment and occurs 2–12 hours after treatment (Figure 12.3). If lymphocytosis is seen during an inflammatory disease, this suggests a more chronic process in which an immune stimulus has caused lymphoid hyperplasia. Lymphocytosis is seen with chronic fungal, bacterial or protozoal infections (Schultze, 2000). Lymphocytosis may be as high as 17–30 × 10^9/l with *Ehrlichia canis* infection or 9 × 10^9/l in *Toxoplasma gondii* infection in cats (Avery and Avery, 2007). Lymphocytosis may be milder (e.g. 4.5 × 10^9/l) during later phases of the recovery from *Anaplasma phagocytophilum* infection in dogs. Despite these examples, Avery and Avery (2007) described lymphocytosis as not being common in chronic infections in dogs and cats. Lymphocytosis up to 20 × 10^9/l was seen in 9 of 22 cats with immune-mediated haemolytic anaemia (IMHA), but not in canine cases of this disease. Lymphocytosis up to 13 × 10^9/l and 9 × 10^9/l may be seen in dogs and cats, respectively, with hypoadrenocorticism, although lymphocytosis occurs in only 5–10% of such patients (Avery and Avery, 2007). Lymphocytosis is seen with the adrenaline-related fear response in young, healthy cats and with various lymphoid neoplasms and leukaemia, and it is therefore not specific for chronic immune stimulation. The maximal values for the above examples of lymphocytosis should not be taken to be commonly expected values. Lymphocytosis is more often closer to the upper limits of the reference values. Maximal values are useful, however, in avoiding a diagnosis

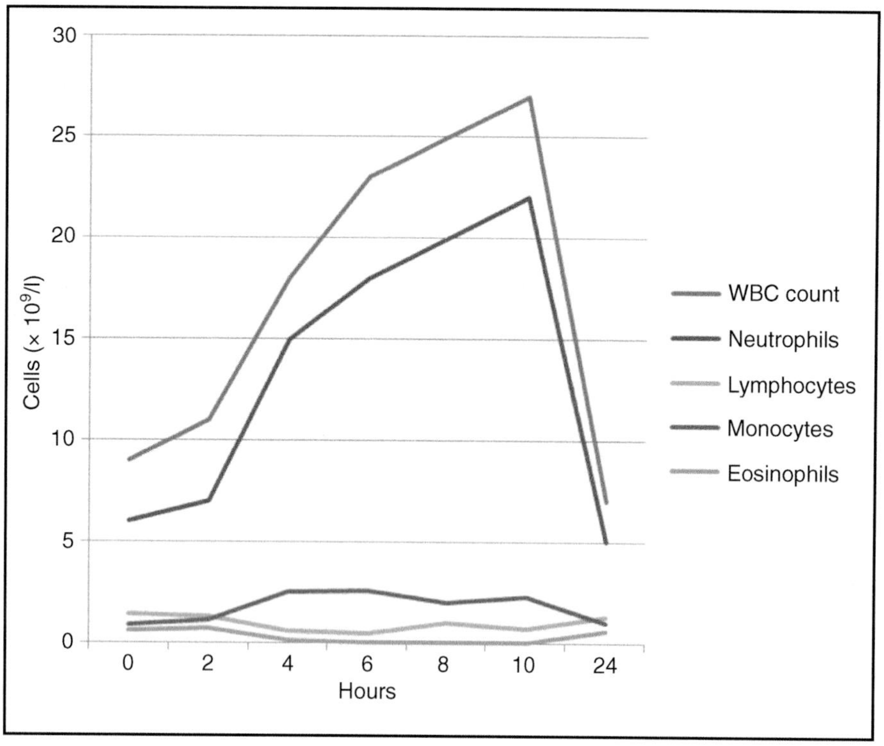

12.3 Responses of leucocytes (cells × 10^9/l on *y* axis) over time (hours on *x* axis) following administration of a single dose of 20 mg prednisolone (2.2 mg/kg) to a dog. Leucocytosis, neutrophilia, monocytosis, lymphopenia and eosinopenia occurred for 2–10 hours after treatment, with a return to baseline values at 24 hours. (Created with data from Jasper, 1965)

of lymphoid leukaemia in patients with lymphocytosis, but without neoplasia.

Reactive lymphocytes

Reactive lymphocytes appear larger, more immature and usually have much darker blue cytoplasm than routine lymphocytes. These may be called variant lymphocytes, blast transformed, atypical, virocytes or immunocytes. Reactive lymphocytes are commonly seen in small numbers in the blood of patients. They reflect immune stimulation, but unfortunately the presence and number of reactive lymphocytes does not seem to be correlated consistently with the degree of immune stimulation. Certainly there are often increased numbers of very reactive lymphocytes in the blood of patients with severe infections and toxaemia. Even asymptomatic dogs and cats can have several reactive lymphocytes. Reactive lymphocytes unfortunately make blood smear evaluation a non-specific and insensitive test for the detection of malignant lymphoma and leukaemia. Reactive lymphocytes are often immature and have other atypical morphology; therefore when found in low numbers (e.g. two to seven per blood smear) they cannot be used to suggest lymphoma in patients with clinical suspicion of lymphoma. Certain diagnosis of lymphoid leukaemia requires either a very large number of lymphocytes (> 30–40 × 10^9/l) or, if they are at least moderate in number, then most or all of them should clearly be very immature. If the lymphoid population appears very monotonous in appearance, that too supports a monoclonal proliferation and is likely to indicate leukaemia.

Prognostic indicators

The prognosis depends on which tissue or organ is affected and the cause of inflammation, but prognosis is also determined by the haematological characteristics of the leucocyte response:

- If the leucocytosis and left shift are mild to moderate and fairly typical in magnitude for the species, then the conclusion is that inflammation is present, without any strong reason to have a poor prognosis attached
- If the degree of left shift or leucocytosis is unusually high or low, this indicates a poor prognosis.

Leucopenia is unexpected in a dog or cat with most inflammatory diseases. Dogs and cats have very responsive bone marrow with a storage pool of about 5 normal days of neutrophil consumption and can release increased numbers of neutrophils within minutes to hours. Thus, leucopenia (or a degenerative left shift) indicates a poor prognosis. A leucopenia indicates an unusually great utilization of neutrophils, and possibly an additional problem with bone marrow production of neutrophils. Concurrent lymphopenia in the stressed animal usually contributes to the severity of leucopenia. One of the more common causes of leucopenia and neutropenia in dogs is parvovirus enteritis, in which there is loss of neutrophils into the inflamed intestine plus an effect of the virus on the bone marrow. An improved prognosis is indicated by a rapid disappearance of the left shift and toxic changes in neutrophils and return of the number of neutrophils and lymphocytes towards normal values.

Leukaemoid response

An excessive leucocyte response to inflammation is called a leukaemoid (leukaemia-like) response because the increase in leucocyte count is so great

(> 50–100 × 10^9/l in the dog and 30–75 × 10^9/l in the cat) that leukaemia needs to be considered. Inflammation commonly causes leucocytosis of about 20–30 × 10^9/l in the dog and cat. Excessive responses indicate something unusual and thus a worse prognosis.

Even in the presence of huge numbers of neutrophils, the primary problem is not being corrected for some reason. This may be an anatomical problem such as pyometra or an abscess from which the infection and pus are not able to drain, or that antibiotics fail to reach the centre of the lesion. In canine leucocyte adhesion deficiency (CD11/CD18 deficiency) the neutrophils cannot kill bacteria, even in the presence of massive numbers of neutrophils, as they are unable to exit the bloodstream. Extreme leucocytosis may occur in haemolytic anaemias such as in IMHA, or with infections by *Babesia canis* and *Mycoplasma haemofelis*. This may be caused by inflammatory mediators released from macrophages in response to necrosis in tissues deprived of oxygen. *Hepatozoon* infections uniquely stimulate leukaemoid reactions in dogs.

Leukaemoid reactions are difficult to differentiate from chronic myelogenous leukaemia in the absence of a typical cause of a leukaemoid reaction. Chronic myelogenous leukaemia also mainly involves the more mature stages of the neutrophil lineage. Paraneoplastic syndromes of various neoplasms are rare causes of leukaemoid reactions.

Leucocyte morphology

The prognosis is also affected by the morphology of leucocytes. A specific grading scale for reporting the severity of toxic change has been reported (Aroch, 2005). Simpler guidelines include the presence of Döhle bodies (small dull blue cytoplasmic inclusions) in cases with mild toxicity, especially in cats. An advantage of the detection of Döhle bodies is that they are not an artefact of stored EDTA blood, so their presence is a definitive toxic change. Neutrophils in stored EDTA blood do develop vacuoles and a more blue-staining cytoplasm, which may be misclassified as toxic change. Moderate toxicity is indicated by increasing cytoplasmic basophilia and foaminess. The foamy cytoplasm is known as toxic vacuolation, but there are no distinct membrane-bound vacuoles. Instead, this toxic change relates to irregular clearing of the darker blue cytoplasm. Distinct cytoplasmic vacuoles are artefacts of storage of EDTA blood. Severe toxicity is recognized when neutrophils become too toxic to distinguish from reactive lymphocytes and reactive monocytes.

Toxic change in neutrophils is an indicator of poor prognosis. Case fatality, hospitalization length, and treatment cost were significantly higher in dogs with neutrophil toxicity (Aroch, 2005). Dogs with toxic neutrophils and leucopenia (< 5.0 × 10^9/l) had a significantly higher case fatality rate when compared with dogs with normal or high leucocyte counts.

Toxic change in feline neutrophils was associated with more severe clinical signs (e.g. fever, vomiting, diarrhoea and depression) than in cats without toxic change (Segev *et al.*, 2006). Cats with toxic neutrophils had severe diseases such as pneumonia, peritonitis, upper respiratory tract infections, shock and sepsis as well as haematological changes of inflammation such as left shift, leucocytosis, neutrophilia or leucopenia. Toxic change in neutrophils indicated more severe disease, longer hospitalization and a greater likelihood of bacterial infection in both cats and dogs. Dogs had even more severe changes than cats, suggesting that toxic neutrophils in cats are associated with milder diseases. About half of the cats reported by Segev *et al.* (2006) with toxic neutrophils had normal WBC and neutrophil counts, therefore toxic neutrophils may be the only haematological marker of inflammation and infection. Veterinary surgeons should not rely only on the results from automated haematology instruments, especially those with only a 'three part differential', to differentiate normal from seriously ill animals consistently. Subjective information from a blood smear adds greatly to diagnostic sensitivity.

Eosinophilia

Eosinophilia is defined as an increase in eosinophils above reference values, which vary from 0–0.8 × 10^9/l to 0–1.3 × 10^9/l. Reference values can be affected by subclinical parasite infestations in the reference population, or the fact that the distribution of absolute eosinophil numbers in normal animals is skewed to the right and is not normal. The estimation of a 95% interval for reference values requires omitting high eosinophil counts from apparently normal animals in the reference population or classifying these high values as 'outliers'. Eosinophilia may be seen in asymptomatic animals. Eosinopenia is difficult to detect because a 100 cell manual differential leucocyte count often fails to include any eosinophils. Reference values are therefore often reported as 0 to an upper limit. Variation in eosinophil peroxidase activity may adversely affect detection of eosinophils by automated instruments. Stress and glucocorticoid treatment cause a decrease in eosinophil numbers, which may obscure or diminish eosinophilia in diseases that cause eosinophilia. Decreased blood cortisol in hypoadrenocorticism may lead to the opposite effect of eosinophilia and lymphocytosis.

Eosinophilic inflammation may cause eosinophilia. Eosinophils kill parasites, therefore many parasitic diseases cause eosinophilia. Eosinophils suppress immune responses as well as causing severe tissue damage in immune responses. However, the list of causes of eosinophilic inflammation and eosinophilia is very long, diverse and includes many diseases that are not associated with parasitism or allergy (Lilliehook and Tvedten, 2003). Hypereosinophilia is defined as eosinophils > 5 × 10^9/l and eosinophil leukaemoid reactions as > 25–30 × 10^9/l. Thus eosinophilia can cause leucocytosis. Hypereosinophilic syndrome, eosinophil leukaemia and paraneoplastic syndromes with eosinophilia all contribute to confusion in the diagnosis of causes of eosinophilia. Eosinopenia is common during different types of inflammation, but this is usually not noticed because normal animals have few eosinophils and other changes distract attention from any eosinopenia.

Monocytosis

Monocytes are the immature blood form of tissue macrophages, and monocytosis can occur in chronic inflammatory diseases that involve tissue infiltration by macrophages. Such granulomatous inflammation is associated with necrosis, malignant neoplasia, haemolytic anaemia (e.g. IMHA where large numbers of damaged red blood cells (RBCs) are removed by macrophages) and infections (e.g. with fungi). Many of these processes are more chronic, so some veterinary surgeons interpret monocytosis to indicate chronic inflammation, but glucocorticoid treatment commonly induces monocytosis with a peak at about 8–10 hours in dogs (see Figure 12.3).

Basophilia

Basophils are so rare in normal dogs and cats that the mention of any basophils on a haematology report indicates basophilia. Basophilia is not rare in dogs. In an unpublished study of 108 canine patients we found 1–17.5% basophils in 8 of the 108 dogs. Basophilia is unlikely to cause leucocytosis. Basophilia is usually associated with eosinophilia, and interpretation in these cases is based mainly on the eosinophilia. Basophilia alone may be associated with lipaemia and disorders of lipid metabolism because heparin from basophils has a role in clearing fat from blood. Basophils can kill ticks attached to the skin (at least in cattle). Basophilia may be seen in animals with neoplasia (e.g. mast cell tumours and myeloproliferative diseases).

Basophil counts are often erroneous. Basophils in canine blood smears are often misidentified as monocytes because their granules often do not stain well. Basophils in feline blood smears are often misidentified as eosinophils with pale granules. Basophils are not detected at all in automated differential counts made by the current veterinary haematology analysers (listed earlier).

Non-inflammatory causes of leucocytosis

Two common non-inflammatory causes of leucocytosis are the glucocorticoid-associated stress response and the adrenaline-associated fear response. The former is mediated by glucocorticoids either given therapeutically (exogenous) or derived from the adrenal cortex during stress (endogenous). Stress may also be caused by inflammation and other severe diseases.

Glucocorticoid-associated stress response

Both dogs and cats have a similar response to glucocorticoids, although the feline response is milder and the monocytosis is not as pronounced (see Figures 12.3 and 12.4; Jasper and Jain, 1965; Jain, 1986). The glucocorticoid-associated stress response may be triggered by treatment with a glucocorticoid. Responses to prednisolone, dexamethasone and adrenocorticotropic hormone (ACTH) seem to be similar, suggesting a general trigger to the response instead of an effect related to the dose or type of glucocorticoid. The release of ACTH mimics the endogenous stress response in the animal. Chronic stress or repeated, long-term treatment with a glucocorticoid gives a different leucocyte response that is mainly characterized by persistent lymphopenia and

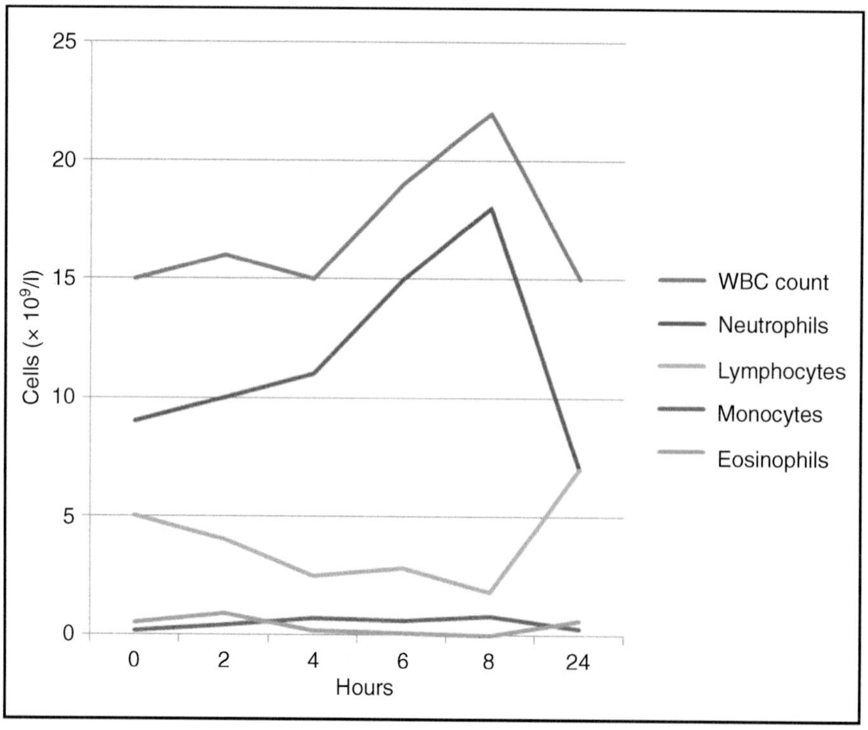

12.4 Responses of leucocytes (cells × 10^9/l on *y* axis) over time (hours on *x* axis) following administration of a single dose of 5 mg of prednisolone to a cat. Leucocytosis, neutrophilia and lymphopenia occurred for 2–8 hours after treatment, with a return to baseline values at 24 hours. Eosinophils and monocytes remained within reference values with a tendency toward eosinopenia and monocytosis. (Created with data from Jain, 1986)

eosinopenia. Eosinopenia is hard to detect, so this means that lymphopenia is more important in indicating chronic stress or glucocorticoid treatment.

The canine glucocorticoid-associated stress response has maximal effect at about 8–12 hours and typically includes a moderate leucocytosis (15–25 × 10^9/l; rarely 40 × 10^9/l) that reflects mainly a mature neutrophilia without left shift and is partially due to a monocytosis (1.5–2.5 × 10^9/l) with a lymphopenia and eosinopenia (see Figures 12.3 and 12.4). The feline response is similar, although milder and often without a noticeable monocytosis. Rarely cats may have WBC counts up to 30 × 10^9/l. The absence of a left shift helps to differentiate the glucocorticoid-associated stress response from an acute inflammatory response. Both typically involve lymphopenia. Hypersegmentation may be seen with the glucocorticoid-associated stress response, reflecting a longer half-life of neutrophils in the blood. Glucocorticoid treatment does increase bone marrow release of neutrophils, but usually not enough to cause a left shift because the storage pool is usually sufficient to provide mature neutrophils.

Adrenaline-associated fear response

The adrenaline-associated fear response (physiological leucocytosis) is seen most often in healthy, and especially young, cats and is a transient effect. Adrenaline (epinephrine) release causes contraction of the spleen, increased blood pressure and leucocytes to be less adherent, all of which cause a redistribution of cells (lymphocytes, neutrophils and erythrocytes) into the circulating pool (see Figure 12.2), which is reflected by the cells present in the EDTA blood sample. The lymphocytosis of the adrenaline-associated fear response helps to differentiate it from the glucocorticoid-associated stress response and an acute inflammatory response, in which there would typically be lymphopenia. The response occurs immediately, before a blood sample can be taken. It probably dissipates over 20–60 minutes, but this is difficult to study when fear is a major stimulus of the response. The leucocytosis of the adrenaline-associated fear response is so mild in the dog that it is unlikely to be detected, but it may be noted in research studies with repeated sampling of dogs. Dogs have a more contractile spleen than cats, so the increase in haematocrit (Hct) is more prominent in dogs. About 20% of the blood volume is stored in the spleen, so splenic contraction can cause polycythaemia. Lymphocytes come from the splenic contraction and lymphocytosis may be more prominent than neutrophilia. Cats often have leucocytosis of about 20 × 10^9/l with lymphocyte counts of 6–15 × 10^9/l. Rare examples of the adrenaline-associated fear response can have absolute lymphocyte counts up to 20 × 10^9/l (Cowell and Decker, 2000). This marked lymphocytosis could in an individual blood sample be confused with chronic lymphocytic leukaemia or a marked chronic immune response. The adrenaline-associated fear response may be the reason that reference values for young cats have higher lymphocyte counts than in adults.

Leucopenia

Leucopenia has been discussed above under Inflammation, but it may also be caused by a variety of bone marrow problems. If bicytopenia or especially pancytopenia is present, it is highly likely that bone marrow production is abnormal. Aplastic pancytopenia of bone marrow origin should have anaemia that is non-regenerative and neutropenia without a left shift. Interpretation is affected by time, in that a bone marrow-induced leucopenia and neutropenia will precede a septicaemia by some days. If a serious infection has caused the neutropenia the animal should concurrently have severe clinical signs. Interpretation is more difficult in a seriously ill animal, because inflammation and infection may cause hypercoagulopathy with secondary thrombocytopenia and non-regenerative anaemia caused by inflammation.

Bone marrow aspiration in leucopenia and pancytopenia may be difficult if the bone marrow is very hypocellular (i.e. fatty marrow). The most important distinction is to determine whether the lack of cells in the sample reflects a poor quality sample or a real reduction in the number of cells in the bone marrow. For this reason it is often useful to take a core biopsy specimen from animals with pancytopenia in which the bone marrow may consist mainly of fat. However, bone marrow biopsy is no guarantee of a successful diagnosis because many biopsy samples are non-diagnostic and do not contain bone marrow. Aspiration and biopsy may provide a definite diagnosis in conditions such as leukaemia, aplastic pancytopenia, myelodysplastic syndrome or myelofibrosis. A common and confusing conclusion from bone marrow evaluation is 'ineffective haemopoiesis,' which is often reported when the bone marrow has normal to increased numbers of haemopoietic cells and the haemopoietic cells appear morphologically normal, but there is pancytopenia, bicytopenia or deficiency of a single cell type in the blood. This means that cells produced in the marrow die in the marrow (probably via apoptosis) and are not effectively released into the blood. The causes of ineffective haemopoiesis are often not obvious, but can include adverse affects of different types of medication, infections or myelodysplasia.

Nucleated erythrocytes

Nucleated red blood cells (nRBCs) are not leucocytes but, as nucleated cells, they are included in the total nucleated cell count (TNCC). The TNCC is reported as the total WBC count by most haematology instruments.

The nRBCs, when present, are often in low numbers (e.g. < 5 nRBC/100 WBC) and thus do not affect the clinical interpretation of leucocyte numbers in blood. Occasionally, nRBCs are present in large numbers (this is termed normoblastaemia).

Most automated haematology instruments do not differentiate nRBCs from WBCs and therefore a manual differential leucocyte count is used to determine the number of nRBCs per 100 WBCs. The proportion is used to determine a corrected WBC count (cWBC) that reflects only the number of leucocytes:

$$\frac{\text{TNCC}}{(100 + \text{nRBC})} = \frac{\text{cWBC}}{100}$$

where TNCC = instrument's displayed WBC count, cWBC = corrected leucocyte count, and nRBC = number of nRBCs observed while counting 100 WBCs in a manual differential leucocyte count.

More commonly, the equation is presented as:

$$\text{Corrected WBC} = \text{TNCC} \times 100/(100 + \text{nRBC})$$

The nRBCs are seen routinely as part of the regenerative response to anaemia, but should be evaluated critically when increased in the absence of reticulocytosis and polychromasia. Causes of increased nRBCs include factors that affect the endothelial lining of the bone marrow (e.g. sepsis, toxaemia and heat stroke) and factors that affect the spleen (e.g. hyperadrenocorticism and extramedullary haemopoiesis). Myeloproliferative disorders may cause large increases in nRBCs, and other causes include haemangiosarcoma and hepatic lipidosis. The nRBCs are usually reported as nRBC/100 WBC, but this is a relative number and affected by the total WBC count. Sepsis and endotoxaemia also cause leucopenia, so the relative ratio of NRBC/100 WBC may seem very high. The absolute number of nRBCs $\times 10^9$/l is easily determined from the correction of the TNCC to corrected WBC count. The TNCC minus the corrected WBC count equals the absolute nRBC count $\times 10^9$/l. Absolute cell counts are always easier to interpret than ratios and percentages (relative counts).

Leukaemia

Leukaemia is discussed in detail in Chapter 16. Briefly, leukaemia can be classified as leukaemic, subleukaemic and aleukaemic. Leukaemia is a proliferation of neoplastic cells in the bone marrow. The neoplastic cells may be retained in the marrow and not released into peripheral blood. Leukaemic leukaemia has a prominent increase of neoplastic cells in the peripheral blood. Subleukaemic leukaemia has a few neoplastic cells in the peripheral blood, and aleukaemic leukaemia has no leukaemic cells in peripheral blood. This means that leucocytosis may be seen in leukaemic leukaemia, but not in subleukaemic or aleukaemic leukaemia. Routine haematology will not detect aleukaemic leukaemia. Given that many sick patients without leukaemia will have a few to moderate numbers of immature reactive lymphocytes (or even myeloid cells or erythroid cells), the detection of a few immature cells in peripheral blood is not specific proof of leukaemia. Haematology is not a sensitive test for the diagnosis of malignant lymphoma. The diagnosis is much more likely to be made from cytological examination of enlarged lymph nodes or other solid tumours.

Drug treatments

Drug treatments may affect leucocyte numbers by causing leucopenia, leucocytosis or changes in individual cell types. Bone marrow toxicity is a common reason why promising drugs never reach the market. Cytopenia can be a direct toxic effect, or an immune-mediated or other indirect effect. A potential drug effect that causes haematological changes in patients being treated with that drug should be considered, with possible withdrawal of the drug to check for improvement. There are too many adverse drug effects to list here, but some common examples of drugs that cause leucopenia and neutropenia are phenylbutazone, chloramphenicol, griseofulvin, oestrogen, trimethoprim/sulfadiazine, phenobarbital and the chemotherapeutic drugs.

References and further reading

Aroch I, Klement E and Segev G (2005) Clinical, biochemical and hematological characteristics, disease prevalence and prognosis of dogs presenting with neutrophil cytoplasmic toxicity. *Journal of Veterinary Internal Medicine* **19**, 64–73

Avery AC and Avery PC (2007) Determining the significance of persistent lymphocytosis. *Veterinary Clinics of North America: Small Animal Practice* **37**, 267–282

Cowell RL and Decker LS (2000) Interpretation of feline leucocyte responses. In: *Schalm's Veterinary Hematology, 5th edn*, ed. BF Feldman, JG Zinkl and NC Jain, pp. 382–390. Lippincott Williams & Wilkins, Philadelphia

Jain NC (1986) The dog: Normal haematology with comments on response to disease. In: *Schalm's Veterinary Hematology, 4th edn*, pp.103–125. Lea & Febiger, Philadelphia

Jasper DE and Jain NC (1965) The influence of adrenocorticotropic hormone and prednisolone upon the marrow and circulation leucocytes in the dog. *American Journal of Veterinary Research* **26**, 844

Kjelgaard-Hansen M and Jensen AL (2006) Is the inherent imprecision of manual leucocyte differential counts acceptable for quantitative purposes? (Letter) *Veterinary Clinical Pathology* **35**, 268–269

Lilliehook I and Tvedten H (2003) Investigation of hypereosinophilia and potential treatments. *Veterinary Clinics of North America: Small Animal Practice* **33**, 1359–1378

Prasse KW, Kaeberle ML and Ramsey FK (1973) Blood neutrophilic granulocyte kinetics in cats. *American Journal of Veterinary Research* **34**, 1021

Rumke CL (1978) The statistically expected variability in differential leucocyte counting. In: *Differential Leucocyte Counting*, ed. JA Koepke, pp. 69–80. College of American Pathologists, Stokie, Illinois

Schultze AE (2000) Interpretation of canine leucocyte responses In: *Schalm's Veterinary Hematology, 5th edn*, ed. BF Feldman, JG Zinkl and NC Jain, pp. 366–381. Lippincott Williams & Wilkins, Philadelphia

Segev G, Klement E and Aroch I (2006) Toxic neutrophils in cats: Clinical and clinicopathologic features, and disease prevalence and outcome – A retrospective case control study. *Journal of Veterinary Internal Medicine* **20**, 20–31

13

Disorders of leucocyte function

Michael J. Day†

Introduction

This chapter considers disorders in which persistent inflammatory or infectious disease is associated with functionally defective peripheral blood leucocytes. Such leucocyte function disorders may be divided broadly into those that are acquired in adult animals and congenital diseases of younger animals that are likely to have an inherited basis. The former are relatively more common and occur as part of a wide spectrum of metabolic or infectious diseases, or secondary to drug therapy. By contrast, congenital leucocyte function defects are rarely encountered in small animals.

The apparent rarity of such diseases may in part reflect the lack of widely available means to diagnose them. Leucocyte function tests are generally only available in a research setting and access to them by veterinary surgeons in general practice is restricted. Despite this, it is generally inadvisable to submit samples from animals to laboratories that deal primarily with human diagnosis. There are specific requirements for the isolation of small animal leucocytes and the performance of *in vitro* testing, and the interpretation of such assays, is best performed by a veterinary immunologist. The laboratory will advise on the type of blood sample required and the volume of blood needed. In most instances the laboratory will require control samples from one or two clinically normal, age-matched animals that will be run in parallel with the test samples.

This chapter considers the range of *in vitro* assays established for the assessment of the function of neutrophils, monocyte–macrophages and lymphocytes in small animals. The situations in which abnormal function may reflect an acquired problem will be reviewed and the known primary, congenital leucocyte function defects discussed.

Tests of leucocyte function

The range of tests available for leucocyte function is summarized in Figure 13.1.

Tests of neutrophil function
• Neutrophil chemotaxis • Neutrophil phagocytosis and killing • Neutrophil respiratory burst after phagocytosis
Tests of monocyte/macrophage function
• Macrophage phagocytosis and killing
Tests of lymphocyte function
• Mitogen-driven lymphocyte proliferation • Antigen-driven lymphocyte proliferation • Cytokine protein or mRNA production by stimulated lymphocyte cultures • Antibody production by stimulated lymphocyte cultures • Cytotoxic killing of labelled target cells

13.1 Tests of leucocyte function.

Tests of neutrophil function

The neutrophil undertakes a variety of activities whilst participating in the inflammatory response *in vivo*. These cells must be mobilized from the bloodstream into extravascular tissue via molecular interactions mediated by adhesion molecules, attracted along chemotactic gradients to sites of inflammation, phagocytose appropriately opsonized particles or microorganisms and perform intracellular killing of such organisms via metabolic pathways involving oxygen-dependent and independent mechanisms. Each of these major neutrophil functions can be assessed by *in vitro* assays.

Isolation of peripheral blood neutrophils

A variety of methods have been described for the isolation of neutrophils from peripheral blood. One study has compared the viability and yield of neutrophils obtained following percoll gradient centrifugation, dextran sedimentation followed by centrifugation over ficoll or centrifugation through commercially available neutrophil isolation medium. The optimum protocol was dextran sedimentation followed by ficoll centrifugation, which yielded approximately 65% of the total number of neutrophils in the blood sample with a viability of 98% and neutrophil purity of 99% (Shearer and Day, 1997).

Neutrophil chemotaxis

Isolated neutrophils can migrate along chemotactic gradients established *in vitro* by various chemical agents, serum, cytokines, complement components or other inflammatory mediators. The most common means of assessing chemotaxis involve use of the

Boyden chamber or the under-agarose assay. In the former, neutrophils are placed into one side of a chamber separated from the chemotactic agent by a millipore filter through which the agent will diffuse. Neutrophils migrate towards, and are trapped within, the filter, which can be stained and examined microscopically. In the under-agarose assay, neutrophils placed into one well in an agarose gel migrate towards chemoattractant placed in a second well by moving beneath the gel. This movement is assessed microscopically.

Neutrophil phagocytosis and killing assays

In these assays, isolated neutrophils are incubated under specific conditions with a known number of particles (e.g. latex beads, yeast, bacteria) which have been opsonized previously with serum antibody and/or complement. Autologous serum (i.e. from the same animal) should be used in parallel with normal serum in order to detect any deficiency in the presence of opsonins. After a period of incubation, phagocytosis can be assessed by stopping the reaction and examining a stained preparation of cytocentrifuged cells. The number of neutrophils containing ingested particles or the number of particles per neutrophil can be measured. As an example, the effect of opsonization on the phagocytosis of *Staphylococcus intermedius* by canine neutrophils is shown in Figure 13.2 (Shearer and Day, 1997). Tests of phagocytosis may also be performed using a flow cytometer. Particles are labelled with a fluorescent marker and, following incubation with neutrophils, the cells are passed dropwise through the machine. Each cell is 'interrogated' by a laser beam and if the cell contains phagocytosed particles a burst of light will be emitted and recorded. Typically, the machine will evaluate 10,000 cells and report the percentage that has phagocytosed the target particles (Eickhoff *et al.*, 2004).

In vitro assays for the intracellular killing ability of canine neutrophils are also reported. Purified canine neutrophils are incubated with a known number of opsonized *S. intermedius* over a 90-minute time course. After phagocytosis has occurred (10 minutes), extracellular bacteria are lysed by the addition of specific enzyme (lysostaphin), and at various time points thereafter (0, 30, 60 and 90 minutes using quadruplicate samples) intracellular bacteria are released by osmotic lysis of the neutrophils. Serial dilutions of the viable intracellular bacteria are then plated onto nutrient agar and the number of colonies determined. The number of viable intracellular organisms at each time point is defined in terms of a fraction of the original number of phagocytosed organisms (100%), allowing a curve of intracellular killing kinetics to be produced (Figure 13.3).

Assessment of neutrophil respiratory burst

The respiratory burst of neutrophils following phagocytosis of particles can be assessed using the nitroblue tetrazolium (NBT) test or chemiluminescence assay. In the former, there is reduction of the colourless dye NBT to dark blue formazan, which can be assessed spectrophotometrically, and in the latter, the release of light during the oxidative burst is measured by a chemiluminometer or scintillation counter.

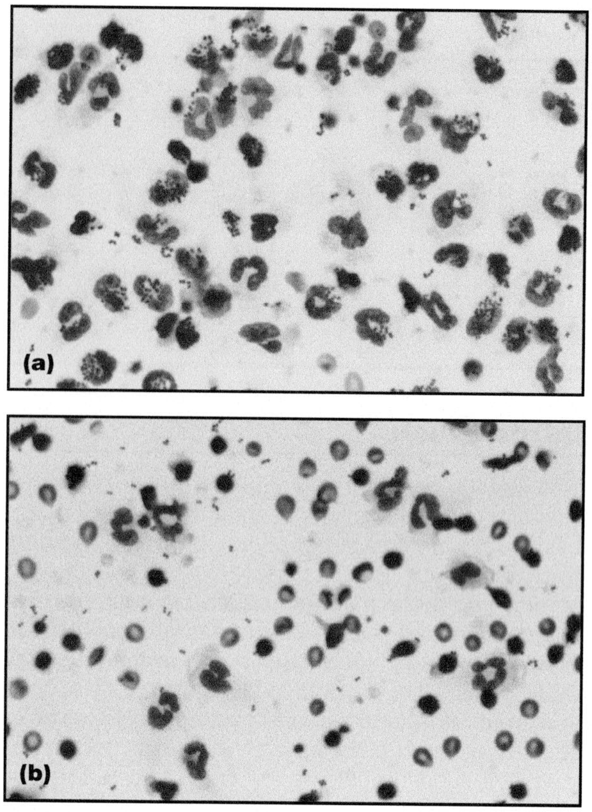

13.2 Neutrophils isolated from the peripheral blood of a normal dog were incubated with **(a)** *Staphylococcus intermedius* opsonized by fresh dog serum or **(b)** *S. intermedius* without prior serum opsonization. After 10 minutes the reactions were stopped by the addition of formal saline and the preparations cytocentrifuged. The neutrophils effectively phagocytose large numbers of opsonized organisms in (a), with a high proportion of neutrophils containing staphylococci and a significant number of staphylococci per neutrophil. By contrast, the unopsonized staphylococci in (b) are poorly phagocytosed.

Tests of monocyte–macrophage function

Peripheral blood monocytes will differentiate to become adherent macrophages during *in vitro* culture. The ability of these macrophages to phagocytose and kill organisms can be examined in a similar manner to the neutrophil assays described above. An *in vitro* assay for the ability of canine macrophages to phagocytose and kill the spores of *Aspergillus* was described (Day, 1987). Peripheral blood mononuclear cells were obtained by density gradient centrifugation and plated onto glass in culture medium. After 5–10 days of culture the adherent population were pure macrophages. Equal numbers of fungal spores and macrophages were co-cultured for 2 hours, following which extracellular spores were removed by aspiration and osmotic lysis of macrophages was performed to release adherent and phagocytosed spores. The percentage killing was then calculated. A similar phagocytic

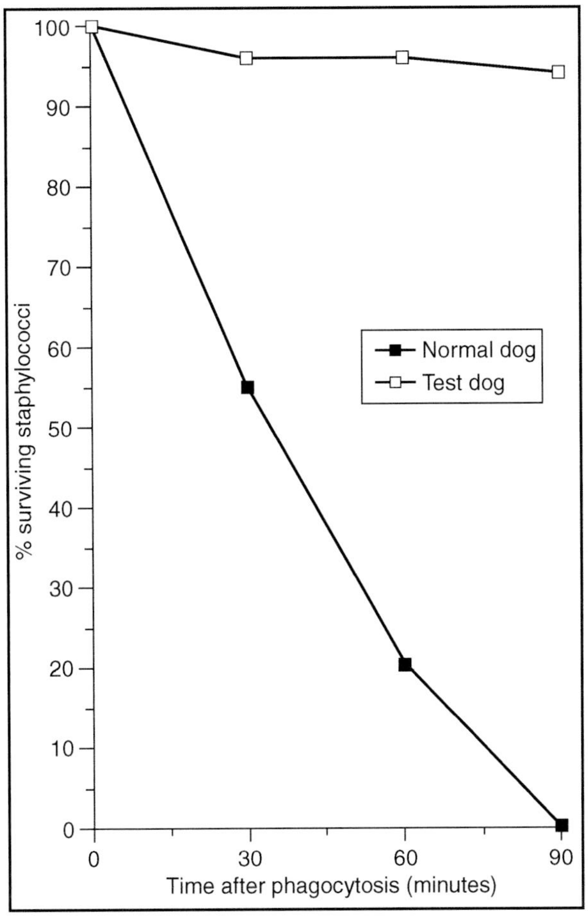

13.3 Assessment of *in vitro* neutrophil killing of *Staphylococcus intermedius*. Opsonized *S. intermedius* were incubated with neutrophils from a normal dog and a dog with a suspected neutrophil function defect (test dog). Phagocytosed organisms were killed progressively by the normal dog neutrophils over a 90-minute time course, but defective neutrophils were unable to kill the phagocytosed staphylococci.

assay using *Candida albicans* has been described for canine macrophages (DeBowes and Anderson, 1991).

Tests of lymphocyte function

Isolation of peripheral blood lymphocytes

Mononuclear cells can be isolated from peripheral blood by the process of density gradient centrifugation, which involves layering diluted blood on to medium such as ficoll–hypaque (Figure 13.4). The cells collected from the resulting interface are a mixture of T and B lymphocytes and monocytes, and the relative proportions of each can be assessed by flow cytometry following labelling with monoclonal antibodies specific for unique surface markers of these cells (Day, 2008). These populations can also be used for *in vitro* functional studies. In the first instance it is normal to perform preliminary assays on whole unfractionated mononuclear cell preparations and some assays have also been adapted for whole blood culture, eliminating the need for prior mononuclear cell enrichment. For more refined assays, it is possible to purify T and B lymphocytes or subsets of these cells selectively by methods such as panning, passage through nylon wool or immunoglobulin (Ig)–anti-Ig columns, erythrocyte rosetting, magnetic bead separation, cytotoxic depletion or cell sorting using the flow cytometer.

Lymphocyte proliferation assays

These assays assess the ability of lymphocytes to respond to *in vitro* stimulation by mitogens or antigens by measuring the incorporation of radiolabelled thymidine (^{3}H-thymidine) into the DNA of dividing cells. Mitogens are substances (often plant derived) that stimulate multiple clones of lymphocytes non-specifically by binding to surface carbohydrate molecules. Some mitogens appear to activate T lymphocytes preferentially (concanavalin A (ConA), phytohaemagglutinin (PHA)) whereas others will have an effect primarily on B lymphocytes (pokeweed mitogen (PWM), bacterial lipopolysaccharide (LPS), staphylococcal protein A). Lymphocytes are cultured with mitogen for a period of 48–72 hours and ^{3}H-thymidine is added to the cultures during the final 18 hours. The cells are

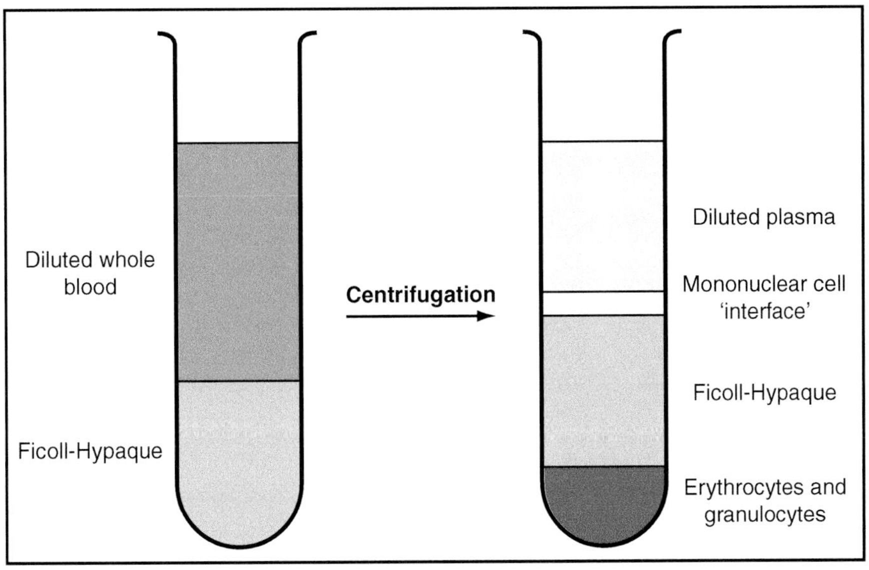

13.4 Isolation of peripheral blood mononuclear cells by separation over Ficoll–Hypaque. A diluted blood sample is overlaid on to density gradient medium (Ficoll–Hypaque, typical specific gravity 1.077). After centrifugation, there is separation as shown and the mononuclear cells at the interface can be aspirated with a Pasteur pipette.

harvested and the proportion of radiolabel taken up by dividing cells is determined, to give an index of stimulation relative to control cultures of mononuclear cells from clinically normal animals.

Such assays have been extended to enable *in vitro* stimulation using specific antigens that will activate antigen-specific lymphocyte clones selectively through recognition of peptide antigen presented by accessory cells to the T cell receptor. The kinetics of such cultures can be examined in order to determine whether a primary or secondary (memory) immune response has been made. Other indicators of cellular activation may be assessed by phenotypic analysis of the stimulated cells after culture. For example, by the use of flow cytometry it may be determined whether the stimulus has preferentially activated T lymphocytes bearing CD4 or CD8.

Release of cytokines or immunoglobulins by stimulated lymphocytes

When T lymphocytes are stimulated in culture, they will release soluble factors (cytokines) to the culture medium, which can be harvested by collection of the culture supernatant and quantified by enzyme-linked immunosorbent assay (ELISA) or bioassay. The latter involves the ability of the supernatant to support the growth of a cytokine-dependent cell line. Cytokines such as interleukin (IL)-1, IL-2, IL-6, tumour necrosis factor (TNF) and interferon gamma (IFN-γ) have been measured in the cat (Lawrence *et al.*, 1995; Rottman *et al.*, 1995) and dog (Mizuno *et al.*, 1993; Yamahita *et al.*, 1994; Rivas *et al.*, 1995) by this method. This traditional methodology is now complemented by the availability of commercial ELISAs for the detection of canine and feline cytokine molecules in tissue culture supernatants or serum. Assays for canine IL-4, IL-10 and IFN-γ are available and one company now markets a multiplex bead-based assay that claims to detect a broad panel of canine cytokines (Boggiatto *et al.*, 2010). These methodologies have not been rigorously independently validated and different research groups claim variable success with their application.

Alternatively, the cells can be collected from culture after stimulation and the presence of cytokine-specific mRNA within the cytoplasm determined by quantitative real-time reverse transcriptase polymerase chain reaction (RT-PCR). RT-PCR assays have been developed for determining gene expression for a wide range of canine and feline cytokine and chemokine molecules (Peeters *et al.*, 2007; Tagliner *et al.*, 2008). There is not necessarily a correlation between the identification of cytokine mRNA and secretion of the mature protein product. Such information provides an assessment of the normal functioning of lymphocytes *in vitro* and whether there is preferential activation of particular lymphocyte subsets (e.g. T helper (Th) 1, Th2 or T regulatory cells) upon challenge with a specific antigen.

In the case of B lymphocytes, *in vitro* stimulation may lead to differentiation to plasma cells and release of Ig into the culture medium. Such antibody production can be detected by examination of the culture supernatant by ELISA (Rivas *et al.*, 1995).

Assessment of cytotoxic function

The function of cytotoxic lymphocytes or natural killer (NK) cells can be assessed *in vitro* by culturing peripheral blood lymphoid cells with specific radiolabelled (^{51}Cr is often used) target cell populations, which may include cell lines of known susceptibility to NK cells, virally infected, histoincompatible or tumour cells. Specific ratios of target cells to cytotoxic cells are used, and the release of radioisotope by damaged targets is measured after a period of culture.

Acquired defects of leucocyte function

The acquired defects of leucocyte function recognized in small animals are summarized in Figure 13.5.

Physiological factors
• Age of animal • Diurnal variation • Dietary factors • Hormonal factors (e.g. endogenous corticosteroid, pregnancy hormones)
Drug therapy
• Immunosuppressive drugs
Chronic disease
• Demodicosis • Deep pyoderma • Anal furunculosis • Viral infection • Neoplasia • Deficiency of opsonins (e.g. immunoglobulin, complement)

13.5 Acquired defects of leucocyte function.

Physiological

Leucocyte function tests should be interpreted in light of the age, breed and sex of the animal and with a view to temporal factors. It has been shown that mitogen-driven lymphocyte proliferation varies with the age of dog, the season, and that there is apparent diurnal variation in the responsiveness of lymphoid cells. Dietary factors, particularly vitamin intake, may affect lymphocyte responses to mitogens. The hormonal effects of pregnancy on leucocyte function have not been well characterized in small animals.

Drug therapy

Immunosuppressive and immunomodulatory drugs have pronounced effects on the immune system and these may be mirrored in the results of *in vitro* functional testing of leucocytes. For this reason, it is optimal to have withdrawn such treatment for several weeks before taking samples for functional studies. Glucocorticoid will have wide-ranging effects on granulocyte, monocyte and lymphocyte function and ciclosporin can have potent suppressive effects on lymphocyte proliferation, even after absorption following topical administration for keratoconjunctivitis sicca (Gilger *et al.*, 1995).

CD4⁺ T lymphocyte balance

Studies in experimental animal models have demonstrated that polarization of immune responses towards humoral (antibody mediated) or cell-mediated activity is regulated by the preferential activation of subsets of the $CD4^+$ T cell population (Th2 and Th1, respectively). This phenomenon of 'immune deviation' also holds for particular disease states in domestic animals. For example, dogs that are susceptible to visceral leishmaniasis make high levels of antibody but weak cell-mediated responses, with reduced *in vitro* production of the key cytokine IFN-γ (Boggiatto *et al.*, 2010). Dogs resistant to the disease have the reverse profile of immunological activity. By contrast, dogs with atopic dermatitis have an immunological profile dominated initially by Th2 immunity (Nuttall *et al.*, 2002) with a reduction in the effects of T regulatory cells producing IL-10 (Keppel *et al.*, 2008). Such preferential activation of specific facets of the immune response may be driven by factors including the nature, dose and route of antigen exposure, and the local tissue milieu (hormones and cytokines) at the site of exposure.

Chronic disease

Animals with chronic infectious, inflammatory or neoplastic disease will often show reduced leucocyte function *in vitro*. In the past, this has sometimes been attributed to a primary leucocyte defect that predisposes the animal to expression of the disease, but it is now considered more likely that the inflammatory and immune responses active in chronic disease themselves cause depression of leucocyte function. Dogs with demodicosis often have depressed lymphocyte proliferation and early studies suggested that this was related to a suppressive factor found in autologous serum. This serum factor may in turn be associated with concurrent bacterial pyoderma and it has been proposed that serum immune complexes of antibody and staphylococcal antigen may act in this manner. Other work has extended these observations by showing decreased IL-2 production and IL-2 receptor expression by stimulated lymphocytes from dogs with demodicosis (Lemarie *et al.*, 1994). Similarly, decreased neutrophil chemotaxis has been shown when normal dog neutrophils were incubated with serum from dogs with demodicosis. Serum factors able to suppress autologous lymphocyte proliferative responses have also been identified in Basenjis with immunoproliferative small intestinal disease and in dogs with a range of other disorders.

Some breeds of dog are susceptible to deep pyoderma, and immunodeficiency has been proposed as an underlying cause. Such animals do often have decreased lymphocyte proliferation, but this is unlikely to be a primary event. Studies have suggested that more subtle leucocyte abnormalities such as failure of cutaneous T lymphocyte homing (Day, 1994) or CD4:CD8 imbalance (Chabanne *et al.*, 1995) may occur in susceptible dogs. Decreased neutrophil chemotaxis has been demonstrated as a secondary event in dogs with pyoderma.

Similarly, dogs with anal furunculosis may have depression of mitogen-induced lymphocyte proliferation, but these responses return to normal after recovery from disease. German Shepherd Dogs with nasal or disseminated aspergillosis have depressed lymphocyte proliferation (Day *et al.*, 1986; Day, 1987) and neutrophil NBT reduction (Day *et al.*, 1986) but these observations are again likely to be due to chronic depression of cell-mediated immunity (Figures 13.6 and 13.7).

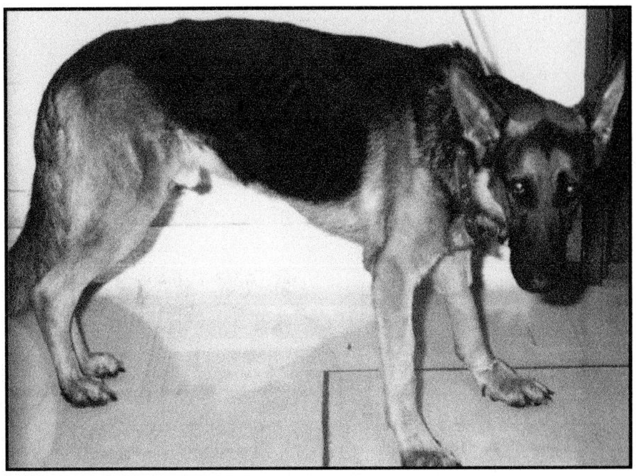

13.6 German Shepherd Dog with late stage disseminated aspergillosis. Such animals may have depression of function of lymphocytes and neutrophils *in vitro*, however these findings are likely to be secondary to chronically high levels of inflammatory mediators and cytokines, or to the release of fungal immunosuppressive metabolites (Day, 1987).

Viral infection may cause acquired abnormalities of leucocyte function. Cats with feline immunodeficiency virus infection have a depressed response of peripheral blood mononuclear cells to T and B cell mitogens associated with reduced IL-2 production (Lawrence *et al.*, 1995) and there is reduced ability of these cells to respond to primary or secondary stimulation with antigens *in vitro*. Canine distemper virus, canine parvovirus and feline leukaemia virus infections may also suppress lymphocyte proliferative responses to mitogens.

In the case of neutrophils and macrophages, apparent dysfunction of chemotaxis or phagocytosis may be attributable to underlying deficiency of opsonins such as serum Ig or complement. Serum from dogs with deficiency of the third component of complement (C3) was inefficient at opsonizing *Pneumococcus* for phagocytosis by normal dog neutrophils and failed to attract such neutrophils effectively after zymosan activation (Winkelstein *et al.*, 1982). The adherence of canine neutrophils to

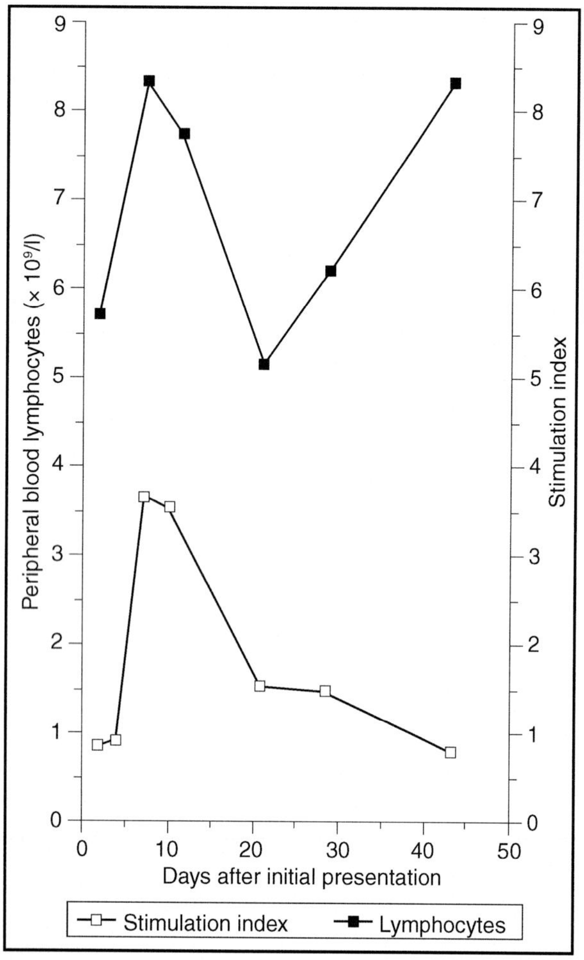

13.7 Data from a German Shepherd Dog with disseminated aspergillosis showing serial monitoring of blood lymphocyte count and response to stimulation of purified mononuclear cells with phytohaemagglutinin *in vitro*. There is persistent lymphocytosis with total lymphocyte count fluctuating between 5.0 and 8.5 × 10^9/l (normal 1.0–4.8 × 10^9/l). The stimulation index (SI) relative to cultures of control dog lymphocytes is initially normal but decreases terminally, despite rising peripheral blood lymphocyte number. This terminally depressed lymphocyte function is likely to be a reflection of the presence of chronic multisystemic inflammation.

nylon wool decreases in dogs suffering from poorly controlled diabetes mellitus (Latimer and Mahaffey, 1984) and this may have a role in the occurrence of secondary infections in this disease. A granulocyte myeloperoxidase deficiency has been documented in lead-intoxicated dogs (Caldwell *et al.*, 1979).

Congenital leucocyte function disorders

The congenital leucocyte function disorders recognized in small animals are summarized in Figure 13.8. These diseases represent one part of the spectrum of congenital immunodeficiency disorders – some of which involve reduced leucocyte number (rather than function) or abnormalities in other aspects of immune function.

- Immunodeficiency of Weimaraner dogs
- Canine leucocyte adhesion deficiency
- Neutrophil defects in Dobermanns
- Canine cyclic haemopoiesis
- Pelger–Huët anomaly
- Chédiak–Higashi syndrome
- X-linked combined immunodeficiency
- Immunodeficiency syndrome of Irish Wolfhounds
- Lethal acrodermatitis of Bull Terrier dogs
- Pneumocystis pneumonia of Miniature Dachshunds
- Disseminated mycobacterial infection in Miniature Schnauzers

13.8 Congenital defects of leucocyte function.

Immunodeficiency of Weimaraner dogs

In 1980 a colony of Weimaraner dogs was described in which there was growth hormone deficiency, thymic aplasia and failure of peripheral blood lymphocytes to respond to T cell mitogens (Roth *et al.*, 1980). Affected dogs had a wasting syndrome and increased susceptibility to infection. Since 1984, an apparently separate syndrome of chronic recurrent infection in young Weimaraner dogs has been recognized in Australia (Studdert *et al.*, 1984; Day, unpublished observations), the United States (Couto *et al.*, 1989), Belgium (Hansen *et al.*, 1995), Israel (Abeles *et al.*, 1999) and the United Kingdom (Day *et al.*, 1997; Foale *et al.*, 2003). These dogs have a left shift neutrophilia with neutrophil-dominated inflammatory lesions at post-mortem examination. The syndrome of hypertrophic osteodystrophy that is recognized in Weimaraner puppies is one presentation of this disorder (Harrus *et al.*, 2002). The clinical signs often appear to be precipitated by vaccination and the syndrome has variable long-term clinical outcome (Harrus *et al.*, 2002; Foale *et al.*, 2003).

A range of immunological tests has been performed on these populations. In the initial series of dogs there was no apparent abnormality in neutrophil or lymphocyte function (Studdert *et al.*, 1984) but subsequent studies by Couto and others (1989) suggested that a primary defect in neutrophil function (chemiluminescence), in the face of normal lymphocyte, monocyte and NK cell function, was present in these dogs. A single case reported by Hansen and others (1995) had defective neutrophil phagocytosis *in vitro* despite normal responses to chemotactic agents. More consistently, reduced serum IgG levels have been documented in these animals (Couto *et al.*, 1989; Hansen *et al.*, 1995; Day *et al.*, 1997; Foale *et al.*, 2003) and IgG quantification has become a useful diagnostic procedure.

Granulocytopathy of Irish Setters

In 1975 an Irish Setter with chronic recurrent infection associated with pyrexia and neutrophilia was investigated for suspected immunodeficiency. Abnormalities in neutrophil bacteriocidal activity following normal phagocytosis were discovered and the disease was reported to be inherited in an autosomal recessive manner (Renshaw *et al.*, 1975, 1977). The disorder was termed canine granulocytopathy syndrome. Subsequent studies demonstrated that neutrophils from the affected dog had reduced glucose oxidation by the hexose monophosphate shunt, but an increased ability to reduce NBT (Renshaw and Davis, 1979). Some years later, an Irish Setter with severe bacterial infections and lack of tissue pus formation in the face of peripheral blood neutrophilia was reported by Giger *et al.* (1987). This animal was shown to have an inherited deficiency in the expression of surface integrin molecules (CD11b and CD18), manifest as inability of neutrophils to adhere to various surfaces *in vitro*, and by extrapolation to vascular endothelium *in vivo*. Neutrophil chemotaxis and aggregation was also impaired. The defect was recognized widely in the breed and was termed the canine leucocyte adhesion deficiency (CLAD) (Trowald-Wigh *et al.*, 1992, 2000). Equivalent disorders occur in humans (LAD) and cattle (BLAD). Inheritance is in an autosomal recessive fashion and the disease is recognized worldwide. The development of a molecular diagnostic test for this disorder has enabled identification of carriers of the defective CD18 gene (Kijas *et al.*, 2000) and the Irish Setter breed associations are working towards eventual elimination of the trait (Jobling *et al.*, 2003). A recent study has reported a litter of crossbred dogs with a CLAD-like disease characterized by reduced neutrophil expression of CD11b/CD18 in the absence of the CLAD mutation in the CD18 gene (Kobayashi *et al.*, 2009).

Neutrophil defects in Dobermanns

In 1987 a series of related Dobermanns with chronic rhinitis and pneumonia was reported. These dogs had defective neutrophil killing of phagocytosed *Staphylococcus* and reduced ability to reduce NBT and produce superoxide after stimulation by opsonized zymosan (Breitschwerdt *et al.*, 1987). The relationship of this syndrome to the granulocytopathy of Irish Setters has not been determined.

Canine cyclic haemopoiesis

Canine cyclic haemopoiesis (also called cyclic neutropenia or grey collie syndrome) is characterized by cyclic (every 12 days) neutropenia in addition to myeloperoxidase deficiency of neutrophils. The dogs have diluted coat colour and display a range of clinical signs during the neutropenic episodes. Cycling of monocytes, reticulocytes and platelets also occurs. The disease is inherited in an autosomal recessive manner and molecular studies have characterized the genetic mutation as lying within the gene encoding the β subunit of the adaptor protein complex 3 – a molecule involved in the movement of neutrophil elastase (Benson *et al.*, 2003).

Pelger–Huët anomaly

This syndrome has been documented in a number of dog breeds, including the American Foxhound and Basenji. There is decreased segmentation of granulocyte nuclei and defective neutrophil chemotaxis in affected dogs; this has been described but not confirmed by later studies. These functional defects appear not to predispose to infection. The anomaly also occurs in the cat, where there is additional abnormality of monocytes and megakaryocytes.

Chédiak–Higashi syndrome

This syndrome is recognized in the Persian cat and is characterized by the presence of abnormal lysosomes and granules within the cytoplasm of granulocytes. This abnormality may be associated with defective neutrophil chemotaxis, degranulation and bactericidal activity. It is accompanied by coat and ocular fundic pigmentation abnormalities and increased susceptibility to infection.

X-linked severe combined immunodeficiency

Severe combined immunodeficiency (SCID) is recognized as an inherited, X-linked recessive trait in Basset Hounds that succumb to severe bacterial and viral infections after loss of maternally derived immunity by 8–16 weeks of age. The dogs have thymic hypoplasia and lymphopenia. Those lymphocytes that are isolated fail to respond to the mitogens PHA and Con A or to recombinant IL-2, but IgM synthesis can be detected following exposure to PWM. These findings are secondary to a mutation in the common γ chain of the receptors for IL-2, IL-4, IL-7, IL-9 and IL-15. A separate mutation in the same gene causes SCID in the Cardigan Welsh Corgi, but this disease is not X-linked (Somberg *et al.*, 1995; Felsburg *et al.*, 1999). Jack Russell Terriers also develop a form of SCID in which the mutation lies in the gene encoding the DNA protein kinase that is involved in the formation of T and B cell receptors. An experimental colony of dogs with this mutation was established by breeding the Jack Russell mutation into laboratory beagles (Meek *et al.*, 2009).

Immunodeficiency syndrome of Irish Wolfhounds

Chronic, recurrent respiratory disease has been recognized in related Irish Wolfhounds in a number of countries, and an underlying immunodeficiency has been proposed. One study of three cases identified subnormal mitogen-driven lymphocyte proliferation in affected dogs, which might be interpreted to suggest an underlying defect of cell-mediated immunity (Leiswitz *et al.*, 1997). By contrast, other research has identified serum IgA deficiency in affected pedigrees, although this was not associated with reduced concentrations of IgA in bronchoalveolar lavage fluid from the same dogs (Clercx *et al.*, 2003).

Lethal acrodermatitis of Bull Terriers

This inherited syndrome of Bull Terriers is characterized by retarded growth, cutaneous hyperkeratosis and infections of the skin and respiratory tract (Jezyk *et al.*, 1986). These dogs have subnormal plasma zinc levels, depletion of T lymphocytes from tissue and depressed lymphocyte proliferative responses to mitogens, in the face of normal neutrophil phagocytosis and killing. Reduced concentrations of serum IgA are also documented (McEwan *et al.*, 2000).

Pneumocystis pneumonia of Miniature Dachshunds

Miniature Dachshunds are predisposed to respiratory infection by *Pneumocystis carinii* and it has been postulated that an underlying immunodeficiency may explain this breed association. It is suggested that a combined defect in T and B cells (common variable immunodeficiency) occurs in these dogs, on the basis of reduced serum IgG, IgM and IgA concentrations, reduced mitogen responsiveness of blood lymphocytes, and an absence of B cells but presence of T cells in lymphoid tissue examined immunohistochemically (Lobetti, 2000).

Disseminated mycobacterial infection in Miniature Schnauzers

Related young Miniature Schnauzers with disseminated infection by organisms of the *Mycobacterium avium* complex have been recognized in a number of countries. Preliminary immunological studies have shown a normal blood CD4:CD8 ratio with elevated B cells and reduced response to mitogen stimulation (Eggers *et al.*, 1997).

Diagnostic approach to suspected leucocyte function disorders

Leucocyte function disorders may be acquired or congenital in nature. Acquired leucocyte function defects occur as secondary phenomena in adult animals and the diagnostic approach should focus on characterization of the underlying disease state. Inherited leucocyte function defects may be considered when young, littermate animals present with chronic, recurrent infections (often involving the skin or respiratory tract) that do not respond to standard antimicrobial therapy or that recur following cessation of therapy. Differential diagnoses include other primary immunodeficiency disorders such as immunoglobulin or complement deficiency, or aplasia of lymphoid tissue with leucopenia. A diagnostic approach to such diseases should include:

- Haematology profile, specifically differential leucocyte count and morphology
- Serum protein analysis, specifically determination of globulin levels
- Characterization of any infectious agent by culture
- Full post-mortem examination of any dead littermates, with histological examination of lymphoid and haemopoietic organs.

Where available, appropriate immunodiagnostic tests would include:

- Quantification of serum Igs and complement
- Ability of peripheral blood lymphocytes to respond to mitogens
- Neutrophil and macrophage function testing.

Such tests are not widely available to veterinary surgeons, although quantification of serum IgG, IgM and IgA (for the dog only) may be sourced through commercial clinical pathology laboratories.

Therapy for leucocyte function disorders

In many of the diseases described above, appropriate antimicrobial therapy may induce clinical improvement, but in the case of most primary, congenital leucocyte defects this will only be a temporary effect because such diseases are often lethal. Although a variety of therapeutic approaches have been used in primary and secondary leucocyte disorders, the effects have been poorly characterized and most agents used are unlicensed. Genetic counselling should be given when inherited leucocyte defects are diagnosed.

Immunomodulatory agents

A range of immunomodulatory agents have been used in therapeutic trials in the dog but their immunological effects are poorly defined. These include products such as staphage lysate (DeBoer *et al.*, 1990), staphoid A-B (Pukay, 1985), killed *Propionibacterium* (Becker *et al.*, 1989) and levamisole (Degen and Breitschwerdt, 1986; Guilford, 1987). The potential for the development of side effects following administration of levamisole is considered to outweigh the usefulness of this agent. Inactivated ovine parapoxvirus has also been used as an immune stimulant for dogs and cats with a range of infectious diseases.

Hormones

Some of the group of Weimaraner puppies with immunodeficient dwarfism reported by Roth *et al.* (1984) were treated with growth hormone and fractions of the thymic hormone thymosin. Although there was clinical improvement, the defective lymphocyte proliferative response in these dogs was not normalized.

Bone marrow transplantation and recombinant cytokines

Cytokines have profound influences on the development and function of leucocytes, and there is potential for therapeutic exploitation of this fact. For example, recombinant canine granulocyte-colony stimulating factor (G-CSF) and recombinant canine stem cell factor have been used successfully in the treatment of cyclic haemopoiesis (Mishu *et al.*, 1992; Dale *et al.*, 1995) and, latterly, delivery of the G-CSF gene by lentivirus vector has been employed to treat the same disease (Yanay *et al.*, 2003). Bone marrow transplantation has also been attempted successfully in dogs with cyclic haemopoiesis (Dale *et al.*, 1995) and X-SCID (Meek *et al.*, 2009). One X-SCID dog was also treated successfully by transplantation of bone marrow stem cells from a histocompatible donor after irradiation and medical immunosuppression to ablate its own immune system (Suter *et al.*, 2007).

Genetic approaches

When leucocyte function defects are attributed to specific monogenic abnormalities, the therapeutic use of gene replacement therapy becomes possible. Experimental gene transfer has already been performed in Basset Hounds with X-SCID by delivering a 'correct' copy of the defective IL-2 receptor γ chain gene with a retrovirus vector (Ting-De Ravin *et al.*, 2006). These studies are performed to investigate the applications of such therapy to human patients and it is unlikely that such therapies will (or should) ever become available in general veterinary practice.

References and further reading

Abeles V, Harrus S, Angles JM *et al.* (1999) Hypertrophic osteodystrophy in six Weimaraner puppies associated with systemic signs. *Veterinary Record* **145**, 130–134

Becker AM, Janik TA, Smith EK *et al.* (1989) *Propionibacterium acnes* immunotherapy in chronic recurrent pyoderma. *Journal of Veterinary Internal Medicine* **3**, 26–30

Benson KF, Li F-Q, Person RE *et al.* (2003) Mutations associated with neutropenia in dogs and humans disrupt intracellular transport of neutrophil elastase. *Nature Genetics* **35**, 90–96

Boggiatto PM, Ramer-Tait AE, Metz K *et al.* (2010) Immunologic indicators of clinical progression during canine *Leishmania infantum* infection. *Clinical and Vaccine Immunology* **17**, 267–273

Breitschwerdt EB, Brown TT, DeBuysscher EV *et al.* (1987) Rhinitis, pneumonia, and defective neutrophil function in the Doberman Pinscher. *American Journal of Veterinary Research* **48**, 1054–1062

Caldwell KC, Taddeini L, Woodburn RL *et al.* (1979) Induction of myeloperoxidase deficiency in granulocytes in lead-intoxicated dogs. *Blood* **46**, 921–930

Chabanne L, Marchal T, Denerolle P *et al.* (1995) Lymphocyte subset abnormalities in German shepherd dog pyoderma (GSP). *Veterinary Immunology and Immunopathology* **49**, 189–198

Clercx C, Reichler I, Peeters D *et al.* (2003) Rhinitis/bronchopneumonia syndrome in Irish Wolfhounds. *Journal of Veterinary Internal Medicine* **17**, 843–849

Couto CG, Krakowka S, Johnson G *et al.* (1989) In vitro immunologic features of Weimaraner dogs with neutrophil abnormalities and recurrent infections. *Veterinary Immunology and Immunopathology* **23**, 103–112

Dale DC, Rodger E, Cebon J *et al.* (1995) Long-term treatment of canine cyclic hematopoiesis with recombinant canine stem cell factor. *Blood* **85**, 74–79

Day MJ (1987) A study of the immune response in canine disseminated aspergillosis. PhD Thesis, Murdoch University, Western Australia

Day MJ (1994) An immunopathological study of deep pyoderma in the dog. *Research in Veterinary Science* **56**, 18–23

Day MJ (2008) Immunodeficiency disease. In: *Clinical Immunology of the Dog and Cat, 2nd edn*, ed. MJ Day, pp.287–314. Manson Publishing, London

Day MJ, Penhale WJ, Eger CE *et al.* (1986) Disseminated aspergillosis in dogs. *Australian Veterinary Journal* **63**, 55–59

Day MJ, Power C, Oleshko J *et al.* (1997) Low serum immunoglobulin concentrations in related Weimaraner dogs. *Journal of Small Animal Practice* **38**, 311–315

DeBoer DJ, Moriello KA, Thomas CB *et al.* (1990) Evaluation of a commercial staphylococcal bacterin for the management of idiopathic recurrent superficial pyoderma in dogs. *American Journal of Veterinary Research* **51**, 636–639

DeBowes LJ and Anderson NV (1991) Phagocytosis and erythrocyte antibody-rosette formation by three populations of mononuclear phagocytes obtained from dogs treated with glucocorticoids. *American Journal of Veterinary Research* **52**, 869–872

Degen MA and Breitschwerdt EB (1986) Canine and feline immunodeficiency – part II. *Compendium on Continuing Education for the Practicing Veterinarian* **8**, 379–386

Eickhoff S, Mironowa L, Carlson R *et al.* (2004) Measurement of phagocytosis and oxidative burst of canine neutrophils: high variation in healthy dogs. *Veterinary Immunology and Immunopathology* **101**, 109–121

Eggers JS, Parker GA, Braaf HA *et al.* (1997) Disseminated *Mycobacterium avium* infection in three miniature Schnauzer littermates. *Journal of Veterinary Diagnostic Investigation* **9**, 424–427

Felsberg PJ, Hartnett BJ, Henthorn PS *et al.* (1999) Canine X-linked severe combined immunodeficiency. *Veterinary Immunology and Immunopathology* **69**, 127–135

Foale RD, Herrtage ME and Day MJ (2003) Retrospective study of 25 young Weimaraners with low serum immunoglobulin concentrations and inflammatory disease. *Veterinary Record* **153**, 553–558

Giger U, Boxer LA, Simpson PJ *et al.* (1987) Deficiency of leukocyte surface glycoproteins Mo1, LFA-1, and Leu M5 in a dog with recurrent bacterial infections: an animal model. *Blood* **69**, 1622–1630

Gilger BC, Andrews J, Wilkie DA *et al.* (1995) Cellular immunity in dogs with keratoconjunctivitis sicca before and after treatment with topical 2% cyclosporine. *Veterinary Immunology and Immunopathology* **49**, 199–208

Guilford WG (1987) Primary immunodeficiency diseases of dogs and cats. *Compendium on Continuing Education for the Practicing Veterinarian* **9**, 641–650

Hansen P, Clercx C, Henroteaux M *et al.* (1995) Neutrophil phagocyte dysfunction in a Weimaraner with recurrent infections. *Journal of Small Animal Practice* **36**, 128–131

Harrus S, Waner T, Aizenberg I *et al.* (2002) Development of hypertrophic osteodystrophy and antibody response in a litter of vaccinated Weimaraner puppies. *Journal of Small Animal Practice* **43**, 27–31

Jezyk PF, Haskins ME, MacKay-Smith WE *et al.* (1986) Lethal acrodermatitis in bull terriers. *Journal of the American Veterinary Medical Association* **188**, 833–839

Jobling AJ, Ryan J and Augusteyn RC (2003) The frequency of canine leukocyte adhesion deficiency (CLAD) allele within the Irish Setter population of Australia. *Australian Veterinary Journal* **81**, 763–765

Keppel KE, Campbell KL, Zuckermann FA *et al.* (2008) Quantitation of canine regulatory T cell populations, serum interleukin-10 and allergen-specific IgE concentrations in healthy control dogs and canine atopic dermatitis patients receiving allergen-specific immunotherapy. *Veterinary Immunology and Immunopathology* **123**, 337–344

Kijas JMH, Juneja RK, Gafvert S *et al.* (2000) Detection of the causal mutation for canine leukocyte adhesion deficiency (CLAD) using pyrosequencing. *Animal Genetics* **31**, 326–328

Kobayashi S, Sato R, Abe Y *et al.* (2009) Canine neutrophil dysfunction caused by downregulation of ß2-integrin expression without mutation. *Veterinary Immunology and Immunopathology* **130**, 187–196

Latimer KS and Mahaffey EA (1984) Neutrophil adherence and movement in poorly and well-controlled diabetic dogs. *American Journal of Veterinary Research* **45**, 1498–1500

Lawrence CE, Callanan JJ, Willett BJ *et al.* (1995) Cytokine production by cats infected with feline immunodeficiency virus: a longitudinal study. *Immunology* **85**, 568–574

Leiswitz AL, Spencer JA, Jacobson LS *et al.* (1997) Suspected primary immunodeficiency syndrome in three related Irish wolfhounds. *Journal of Small Animal Practice* **38**, 209–212

Lemarie SL, Foil CS and Horohov DW (1994) Evaluation of interleukin-2 production and interleukin-2 receptor expression in dogs with generalised demodicosis. *Proceedings of the American Academy of Veterinary Dermatology*, p. 26Lobetti R (2000) Common variable immunodeficiency in miniature dachshunds affected with *Pneumocystis carinii* pneumonia. *Journal of Veterinary Diagnostic Investigation* **12**, 39–45

McEwan NA, McNeil PE, Thompson H *et al.* (2000) Diagnostic features, confirmation and disease progression in 28 cases of lethal acrodermatitis of Bull Terriers. *Journal of Small Animal Practice* **41**, 501–507

Meek K, Jutkowitz A, Allen L *et al.* (2009) SCID dogs: similar transplant potential but distinct intra-uterine growth defects and premature replicative senescence compared with SCID mice. *Journal of Immunology* **183**, 2529–2536

Mishu L, Callahan G, Allebban Z *et al.* (1992) Effects of recombinant canine granulocyte colony-stimulating factor on white blood cell production in clinically normal and neutropenic dogs. *Journal of the American Veterinary Medical Association* **200**, 1957–1964

Mizuno S, Fujinaga T and Hagio M (1993) Characterization of dog interleukin-2 activity. *Journal of Veterinary Medical Science* **55**, 925–930

Nuttall TJ, Knight PA, McAleese SM *et al.* (2002) Expression of Th1, Th2 and immunosuppressive cytokine gene transcripts in canine

atopic dermatitis. *Clinical and Experimental Allergy* **32**, 789–795
Peeters D, Peters IR, Helps CR *et al.* (2007) Distinct tissue cytokine and chemokine mRNA expression in canine sino-nasal aspergillosis and idiopathic lymphoplasmacytic rhinitis. *Veterinary Immunology and Immunopathology* **117**, 95–105
Pukay BP (1985) Treatment of canine bacterial hypersensitivity by hyposensitization with *Staphylococcus aureus* bacterin-toxoid. *Journal of the American Animal Hospital Association* **21**, 479–483
Renshaw HW, Chatburn C, Bryan GM *et al.* (1975) Canine granulocytopathy syndrome: neutrophil dysfunction in a dog with recurrent infections. *Journal of the American Veterinary Medical Association* **166**, 443–447
Renshaw HW and Davis WC (1979) Canine granulocytopathy syndrome: an inherited disorder of leukocyte function. *American Journal of Pathology* **95**, 731–744
Renshaw HW, Davis WC and Renshaw SJ (1977) Canine granulocytopathy syndrome: defective bactericidal capacity of neutrophils from a dog with recurrent infections. *Clinical Immunology and Immunopathology* **8**, 385–395
Rivas AL, Kimball ES, Quimby FW *et al.* (1995) Functional and phenotypic analysis of in vitro stimulated canine peripheral blood mononuclear cells. *Veterinary Immunology and Immunopathology* **45**, 55–71
Roth JA, Kaeberle ML, Grier RL *et al.* (1984) Improvement in clinical condition and thymus morphological features associated with growth hormone treatment of immunodeficient dwarf dogs. *American Journal of Veterinary Research* **45**, 1151–1155
Roth JA, Lomax LG, Altszuler N *et al.* (1980) Thymic abnormalities and growth hormone deficiency in dogs. *American Journal of Veterinary Research* **41**, 1256–1262
Rottman JB, Freeman EB, Tonkonogy S *et al.* (1995) A reverse transcription-polymerase chain reaction technique to detect feline cytokine genes. *Veterinary Immunology and Immunopathology* **45**, 1–18
Shearer DH and Day MJ (1997) An investigation of phagocytosis and intracellular killing of *Staphylococcus intermedius* by canine neutrophils in vitro. *Veterinary Immunology and Immunopathology* **58**, 219–230
Somberg RL, Pullen RP, Casal ML *et al.* (1995) A single nucleotide insertion in the canine interleukin-2 receptor gamma chain results in X-linked severe combined immunodeficiency disease. *Veterinary Immunology and Immunopathology* **47**, 203–213
Studdert VP, Phillips WA, Studdert MJ *et al.* (1984) Recurrent and persistent infections in related Weimaraner dogs. *Australian Veterinary Journal* **61**, 261–263
Suter SE, Gouthro TA, O'Malley T *et al.* (2007) Marking of peripheral T-lymphocytes by retroviral transduction and transplantation of $CD34^+$ cells in a canine X-linked severe combined immunodeficiency model. *Veterinary Immunology and Immunopathology* **117**, 183–196
Taglinger K, Nguyen Van N, Helps CR *et al.* (2008) Quantitative real-time RT-PCR measurement of cytokine mRNA expression in the skin of normal cats and cats with allergic skin disease. *Veterinary Immunology and Immunopathology* **122**, 216–230
Ting-De Ravin SS, Kennedy DR, Naumann N *et al.* (2006) Correction of canine X-linked severe combined immunodeficiency by in vivo retroviral gene therapy. *Blood* **107**, 3091–3097
Trowald-Wigh G, Ekman S, Hansson K *et al.* (2000) Clinical, radiological and pathological features of 12 Irish Setters with canine leukocyte adhesion deficiency. *Journal of Small Animal Practice* **41**, 211–217
Trowald-Wigh G, Hakansson L, Johannisson A *et al.* (1992) Leucocyte adhesion protein deficiency in Irish setter dogs. *Veterinary Immunology and Immunopathology* **32**, 261–280
Winkelstein JA, Johnson JP, Swift AJ *et al.* (1982) Genetically determined deficiency of the third component of complement in the dog: *in vitro* studies on the complement system and complement-mediated serum activities. *Journal of Immunology* **129**, 2598–2602
Yamahita K, Fujinaga T, Hagio M *et al.* (1994) Bioassay for interleukin-1, interleukin-6, and tumour necrosis factor-like activities in canine sera. *Journal of Veterinary Medical Science* **56**, 103–107
Yanay O, Barry SC, Katen LJ *et al.* (2003) Treatment of canine cyclic neutropenia by lentivirus-mediated G-CSF delivery. *Blood* **102**, 2046–2052

14

Neutropenia

Anthony Abrams-Ogg

Introduction

Neutropenia results from impaired granulopoiesis (myelosuppression) and/or overwhelming infection, where tissue demands exceed granulopoiesis. It may be an incidental laboratory finding or discovered in the work-up of a sick animal, and it may be an isolated haematological abnormality or a feature of pancytopenia. There are no clinical signs associated with neutropenia in itself – the signs are due to the underlying disease and secondary infection. Neutropenic animals are at increased risk of bacterial and fungal infections, and established infections in neutropenic patients are more difficult to eradicate with appropriate antimicrobial treatment. Such infections may be caused either by organisms that are normally considered to be pathogenic or by opportunistic pathogens. In most cases of infection secondary to transient myelosuppression, early therapy with antibiotics and good supportive care will result in a successful outcome.

Pathophysiology and consequences

Specific causes of neutropenia in the dog and cat are listed in Figure 14.1. The critical clinical consequence of neutropenia is secondary infection.

When a septic neutropenic animal is presented, there are three possible scenarios:

- Primary bacterial sepsis, where the tissue demands overwhelm marrow granulocyte reserve and production (e.g. septic peritonitis). Prior to illness the marrow was normal
- Primary impairment of granulopoiesis (e.g. feline leukaemia virus (FeLV) infection) and therefore an increased susceptibility to infection. Secondary sepsis occurs, which in turn exacerbates neutropenia. Impairment of granulopoiesis is usually a facet of acquired generalized impairment of haemopoiesis, but neutropenia is the first peripheral blood abnormality to appear because of the short lifespan of the neutrophil
- Concurrent tissue injury promoting sepsis and impaired granulopoiesis (e.g. parvoviral infections and cytotoxic chemotherapy).

Several factors determine the risk, severity and outcome of neutropenic sepsis:

- Severity and duration of neutropenia
- Disruption of natural barriers and immunosuppression
- Tumour type and biological stage in patients with cancer
- Microbial organisms involved and site of infection.

Severity and duration of neutropenia

The severity of neutropenia is the most important risk factor for developing an infection. The risk increases exponentially with increasing severity of neutropenia (Figure 14.2). As the neutrophil count decreases, the duration of neutropenia becomes an increasingly important factor.

The duration of neutropenia is the most important risk factor in determining the outcome of an infection. When neutropenia is of short duration (< 7 days) most infections can be controlled with appropriate antimicrobial therapy. Infections that complicate neutropenia of moderate duration (7–14 days) are more difficult to treat. Infections in patients with prolonged neutropenia (> 14 days) are even more difficult to treat, especially if the neutrophil count is less than 0.2×10^9/l. The likelihood of clearing an established infection with antimicrobial therapy decreases in neutropenia because antimicrobial agents act in synergy with host defences to kill invading organisms.

Cats seem to tolerate lower neutrophil counts and neutropenia of longer duration better than dogs. Neutropenic cats are at less risk of developing infections, and their infections are more easily treated.

Disruption of natural barriers and immunosuppression

Disruption of natural physical barriers and suppression of antibody production and cell-mediated immunity increase the risk of infection. Natural barriers are disrupted with gastrointestinal (GI) damage during parvoviral infections and cancer chemotherapy, facilitating invasion by enteric bacteria. Intravenous catheterization increases the risk of infection with cutaneous organisms. Immunosuppression may be present concurrently with myelosuppression, either because of the primary disease (e.g. multiple myeloma), as a result of therapy (e.g. cyclophosphamide) or because of malnutrition secondary to inappetence. The risk of

Inherited
Cyclic haemopoiesis in grey collies Mild asymptomatic neutropenia in some breeds (e.g. Greyhounds, Belgian Tervuren)
Infectious
Canine parvovirus-2 Feline parvovirus Feline leukaemia virus (FeLV) Feline immunodeficiency virus (FIV) *Ehrlichia canis* (and potentially other members of Anaplasmataceae family) Overwhelming sepsis Systemic mycosis
Neoplastic
Lymphocytic leukaemia/leukaemic lymphoma Multiple myeloma Myelogenous leukaemia, myelodysplastic syndrome Metastatic cancer to bone marrow (myelophthisis) Oestrogen-secreting (Sertoli cell) tumour (dog)
Therapeutics
Antineoplastic cytotoxic chemotherapeutic agents and large-field radiation therapy causing predictable myelosuppression Antineoplastic tyrosine kinase inhibitors causing predictable mild neutropenia Drugs with known but unpredictable risk of causing myelosuppression: • Dog: Oestrogens, phenylbutazone • Cat: Chloramphenicol, griseofulvin (especially in FIV-infected cats), propylthiouracil, methimazole, carbimazole, lithium Drugs with reported idiosyncratic reactions causing neutropenia (any drug has the potential to cause neutropenia by immune or direct myelotoxic mechanisms): • Dog: Cephalosporins, sulphonamides, angiotensin-converting enzyme inhibitors, phenobarbital, streptozotocin, fenbendazole, albendazole • Cat: cephalosporins
Toxins
Autumn crocus (colchicine is the toxic principle)
Miscellaneous
Idiopathic Granulocyte-colony stimulating factor deficiency Immune-mediated neutropenia Myelofibrosis Disseminated intravascular coagulation (dog) Hypoadrenocorticism (neutropenia is mild and is not associated with secondary infection)

14.1 Aetiology of neutropenia in the dog and cat.

Neutrophil count	Definition	Risk of infection
2.0×10^9/l to < lower limit of normal	Grade 0 neutropenia	Minimal
1.5×10^9/l to < 2.0×10^9/l	Grade 1 neutropenia	Marginal
1.0×10^9/l to < 1.5×10^9/l	Grade 2 neutropenia	Mild
0.5×10^9/l to < 1.0×10^9/l	Grade 3 neutropenia	Moderate
0.0×10^9/l to < 0.5×10^9/l	Grade 4 neutropenia	High

14.2 Risk of opportunistic infection during neutropenia. For a given grade of neutropenia a higher risk of infection is associated with a falling, rather than a stable, neutrophil count. (Source: Veterinary Co-Operative Oncology Group, 2004)

infection in neutropenic human patients is greater with concurrent lymphopenia and monocytopenia.

Tumour type and biological stage in patients with cancer

Infections secondary to neutropenia are likely to be more severe in human patients with acute compared with chronic haematological malignancies, haematological malignancies in relapse compared with malignancies in remission, and haematological malignancies compared with solid tumours. A recent study in dogs identified an increased risk of neutropenic sepsis in dogs with lymphoma (especially during induction chemotherapy) compared with dogs with solid tumours (Sorenmo *et al.*, 2010).

Microbial organisms involved and site of infection

Infections in neutropenic animals may occur with environmental and hospital-acquired organisms or be acquired from other animals. However, the greatest source of infection is the animal's own flora, especially that of the GI tract, which may translocate to other sites. The organisms isolated most frequently are Gram-negative enteric bacilli (e.g. *Escherichia coli, Klebsiella* spp., *Enterobacter* spp.), followed by Gram-positive cocci (e.g. *Staphylococcus* spp., *Streptococcus* spp.). *Pseudomonas* spp. are isolated less frequently, but are feared because of antimicrobial resistance. Despite being present in large numbers in the GI tract, anaerobic bacteria are not commonly the first invaders in opportunistic infection during neutropenia. It is possible, however, that anaerobic bacteria contribute to sepsis during parvoviral infections because intestinal proliferation of *Clostridium perfringens* has been documented in canine parvovirus-2 infection (Turk *et al.,* 1992).

The most common sites of infection are the bloodstream (bacteraemia) and the lung, and infections at these sites are more difficult to treat in human patients than infections at other sites. Pneumonia may occur as an opportunistic infection caused by upper respiratory flora or more commonly from translocation of GI bacteria. Local cellulitis may occur, manifested as oedema of one or more limbs. Other possible sites of infection include the oral cavity, GI tract, urinary tract, heart and central nervous system (CNS).

Invasive fungal infections with *Candida* spp. and *Aspergillus* spp. have been reported as complications of cytotoxic therapy and parvoviral infections in dogs and cats but the prevalence seems to be low. The risk of fungal infection increases with the duration of neutropenia, duration of antibacterial therapy and concurrent immunosuppressive therapy (e.g. with ciclosporin).

Clinical presentation

Neutrophils are not a major source of endogenous pyrogens, and when secondary infection occurs, most neutropenic animals will develop a fever. Occasionally only lethargy, inappetence and tachycardia occur. This is most likely in elderly animals and in animals treated with anti-inflammatory drugs, which may have blunted febrile responses. Septic animals may also present with vomiting and/or diarrhoea, or may be in shock, which is variably characterized by hypothermia, bradycardia and hypotension. If granulopoiesis is impaired, the signs of local inflammation are subtle, and a site of infection may be difficult to identify. Other clinical signs will vary with the primary disorder.

Diagnosis

Neutropenia is diagnosed from a haemogram. Clots in the sample may result in artificial neutropenia. Haemodilution from aggressive fluid therapy may result in mild depression of leucocyte counts.

Diagnosis of the specific cause of neutropenia is often possible on the basis of the history, physical examination and routine laboratory and serological tests. On a haemogram, a minimal left shift and pancytopenia suggest that granulopoietic failure is contributing to neutropenia. However, many pathophysiological processes affect haematology results and, with the exception of the presence of neoplastic cells or certain microorganisms, there are no pathognomonic patterns for any given cause of neutropenia. Serial evaluation of haemograms may be necessary to explain abnormalities. Bone marrow biopsy should be considered if there is evidence of impaired granulopoiesis.

Diagnosis of the site(s) of, and/or the organism(s) causing, secondary infection relies on diagnostic imaging and microbial cultures of blood, catheters, airway washes, urine, faeces or other tissues or fluids. These are not recommended routinely in animals with parvoviral infections or animals receiving cytotoxic chemotherapy, but are recommended if there are specific signs (e.g. thoracic radiographs and airway wash for an animal with cough or dyspnoea). If there is no obvious site of infection, two simultaneous blood cultures of 5–10 ml each from different veins should be considered. Polymerase chain reaction (PCR) tests for the detection of bacteria and fungi, and β-glucan and galactomanan assays for detection of *Aspergillus* spp., are being used increasingly in human patients. Measurement of galactomanan is unreliable for the diagnosis of sinonasal aspergillosis in dogs and has not been evaluated for the diagnosis of neutropenic invasive aspergillosis in dogs (Billen *et al.*, 2009).

Therapy

In small animal medicine, management of neutropenia usually involves neutropenia of short duration (< 7 days) and/or of mild to moderate severity. Animals with neutropenia of prolonged duration usually have only mildly depressed neutrophil counts. This is in part due to the use of only moderately aggressive cancer chemotherapy and to euthanasia of severely neutropenic animals that have a poor prognosis for prompt recovery. The discussion that follows concerns the management of infection. Underlying diseases should be treated in accordance with standard recommendations, and any drugs that are suspected of causing neutropenia should be withdrawn. Treatment options to control infections are:

- Isolation (to reduce the risk of an increased need for neutrophils)
- Antimicrobial therapy: prophylactic therapy (to reduce the risk for an increased need for neutrophils), empirical treatment of febrile neutropenic patients and therapy of documented infections (to assist existing neutrophils)
- Granulocyte transfusions (to replace neutrophils)
- Haemopoietic drugs (to stimulate neutrophil production and function)
- Removal of the focus of infection (to reduce the existing increased need for neutrophils).

Isolation

Isolation reduces the risk of acquiring infections from the environment and other animals. Neutropenic animals that do not require critical care should be maintained at home and confined to the house and garden or yard. The feeding of table scraps should be avoided and only canned foods offered to dogs and cats with severe neutropenia. In the veterinary hospital, contact with the general patient population should be avoided. Staff should wash their hands thoroughly and change laboratory coats before handling neutropenic animals. The use of gloves and isolation gowns should be considered for severely neutropenic cases. Body temperature should be measured with a thermometer restricted to use in a particular patient.

Antimicrobial therapy

Antimicrobial therapy is the cornerstone of the management of neutropenia. It may be divided into three categories:

1. Prophylactic therapy (of an animal that is not showing signs of infection):
   - Prophylactic therapy where neutropenia is present
   - Prophylactic therapy where neutropenia is anticipated
2. Empirical treatment during febrile episodes
3. Treatment of documented infections (where the sites of infection and/or infecting organisms are known).

Prophylactic therapy

Antimicrobial prophylaxis in the asymptomatic patient should be started with the occurrence of grade 4 neutropenia, should be considered with grade 3 neutropenia, and should be considered when grade 3–4 neutropenia is anticipated (see Figure 14.2). Antimicrobial therapy is directed at the GI flora, with the principal objective of reducing the aerobic organisms most often responsible for infections. The GI anaerobic population is left relatively undisturbed because it contributes to resistance to fungal overgrowth and colonization by pathogenic organisms. A second objective of prophylactic therapy is to provide sufficient tissue drug levels to contain an incipient bacterial infection. Drug choices for prophylactic therapy are presented in Figure 14.3.

Antimicrobial prophylaxis during cancer chemotherapy is controversial. Potential advantages include a reduction in the infection rate, increased time to onset of infection, and reduced speed at which an incipient infection develops into overwhelming sepsis. These benefits facilitate home management of neutropenic animals and improve quality of life. Potential disadvantages include drug-induced inappetence and vomiting, and development of resistant organisms. Antimicrobial prophylaxis may also be an unnecessary expense, although treating sepsis is usually more expensive than preventing it. In two studies of veterinary cancer patients receiving doxorubicin, trimethoprim–sulphonamide prophylaxis reduced various treatment-associated adverse effects (Couto, 1990; Chretin *et al.*, 2007).

Routine antimicrobial prophylaxis during cancer chemotherapy is not used in the author's hospital if the owner can observe the animal closely for signs of infection and if the anticipated neutropenia is of short duration, such as occurs with many commonly used chemotherapeutic protocols. Prophylactic therapy is discouraged in cats, which are at less risk of infection than dogs, harder to give medication to, and at more risk of antimicrobial-induced GI disorders (Kunkle *et al.*, 1995).

If grade 3–4 neutropenia has occurred during a previous treatment, prophylaxis is given for a 5–7 day period to bridge the anticipated neutrophil nadir (e.g. from day 5 to day 10 after doxorubicin). If neutropenia is noted on a pre-treatment haemogram, the chemotherapy is not given, and antimicrobial prophylaxis is started with grade 3–4 neutropenia. The animal is returned for its next chemotherapy treatment 4–7 days later, by which time the neutrophil count has usually recovered. In the event that chemotherapy is delayed again because the neutrophil count has not recovered sufficiently, antimicrobial prophylaxis is discontinued if the severity of neutropenia has lowered to grade 1–2.

Antimicrobial prophylaxis is recommended if severe prolonged neutropenia is anticipated, such as with pancytopenia caused by oestrogen toxicosis in dogs.

Empirical treatment of febrile neutropenic patients

Asymptomatic animals with neutropenia and animals at risk for neutropenia should have their body temperature monitored. Depending on the anticipated risk, this may vary from measuring temperature when there are signs of lethargy or inappetence to routine monitoring 2–4 times a day.

Antimicrobial agent	Dose	Comments
Sulphonamides		
Trimethoprim/sulfamethoxazole	15 mg/kg (combined dose) q12h	Inexpensive. No prophylaxis against *Pseudomonas* spp. Risk of keratoconjunctivitis sicca and cutaneous, haematological and other immune-mediated abnormalities. May retard marrow recovery following severe myelosuppression
Trimethoprim/sulfadiazine	30 mg/kg (combined dose) q12–24h	
Fluoroquinolones		
Enrofloxacin	5–20 mg/kg q24h (dogs)	Dose > 10 mg/kg needed to achieve tissue levels effective against *Pseudomonas* spp. Relatively more expensive
Ciprofloxacin	10–30 mg/kg q24h (dogs)	Relatively more expensive
Orbifloxacin	2.5–7.5 mg/kg q24h (dogs)	Relatively more expensive
Marbofloxacin	2.5–5 mg/kg q24h (dogs and cats)	Least risk for retinopathy in cats. Relatively more expensive
Difloxacin	5–10 mg/kg q24h (dogs)	Relatively more expensive
Beta-lactam antibiotics		
Cefalexin	30 mg/kg q12h (dogs)	Relatively more expensive. No prophylaxis against *Pseudomonas* spp.
Amoxicillin	10–20 mg/kg q12h (dogs and cats)	Inexpensive. No prophylaxis against *Pseudomonas* spp. More disturbance of gut flora than cefalexin. First choice for cats
Amoxicillin/ clavulanate	12.5–25 mg/kg q12h	As for amoxicillin. Increased activity against *Staphylococcus* spp., *Klebsiella* spp., *Escherichia coli* and *Bacteroides* spp. compared with amoxicillin
Combinations		
Fluroquinolone + beta-lactam	See above	Reserved for animals with severe prolonged neutropenia

14.3 Choices for prophylactic oral antimicrobial therapy for the asymptomatic dog and cat with anticipated or existing grade 3–4 neutropenia. (Modified from Abrams-Ogg and Kruth, 2006. Doses adapted from Allen *et al.*, 2005; Greene *et al.*, 2006 and Plumb, 2008)

Axillary temperature measurements facilitate home monitoring and are 0.5–1°C lower than rectal temperature measurements. A rectal temperature above 39.0°C in dogs and above 39.2°C in cats should be regarded with suspicion. A temperature above 39.5°C in most cases represents a true fever.

Fever and/or unexplained depression and inappetence in a neutropenic animal should be considered infectious in origin until proven otherwise, and empirical antimicrobial therapy should be initiated promptly while awaiting any culture results. Previous culture results, localizing signs, cytological examination of body fluid and the antimicrobial susceptibility pattern of a suspected nosocomial pathogen may assist in antimicrobial selection. If there is a history of prophylactic therapy with a fluoroquinolone, a febrile episode is most likely due to a Gram-positive organism. The antibiotics chosen should ideally be bactericidal, have limited marrow toxicity and be active against Gram-negative enteric bacilli, *Pseudomonas* spp. and Gram-positive cocci. Standard recommended drug doses are employed. A representative selection of antibiotics and doses is presented in Figure 14.4.

Disease	First choice(s) in author's hospital	Alternative choices
Parvoviral infection	Ampicillin 20–40 mg/kg q6–8h, i.v., i.m., s.c. Cefoxitin [a] 20–30 mg/kg q6–8h, i.v., i.m., s.c.	Ampicillin–sulbactam 50 mg/kg q6–8h, i.v., i.m. *Combination therapy:* Ampicillin 20–40 mg/kg q6–8h, i.v., i.m., s.c., ***AND*** Amikacin [b] 15–20 mg/kg q24h, i.v., i.m., s.c., ***OR*** Gentamicin [b] 5–6 mg/kg q24h, i.v., i.m., s.c., ***OR*** Netilmycin [b] 6 mg/kg q24h, i.v., ***OR*** Tobramycin [b] 6 mg/kg q24h, i.v., i.m., s.c. ***OR*** Enrofloxacin (**DOGS** only)[c] 5–10 mg/kg q12–24h i.v., i.m.
Myelosuppression from cytotoxic therapy, toxicoses, FIV/FeLV, neoplasia	**DOGS:** Enrofloxacin [c] 5–10 mg/kg q12–24h i.v., i.m., ***AND*** Cefazolin [a] 20–30 mg/kg q6–8h, i.v., i.m., s.c., ***OR*** Cephalothin [a] 25–40 mg/kg q6–8h, i.v., i.m., s.c.	*Alternative choices for enrofloxacin:* Ciprofloxacin 5–10 mg/kg q12–24h, i.v. (1-hour infusion) Amikacin [b]15–20 mg/kg q24h, i.v. ,i.m., s.c., ***OR*** Gentamicin [b] 5–6 mg/kg q24h, i.v., i.m., s.c., ***OR*** Netilmycin [b] 6 mg/kg q24h, i.v., ***OR*** Tobramycin [b] 6 mg/kg q24h, i.v., i.m., s.c. *Alternative choices for cefazolin and cefalothin:* Ampicillin 20–40 mg/kg q6–8h, i.v., i.m., s.c., ***OR*** Ampicillin–sulbactam 50 mg/kg q6–8h, i.v., i.m., ***OR*** Piperacillin 25–50 mg/kg q6–8h, i.v., i.m., ***OR*** Piperacillin–tazobactam 25–50 mg/kg q6–8h, i.v., i.m. Ticarcillin 40–75 mg/kg q6–8h, i.v., i.m., ***OR*** Ticarcillin–clavulanate 30–50 mg/kg q6–8h i.v., i.m. *Alternative single-agent choices:* Cefoxitin [a] 20–30 mg/kg q6–8h, i.v., i.m., s.c., ***OR*** Imipenem–cilastatin [d] 2–10 mg/kg q6–8, i.v. (1-hour infusion), ***OR*** Meropenem 13–15 mg/kg i.v. q8h; 30 mg/kg s.c. q12h ***OR*** Ceftazidime [a] 25–30 mg/kg i.v., i.m., s.c. q8h
	CATS: Ampicillin 20–40 mg/kg q6–8h, i.v., i.m., s.c. Cefoxitin [a] 20–30 mg/kg q6–8h, i.v., i.m., s.c.	Ampicillin–sulbactam 50 mg/kg q6–8h, i.v., i.m., ***OR*** Cefazolin [a] 20–30 mg/kg q6–8h, i.v., i.m., s.c., ***OR*** Cephalothin [a] 25–40 mg/kg q6–8h, i.v., i.m., s.c. *Combination therapy:* Ampicillin 20–40 mg/kg q6–8h, i.v., i.m., s.c., ***OR*** Cefazolin [a] 20–30 mg/kg q6–8h, i.v., i.m., s.c., ***OR*** Cephalothin [a] 25–40 mg/kg q6–8h, i.v., i.m., s.c., ***AND*** Amikacin [b] 15–20 mg/kg q24h, i.v., i.m., s.c., ***OR*** Gentamicin [b] 5–6 mg/kg q24h, i.v., i.m., s.c., ***OR*** Netilmycin [b] 6 mg/kg q24h, i.v., ***OR*** Tobramycin [b] 6 mg/kg q24h, i.v., i.m., s.c. *Alternative choices for cefoxitin and combinations above:* Imipenem–cilastatin [d] 2–10 mg/kg q6–8, i.v. (1-hr infusion), ***OR*** Meropenem 13–15 mg/kg i.v. q8h; 30 mg/kg s.c. q12h, ***OR*** Ceftazidime [a] 25–30 mg/kg i.v., i.m., s.c. q8h

14.4 Parenteral empirical antibiotic therapy for the febrile neutropenic dog or cat. Intravenous administration is preferred. All i.v. injections are given as a slow push over 15–20 minutes unless indicated otherwise. (Modified from Abrams-Ogg and Kruth, 2006. Doses adapted from Allen *et al.*, 2005; Greene *et al.*, 2006 and Plumb, 2008). [a] Cephalosporins (cefazolin, cefalothin, cefoxitin, ceftazidime) are usually given at 30 mg/kg q8h, i.v.; [b] Avoid use of aminoglycoside antibiotics in animals that are dehydrated or receiving furosemide to reduce the risks of nephrotoxicity; [c] The initial dose of enrofloxacin in dogs is usually 5 mg/kg q12h i.v. Higher doses are reserved for those cases where *Pseudomonas* spp. are suspected or isolated, because of the risk of causing seizures and other neurological signs, especially with repetitive administration to geriatric patients, and those with hypoalbuminaemia or a history of seizures. Enrofloxacin is approved for i.m. use only but the solution is a tissue irritant and i.v. administration is preferred, injected over 20–60 minutes; dilution of 1 part parenteral solution with 9 parts sterile water for injection may be used. The parenteral solution should not be injected s.c. Enrofloxacin may cause cartilage defects in young growing dogs, but clinical experience suggests that use at standard doses for 3–5 days is not associated with long-term sequelae. [d] The standard dose is 5 mg/kg q8h i.v. (1 hour infusion). (continues) ▶

Disease	First choice(s) in author's hospital	Alternative choices
Ehrlichiosis	**Mild–moderately ill:** Doxycycline 5 mg/kg q12h i.v. (1-hour infusion)	Tetracycline 5–10 mg/kg q8h i.v., i.m.
	Severely ill: Doxycycline 5 mg/kg q12h i.v. (1-hr infusion), ***AND*** Enrofloxacin [c] 5–10 mg/kg q12–24h i.v., i.m., ***OR*** Ciprofloxacin 5–10 mg/kg q12–24h, i.v. (1-hour infusion)	Doxycycline 5 mg/kg q12h i.v. (1-hour infusion), ***OR*** Tetracycline 5–10 mg/kg q8h i.v., i.m., ***AND*** Cefoxitin [a] 20–30 mg/kg q6–8h, i.v., i.m., s.c., ***OR*** Amikacin [b] 15–20 mg/kg q24h, i.v., i.m., s.c., ***OR*** Gentamicin [b] 5–6 mg/kg q24h, i.v., i.m., s.c., ***OR*** Netilmycin [b] 6 mg/kg q24h, i.v., ***OR*** Tobramycin [b] 6 mg/kg q24h, i.v., i.m., s.c.
Neutropenia of unknown cause	Mild–moderately ill: As per myelosuppression	As per myelosuppression
	Severely ill: Imipenem [d] 2–10 mg/kg q6–8, i.v. (1-hr infusion) Cilastatin, ***OR*** Meropenem 13–15 mg/kg i.v. q8h; 30 mg/kg s.c. q12h	As per myelosuppression *Alternative beta-lactam combination therapy choices:* Ampicillin 20–40 mg/kg q6–8h, i.v., i.m., s.c., ***OR*** Ampicillin–sulbactam 50 mg/kg q6–8h, i.v., i.m., ***OR*** Cefazolin [a] 20–30 mg/kg q6–8h, i.v., i.m., s.c., ***OR*** Cephalothin [a] 25–40 mg/kg q6–8h, i.v., i.m., s.c., ***AND*** Piperacillin 25–50 mg/kg q6–8h, i.v., i.m., ***OR*** Piperacillin–tazobactam 25–50 mg/kg q6–8h, i.v., i.m. Ticarcillin 40–75 mg/kg q6–8h, i.v., i.m., ***OR*** Ticarcillin–clavulanate 30–50 mg/kg q6–8h i.v., i.m., ***OR*** Ceftazidime [a] 25–30 mg/kg i.v., i.m., s.c. q8h, ± Cefoxitin [a] 20–30 mg/kg q6–8h, i.v., i.m., s.c., ***OR*** Metronidazole 10–15 mg/kg q8h i.v. (1-hr infusion), ***OR*** Clindamycin 10 mg/kg q12h i.v., s.c.
Overwhelming sepsis	Imipenem-cilastin [d] 2–10 mg/kg q6–8, i.v. (1-hr infusion), ***OR*** Meropenem 13–15 mg/kg i.v. q8h; 30 mg/kg s.c. q12h	Enrofloxacin (dogs) [c] 5–10 mg/kg q12–24h i.v., i.m., ***OR*** Ciprofloxacin (dogs) 5–10 mg/kg q12h, i.v. (1-hr infusion), ***OR*** Amikacin [b] 15–20 mg/kg q24h, i.v., i.m., s.c., ***OR*** Gentamicin [b] 5–6 mg/kg q24h, i.v., i.m., s.c., ***OR*** Netilmycin [b] 6 mg/kg q24h, i.v., ***OR*** Tobramycin [b] 6 mg/kg q24h, i.v., i.m., s.c., ***AND*** Ampicillin 20–40 mg/kg q6–8h, i.v., i.m., s.c., ***OR*** Cefazolin [a] 20–30 mg/kg q6–8h, i.v., i.m., s.c., ***OR*** Cefalothin [a] 25–40 mg/kg q6–8h, i.v., i.m., s.c., ± Metronidazole 10–15 mg/kg q8h i.v. (1-hr infusion), ***OR*** Clindamycin 10 mg/kg q12h i.v., s.c. *Alternative beta-lactam based combination therapy choices:* As per neutropenia of unknown cause

14.4 (continued) Parenteral empirical antibiotic therapy for the febrile neutropenic dog or cat. Intravenous administration is preferred. All i.v. injections are given as a slow push over 15–20 minutes unless indicated otherwise. (Modified from Abrams-Ogg and Kruth, 2006. Doses adapted from Allen *et al.*, 2005; Greene *et al.*, 2006 and Plumb, 2008). [a] Cephalosporins (cefazolin, cefalothin, cefoxitin, ceftazidime) are usually given at 30 mg/kg q8h, i.v.; [b] Avoid use of aminoglycoside antibiotics in animals that are dehydrated or receiving furosemide to reduce the risks of nephrotoxicity; [c] The initial dose of enrofloxacin in dogs is usually 5 mg/kg q12h i.v. Higher doses are reserved for those cases where *Pseudomonas* spp. are suspected or isolated, because of the risk of causing seizures and other neurological signs, especially with repetitive administration to geriatric patients, and those with hypoalbuminaemia or a history of seizures. Enrofloxacin is approved for i.m. use only but the solution is a tissue irritant and i.v. administration is preferred, injected over 20–60 minutes; dilution of 1 part parenteral solution with 9 parts sterile water for injection may be used. The parenteral solution should not be injected s.c. Enrofloxacin may cause cartilage defects in young growing dogs, but clinical experience suggests that use at standard doses for 3–5 days is not associated with long-term sequelae. [d] The standard dose is 5 mg/kg q8h i.v. (1 hour infusion).

Combination therapy has historically been preferred over monotherapy to increase the antibacterial spectrum, take advantage of additive and synergistic effects while minimizing toxicity, and to reduce the development of resistance. Historically most approaches combined an aminoglycoside with a beta-lactam, but newer approaches have been developed to avoid aminoglycoside nephrotoxicity and to improve efficacy. When fluoroquinolones are used it should be noted that they seem to have a limited activity against Gram-positive organisms in neutropenic patients. For infections complicating the episodes of neutropenia most commonly encountered by veterinary surgeons, the various protocols are probably of equivalent efficacy. The author currently uses enrofloxacin plus cefazolin in cancer patients, ampicillin plus gentamicin or enrofloxacin, or cefoxitin alone, in animals with parvoviral diseases, and meropenem for initial therapy in animals with overwhelming sepsis associated with severe neutropenia of undetermined cause. Intravenous antibiotic administration is preferred, but there must be strict adherence to asepsis during catheter placement and use.

After starting antibiotic therapy, reduction of fever is expected within 72 hours and the animal should appear more alert. Increased depression accompanying a decreasing temperature may be a sign of impending septic shock. Therapy should continue for 1–7 days after the animal's neutrophil count increases to more than 1.0–2.0 × 10^9/l and the fever resolves. If the fever has resolved, but prolonged neutropenia is anticipated, consideration may be given to changing to oral therapy with the same agents as used for antimicrobial prophylaxis (see Figure 14.3).

Pyrexia may not resolve promptly if:

- It is not bacterial in origin (and this should be reconsidered)
- The organism is not sensitive to the antimicrobial agents
- Drug doses are too low (uncommon)
- Host defences are so severely compromised that the infection and associated fever will not resolve with any antimicrobial agent until defences are repaired.

Initial culture results may assist therapeutic decision-making with unresponsive fever, but often another empirical judgement will be necessary. If the animal is clinically stable the current medication may be continued until the fever resolves and the neutrophil count improves as previously discussed. If the animal is deteriorating, new antimicrobials should be employed. In most cases it is preferable to use new drugs in addition to, rather than as a substitute for, existing therapy. The choice of additional drugs depends on which antibiotics were used for initial therapy. Failure of response to empirical therapy with cefoxitin or an aminoglycoside plus a first-generation cephalosporin would prompt additional therapy against *Pseudomonas* spp. with ticarcillin, piperacillin, ceftazidime or a carbapenem. If a resistant Gram-negative enteric organism is suspected (e.g. with signs of intestinal injury or pneumonia), choices for additional therapy include an aminoglycoside, fluoroquinolone, second- or third-generation cephalosporin, or a carbapenem. If a resistant Gram-positive cutaneous organism is suspected (e.g. with catheter-associated phlebitis or pneumonia), the animal should be treated with clindamycin at 10 mg/kg i.v., i.m. or s.c. q12h. A non-responding fever may also be due to an anaerobic organism. Additional therapy could include metronidazole (10–15 mg/kg i.v., 1-hour infusion, q8h), clindamycin, cefoxitin or a carbapenem. Although carbapenems are expensive, they may be less expensive than triple coverage with enrofloxacin, cefazolin and metronidazole and may be substituted for the latter. If initial therapy is with enrofloxacin plus cefazolin, the author currently intensifies therapy with ceftazidime or metronidazole or changes to a carbapenem.

The preceding recommendations are appropriate for many cases, but may not be feasible because of cost or the inability of the owner to return the animal to the hospital. In such cases, initial therapy with oral antimicrobial therapy may be warranted. In addition, oral antimicrobial agents may be sufficient for the initial treatment of neutropenic animals that have been febrile and clinically stable for several days. A fluoroquinolone plus a first-generation cephalosporin or aminopenicillin will provide broad-spectrum antibacterial activity similar to the injectable combinations discussed previously and is recommended if oral therapy is elected in animals with grade 3–4 neutropenia. For clinically stable animals with grade 1–2 neutropenia and mild pyrexia, treatment as described in Figure 14.3 may suffice. Treatment for *Ehrlichia canis* infection with oral tetracyclines may also control infection secondary to neutropenia. Doxycycline is preferred when a dog with ehrlichiosis is neutropenic because it causes less disturbance of the GI flora than do tetracycline and oxytetracycline. In all cases of oral therapy the animal should be observed closely for deterioration, and arrangements made to initiate parenteral therapy. Oral antimicrobial therapy is not appropriate when the animal is dehydrated or vomiting, or when there is disruption of the intestinal mucosa.

Empirical antifungal therapy is used in human patients, but is not recommended in dogs or cats. If neutropenia and antibacterial therapy persist beyond 10 days, monitoring of faeces by cytology or culture for overgrowth of *Candida* spp. should be considered, especially if antibacterial agents are being used that disturb the GI flora (e.g. amoxicillin, cefoxitin, metronidazole).

Treatment of documented infections

Treatment of documented bacterial infections should consist of bactericidal antibiotics with the choices based upon susceptibility testing. The trend in human medicine is towards monotherapy. Treatment of bacteraemia without evidence of other organ involvement should continue for 1–7 days after the animal's neutrophil count increases above 1.0–2.0 × 10^9/l and the fever resolves. Treatment of pneumonia and urinary tract and soft tissue infections should continue for at least 7 days after the animal's neutrophil count increases above 1.0–2.0 × 10^9/l and clinical and radiographic signs resolve. The infection may transiently seem to become worse as the neutrophil count increases, but fever should be decreasing if antimicrobial therapy is appropriate.

Amphotericin B was previously the drug of choice for invasive fungal infections in neutropenic human patients, but it is being replaced by voriconazole for aspergillosis and by echinocandins for candidiasis. Ketoconazole, itraconazole or fluconazole may also be adequate to treat candidiasis.

Granulocyte transfusions

The lifespan of transfused neutrophils is only a few hours in a neutropenic septic patient. Nevertheless, the transient increase in neutrophils may help to control sepsis. Neutrophil transfusion in human patients is most beneficial in the treatment of severe, especially prolonged, neutropenia, and in neonatal sepsis. Neutrophils are transfused as granulocyte concentrates prepared by leucophoresis. Technical difficulties, expense, immunological sensitization from repetitive transfusions, and the need to irradiate granulocyte concentrates to prevent transfusion-related graft-versus-host disease make such transfusion impractical in most veterinary clinics. Fresh whole blood transfusion (22 ml/kg) is anecdotally reported to be beneficial in treating severe parvovirus infection in kittens (Kowall, 1974). This benefit may be in part attributable to transfused neutrophils. For further information, the reader is referred to Abrams-Ogg, 2010.

Haemopoietic stimulant drugs

The haemopoietic cytokines granulocyte colony-stimulating factor (G-CSF) and granulocyte–monocyte colony-stimulating factor (GM-CSF) stimulate granulocyte progenitor cells and mature neutrophils, thereby enhancing neutrophil production, differentiation, marrow release and function. Several recombinant human (rHu) cytokines are now available as commercial drugs, with availability varying by country. These include filgrastim and lenograstim (rHuG-CSF), pegfilgrastim (pegylated (long-acting) rHuG-CSF), and sargramostim and molgramostin (rHuGM-CSF). Recombinant canine and feline GM-CSF are available commercially as laboratory reagents.

Haemopoietic cytokines are most useful in human patients when given prophylactically after cytotoxic therapy to reduce the duration and severity of neutropenia, and such use is now the standard of care in aggressive cancer treatment protocols. They are less useful in established neutropenia caused by cytotoxic therapy with or without sepsis, because progenitor cells may be exhausted and/or endogenous cytokine levels are already increased. They are of limited utility in aplastic anaemia (immune-mediated pancytopenia) because endogenous cytokine levels are often markedly increased. The utility of cytokine therapy for neutropenia caused by drug reaction varies with the mechanism of toxicosis. Cytokine therapy also reduces the severity of cyclic neutropenia and certain other idiopathic neutropenic conditions and may be beneficial in human patients with acquired immunodeficiency syndrome. The role of cytokine therapy in established sepsis is not clear – it is potentially beneficial, of no benefit, or even detrimental depending on the circumstances. The benefits of prophylactic cytokine therapy and therapy of established neonatal sepsis are controversial. Side effects of G-CSF in human patients include bone pain and, rarely, side effects from overproduction of neutrophils. Side effects of GM-CSF also include influenza-like syndromes and capillary leak syndrome.

A form of rHuG-CSF (Neupogen; Amgen, Thousand Oaks, California, USA) has been used the most in dogs and cats. It is a potent stimulator of granulopoiesis, but the effect is transient in normal animals because of the formation of neutralizing antibody. Increased neutrophil counts begin to decline after 2–3 weeks of daily treatment, and neutropenia will occur if treatment is continued because of antibody cross-reactivity with endogenous G-CSF. Veterinary surgeons have used rHuG-CSF successfully to ameliorate myelosuppression in dogs and cats receiving cancer chemotherapy. Typically the drug is given at a dose of 5 μg/kg s.c. q24h to febrile neutropenic animals, prophylactically with grade 3–4 neutropenia, or beginning 5 days after chemotherapy, and it is continued until the neutrophil count increases above 1.0–2.0 × 10^9/l. This is later than the typical use in human patients, where rHuG-CSF is started 1–2 days after chemotherapy. The normal recommendation is that the drug should not be given within 24 hours before or after chemotherapy because this will increase injury to cytotoxic progenitor cells. This recommendation, however, has been challenged, and haemopoietic protection from cytokine therapy prior to cytotoxic therapy has also been reported. Neupogen is supplied as a 300 μg/ml preservative-free solution in a single-use vial. Given the cost of the product, veterinary surgeons typically use the vial for multiple doses. It is essential that the vial be penetrated aseptically and stored under refrigeration. To facilitate the measurement of small doses, a diluted solution may be prepared by a compounding pharmacy. The short courses of therapy and possible concurrent immunosuppression from cytotoxic chemotherapy reduce the antibody effect and permit repeated use (Henry *et al.,* 1995). Stimulation of granulopoiesis may result in a left shift and toxic changes in the neutrophils that may be confused with a response to infection. Side effects other than antibody formation are rare. The use of rHuG-CSF is expensive and the cost–benefit ratio compared with the risk of developing and the cost of treating sepsis in dogs and cats is not known. Similarly, although the use of rHuG-CSF may prevent dose reduction and may permit dose escalation of anticancer drugs in dogs and cats, the benefits for improved tumour control and patient survival are not known. Although the drug has been used in dogs and cats for over 15 years, its use has not become routine in veterinary oncology, and nor is this encouraged. Therapy with rHuG-CSF has been reportedly or anecdotally beneficial in cases with myelosuppression caused by oestrogen or phenobarbital toxicosis in dogs and griseofulvin toxicosis in cats.

The routine use of rHuG-CSF in parvoviral infections and other causes of sepsis in dogs and cats is not recommended (Kraft and Kuffer, 1995; Rewerts *et al.*, 1998; Mischke *et al.*, 2001; Duffy *et al.*, 2010), although use in septic neonates should be considered. Cats with FeLV-induced myelosuppression have been anecdotally reported to be treated with rHuG-CSF with variable results, but the drug is effective in increasing neutrophil counts in cats infected experimentally with feline immunodeficiency virus (FIV; Phillips *et al.*, 2005). Although cats with FeLV and FIV infections are immunosuppressed, neutralizing antibodies will develop. The neutrophilic effect of rHuGM-CSF is not as strong in cats with retroviral infection, and the drug increases FIV viral load (Arai *et al.*, 2000).

Dogs have also been treated with rHuGM-CSF. Stimulation of granulopoiesis is lower than with rHuG-CSF. Given the lower efficacy and greater potential for side effects, the use of rHuGM-CSF is in general not recommended for the treatment of neutropenia in dogs and cats.

Lithium carbonate is a non-specific haemopoietic stimulant that causes a mild increase in neutrophil counts in normal dogs. It has limited utility in treating chemotherapy-induced myelosuppression in dogs, and any reported association with recovery from myelosuppression due to other causes may have been coincidental (Abrams-Ogg, 2010; Leclerc *et al.*, 2010). The drug is inexpensive, but serum blood levels must be monitored, which increases expense. Side effects include depression, seizures and nephrogenic diabetes insipidus. The drug may be myelosuppressive in cats (Dieringer *et al.*, 1992).

Removal of the focus of infection

Acknowledging the anaesthetic concerns with a critical patient, excision or debridement of the site of infection should be considered in animals with neutropenia associated with overwhelming sepsis, or in animals with primary neutropenia where a secondary infection has localized in soft tissue and is not responding to antimicrobial therapy alone.

Other treatments

Other therapeutic strategies in the management of sepsis have been reviewed (DeClue, 2010).

References and further reading

Abrams-Ogg ACG (2006) Neutropenia. In: *Veterinary Emergency and Critical Care Manual, 2nd edn,* ed. KA Mathews, pp. 435–442. Lifelearn Inc., Guelph

Abrams-Ogg ACG (2010) Platelet and granulocyte transfusion. In: *Schalm's Veterinary Hematology, 6th edn,* ed. D Weiss and KJ Wardrop, pp. 751–756. Blackwell Publishing, Ames

Abrams-Ogg ACG (2011) The use of lithium carbonate to prevent lomustine-induced myelosuppression in dogs: a pilot study. *Canadian Journal of Veterinary Research* **75**, 73–76

Abrams-Ogg ACG and Kruth SA (2006) Infections associated with neutropenia in the dog and cat. In: *Antimicrobial Therapy in Veterinary Medicine, 4th edn*, ed. S Giguere, J Prescott, J Baggot, R Walker and P. Dowling, pp. 344–356. Blackwell Publishing, Ames

Allen DG, Dowling PM and Smith DA (2005) *Handbook of Veterinary Drugs, 3rd edn,* ed. DG Allen, PM Dowling and DA Smith, pp. 5–54. Lippincott Williams & Wilkins, Philadelphia

Anderson PG and Pidgeon G (1987) Candidiasis in a dog with parvoviral enteritis. *Journal of the American Animal Hospital Association* **23**, 27–30

Arai M, Darman J, Lewis A and Yamamoto JK (2000) The use of human hematopoietic growth factors (rhGM-CSF and rhEPO) as a supportive therapy for FIV-infected cats. *Veterinary Immunology and Immunopathology* **77**, 71–92

Billen F, Clercx C, Le Garérrès A *et al.* (2009) Comparison of the value of measurement of serum galactomannan and *Aspergillus*-specific antibodies in the diagnosis of canine sino-nasal aspergillosis. *Journal of Small Animal Practice* **50**, 67–72

Chretin JD, Rassnick KM, Shaw NA *et al.* (2007) Prophylactic trimethoprim-sulfadiazine during chemotherapy in dogs with lymphoma and osteosarcoma: a double-blind, placebo-controlled study. *Journal of Veterinary Internal Medicine* **21**, 141–148

Couto CG (1990) Management of complications of cancer chemotherapy. *Veterinary Clinics of North America: Small Animal Practice* **20**, 1037–1053

Daly M, Sheppard S, Cohen N *et al.* (2011) Safety of masitinib mesylate in healthy cats. *Journal of Veterinary Internal Medicine* **25**, 297–302

DeClue A (2010) Sepsis and the systemic inflammatory response syndrome. In: *Textbook of Veterinary Internal Medicine 7th edn,* ed. SJ Ettinger and EC Feldman, pp. 523–527. Saunders Elsevier, St. Louis

Dieringer TM, Brown SA, Rogers KS *et al.* (1992) Effects of lithium carbonate administration to healthy cats. *American Journal of Veterinary Research* **53**, 721–726

Diniz PP, Schulz BS, Hartmann K and Breitschwerdt EB (2011) 'Candidatus Neoehrlichia mikurensis' infection in a dog from Germany. *Journal of Clinical Microbiology* **49**, 2059–2062

Dow SW, Curtis CR, Jones RL and Wingfield WE (1989) Bacterial culture of blood from critically ill dogs and cats. *Journal of the American Veterinary Medical Association* **195**, 113–117

Duffy A, Dow S, Ogilvie G, Rao S and Hackett T (2010) Hematologic improvement in dogs with parvovirus infection treated with recombinant canine granulocyte-colony stimulating factor. *Journal of Veterinary Pharmacology and Therapeutics* **33**, 352–356

Greene CE, HartmannK and Calpin J (2006) Antimicrobial drug formulary. In: *Infectious Diseases of the Dog and Cat, 3rd edn,* ed. C.E. Greene, pp. 1186–1333. Elsevier, Philadelphia

Henry CJ, Buss MS and Lothrop CD (1998) Veterinary uses of recombinant human granulocyte colony-stimulating factor. Part I. Oncology. *Compendium on Continuing Education for the Practicing Veterinarian* **20**, 728–734

Henry CJ, Lothrop CD and Goodman S (1995) Dogs receiving mitoxantrone and cyclophosphamide do not produce clinically significant antibody titers to rhG-CSF. *Journal of Veterinary Internal Medicine* **9**, 205

Kowall NL (1974) Feline panleukopenia. In: *Current Veterinary Therapy V: Small Animal Practice,* ed. RW Kirk, pp. 957–959. WB Saunders, Philadelphia

Kraft W and Kuffer M (1995) Behandlung schwerer neutropenien bei hund und katze mit filgrastim. *Tierarztliche Praxis* **23**, 609–613

Kunkle GA, Sundlof S and Keisling K (1995) Adverse effects of oral antibacterial therapy in dogs and cats: an epidemiologic study of pet owners' observations. *Journal of the American Animal Hospital Association* **31**, 46–55

Leclerc A, Abrams-Ogg ACG, Kruth SA and Bienzle D (2010) Effects of lithium carbonate on carboplatin-induced thrombocytopenia in dogs. *American Journal of Veterinary Research* **71**, 555–563

Lobetti RG, Joubert KE, Picard J, Carstens J and Pretorius E (2002) Bacterial colonization of intravenous catheters in young dogs suspected to have parvoviral enteritis. *Journal of the American Veterinary Medical Association* **220**, 1321–1324

Mischke R, Barth T, Wohlsein P, Rohn K and Nolte I (2001) Effect of recombinant human granulocyte colony-stimulating factor (rhG-CSF) on leukocyte count and survival rate of dogs with parvoviral enteritis. *Research in Veterinary Science* **70**, 221–225

Phillips K, Arai M, Tanabe T *et al.* (2005) FIV-infected cats respond to short-term rHuG-CSF treatment which results in anti-G-CSF neutralizing antibody production that inactivates drug activity. *Veterinary Immunology and Immunopathology* **108**, 357–371

Plumb DC (2008) *Plumb's Veterinary Drug Handbook, 6th edn.* Blackwell Publishing, Ames

Rewerts JM, McCaw DL, Cohn LA, Wagner-Mann C and Harrington D (1998) Recombinant human granulocyte colony-stimulating factor for treatment of puppies with neutropenia secondary to parvovirus infection. *Journal of the American Veterinary Medical Association* **213**, 991–992

Rosenthal RC (1988) Autologous bone marrow transplantation for lymphoma. *Proceedings of the 6th Annual Veterinary Medical Forum of the American College of Veterinary Internal Medicine*, pp. 397–399

Rubin RH and Young LS (2011) *Clinical Approach to Infection in the Compromised Host, 5th edn*, ed. RH Rubin and LS Young. Springer Publishing Company, New York

Sorenmo KU, Harwoood LP, King LG and Drobatz KJ (2010) Case-control study to evaluate risk-factors for the development of sepsis (neutropenia and fever) in dogs receiving chemotherapy. *Journal of the American Veterinary Medical Association* **236**, 650–656

Suter SE (2010) Clinical use of hematopoietic growth factors. In: *Schalm's Veterinary Hematology, 6th edn,* ed. D Weiss and KJ Wardrop, pp. 790–796. Blackwell Publishing, Ames

Turk J, Fales W, Miller M *et al.* (1992) Enteric *Clostridium perfringens* infection associated with parvoviral enteritis in dogs: 74 cases (1987–1990). *Journal of the American Veterinary Medical Association* **200**, 991–994

Turk J, Miller M, Brown T *et al.* (1990) Coliform septicemia and pulmonary disease associated with canine parvoviral enteritis: 88 cases (1987–1988). *Journal of the American Veterinary Medical Association* **196**, 771–773

Vail DM (2009) Supporting the veterinary cancer patient on chemotherapy: neutropenia and gastrointestinal toxicity. *Topics in Companion Animal Medicine* **24**, 122

Veterinary Co-Operative Oncology Group (2004) Veterinary co-operative oncology group – common terminology criteria for adverse events (VCOG-CTCAE) following chemotherapy or biological antineoplastic therapy in dogs and cats v1.0. *Veterinary and Comparative Oncology* **2**, 194–213

15

Eosinophilia

Caroline Mansfield

Introduction

Eosinophils are important components of the immune system, and are often involved in hypersensitivity disorders and parasitic infestations. They are particularly induced by parasites that have a long tissue contact time.

Eosinophilia is defined as an increase in the total eosinophil count in blood or tissue. Although the upper reference interval for the blood concentration of eosinophils in dogs is 0.75×10^9/l, significant circulating eosinophilia is considered to be present when the count exceeds 2.2×10^9/l. This occurs most commonly as a leukaemoid response, or when eosinophil counts increase in response to an underlying cause (Figure 15.1). Idiopathic eosinophilic diseases also occur, affecting specific organ systems or as part of a generalized syndrome.

Pathophysiology

The exact mechanisms for eosinophil production are unknown, but interleukin (IL)-5, IL-3 and granulocyte–monocyte colony-stimulating factor (GM-CSF) all inhibit eosinophil apoptosis and there are specific receptors for these cytokines on eosinophils. Basophils are also primed by IL-3, and therefore basophilia often accompanies eosinophilia. Canine eosinophilic bronchopneumopathy is associated with an increased ratio of $CD4^+$ to $CD8^+$ T lymphocytes in bronchioalveolar lavage fluid (BALF), which suggests that T helper cells may have a role in mediating this eosinophil-dominated inflammatory reaction. Certain tumours (e.g. mast cell tumours and lymphoma) are characterized by an infiltration of eosinophils that is thought to be induced when the neoplastic cells produce eosinophil-stimulating cytokines such as IL-5. Further investigations of the molecular signalling mechanisms that underlie eosinophilia in animals is warranted, because this may allow the establishment of diagnostic criteria that differentiate between allergic, parasitic, idiopathic and neoplastic causes.

Eosinophils are attracted into tissues by local chemoattractant molecules (chemokines) derived from cells such as Th2 lymphocytes. Tissue recruitment of eosinophils is an appropriate response to the presence of migrating parasites because these cells play a role in the immunological destruction of the organisms. Eosinophils contain many toxic inflammatory mediators. Eosinophil cationic protein, in particular, appears to promote the activity of other toxic mediators in target tissue as well as triggering mast cell degranulation and inciting thrombosis. In addition, eosinophils produce leucotrienes that are capable of increasing vascular permeability, and stimulating mucus secretion and smooth muscle contraction. Eosinophil peroxidase may enhance fibrosis by production of oxygen free radical species. If eosinophilia is stimulated inappropriately (i.e. in the absence of helminths), the accumulation of eosinophils has the potential to cause significant damage to the target organs. Target organs include the respiratory, central nervous and intestinal systems.

Causes of eosinophilia

The most common underlying causes for eosinophilic leukaemoid responses in humans are atopy and helminth infestation. This does not appear to be the case in dogs or cats (Figure 15.1).

Breed predispositions

Dogs may have significant tissue infiltration with eosinophils (e.g. eosinophilic stomatitis or eosinophilic meningoencephalomyelitis) in the absence of circulating eosinophilia. This may be due to the short circulating half-life of eosinophils or sequestration of these cells in the organ involved. Diurnal variation may also play a role, because circulating eosinophil numbers in healthy dogs have been shown to peak in late evening, and to be at their lowest at noon. Rottweilers are predisposed to eosinophilic disease, including hypereosinophilic syndrome. German Shepherd Dogs also appear to have an increased incidence of exaggerated eosinophil responses to normal stimuli. Cavalier King Charles Spaniels appear predisposed to eosinophilic stomatitis and other tissue eosinophilic inflammatory diseases, whilst Alaskan Malamutes and Siberian Huskies are over-represented in reports of eosinophilic intestinal and airway disease.

Cats show eosinophilia most commonly in response to flea allergy dermatitis and gastrointestinal disease. They are also frequently reported to have eosinophilia in association with systemic mastocytosis, lymphoma and feline bronchial disease.

Parasitic

- Ancylostomiasis (D)
- **Dirofilariasis (D, C)**
- **Dipetalonemaisis (D)**
- **Ctenophalidiasis (D, C)**
- Filaroidiasis (C)
- Aelurostrongylosis (C)
- Angiostrongylosis (D)
- Ascariasis (D, C)
- Paragonimiasis (D, C)
- ***Sarcoptes scabiei* (D)**
- *Pneumomonyssoides caninum* (D?)

Hypersensitivity

- **Atopy (D, C)**
- **Flea allergy dermatitis (D, C)**
- **Food allergy (D, C)**

Eosinophilic infiltrative disorders

- **Feline bronchial asthma (C)**
- **Eosinophilic bronchopneumopathy (D)**
- Eosinophilic gastroenteritis/colitis (D, C)
- Hypereosinophilic syndrome (D, C)

Infectious diseases

- Upper respiratory tract viral disorders (C?)
- Feline panleucopenia (C?)
- Feline infectious peritonitis (C?)
- Toxoplasmosis (C)
- Suppurative processes (chronic upper respiratory disease, pneumonia, metritis, mastitis, lower urinary tract infection) (D, C)

Neoplasia

- **Mast cell tumour (D, C)**
- **Lymphoma (D, C)**
- Myeloproliferative disorders
- Solid tumours (D, C) (myxosarcoma, basal cell tumour, squamous cell carcinoma, salivary gland adenocarcinoma, sweat gland adenocarcinoma)
- Haemangiosarcoma (D)

Other

- Soft tissue trauma (D, C?)
- Feline urological syndrome (C?)
- Cardiomyopathy (D, C?)
- Renal failure (D, C?)
- Hyperthyroidism (C?)
- Oestrus (D?)
- Pemphigus foliaceus (D?, C?)
- Snake bite (D?)
- Hypoadrenocorticism (D?)
- Immune-mediated haemolytic anaemia (D?)
- Hepatopathy (D?)
- Chronic renal failure (D?)
- Arthrosis (D?)
- Hypocalcaemia (D?)
- Pulmonary oedema (D?)
- Constipation (D?)
- Diabetes mellitus (D?)
- Hypoparathyroidism (D?)
- Juvenile nephropathy (D?)
- Hydrothorax (D?)
- Panosteitis (D?)

15.1 Reported differential diagnoses for peripheral eosinophilia in dogs (D) and cats (C). Those diseases that are commonly associated with eosinophilia are shown in bold, and those speculatively associated are followed by '?'. Note that eosinophilic infiltrative disorders such as eosinophilic stomatitis, eosinophilic granuloma complex or eosinophilic meningoencephalomyelitis are not commonly associated with peripheral eosinophilia.

Inflammatory disease

Inflammatory disease of organs with large epithelial surface areas (e.g. the intestine or lungs) is most commonly associated with peripheral eosinophilia. Circulatory eosinophilia may also accompany canine sarcoptic mange, but is not a common feature of atopic dermatitis or eosinophilic dermatitis. Dogs with *Angiostrongylus vasorum* (lungworm) or *Dirofilaria immitis* (heartworm) infections may have significant eosinophilia; however, the presence of low numbers of intestinal parasites does not cause significant eosinophilia.

Paraneoplastic disease

Paraneoplastic eosinophilia is commonly reported in both dogs and cats. Round cell tumours (e.g. mast cell tumours and lymphoma) are implicated most frequently, but other solid tumours may also cause eosinophilia (see Figure 15.1). The severity of eosinophilia associated with tumours is highly variable, and can range from mild to extremely severe.

Eosinophilic bronchopneumopathy

Eosinophilic bronchopneumopathy (EBP; previously known as pulmonary infiltration of eosinophils (PIE)) is commonly astsociated with peripheral eosinophilia. The clinical presentation is variable and can range from a soft cough to dyspnoea. Radiographic changes are also variable, ranging from diffusely increased interstitial lung patterns (Figure 15.2), to coalescing diffuse alveolar lung patterns (Figure 15.3). The diagnosis of EBP is dependent on demonstration of a high percentage of eosinophils (generally > 20%) within BALF with no identifiable parasitic cause.

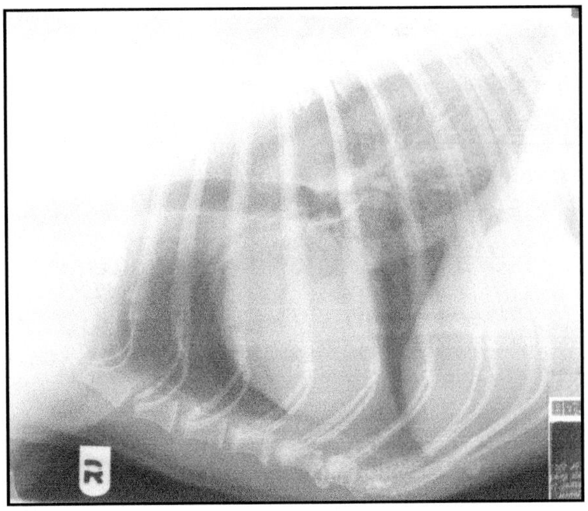

15.2 Lateral thoracic radiograph from a 4-year-old neutered female German Shepherd Dog presented with vague signs of lethargy. The resting respiratory rate was mildly increased (40 breaths per minute), and the peripheral eosinophil count was 2.8 × 10^9/l. The lateral radiograph of the thorax shows a mild increase in interstitial opacity. Bronchoalveolar lavage demonstrated a high eosinophil count (35%) and parasitic testing was negative. The dog responded well to prednisolone treatment.

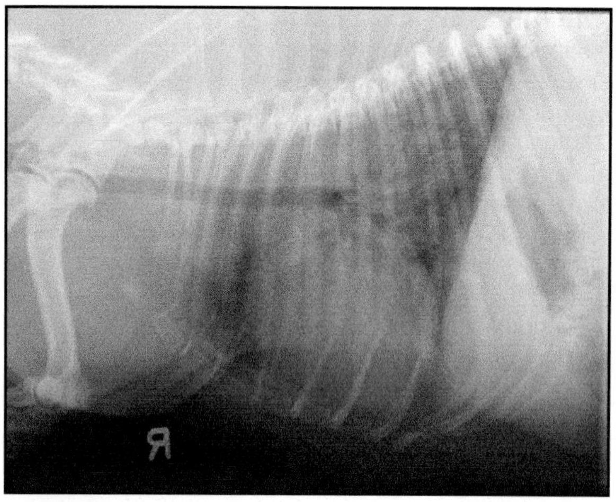

15.3 Lateral thoracic radiograph from a 3-year-old male Staffordshire Bull Terrier. The dog had a history of coughing for 1 week, and had presented with severe dyspnoea and haemoptysis. The resting respiratory rate was 55 breaths per minute and there were some abnormal lung sounds on auscultation. There was marked circulating eosinophilia (7.5×10^9/l) and a significant proportion of eosinophils in bronchoalveolar lavage fluid. No other organ system appeared to be involved and parasite testing was negative. The dog initially responded well to prednisolone treatment, but relapsed upon discontinuation and deteriorated rapidly.

Eosinophilic gastroenteritis

Eosinophilic gastritis, enteritis and colitis occur infrequently, but when they do many affected animals exhibit peripheral eosinophilia. Young, purebred dogs, including German Shepherd Dogs, appear to be predisposed and a hypersensitivity basis is suspected. The intestinal mucosa always contains a baseline number of eosinophils and discrimination between normal and eosinophilic inflammation is challenging. The World Small Animal Veterinary Association (WSAVA) Gastrointestinal Standardization Group has produced guidelines that assist in making this distinction and in grading the severity of eosinophilic enteritis (Day *et al.*, 2008). Again, elimination of underlying parasitic or neoplastic disease is important.

Eosinophilic pleocytosis of cerebrospinal fluid

Eosinophilic pleocytosis of cerebrospinal fluid (CSF) is defined when the total nucleated cell count exceeds 3/μl, and > 20% of the nucleated cells are eosinophils. This change is most commonly idiopathic (i.e. eosinophilic meningoencephalomyelitis), but infectious conditions such as protothecosis, neosporosis and cryptococcosis should be ruled out. Uncommonly, parasitic migration through the central nervous system (CNS) may be associated with the presence of eosinophils in the CSF. Generally idiopathic eosinophilic meningoencephalomyelitis is not associated with peripheral eosinophilia, so the presence of eosinophilia in an animal with eosinophil pleocytosis in the CSF should alert the clinician to the possibility of parasitic involvement.

Hypereosinophilic syndrome

Hypereosinophilic syndrome (HES) is a rare syndrome that has been described in humans, cats and less commonly in dogs. Rottweilers are over-represented in the published reports. The criteria for the definition of idiopathic HES in humans are an eosinophil count persistently > 1.5×10^9/l, damage to end-organs (e.g. the heart and lungs), no ascertainable cause for the eosinophilia and no evidence of clonality. In all reported cases of HES in dogs and cats the eosinophil count has exceeded 4.0×10^9/l. It would be extremely unlikely to diagnose HES in an animal with a mild to moderate eosinophilia (i.e. < 4.0×10^9/l). Paraneoplastic HES has also been reported in a cat, associated with T-cell lymphoma. Other tumours may also cause significant eosinophilia, with some reports of massive eosinophilia ($40–60 \times 10^9$/l). Again, HES should be considered a diagnosis of exclusion and all body systems evaluated for possible neoplasia.

The prognosis for HES is considered universally poor. However there have been individual reports of good survival times with spontaneous clinical remission, as well as resolution with hydroxycarbamate (hydroxyurea) and prednisolone treatment. This suggests that there may be a similar form to the 'benign HES' type identified in humans. Differentiation of HES from eosinophilic leukaemia (EL) is clinically difficult, but in the latter disease there are generally > 5% blast cells in the bone marrow or a large number of clonal karyotype abnormalities, as well as the presence of other cytopenias.

Diagnosis

Given that Rottweilers seem to be predisposed to higher eosinophil counts, circulating eosinophil counts > 0.75×10^9/l may be considered normal in that breed. Owing to the large list of conditions associated with eosinophilia, it is important to verify whether there could be any known underlying disease in an animal that has eosinophilia. This is most important when considering mild to moderate eosinophilia ($0.75–4.0 \times 10^9$/l). Underlying disease may be easily evident on physical examination (e.g. the presence of pruritic skin lesions or ectoparasitic infestation). Skin scrapings may be necessary to rule out mite infestation. Alternatively, the presenting problem may provide further information about the potential organ system involved (e.g. coughing, diarrhoea or neurological signs). In this situation, imaging and then cytological evaluation of that specific organ system is warranted. At all times, parasitic and neoplastic causes must be ruled out before diagnosing an idiopathic eosinophilic syndrome.

If there is no obvious external cause, then specific parasitic testing could be considered in endemic areas. Faecal analysis for *Angiostrongylus vasorum* and *Aelurostrongylus abstrusus* infection may be indicated, especially if there are pulmonary or coagulopathic signs. Heartworm (*Dirofilaria immitis*) should also be ruled out in endemic regions.

If the eosinophilia is only mild in dogs, and the clinical signs are non-specific, then atypical hypoadrencorticism should be considered. Diagnosis (or exclusion) is made by an adrenocorticotropic hormone (ACTH) stimulation test, showing a lack of adrenal response to external stimuli. A lack of endogenous glucocorticoids results in circulating eosinophilia, which is an unexpected finding in a sick animal.

Paraneoplastic conditions, especially round cell tumours, should be considered, especially in cases of moderate to severe eosinophilia. Dependent on the physical examination findings, fine-needle aspiration of peripheral lymph nodes, dermal masses or enlarged mesenchymal organs (e.g. the spleen) may be indicated.

If multiple organ systems are involved, or HES is suspected, then a thorough systematic review is indicated. This includes serum biochemistry, thoracic radiography and abdominal imaging. BALF and ideally bone marrow aspirates should be obtained for cytological examination. Owing to the possibility of paraneoplastic HES, fine-needle aspiration of any enlarged abdominal organs, dermal masses and lymph nodes should also be performed. A diagnostic approach to eosinophilia is shown in Figure 15.4.

Treatment

If an infectious or parasitic cause is identified, this needs to be treated specifically. When there is eosinophilic inflammation of the intestine, treatment with a broad anti-parasitic drug such as fenbendazole (50 mg/kg q24h for 3–5 days) may be indicated prior to other treatment modalities. It is generally recommended that when an eosinophilic enteropathy is present a hypoallergenic diet should be fed in case hypersensitivity has contributed to the process.

With most idiopathic eosinophilic diseases, prednisolone is the cornerstone of management. Prednisolone has profound effects on inflammation, by inhibiting fibroblast proliferation and lymphocyte sensitization, and down-regulating inflammatory cytokine production. Initial management of eosinophilic disease justifies the use of immunosuppressive doses (1–2 mg/kg/day in dogs and 2–4 mg/kg/day in cats), reducing to effect.

In many cases of idiopathic eosinophilic disease or even HES, an initial course of prednisolone may be sufficient to attain remission. Tapered withdrawal of prednisolone is necessary to avoid side effects associated with hypercortisolaemia.

In severe cases, or when prednisolone fails to attain remission, alternative immunosuppressive drugs should be considered. Ciclosporin is used extensively for the treatment of atopy in both dogs

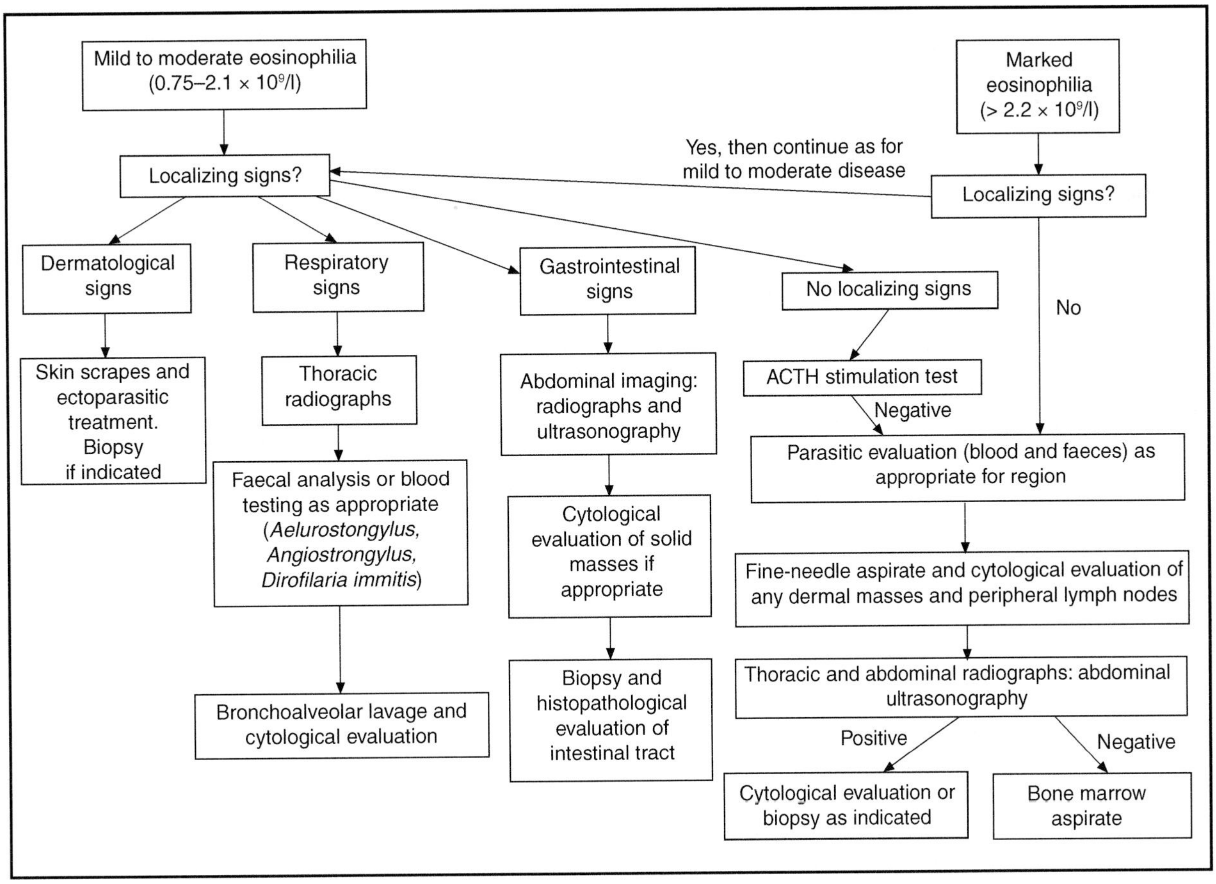

15.4 Diagnostic flow chart for eosinophilia.

and cats and may also be useful in eosinophilic diseases. This drug targets T helper lymphocytes and inhibits their ability to produce a range of cytokines. The bioavailability and dosage of ciclosporin is dependent on the formulation and the licensed veterinary product should be used by choice. Absorption can be erratic and idiosyncratic, so monitoring of trough levels is recommended. Reduction of the dose is also desirable because of the expense and the range of side effects associated with the drug. In some situations (e.g. atopy), oral ketoconazole has been given to reduce the dosage of ciclosporin by interfering with the hepatic microsomal P450 enzymes involved in its metabolism. Recrudescence of toxoplasmosis is a significant risk in the use of ciclosporin in cats, and care should always be taken to check for drug interactions.

Hydroyxcarbamide has also been reported to be effective in the treatment of HES in dogs, although it is possible that the disease in these dogs may have resolved spontaneously without treatment. It is also possible that interferon (IFN)-γ may have some efficacy against eosinophilic diseases. IFN-γ causes a shift from a Th2 to a Th1 response, which directly inhibits IgE. This has not been evaluated in veterinary patients.

References and further reading

Aroch I, Perl S and Markovics A (2001) Disseminated eosinophilic disease resembling idiopathic hypereosinophilic syndrome in a dog. *Veterinary Record* **149**, 386–389

Barcante JM, Barcante TA, Ribeiro VM *et al.* (2008) Cytological and parasitological analysis of bronchoalveolar lavage fluid for the diagnosis of *Angiostrongylus vasorum* infection in dogs. *Veterinary Parasitology* **158**, 93–102

Barrs VR, Beatty JA, McCandlish IA and Kipar A (2002) Hypereosinophilic paraneoplastic syndrome in a cat with intestinal T cell lymphosarcoma. *Journal of Small Animal Practice* **43**, 401–405

Bloom PB (2006) Canine and feline eosinophilic skin diseases. *Veterinary Clinics of North America: Small Animal Practice* **36**, 141–160, vii

Clercx C, Peeters D, German A *et al.* (2002) An immunologic investigation of canine eosinophilic bronchopneumopathy. *Journal of Veterinary Internal Medicine* **16**, 229–237

Day MJ, Bilzer T, Mansell J *et al.* (2008) Histopathological standards for the diagnosis of gastrointestinal inflammation in endoscopic biopsy samples from the dog and cat: a report from the World Small Animal Veterinary Association Gastrointestinal Standardization Group. *Journal of Comparative Pathology* **138**, S1–S43

Gelain ME, Antoniazzi E, Bertazzolo W, Zaccolo M and Comazzi S (2006) Chronic eosinophilic leukemia in a cat: cytochemical and immunophenotypical features. *Veterinary Clinical Pathology* **35**, 454–459

German AJ, Holden DJ, Hall EJ and Day MJ (2002) Eosinophilic diseases in two Cavalier King Charles spaniels. *Journal of Small Animal Practice* **43**, 533–538

James FE and Mansfield CS (2009) Clinical remission of idiopathic hypereosinophilic syndrome in a Rottweiler. *Australian Veterinary Journal* **87**, 330–333

Lilliehook I, Gunnarsson L, Zakrisson G and Tvedten H (2000) Diseases associated with pronounced eosinophilia: a study of 105 dogs in Sweden. *Journal of Small Animal Practice* **41**, 248–253

Lyles SE, Panciera DL, Saunders GK and Leib MS (2009) Idiopathic eosinophilic masses of the gastrointestinal tract in dogs. *Journal of Veterinary Internal Medicine* **23**, 818–823

Marchetti V, Benetti C, Citi S and Taccini V (2005) Paraneoplastic hypereosinophilia in a dog with intestinal T-cell lymphoma. *Veterinary Clinical Pathology* **34**, 259–263

Mauldin EA, Palmeiro BS, Goldschmidt MH and Morris DO (2006) Comparison of clinical history and dermatologic findings in 29 dogs with severe eosinophilic dermatitis: a retrospective analysis. *Veterinary Dermatology* **17**, 338–347

Muir P, Gruffydd-Jones TJ and Brown PJ (1993) Hypereosinophilic syndrome in a cat. *Veterinary Record* **132**, 358–359

Peeters D, Peters IR, Clercx C and Day MJ (2006) Real-time reverse-transcriptase PCR quantification of mRNA encoding cytokines, cc chemokines and CCR3 in bronchial biopsies from dogs with eosinophilic bronchopneumopathy. *Veterinary Immunology and Immunopathology* **110**, 65–77

Perkins M and Watson A (2001) Successful treatment of hypereosinophilic syndrome in a dog. *Australian Veterinary Journal* **79**, 686–689

Sharifi H, Nassiri SM, Esmaelli H and Khoshnegah J (2007) Eosinophilic leukaemia in a cat. *Journal of Feline Medicine and Surgery* **9**, 514–517

Sykes JE, Weiss DJ, Buoen LC, Blauvelt MM and Hayden DW (2001) Idiopathic hypereosinophilic syndrome in 3 Rottweilers. *Journal of Veterinary Internal Medicine* **15**, 162–166

Windsor RC, Sturges BK, Vernau KM and Vernau W (2009) Cerebrospinal fluid eosinophilia in dogs. *Journal of Veterinary Internal Medicine* **23**, 275–281

16

Leukaemia

Elizabeth Villiers, Joanna Morris and Jane Dobson

Introduction

Leukaemia is a malignant transformation of cells of the haemopoietic system and is characterized by an abnormal proliferation of blood cells, usually white blood cells. Leukaemia is a broad term covering a spectrum of diseases that includes acute leukaemia (myeloid and lymphoblastic), chronic leukaemia (myeloid and lymphoid) and the leukaemic phase of lymphoma. Although leukaemia is not a common condition (much less frequent than lymphoma), it is important because of the diagnostic challenges in distinguishing the different types, which have varying treatment outcomes and prognoses.

Leukaemia usually arises in the bone marrow, with neoplastic cells spilling out into the blood and sometimes infiltrating other organs, including the spleen, liver and lymph nodes. However, some types of leukaemia, such as T cell chronic lymphoid leukaemia (CLL), arise in the spleen. Different types of leukaemia have very different prognoses and are treated with different drug protocols and so it is important to make an accurate diagnosis.

Traditionally, diagnosis has been based on examination of cell morphology, sometimes with the use of cytochemical stains. This has many limitations because there is overlap in the morphological appearance of different types of leukaemia and there is a limited number of cytochemical stains, with inconsistent staining for different subtypes. In recent years there has been increasing use of immunophenotyping by flow cytometry, which, when combined with cell morphology, enables clinical pathologists to classify leukaemia more accurately. A recent study using flow cytometry and morphology to classify leukaemia found that 40% of cases were acute leukaemia, 29% were CLL and 31% were the leukaemic phase of high grade lymphoma (Tasca *et al.*, 2009). There were no chronic myeloid leukaemias in this study, which is probably because these leukaemias are usually identified readily using cell morphology, and immunophenotyping does not provide additional information.

The haemopoietic system – leucocyte lineages

An understanding of leukaemia requires an appreciation of the structure and function of bone marrow. Pluripotent stem cells in the marrow give rise to differentiating progenitor cells, which further divide and differentiate into functional mature blood cells (Figure 16.1). In the early stages of haemopoiesis the stem and progenitor cells remain relatively undifferentiated and retain the capacity for cell division and multiplication. As the cells become more differentiated and committed to a certain cell lineage, the capacity for replication is progressively diminished and it is ultimately lost in the mature cell lines seen in peripheral blood. Hence, for each cell lineage there is a pyramidal arrangement of cells within the bone marrow, with dividing undifferentiated cells at the apex and non-dividing mature cells at the base (Figure 16.2). Myeloid cells are fully functional once mature, but lymphocytes released from the bone marrow may require processing by other lymphoid tissues before they are capable of assuming the functions of mature T and B cells.

Neoplastic transformation may occur at several levels of this proliferative/maturation process. Transformation of stem cells or early precursors causes a massive proliferation of undifferentiated cells that are incapable of maturation, resulting in acute leukaemia. Transformation of late precursor cells or mature lymphocytes causes an overproduction of mature differentiated cells, resulting in chronic leukaemia (Figure 16.3).

Aetiology

The cause of leukaemia in dogs and cats is not known in most cases, but genetic changes and environmental factors such as exposure to ionizing radiation (which causes myeloproliferative disease in dogs) may play a role.

Viral infection

Despite one demonstration of virus-like particles and the isolation of a novel retrovirus, there is little strong evidence to suggest that viruses cause canine leukaemia.

In the cat, however, the oncogenic retrovirus feline leukaemia virus (FeLV) causes both lymphoproliferative (LPD) and myeloproliferative diseases (MPD) by insertion of the provirus into the cat's genome and consequent alteration of cellular oncogene function, a process known as insertional

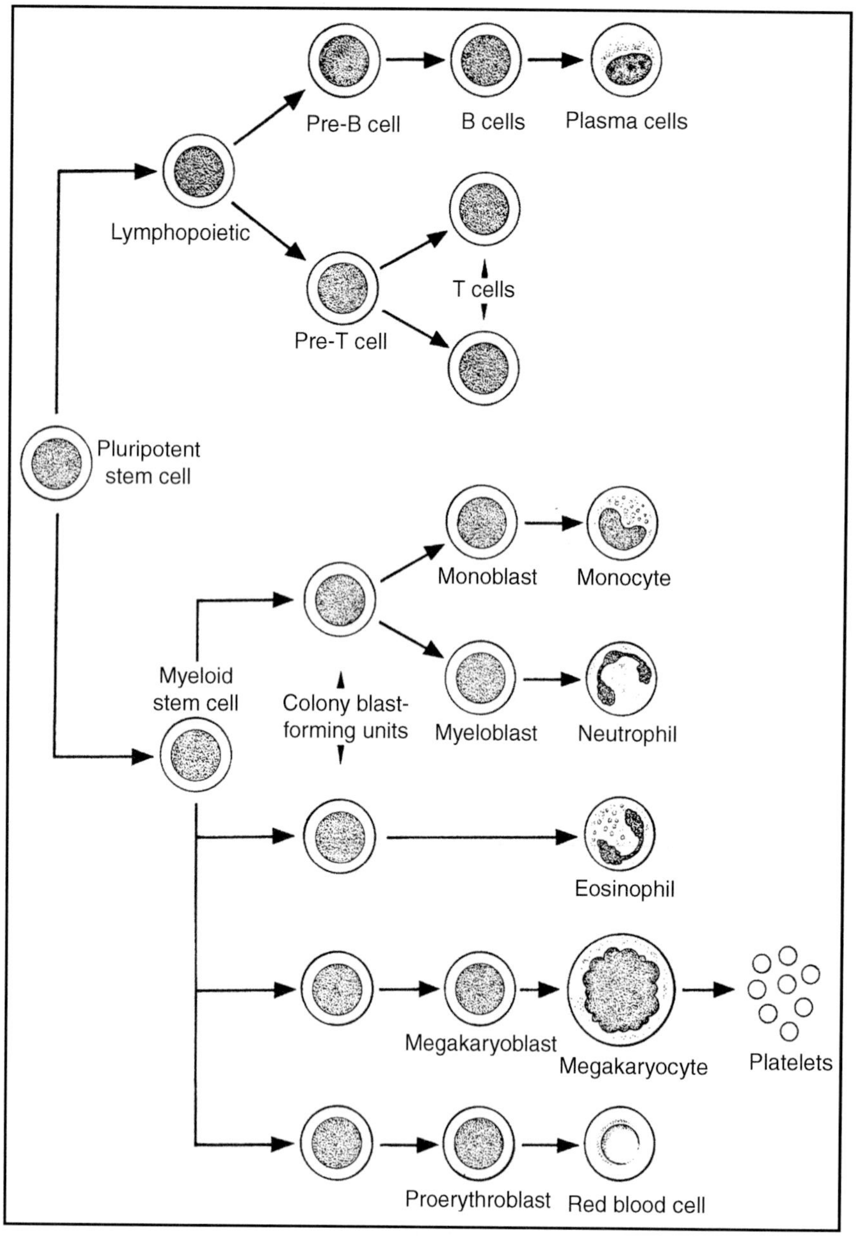

16.1 Schematic diagram depicting haemopoiesis in the bone marrow. The different cell lineages recognized in peripheral blood are the progeny of pluripotential stem cells.

mutagenesis. Alternatively, the FeLV virus may acquire a cellular oncogene by recombination, a process known as transduction. Such recombinant viruses induce rapid tumour development. In the 1970s, between 60 and 90% of cats with LPD or MPD were reported to be FeLV-positive. However, in recent years, following successful test and elimination programmes and vaccination, the percentage of FeLV-positive cats with lymphoma/leukaemia is considerably lower. Feline immunodeficiency virus (FIV) may also cause the development of LPD and MPD as it integrates into the genome and persistently infects lymphoid and myelomonocytic cells (Dunham and Graham, 2008).

Cytogenetics

In humans, many leukaemias arise when the genome is disrupted by structural rearrangements of chromosomes, e.g. translocations and insertions. In many cases a single chromosome rearrangement is consistently identified with a particular type of leukaemia. Many translocations that occur in lymphoid leukaemias involve the loci encoding immunoglobulins and T cell receptors (TCRs), and are thought to originate during normal maturation of B and T cells, as the various receptor subunits on different chromosomes rearrange. In chronic myeloid leukaemia (CML), a translocation between chromosomes 9 and 22 leads to a shortened chromosome 22, which is readily identified cytogenetically and known as the 'Philadelphia chromosome'. At the translocation break points, the genes for the B cell receptor (*BCR*) and Abelson murine leukaemia (*ABL*) are brought together to form a fusion product, BCR–ABL, which acts as a tyrosine kinase and is crucial for the oncogenic effect.

Given that different chromosome numbers exist in different animal species, it is difficult to make direct comparisons, but translocations corresponding to the same gene regions as the human t(9;22)

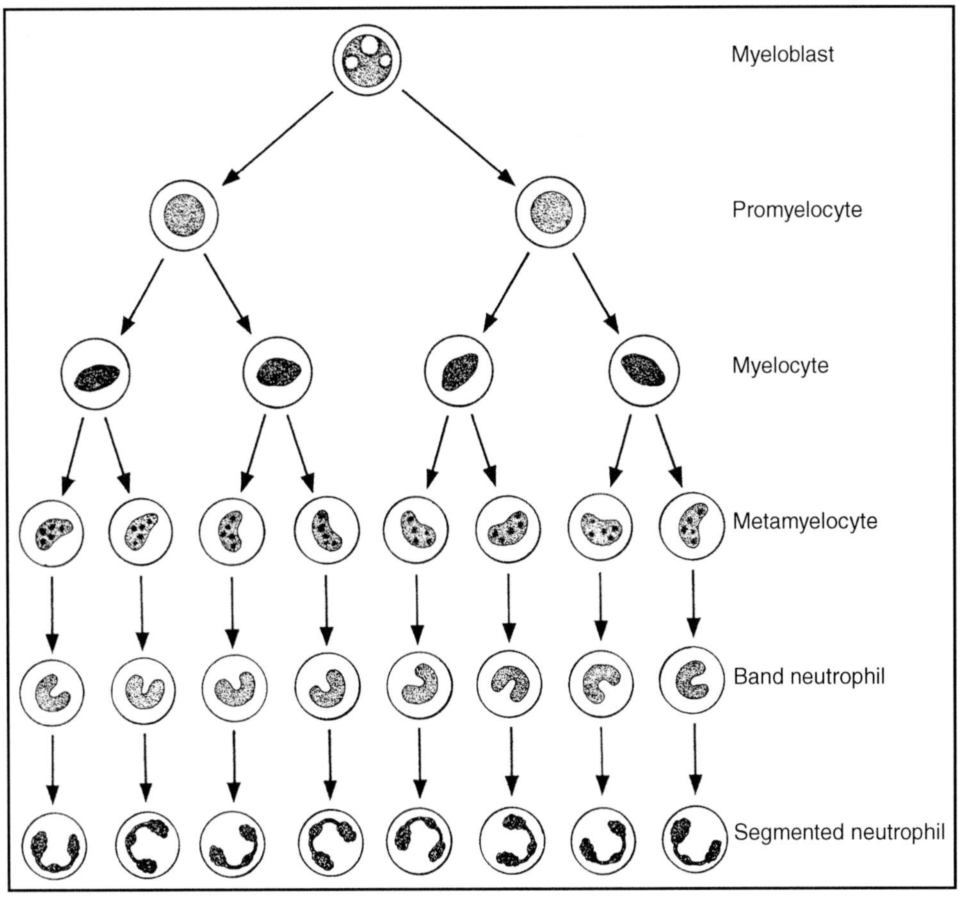

16.2 Schematic diagram of the normal maturation process of bone marrow showing the pyramidal arrangement, with the dividing cells at the apex and non-dividing mature cells at the base.

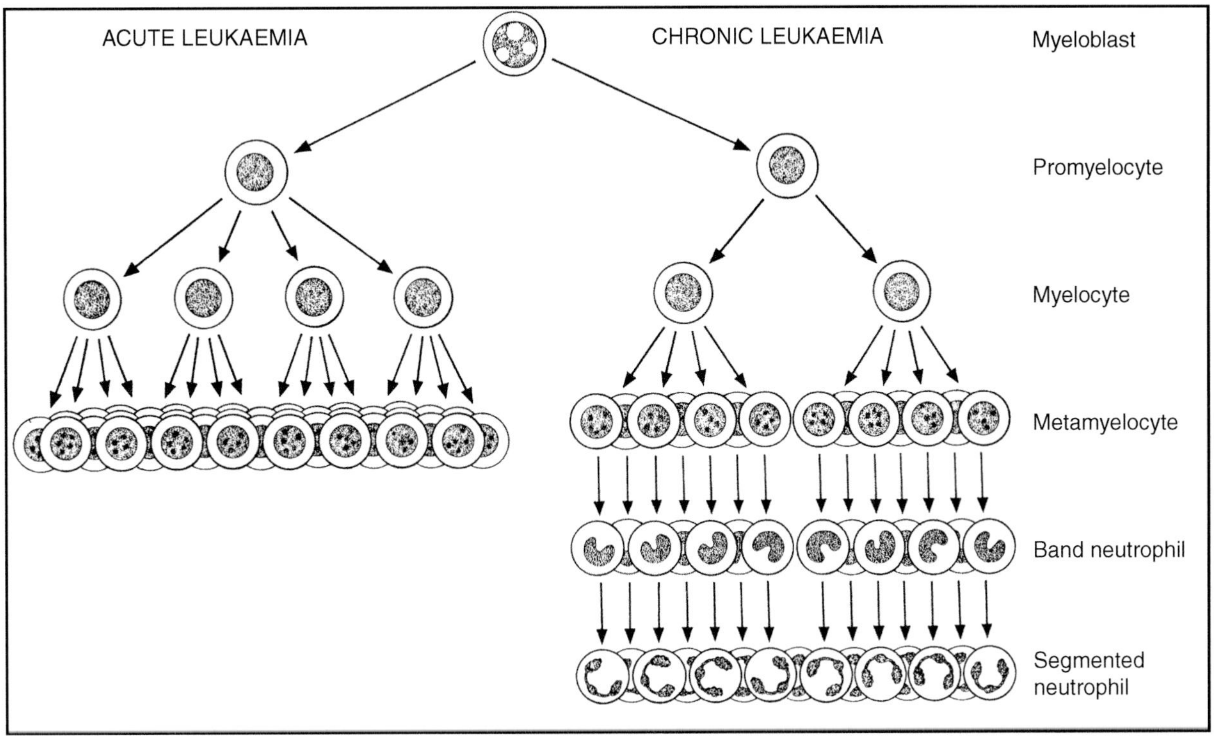

16.3 Schematic diagram of bone marrow depicting the difference between acute and chronic leukaemia in the level of transformation and outcome. In acute leukaemia, transformation of early precursors results in a massive proliferation of undifferentiated cells. In chronic leukaemia, transformation at a later stage results in an overproduction of mature differentiated cells.

of CML and the BCR–ABL fusion product have been identified recently in a few cases of canine CML. In addition, deletions of canine chromosome 22 containing the retinoblastoma gene (*RB1*) have been demonstrated in cases of CLL (Breen and Modiano, 2008), which suggests that the same cytogenetic changes exist in canine and human leukaemias. At the sub-chromosome level, the genes most commonly affected in human leukaemia are also altered in canine leukaemia. In one study, 61% of acute canine leukaemias harboured mutations in *N/K-Ras*, *FLT3*, or *C-KIT* (Usher *et al.*, 2008). In the cat, chromosome translocations occur in both FeLV-positive and FeLV-negative cats, suggesting that the virus itself is not responsible for the chromosome alterations.

Acute leukaemia

Acute leukaemia arises as a result of the neoplastic transformation of early precursors in the bone marrow. In the case of lymphoblastic leukaemia these are committed B or T precursor lymphoblasts, while in acute myeloid leukaemia (AML) they are committed myeloblasts, monoblasts, proerythroblasts, etc. (Figure 16.4). These blasts proliferate in an uncontrolled way in the bone marrow and usually show arrested maturation (there may be a degree of maturation with AML). Proliferation is rapid and the bone marrow quickly becomes crowded with blast cells, which compete with normal haemopoietic cells for nutrients and also release inhibitory substances that lead to failure of the production of stimulatory factors by marrow stroma. The result is reduced normal haemopoiesis, which manifests first as neutropenia (owing to the short circulating half-life of neutrophils), then thrombocytopenia. Neutropenia may lead to sepsis while thrombocytopenia may lead to petechial and ecchymotic haemorrhages, melaena and epistaxis.

Acute leukaemias	Chronic leukaemias
Aggressive	Tend to be less aggressive
Rapidly progressive	Slowly progressive
Excessive numbers of abnormal undifferentiated or 'blast' cells in bone marrow and peripheral blood	Excessive numbers of mature differentiated cells in bone marrow and peripheral blood
Accompanied by severe non-regenerative cytopenias	May or may not be accompanied by cytopenia in other cell lines. If cytopenia present, usually less severe than in acute leukaemia

16.4 Differences between acute and chronic leukaemias.

Because red cells have a long circulating lifespan (110 days in dogs, 70 days in cats) anaemia develops later in the disease course and so may not be present at the time of presentation. Anaemia may develop sooner as a result of haemorrhage associated with thrombocytopenia, or may result from secondary immune-mediated haemolytic anaemia (IMHA). The latter is more likely to occur with lymphoblastic leukaemia.

Blast cells are usually released into the blood, sometimes in large numbers, which may cause hyperviscosity. This may manifest as neurological signs (e.g. seizures, depression, ataxia), retinal haemorrhage or detachment, renal impairment and thromboembolic disease. Blast cells may also infiltrate the spleen, often leading to prominent splenomegaly, and also lymph nodes, usually manifesting as mild to moderate lymphadenopathy (in contrast to the marked lymphadenopathy seen in lymphoma). Other potential sites for infiltration include the liver, central nervous system (CNS) and skin.

Clinical signs

The clinical signs of acute leukaemia may be vague and non-specific with malaise and inappetence, or may be more dramatic, as a result of cytopenias or hyperviscosity, as described above. On examination there may be mild lymphadenopathy and mild or moderate splenomegaly, evidence of bleeding, pallor or pyrexia. There is usually a short period of illness before presentation. Although lymphoid and myeloid leukaemias cannot be distinguished reliably on the basis of the physical examination, subtle differences do exist. For example, pyrexia, shifting lameness (caused by bone pain), ocular lesions and disseminated intravascular coagulation (DIC) are more common in AML, whereas neurological signs and mild lymphadenopathy are more common with acute lymphoblastic leukaemia (ALL).

Hypercalcaemia may occur in ALL and leads to polydipsia, polyuria and potentially azotaemia. Pseudohyperkalaemia may occur as a result of *in vitro* release of potassium from blast cells.

Acute lymphoblastic leukaemia

In dogs ALL, also known as precursor lymphoblastic leukaemia, appears to be more common than AML (Adam *et al.*, 2009; Tasca *et al.*, 2009; and authors' personal observations), and comprises 56–67% of cases of acute leukaemia. It usually affects middle-aged dogs (mean age 7 years) although the reported age range is wide (2–12 years). It may affect many pure breeds of dog as well as cross breeds, but it is more common in large and giant breeds. Golden Retrievers are over-represented. There is no sex predilection. More than 90% of dogs with ALL have at least one cytopenia at the time of presentation and many have pancytopenia. B cell ALL is much more common than T cell ALL, reflecting the site at which these precursors develop. B cell precursors develop in the bone marrow, while T cell precursors move from the bone marrow to the thymus. Malignant proliferations of precursor T lymphoblasts manifest more frequently as lymphoblastic lymphoma with mediastinal involvement rather than lymphoblastic leukaemia, but many of these cases are probably classified non-specifically as high grade lymphoma. In humans, precursor T lymphoblastic lymphoma and precursor T lymphoblastic leukaemia are regarded as different manifestations of the same disease, which is classified arbitrarily depending on the location of the bulk of the disease. Hence if the disease is confined to a mass lesion without or with minimal evidence of blood and bone marrow involvement, the diagnosis is lymphoblastic lymphoma. If there is extensive blood and marrow involvement ALL is the appropriate term. However, these two forms are treated in the same way and have a similar prognosis. Increasing use of flow cytometry in dogs will no doubt help to identify this form of T cell lymphoma/ leukaemia because precursor cells express a stem cell marker (CD34), which is not expressed by other forms of lymphoma or by chronic leukaemia.

ALL is diagnosed on the basis of morphological identification of blasts in the blood and bone marrow together with immunophenotyping. The blast cells are usually intermediate in size (approximately twice the diameter of a red blood cell (RBC; i.e. smaller than myeloblasts or monoblasts) with a round nucleus containing stippled chromatin but no nucleoli and sparse cytoplasm (Figure 16.5). In some cases, the cells are larger with irregularly shaped nuclei, one or more prominent nucleoli and more cytoplasm. Immunophenotyping, which is best performed by flow cytometry, allows the identification of specific cluster of differentiation (CD) antigens expressed on the cell surface (Figures 16.6 and 16.7) and thus enables different types of cell (and thus types of leukaemia) to be recognized. In B cell ALL there may be an associated monoclonal gammopathy, while in T cell ALL there may be hypercalcaemia.

Acute myeloid leukaemia

AML may arise from granulocyte precursors, erythroid precursors or megakaryocyte precursors. It is classified according to which precursor is involved and the degree of differentiation, as shown in Figure 16.8 (McManus, 2005). In dogs, AML-M5 (arising from monocyte precursors) is most common, followed by AML-M1 (arising from neutrophil precursors) and M4 (arising from a shared precursor of monocytes and neutrophils). AML-M0 (undifferentiated AML) and M7 (megakaryoblastic leukaemia) are seen infrequently and AML-M6 (erythroid leukaemia) is extremely rare. In cats AML-M1 and AML-M2 are most common, but erythroid leukaemia is also common, accounting for approximately one third of cases of AML. The clinical/prognostic relevance of this classification system to veterinary medicine has yet to be established.

AML has a peak incidence in dogs at 5 years of age (slightly younger than ALL), but again there is a wide age range (2–12 years). Many different breeds are affected, but German Shepherd Dogs may be over-represented. In cats there is a similar wide age range with a median age of 4 years. Early studies performed prior to FeLV vaccination showed that 90% of cats with AML were FeLV positive, but the current incidence of FeLV in cases of AML is unknown.

There is a high incidence of cytopenias in AML, as with ALL, although sometimes a neutrophilia or occasionally a thrombocytosis is seen. There is a lower incidence of circulating leukaemic cells in AML compared with ALL, perhaps because blasts in AML tend to undergo neoplastic transformation at an earlier stage and so do not develop adhesion molecules, which are required for passage into the vasculature.

AML is diagnosed when there are > 20% blasts in the bone marrow that are identified as myeloid in origin using flow cytometry. Myeloblasts tend to be approximately three times the diameter of canine RBCs (i.e. slightly larger than lymphoblasts), with more abundant light basophilic cytoplasm that may contain pink granules. The large nuclei contain one or more nucleoli. There may be evidence of maturation to metamyelocytes, or band and segmented neutrophils. Monoblasts may be slightly larger and often have irregularly shaped nuclei and cytoplasmic vacuoles (Figure 16.5). Again, there may be evidence of maturation to promonocytes and monocytes. Megakaryoblasts often have blebbed cytoplasm and may be binucleated. Rubriblasts (erythroid precursors) have dark blue cytoplasm and their nuclei have coarse chromatin. Blast cells and developing precursors may be atypical. There is overlap in the appearance of lymphoblasts and myeloblasts/monoblasts, hence the requirement for immunophenotyping to obtain an accurate diagnosis.

Leukaemic phase of high grade lymphoma (LHGL)

High-grade lymphomas arise as a result of clonal expansion of B and T cells (not their precursors) in peripheral lymphoid tissue, usually lymph nodes and sometimes the spleen, intestinal tract or other extranodal site. Most high grade B cell lymphomas arise from lymphoid cells at various stages of differentiation in the germinal centre of a lymph node follicle, with centroblastic/diffuse large lymphoma being the most common subtype. With the exception of lymphoblastic lymphoma, T cell lymphomas arise from post-thymic T cells in lymph (see the discussion of lymphoblastic leukaemia/lymphoma above). These neoplastic lymphoid cells can infiltrate the bone marrow and blood, leading to the so-called leukaemic phase of lymphoma. Affected animals usually have marked lymphadenopathy, in contrast to the mild to moderate lymphadenopathy seen in acute leukaemia, although in advanced ALL lymphadenopathy may be quite marked. Bone marrow infiltration can lead to cytopenias, with anaemia being most common, followed by thrombocytopenia. Neutropenia is less common and in fact neutrophilia is more frequent in LHGL. Chronic inflammation associated with neoplastic involvement of different tissues may explain the neutrophilia and also could explain mild to moderate anaemia (anaemia of chronic inflammatory disease).

LHGL is a common cause of circulating 'blast' cells and in one study accounted for 31% of cases of dogs with a leukaemic blood picture (Tasca *et al.*,

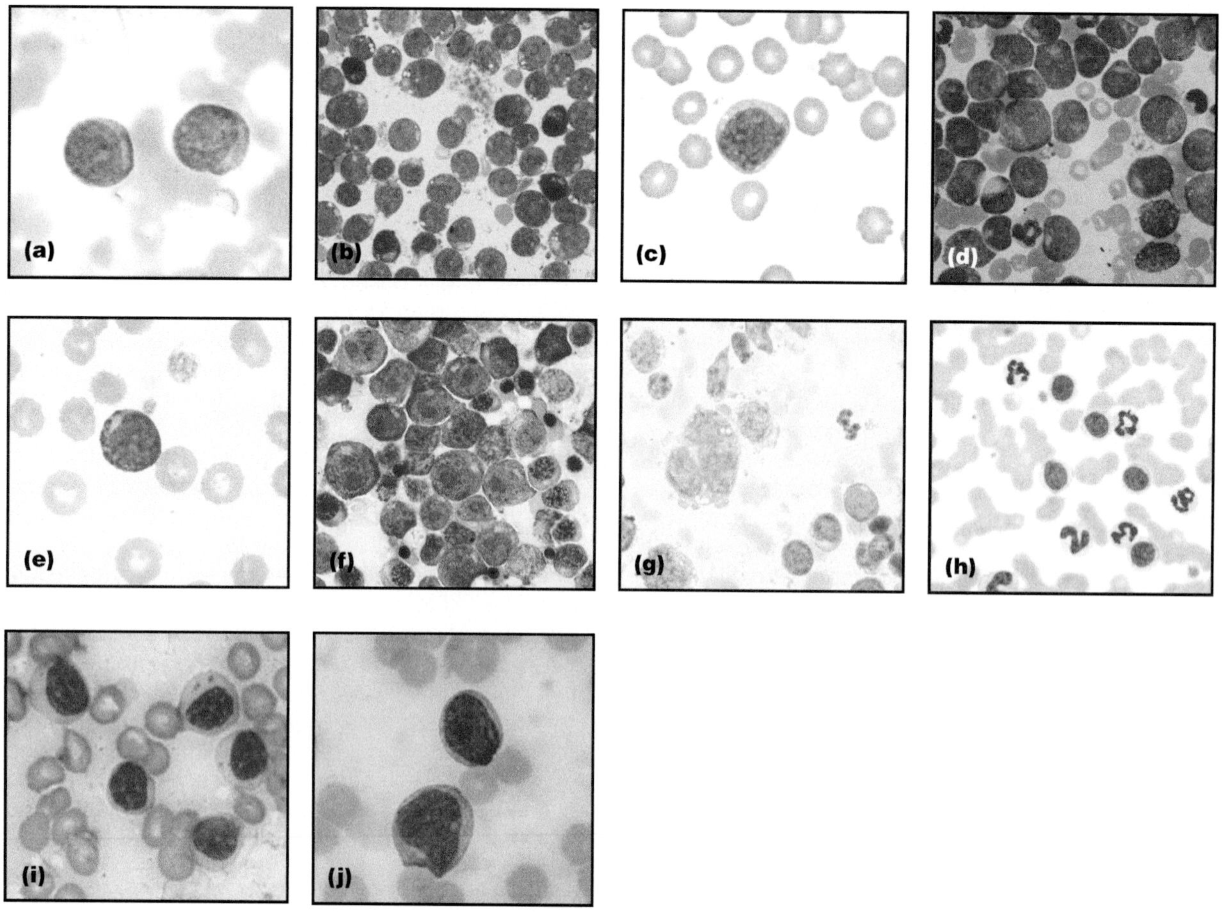

16.5 Cellular morphology in acute and chronic leukaemia. **(a)** Two lymphoblasts in a case of B cell acute lymphoblastic leukaemia (ALL). The blasts are 2.5 times the diameter of red blood cells (RBCs), have round nuclei containing stippled chromatin and an indistinct nucleolus. Cytoplasm is sparse. **(b)** Bone marrow from a dog with B cell ALL. There are numerous lymphoblasts with round nuclei, stippled chromatin and sparse basophilic cytoplasm, sometimes containing vacuoles. There are a few plasma cells. Haemopoietic precursors are not present because the marrow has been ablated by leukaemic cells. **(c)** Blast cell from a dog with acute myeloid leukaemia (AML-M1). The myeloblast is three times the diameter of an RBC, with a round nucleus containing stippled chromatin and sparse cytoplasm. It is very similar to the lymphoblasts shown in (a), illustrating the need for immunophenotyping. **(d)** Bone marrow from a dog with acute monoblastic leukaemia (AML-M5a). These blast cells often have irregular indented nuclei, sometimes containing nucleoli. They have more abundant basophilic cytoplasm with the nucleus positioned eccentrically in the cell. The cytoplasm sometimes contains small clear vacuoles and occasionally contains pink granules. **(e)** Blast cell in blood from a dog with acute monoblastic leukaemia (AML-M5a). This blast cell has a round nucleus with sparse cytoplasm, which contains prominent pink cytoplasmic granules. Such granules may be seen in both lymphoid and myeloid leukaemia. **(f)** Bone marrow from a cat with erythroleukaemia (AML-M6). There are many large rubriblasts with a large nucleus containing quite coarse chromatin and a prominent large nucleolus. The blasts have abundant basophilic cytoplasm. There are also some developing RBC precursors. (Courtesy of Robin Allison, Oklahoma State University) **(g)** Bone marrow from a dog with acute megakaryoblastic leukaemia (AML-M7). There are some mononuclear blast cells and in the centre a trinucleated blast cell with prominent blebs of cytoplasm protruding from the cell surface. **(h)** Small lymphocytes from a dog with chronic lymphoblastic leukaemia (CLL). The cells are slightly smaller than neutrophils, have round nuclei with clumped chromatin (tortoise-shell pattern) and no nucleoli. **(i)** Large granular lymphocytes in a case of T cell LGL CLL. These cells have mildly enlarged nuclei containing mature clumped chromatin and have abundant light staining cytoplasm with several pink granules positioned on one side of the nucleus. **(j)** Leukaemic phase of high-grade lymphoma. These large lymphoid cells are difficult to distinguish from the cells in ALL. (All smears stained with Modified Wright's stain.)

2009). The lymphoblasts in LHGL are often larger and have more prominent nucleoli than the precursor lymphoblasts of ALL, although morphology alone often cannot distinguish LHGL from ALL or AML (Figure 16.5). These diseases can be distinguished on the basis of the clinical presentation (marked or mild lymphadenopathy, mild or severe cytopenias) together with flow cytometric immunophenotyping (see below).

Chronic leukaemia

Chronic leukaemias are characterized by proliferations of mature, differentiated lymphoid or myeloid cells (see Figures 16.3 and 16.4).

Chronic lymphoid leukaemia

This disease results from neoplastic transformation of differentiated, mature T or B lymphocytes. In B

Antibody	Specificity	Leukaemias showing positive labelling
CD3e Intracellular CD3	T cell precursors and mature T cells	T-ALL, T-LHGL, T-CLL, large granular T-CLL
CD3 Surface CD3	T cells (not primitive precursors in T-ALL)	T-LHGL, T-CLL, large granular T-CLL
CD4	Helper T cells, canine neutrophils and neutrophil precursors	T-LHGL$^{+/-}$, T-CLL$^{+/-}$, AML$^{+/-}$, CML
CD5	T cell precursors and mature T cells, subset of B cells including early precursors	T-ALL, B-ALL$^{+/-}$, T-LHGL, T-CLL
CD8	Cytotoxic T cells, large granular lymphocytes	T-LHGL$^{+/-}$, T-CLL, large granular T-CLL
CD11d	Large granular lymphocytes and subset of monocytes	Large granular T-CLL
CD14	Monoblasts and mature monocytes	AML-M4, AML-M5, CMoL
CD21	Mature B cells (not expressed in B-ALL)	B-LHGL, B-CLL
CD79a	B cells including early precursors	B-ALL, B-LHGL, B-CLL
MPO (myeloperoxidase)	Myeloblasts through to neutrophils Weak staining of monoblasts and monocytes	AML-M1, M2, M4, M5$^{+/-}$, CML
MAC387	Neutrophils and monocytes/macrophages and their precursors	AML-M1 AML-M1$^{+/-}$, M2, M4, M5$^{+/-}$, CML
Neutrophil specific antibody	Neutrophils, not usually immature precursors	AML-M1, M2, M4, M5$^{+/-}$, CML
CD41	Platelets and their precursors	AML-M7
CD34	Stem cells and early committed myeloid and lymphoid progenitors in acute leukaemia (not chronic leukaemia or LHGL)	B-ALL, T-ALL, AML (vast majority of cases)

16.6 Antibodies commonly used in flow cytometric evaluation of canine leukaemia. ALL, acute lymphoblastic leukaemia; AML, acute myeloid leukaemia; CLL, chronic lymphoid leukaemia; CML, chronic myeloid leukaemia; LHGL, leukaemic phase of high grade lymphoma; $^{+/-}$ indicates that labelling may be positive or negative.

Type of leukaemia	Typical immunophenotype
T cell ALL	CD3e$^+$, CD34$^+$, CD5$^+$, CD45$^+$
B cell ALL	CD79a$^+$, CD34$^+$, CD5$^{+/-}$
B cell LHGL	CD79a$^+$, CD21$^+$
T cell LHGL	CD3e$^+$, CD3$^+$, CD5$^+$, either CD4$^+$/CD8$^-$ or CD4$^-$/CD8$^+$ or CD4$^-$/CD8$^-$ or CD4$^+$/CD8$^+$
AML-M1,-M2	CD34$^+$, MPO$^+$, MAC387$^{+/-}$, CD4$^{+/-}$, NSA$^{+/-}$
AML-M4, -M5	CD34$^+$, CD14$^+$, MPO$^+$, CD4$^{+/-}$, MAC387$^{+/-}$, CD4$^{+/-}$
AML-M7	CD34$^+$, CD41$^+$
B-CLL	CD79a$^+$, CD21$^+$
Large granular lymphocyte CLL	CD3e$^+$, CD3$^+$, CD5$^+$, CD8$^+$, CD11d$^+$
Non-granular T cell CLL	CD3e$^+$, CD3$^+$, CD5$^+$, either CD4$^+$/CD8$^-$ or CD4$^-$/CD8$^+$
CML	MPO$^+$, NSA$^+$, MAC387$^+$, CD4$^+$, CD14$^{+/-}$

16.7 Typical immunophenotye in lymphoid and myeloid leukaemia in the dog. ALL, acute lymphoblastic leukaemia; AML, acute myeloid leukaemia; CLL, chronic lymphoid leukaemia; CML, chronic myeloid leukaemia; LHGL, leukaemic phase of high grade lymphoma; $^{+/-}$ indicates that labelling may be positive or negative.

cell CLL these are probably naïve B cells, which proliferate in the marrow and spill out into the blood. Lymph node and splenic infiltration are not uncommon. Small lymphocytic lymphoma (SLL) describes a proliferation of small, mature lymphocytes in lymph nodes without leukaemia. In humans, B cell SLL and CLL are regarded as different manifestations of one disease, which are classified as CLL or SLL based on the location of the bulk of disease, but which are treated similarly. It would seem logical to apply this approach to dogs and cats.

In T cell CLL of dogs, the proliferating lymphoid cells are usually a subset of CD8$^+$ CD11d$^+$ T cells known as large granular lymphocytes (LGLs), which proliferate in the spleen rather than the bone marrow (Vernau and Moore, 1999). These have a distinctive morphology with a slightly enlarged nucleus containing mature chromatin and with abundant light staining granules, which are clustered together on one side of the nucleus (see Figure 16.5). T cell CLL arises less commonly from non-granular lymphocyte T cells. In dogs, T-CLL is much more common that B-CLL, but unlike the situation in high grade lymphoma, the T cell phenotype does not carry a worse prognosis and patients with both B- and T-cell CLLs can have prolonged survival and be treated successfully with chemotherapy. In cats, CLL is less well documented but appears to be more commonly T cell in nature, and usually arises from CD4$^+$ T cells rather than LGLs.

Subtype	Precursor	Degree of differentiation in marrow
AML-M0	Committed myeloid stem cells	None – all blast cells
AML-M1	Myeloblasts (neutrophil precursors)	Minimal differentiation with > 90% myeloblasts
AML-M2	Myeloblasts (neutrophil precursors)	20–90% of marrow cells are blasts with evidence of maturation to neutrophils and with > 10% neutrophils
AML-M3	Promyelocytes	Not reported in dogs and cats
AML-M4	Myeloblasts and monoblasts	> 20% of marrow cells are blasts, with evidence of maturation of both neutrophils and monocytes
AML-M5a AML-M5b	Monoblasts	> 80% monoblasts 20–80% monoblasts with evidence of monocyte maturation
AMl-M6a	Erythroblasts and myeloblasts	> 50% erythroid precursors, > 20% of non-erythroid cells are myeloblasts
AML-M6b	Erythroblasts	> 80% erythroid cells of which > 20% are erythroblasts
AML-M7	Megakaryoblasts	20–90% megakaryoblasts with evidence of maturation to megakaryocytes

16.8 Classification of acute myeloid leukaemia (McManus, 2005).

CLL tends to affect older animals, with a mean age of about 10 years in dogs, although there is a wide reported age range (1.5–15 years). Some studies have suggested a sex predilection for male dogs, but this finding is not consistent. Golden Retrievers and German Shepherd Dogs may be over-represented. The disease affects elderly cats with a mean age of 14 years and a range of 6–19 years (Workman and Vernau, 2003).

CLL may not cause clinical signs and so is sometimes identified as an incidental finding. Alternatively it may cause vague signs such as lethargy, decreased appetite and weight loss. On clinical examination there may be lymphadenopathy, splenomegaly, hepatomegaly and occasionally pyrexia. Hyperviscosity is uncommon because the neoplastic cells are small, although B cell CLL can lead to a monoclonal gammopathy, which can contribute to hyperviscosity and can lead to associated clinical signs.

The primary haematological abnormality is a persistent lymphocytosis, consisting of mature lymphocytes, which may be mild to very marked (6–200 $\times$ 10^9/l). The lymphocyte count may fluctuate but generally increases steadily over time. Anaemia is seen in more than 50% of affected dogs and is usually mild or moderate, but is occasionally severe. Neutropenia is very uncommon, although a mature neutrophilia is often present. There may be a mild to moderate thrombocytopenia. In B cell CLL the bone marrow contains > 30% small lymphocytes and identical cells may be identified in the spleen and lymph nodes (although they are not readily distinguishable cytologically from normal small lymphocytes in these sites). Since large granular T cell CLL originates in the spleen, the bone marrow is not usually infiltrated, unless there is advanced disease, but these distinctive LGLs are identified in fine-needle aspirates or histological sections from the spleen (see Figure 16.5).

CLL is diagnosed on the basis of the documentation of a persistent mature lymphocytosis consisting of a single population of either B or T cells, identified with flow cytometry, together with evidence of infiltration of the bone marrow or spleen (see Figure 16.5). CLL must be distinguished from a reactive lymphocytosis in which lymphocyte counts as high as 30 $\times$ 10^9/l, but more commonly less than 15 $\times$ 10^9/l may be seen. In dogs, reactive lymphocytosis usually results from infectious disease or hypoadrenocorticism and is seen occasionally in association with thymoma. Notably, ehrlichiosis (caused by *Ehrlichia canis*) can lead to a moderately severe lymphocytosis (up to 30 $\times$ 10^9/l), attributable to increased numbers of LGLs. In cats, a reactive lymphocytosis may be seen with non-regenerative IMHA and pure red cell aplasia (PRCA; which also leads to increased numbers of lymphocytes in the bone marrow), infectious diseases including FIV and toxoplasmosis, thymoma and occasionally hyperthyroidism (Avery and Avery, 2007). A very marked lymphocytosis consisting of mature lymphocytes would only result from CLL, but where there is a mild to moderate lymphocytosis (< 30 $\times$ 10^9/l) investigations are required to distinguish a reactive from a neoplastic cause. These would include testing for infectious diseases, such as polymerase chain reaction (PCR) tests for *E. canis*, serological testing for toxoplasmosis and FIV, imaging to exclude thymoma, and tests for lymphocyte clonality using PCR for antigen receptor rearrangements (PARR; see below). Flow cytometry is used to quantify the proportions of T and B cells present. In healthy animals, approximately 80% of circulating lymphoid cells are T cells and 15% B cells, with the remainder being natural killer (NK) cells. The presence of a single population of B or T cells would be supportive of a diagnosis of CLL (although this finding is not specific and is sometimes seen with certain infections, such as ehrlichiosis), whilst a mixed population would indicate a reactive lymphocytosis. In cats with PRCA and non-regenerative IMHA, bone marrow histology with immunohistochemistry may be useful because the lymphocytes in bone marrow are present in follicles that can be identified histologically, rather than the diffuse infiltration seen in CLL.

Chronic myeloid leukaemia

Chronic leukaemias may arise from neutrophil, monocyte, eosinophil, basophil, platelet or red cell precursors. The latter is known as polycythaemia or primary erythrocytosis (see Chapter 4). Chronic leukaemia arising from platelet precursors is called essential thrombocythaemia. This discussion will focus on leukaemias arising from monocytes and granulocytes as a result of mutations in early precursors (e.g. myeloblasts, monoblasts, eosinoblasts), which leads to excessive proliferation. However, unlike AML, the precursors differentiate into mature leucocytes that are released into the blood, often in high numbers. These leukaemias are rare and there is a paucity of published data, but it appears that neutrophil proliferations are most common. As with CLL, chronic myeloid leukaemias (CMLs) are insidious in onset and usually have vague clinical signs such as lethargy, pyrexia, hepatosplenomegaly and occasionally mild lymphadenopathy.

Chronic granulocytic/neutrophilic leukaemia

CML tends to affect a single cell line rather than leading to an increase in all granulocytes, unlike CML in humans, which is characterized by neutrophilia with varying eosinophilia, basophilia, monocytosis and thrombocytosis. Haematological abnormalities may be confined to an increase in number of the cell line affected. For example, there may be increased neutrophils in chronic neutrophilic leukaemia, which in small animals is also referred to as chronic granulocytic leukaemia or CML, although this is not the same disease as human CML), monocytes in chronic monocytic leukaemia, or eosinophils in chronic eosinophilic leukaemia. The leucocytosis may be very pronounced (up to 300 × 10^9/l). There may be a marked left shift to the metamyelocyte stage, sometimes with a few circulating blasts and promyelocytes present. There are usually no dysplastic features, although atypical morphology is observed in some cases. There is often a mild to moderate non-regenerative anaemia, and less frequently a thrombocytopenia. The cell lineage is generally obvious from morphology alone, and immunophenotyping is not generally helpful because the cells have identical antigen expression to their non-neoplastic counterparts.

The bone marrow shows a marked increase in the proportion of developing myeloid precursors, with a markedly increased myeloid:erythroid ratio, and generally an orderly maturation. Again, there is usually no cell dysplasia, although atypical morphology has been reported in some cases. CML is defined by the presence of < 20% blasts, although in most cases blasts usually account for < 5% of cells. In humans with CML, a higher proportion of blast cells (10–19%) indicates an accelerated phase, which then leads to a blast phase with > 20% blasts, wherein the disease transforms into an acute leukaemia/blast crisis. Similar transformation to aggressive disease can occur in CML in dogs and cats.

Diagnosis of chronic neutrophilic (myeloid) leukaemia rests on excluding a so-called 'leukaemoid reaction' (LR). The latter is a marked non-clonal neutrophilia that can arise as a result of infection (e.g. in pyometra or pyothorax), immune-mediated diseases such as IMHA, tissue necrosis (e.g. associated with neoplasia or pancreatitis) and paraneoplastic neutrophilia, where tumours release cytokines that stimulate granulopoiesis. A thorough clinical examination may demonstrate the cause of LR; alternatively further investigations including imaging studies are performed. The presence of toxic change in neutrophils is supportive of LR, while the presence of circulating myeloblasts or atypical cells would suggest leukaemia. Cytochemical staining with alkaline phosphatase may help to identify CML, because positive staining may be present in CML neutrophils, but is absent from normal neutrophils. However, not all cases of CML exhibit positive staining and so this test lacks sensitivity. Unfortunately there is currently no test available to identify clonality in neutrophils.

Chronic eosinophilic leukaemia and hypereosinophilic syndrome

Eosinophilia may be reactive (in association with allergic, parasitic or infectious disease); may arise due to neoplasia, especially T-cell lymphoma and mast cell tumours; or may be due to chronic eosinophilic leukaemia (CEL) and hypereosinophilic syndrome (HES) (see Chapter 15). Both CEL and HES are characterized by a persistent circulating eosinophilia, with eosinophilic hyperplasia in the bone marrow and multiple organ infiltration by mature eosinophils, but no demonstrable underlying cause. Common sites of organ infiltration include the gastrointestinal (GI) tract, liver, spleen, lymph nodes and lung. These two diseases are very difficult to distinguish in animals. In humans, CEL is distinguished from HES by demonstrating clonality of eosinophils, and in some cases demonstrating specific mutations of genes encoding platelet derived growth factor (PDGF) or fibroblast growth factor (FGF). Eosinophils in HES are non-clonal and do not have these mutations. There is also a lymphocytic variant of HES in which aberrant clones of T cells produce excessive cytokines, especially interleukin (IL)-5, which leads to excessive production of eosinophils and organ infiltration with eosinophils. These aberrant lymphocytes are identified by demonstrating clonality and aberrant antigen expression using multicolour flow cytometry (Vardiman *et al.*, 2009).

Tests for clonality in eosinophils are not available in small animals and specific mutations causing CEL have not been identified. Examination of the bone marrow is sometimes helpful in distinguishing HES and CEL, since HES is characterized by < 5% myeloblasts in the marrow, whilst in CEL there is often > 5% blasts. However, this finding is not absolute and many cases of CEL have fewer than 5% marrow blasts. The differentiation of CEL and HES is consequently often not possible and indeed may not be clinically relevant because treatment strategies for the two conditions are currently similar (although tyrosine kinase inhibitors may have a future role in treating CEL). Diagnostic tests should instead focus on excluding underlying causes of eosinophilia (e.g. parasitic disease and neoplasia). Importantly, T cell lymphoma can lead to paraneoplastic HES because the neoplastic T cells produce large amounts of IL-5, and so investigations should include imaging and aspiration of any enlarged lymph nodes or solid organs, to exclude lymphoma.

Myelodysplastic syndrome

Myelodysplastic syndrome (MDS) results from mutations in haemopoietic stem cells, leading to ineffective haemopoiesis, dysplasia and premature cell death in one or more cell lines. This leads to cytopenias, sometimes confined to anaemia, but often bi- or pancytopenia. The bone marrow is hypercellular, but early precursors do not develop normally into their mature counterparts and exhibit abnormal morphology. Dysplastic features include asynchronous nuclear:cytoplasmic development with immature nuclei and mature cytoplasm, hyper- or hypogranularity in granulocytes, giant nuclei, ring-shaped nuclei in granulocyte precursors, fragmented nuclei and multinucleation. There may be increased numbers of blast cells, but these do not exceed 20%. There are various subtypes of MDS, which vary in severity and disease progression. MDS-refractory anaemia leads to anaemia only, and can have an indolent course, often showing a good response to erythropoietin therapy. MDS-excessive blasts is characterized by a higher proportion of blasts in the bone marrow (5–20%) and leads to bi- or pancytopenia. The prognosis for this form is very poor and survival times range from days to months. Death frequently results from sepsis as a result of neutropenia. This form may progress to AML (Weiss, 2005). Although older reports show a strong association between FeLV and MDS, a more recent study showed that only 36% of cats with MDS were FeLV positive (Weiss, 2006). Secondary dysmyelopoiesis, which may be triggered by underlying diseases such as IMHA and lymphoma, may lead to a similar haematological picture to that of MDS, but it is reversible if the underlying disease process is treated successfully.

General approach to the leukaemic patient

In most cases, the presenting clinical signs and physical examination are non-specific and may not immediately suggest a diagnosis of leukaemia (Figure 16.9). Invariably, a series of laboratory-based investigations are required to reach a definitive diagnosis of leukaemia and to assess the presence and severity of disease-related complications. These include: evaluation of a complete blood count (CBC) and bone marrow, including morphological examination of abnormal cells by a specialist cytopathologist/haematologist; serum biochemistry; urinalysis; haemostasis tests; imaging for staging; flow cytometry; and, possibly, tests for clonality with PARR.

Clinical finding	Underlying causes
Weight loss	Cancer cachexia/anorexia, gastrointestinal upset
Pyrexia	Neutropenia, hypergammaglobulinaemia, cytokine release
Pale mucous membranes	Anaemia
Petechial haemorrhages	Thrombocytopenia
Ecchymotic haemorrhages, other evidence of bleeding	Bleeding diathesis, disseminated intravascular coagulation
Ocular lesions (retinal detachment, tortuous retinal vessels, hypopyon, iris infiltration)	Hyperviscosity syndrome, tumour infiltration
Neurological signs, abnormal cerebral function (disorientation, depression, stupor, paresis)	Hyperviscosity syndrome, infiltration of nerves/central nervous system, intracranial haemorrhage, hypercalcaemia
Lymphadenopathy	Infiltration of lymph nodes
Hepatosplenomegaly	Infiltration of abdominal organs, extramedullary haemopoiesis
Lameness, skeletal pain, muscle weakness	Infiltration of joints, bone lesions, hypercalcaemia

16.9 Clinical findings in leukaemia.

Haematology

Routine haematological assessment of the patient usually provides the first indication of leukaemia. Haematological abnormalities may include:

- Cytopenias:
  - Anaemia (usually non-regenerative)
  - Neutropenia
  - Thrombocytopenia
- Increased cell numbers:
  - Disproportionate increase of one cell lineage
- Abnormal cells:
  - Immature or atypical blood cells in the peripheral circulation. Cells in acute leukaemia may have characteristic morphology or may be less well differentiated, and morphology alone cannot reliably distinguish AML, ALL and LHGL
  - In T cell chronic large granular lymphocytic leukaemia, the cells have medium-sized nuclei with clumped chromatin and no nucleoli. They have abundant light staining cytoplasm with several pink granules clustered together on one side of the cell. Cells in non-granular CLL have sparse cytoplasm and small round nuclei, similar in size or perhaps slightly larger than those of normal lymphocytes, and have characteristic coarsely clumped chromatin, resembling cracked mud.

Figure 16.5 illustrates the typical cell morphology in different types of leukaemia.

Bone marrow histology

Assessment of the bone marrow will help clarify the diagnosis and provide information upon which the prognosis and treatment strategy can be defined, depending on the degree of disruption of normal marrow elements. Bone marrow core biopsy can also be useful to assess the degree of infiltration, and the same sample can be used for immunohistochemistry (see Chapter 2).

Biochemistry

Serum biochemical changes in leukaemic patients may include alterations in:

- Electrolytes: hypercalcaemia can be present in T cell lymphoid leukaemia; elevated potassium and phosphate can result from *in vitro* release from leukaemic cells and are more commonly seen with severe leucocytosis, especially in serum samples because these electrolytes are released from cells as the blood clots
- Urea and creatinine: azotaemia may be associated with hypercalcaemia, may be prerenal or rarely may reflect kidney infiltration
- Liver enzymes may be elevated when there is hepatic infiltration
- Proteins: panhypoproteinaemia may occur with diffuse intestinal infiltration; selectively low albumin may result from hepatic infiltration; hyperglobulinaemia with a monoclonal gammopathy may be seen with acute and chronic B cell leukaemias and with B cell LHGL. Serum protein electrophoresis should be performed to identify monoclonal gammopathy. When globulins are elevated, serum protein electrophoresis should be performed.

Urinalysis

Urinalysis is especially indicated in cases with hypercalcaemia or hypergammaglobulinaemia.

Tests of haemostasis

A haemostatic profile, including one-stage prothrombin time (PT), activated partial thromboplastin time (APTT), and measurement of D dimers should be performed if DIC is suspected.

Diagnostic imaging

Radiography and ultrasonography should be performed in order to assess possible neoplastic infiltration of internal organs, especially the liver, spleen and lung. Skeletal radiography should be performed if the animal presents with lameness or if myeloma is suspected.

Flow cytometry

In this technique, aliquots of leukaemic cells are labelled with a panel of monoclonal antibodies, each being specific for a cell surface antigen. For example, antibodies to CD3 will bind to T lymphocytes, but not to B cells or myeloid cells. These antibodies are tagged with a fluorescent dye (e.g. fluorescein), emission of light from which is detected by the flow cytometer. The flow cytometer has a fluidic system in which sheath fluid flows around the patient's cells, producing a hydrodynamically focused stream of individual cells. This stream of cells is directed through a laser beam, resulting in scattering of the laser light, and when the laser encounters a fluorescent tag bound to a cell, fluorescent light is emitted. Several detectors are aimed at the point where the stream passes through the light beam: one in line with the light beam (detecting forward scatter, which depends on cell size), one perpendicular to it (detecting side scatter, which depends on cell granularity/complexity), and one or more fluorescence detectors. Evaluation of forward and side scatter facilitates identification of the leukaemic population, and evaluation of fluorescence determines whether the population has been labelled with a given antibody. Antibodies may be conjugated to one of several different fluorochromes so cells can be dual- or even triple-labelled. Figure 16.10 shows an example of a scatter plot of blast cells that are labelled with antibodies specific for CD3e (a T cell marker) and CD34 (a marker of acute leukaemia). Figure 16.6 shows commonly used antibodies and their specificity and indicates which leukaemias would label positively with each antibody. In the United Kingdom, flow cytometric evaluation of leukaemia is currently commercially available only for dogs and is now offered by a number of specialist laboratories in the UK and other countries.

The identification of acute leukaemia is based on the expression of CD34, which is found only on early stem cells/haemopoietic precursors and not on more mature cells. CD34 is expressed in the vast majority of acute myeloid and lymphoid leukaemias, but is always negative in lymphoma and CML. This antibody is very useful for distinguishing lymphoma with blood and bone marrow involvement from advanced ALL, in which there may be moderate to marked organomegaly and lymphadenopathy. Figure 16.7 shows the typical pattern of expression in the more common leukaemias in the dog (Villiers *et al.*, 2006, Tasca *et al.*, 2009). Aberrant antigen expression is sometimes seen in both lymphoid and myeloid leukaemias, but appears to be most common in lymphoid leukaemia and LHGL. For example, there may be co-expression of CD79a (a B cell marker) and CD3 (a T cell marker) by neoplastic lymphoid cells (Wilkerson *et al.*, 2005). Weak aberrant expression of CD79a is sometimes seen in myeloid leukaemia (authors' personal observation). In such cases, the immunophenotype can be determined from results of a wide panel of antibodies. If there is positive labelling for several T cell markers and only one B cell marker, the disease is classified as T cell with aberrant expression of a B marker. PARR can also be used to determine the immunophenotype in these cases.

PARR

PARR is a technique that uses PCR to detect antigen receptor rearrangements and to establish whether clonal populations of lymphoid cells are present. It is usually assumed that neoplastic populations of lymphoid cells are clonal expansions and therefore share unique sequences of DNA. The antigen binding region of both immunoglobulin and T cell receptors is encoded by the complementarity determining region (CDR3) of the respective genes. The CDR3 region is produced by recombination of variable (V), diversity (D) and joining (J) genes for B

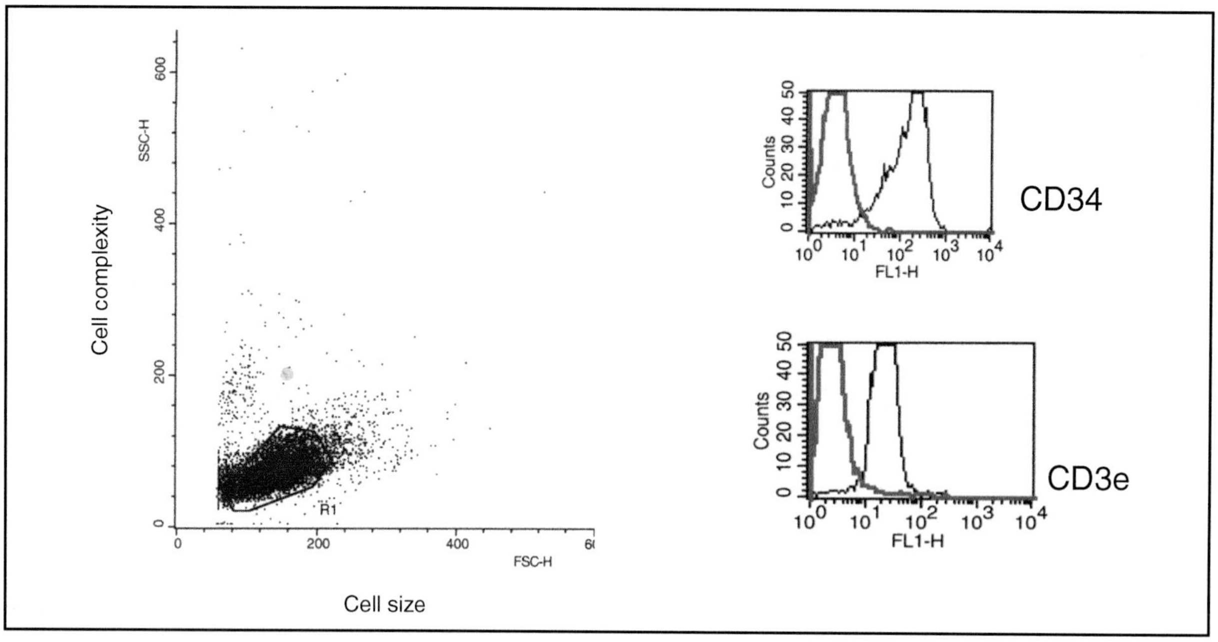

16.10 Flow cytometric analysis of cells from a dog with T cell acute lymphoblastic leukaemia. The dot plot on the left shows a single population of cells with low complexity (granularity) and moderate size. The histogram plots on the right show labelling with two antibodies (CD3e and CD34) in black, overlaid with the low fluorescence of the negative control in red.

cells or just V and J for T cells, and involves the addition of random nucleotides between gene segments to create diversity in sequence and length (Burnett *et al.*, 2003). The final sequence of the receptor CDR3 region is unique to that particular B or T cell. By using primers designed to bind to conserved regions of V and J genes, the PCR can be used to amplify sections of DNA between the primers. The resultant PCR products are separated by gel electrophoresis and the presence of a single dominant band suggests that all the receptors in the cell population are identical (i.e. the population is clonal).

The PARR technique can be used in both cats and dogs to determine whether a cell population is neoplastic or reactive, particularly when this may be difficult to determine by other means. In cases with moderate lymphocyte counts of 30 × 10^9/l or below, where leukaemia is suspected but not obvious, PARR can be very helpful, but accurate interpretation of the result should always take into account other clinical information, and immunophenotyping may also confirm the diagnosis. Given that the limit of detection of the technique is 1 neoplastic lymphocyte in a population of 100 heterogeneous, non-neoplastic lymphocytes (Burnett *et al.*, 2003), the technique is also useful to detect minimum residual disease. It is more sensitive for the detection of neoplastic lymphocytes in peripheral blood than routine or standardized microscopic evaluation (Keller *et al.*, 2004) and therefore provides the opportunity for early diagnosis or for monitoring the response to chemotherapy. Sufficient DNA for the technique can be extracted from relatively few cells, which could be from peripheral blood, lymph nodes, bone marrow or cavity fluids. Formalin-fixed paraffin wax-embedded material can also be used in some cases.

The reported sensitivity of PARR for confirmation of neoplastic transformation ranges between 70 and 80%, but is up to 95% for the detection of epitheliotropic lymphoma in extracts from formalin-fixed and paraffin wax-embedded skin biopsies.

Management of leukaemia

Acute leukaemia

Supportive measures for acute leukaemia include fluid therapy for dehydration, anorexia or hypercalcaemia, blood component therapy for severe loss of red cells or platelets, and antibiotic therapy for secondary infections.

The aim of specific therapy for acute leukaemia is to destroy the leukaemic cells by using chemotherapy, and thereby allow resumption of normal haemopoiesis. However, this is rarely achieved in veterinary medicine (see below), and treatment of acute leukaemia in dogs is not usually successful. Euthanasia is an option that should be considered at the time of diagnosis.

Chemotherapy

In human medicine, allogeneic haemopoietic stem cell transplantation (SCT) applied early in first remission forms the basis of a curative treatment for some acute haematological malignancies, especially in younger patients and those in high-risk groups. The combination of vincristine, prednisolone and crisantaspase (L-asparginase) is one of the standard remission induction regimes in childhood ALL. Children with high-risk disease may also receive additional drugs such as the anthracyclines (doxorubicin or daunorubicin) and/or cyclophosphamide. Standard induction therapy for patients with AML consists of cytarabine (ara-C) and daunorubicin in conventional doses and results in a complete remission rate of 50–60% with 10–12% long-term survival. The duration of remission may also be improved by intensification with etoposide, thioguanine, cytarabine and daunorubicin. Idarubicin and mitoxantrone have been compared with daunorubicin in induction protocols but there is no evidence that either achieves higher remission rates. High-dose cytarabine may be used to maintain remission.

While SCT has not been developed in veterinary medicine, the human experience with drug selection for induction remission regimes largely informs drug selection in the treatment of veterinary patients:

- Drugs recommended for the treatment of ALL are similar to those recommended for lymphoma, that is, vincristine and prednisolone plus an alkylating agent (cyclophosphamide) and an anthracycline (doxorubicin) – i.e. CHOP, although many different protocols exist
- Drugs recommended for the treatment of AML include prednisolone, cytarabine (used because it may encourage differentiation of blast cells) and daunorubicin or doxorubicin.

Induction protocols for acute leukaemia are used until the white blood cell (WBC) count returns to the normal range and blast cells are no longer seen in peripheral blood. In theory, drug doses and frequencies can then be reduced to maintenance levels, but in practice this is rarely achieved. The use of chemotherapy for the treatment of acute leukaemia is severely restricted by the degree of myelosuppression caused by the disease. The inability to preserve sufficient levels of normal blood cells during treatment is a constant problem. Furthermore, the toxicity of cytotoxic agents may be exacerbated by compromised hepatic and renal function. Most animal patients succumb to either overwhelming sepsis secondary to neutropenia, organ failure secondary to infiltration with neoplastic cells or DIC.

Prognosis

Although the diagnosis and classification of canine and feline leukaemias has advanced through use of immunophenotyping, little progress has been made in terms of treatment and improving survival. The prognosis remains poor for acute leukaemias in general, although that for ALL is slightly better than for AML in both species. For ALL, survival times of 1–6 months have been reported in dogs and cats (Presley *et al.*, 2006). For AML, there are no large studies in the literature, only case reports and small case series, but survival times rarely exceed 2–3 months for both dogs and cats. However, one dog with acute megakaryoblastic leukaemia (AML-M7) achieved a survival time of nearly 2 years after repeated cycles of high dose cytarabine (1000 mg/m^2), etoposide and daunorubicin in combination with blood transfusions and antibiotics (Willmann *et al.*, 2009).

Chronic leukaemia

For asymptomatic cases of CLL, there may be no need for treatment, although frequent monitoring and haematological screens are advised.

Chemotherapy

For symptomatic cases of CLL and for all cases of CML, chemotherapy is the treatment of choice. As with acute leukaemia, drug selection for treatment of chronic leukaemia is largely informed by human experience. Primary treatment of human patients with CLL is recommended to be with an oral alkylating agent such as chlorambucil. The addition of corticosteroids to alkylator regimes has not been proven to give any benefit.

In dogs with CLL, the alkylating agent chlorambucil is used with or without prednisolone. More potent alkylating agents such as cyclophosphamide may be used in refractory cases of CLL, where they may also be combined with vincristine and doxorubicin (CHOP).

CML is usually treated with either the alkylating agent busulfan or hydroxycarbamide (hydroxyurea), usually in combination with prednisolone. In both CLL and CML, the aim of treatment is to restore the peripheral blood counts to within the normal range, and response to treatment is monitored by haematological findings. Once remission is achieved, maintenance therapy is continued at reduced doses and frequencies of the appropriate drugs in order to keep the WBC counts within the normal range. Paraneoplastic complications such as hypercalcaemia and hypergammaglobulinaemia may need to be addressed in chronic leukaemia.

Prognosis

The prognosis for chronic leukaemia is much more favourable than for acute leukaemia. Mean and median survival times for CLL in the dog may exceed 1 year (Vernau and Moore, 1999; Presley *et al.*, 2006), but are usually shorter for CML, which has a greater risk of blast cell crisis.

New approaches

The treatment and prognosis for chronic leukaemia in human patients has been revolutionized by the development of new approaches to cancer treatment. The tyrosine kinase (TK) domain in the BCR–ABL fusion protein in CML was one of the first targets identified for the TK inhibitor imatinib. With the sequential advances of imatinib, followed by dasatinib and nilotinib, the treatment approach for CML has been completely rewritten and continues to evolve in the current era of kinase inhibitors. Likewise for CLL, Alemtuzumab (a monoclonal antibody targeting CD52) and Rituximab (anti-CD20) have demonstrated efficacy in patients with CLL. These developments have yet to have an impact on the management of dogs and cats with chronic leukaemia.

Case study 1: An 11-year-old female Golden Retriever weighing 32.0 kg

History
Presented with a 2-week history of progressive inappetence and lethargy.

Clinical examination
Quiet, good body condition. Pyrexia (39.5°C). Heart rate and respiration normal. Pale mucous membranes. No other abnormalities detected.

Routine blood samples were submitted and on the basis of these results, bone marrow aspirates were obtained for cytological interpretation and flow cytometry. Abdominal ultrasonography was also performed.

Haematology results

Parameter	Result	Reference range
Total RBC	2.55	5.5– 8.5 x 10^{12}/l
Hct	0.19	0.37–0.55 l/l
Hb	6.2	12–18 g/dl
MCV	73	60–77 fl
MCH	24.3	19.5–24.5 pg
MCHC	34	32–37 g/dl
Platelets	71	175–500 x 10^9/l

Parameter	Result	Reference range (x 10^9/l)
Total WBC	1.49	6–17
Neutrophils	0.9	3–11.5
Lymphocytes	0.5	1–4.8
Monocytes	0.1	0.2–1.5
Eosinophils	0	0.1–1.3
Basophils	0	0.0–0.5

Smear comments: pancytopenia. Red cells are normocytic and normochromic with no evidence of polychromasia. Platelets appear low. No clumps seen. Leucocytes display normal morphology.

Biochemistry results
Within normal limits except for alkaline phosphatase (402 IU/l; reference range 3–142 IU/l), aspartate aminotransferase (65 IU/l; reference range 20–32 IU/l) and albumin (16 g/l; reference range 25–40 g/l).

Coagulation profile
Within normal limits.

Abdominal ultrasonography
Spleen slightly hyperechoic in appearance.

Bone marrow cytology
Normal maturation sequence disrupted. High numbers of blasts present (approximately 60% of nucleated cell population), which are approximately twice the diameter of small lymphocytes. They have round or occasionally convoluted nuclei, prominent nucleoli, stippled, dispersed chromatin and moderately abundant pale basophilic cytoplasm. Small numbers of small lymphocytes and plasma cells. Low numbers of granulocytic and erythroid precursors.

Comment: The increased proportion of blasts is consistent with an acute leukaemia, however from the morphology alone it is not clear if these are lymphoid or myeloid cells.

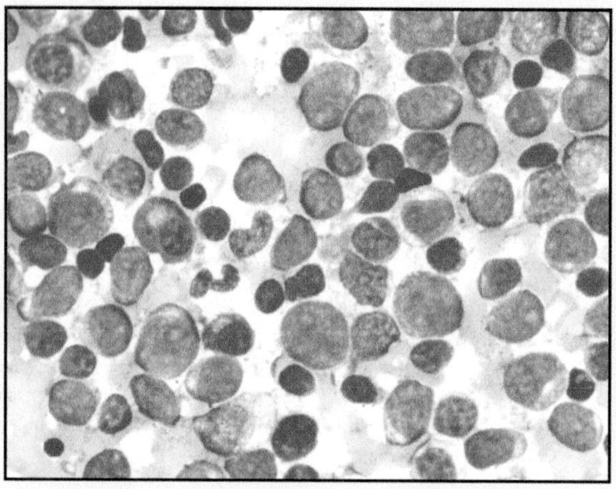

Bone marrow aspirate showing lymphoblast, plasma cells and small lymphocytes. (Modified Wright's stain; original magnification x1000)

continues ▶

Case study 1: An 11-year-old female Golden Retriever weighing 32.0 kg (continued)

Flow cytometry results for bone marrow sample

Antibody	Result	Significance
CD3	Negative	T cells
CD3e	**Positive**	**Intracellular component of CD3**
CD4	Negative	T helper cells and neutrophils
CD5	**15% positive**	**T cells and subset of B cells**
CD8	Negative	Cytotoxic T cells
CD11d	Negative	Large granular lymphocytes
CD14	Negative	Monocytes
CD21	Negative	B cells only (if relatively mature)
CD34	**15% positive**	**Stem cells, primitive leukaemic blast cells**
CD45	Negative	Leucocytes
CD79a	Negative	B cells
CD90/Thy1	**40% positive**	**T cells, subset of B cells, monocytes**
MPO	Negative	Granulocytes
CADO48	Negative	Neutrophils (neutrophil specific antibody)

Diagnosis
On the basis of the proliferation of blasts within the bone marrow, which expressed T cell specific markers on flow cytometry, a diagnosis of **T cell acute lymphoblastic leukaemia** was made. Although a poor prognosis was given, chemotherapy was started.

Treatment
Treatment was begun with cytarabine (100 mg/m^2 s.c. q24h for 4 days) and prednisolone (40 mg/m^2 orally q24h for 7 days then 20 mg/m^2 q48h). Antibiotic therapy (metronidazole 600 mg orally q12h and amoxicillin/clavulanate 500 mg q12h) was given for the first 3 weeks.

Response to treatment
A good response to treatment was seen within 3 weeks, with clinical and haematological improvement (WBC, RBC and platelet parameters). Doxorubicin (30 mg/m^2 i.v. q3 weeks) was commenced at this visit and the response to treatment continued at subsequent visits. The dog is currently clinically well (week 10).

Parameter	Week 3	Week 6	Week 9	Reference values
Total RBC	4.58	5.16	5.06	5.5–8.5 x 10^{12}/l
Hct	0.35	0.383	0.367	0.37–0.55 l/l
Hb	12.1	12.9	12.6	12–18 g/dl
MCV	77	74.2	72.5	60–77 fl
MCH	26.4	25.0	24.9	19.5–24.5 pg
MCHC	34	33.7	34.3	32–37 g/dl
Platelets	170	226	210	175–500x 10^9/l
Total WBC	6.48	10.93	10.58	6–17 x 10^9/l
Neutrophils	4.7	7.89	7.69	3–11.5 x 10^9/l
Lymphocytes	1.7	3.0	2.42	1–4.8 x 10^9/l

Case study 2: A 9.5-year-old neutered female Boxer weighing 30.2 kg

History
Presented with a 3-week history of haematuria, which had responded poorly to symptomatic treatment with antibiotics (amoxicillin/clavulanate), a non-steroidal anti-inflammatory drug (meloxicam) and nutraceuticals. Otherwise fit and well.

Clinical examination
Good body condition, bright and alert. Temperature, pulse and respiration within normal limits; mucous membranes pink and moist with normal capillary refill. Thoracic auscultation normal. Mild hepatosplenomegaly on abdominal palpation. No palpable lymphadenopathy. Mild pedal dermatitis.

Blood samples and urine (cystocentesis) were collected and abdominal ultrasonography was performed. These investigations prompted flow cytometric analysis of the blood and collection of fine-needle aspirates from the liver, spleen and bone marrow.

continues ▶

Case study 2: A 9.5-year-old neutered female Boxer weighing 30.2 kg (continued)

Urinalysis results
Appearance : dark red in colour
Specific gravity: 1.019
pH: 7.0
Protein: +++
Blood/haemoglobin: +++
Glucose, ketones, urobilinogen: negative
Few white cells and bacteria seen on sediment examination
No bacterial growth was present on urine culture, but the dog was on antibiotics.

Haematology results

Parameter	Result	Reference range
Total RBC	5.65	5.5–8.5 x 10^{12}/l
Hct	0.39	0.37–0.55 l/l
Hb	12.9	12–18 g/dl
MCV	70	60–77 fl
MCH	22.8	19.5–24.5 pg
MCHC	33	32–37 g/dl
Platelets	104	175–500 x 10^9/l

Parameter	Result	Reference range (x 10^9/l)
Total WBC	288.9	6–17
Bands		0–0.3
Neutrophils	2.9	3–11.5
Lymphocytes	286.0	1–4.8
Monocytes	0	0.2–1.5
Eosinophils	0	0.1–1.3
Bands		0–0.3

Smear comment: lymphocytosis consisting of small lymphocytes with round nuclei containing condensed clumped nuclear chromatin, no nucleoli and with sparse cytoplasm. No platelet aggregates present. Platelets appear low on film. Red cells are normocytic and normochromic.

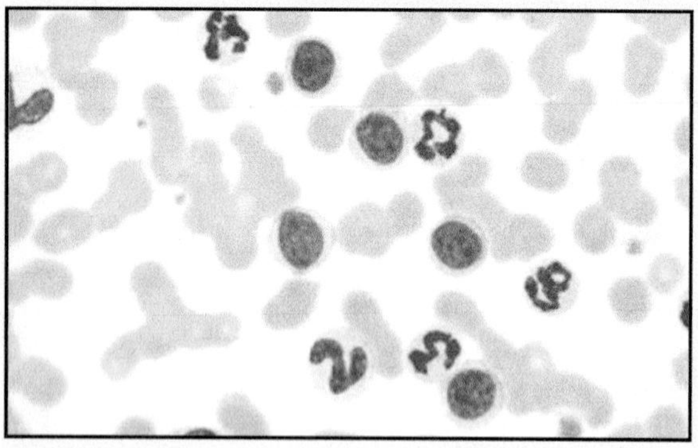

Blood smear showing small lymphocytes with a round nucleus containing condensed chromatin, no nucleoli and sparse cytoplasm. (Modified Wright's stain; original magnification x1000)

Biochemistry results
Within normal limits except for alkaline phosphatase (205 IU/l; reference range 3–142 IU/l), aspartate aminotransferase (40 IU/l; reference range 20–32 IU/l) and glucose (6.7 mmol/l; reference range 3.4–5.3 mmol/l).

Coagulation profile
Within normal limits.

Abdominal ultrasonography
No abnormalities noted with the bladder. Spleen enlarged, heterogeneous and hyperechoic in appearance.

Cytology
Spleen: predominantly red cells and mature small lymphocytes, similar in appearance to those in peripheral blood.
Liver: Scattered normal hepatocytes with no obvious lymphoid infiltrate.

Flow cytometry results

Antibody	Result	Significance
CD3	Negative	T cells
CD3e	Negative	Intracellular component of CD3
CD4	Negative	T helper cells and neutrophils
CD5	Negative	T cells and subset of B cells
CD8	Negative	Cytotoxic T cells
CD11d	Negative	Large granular lymphocytes
CD14	Negative	Monocytes
CD21	**Positive**	**B cells only (if relatively mature)**

continues ▶

Case study 2: A 9.5-year-old neutered female Boxer weighing 30.2 kg (continued)

Antibody	Result	Significance
CD34	Negative	Stem cells, primitive leukaemic blast cells
CD45	**Positive**	**Leucocytes**
CD79a	**Positive**	**B cells**
CD90/Thy1	Negative	T cells, subset of B cells, monocytes
MPO	Negative	Granulocytes
CADO48	Negative	Neutrophils (neutrophil specific antibody)

Bone marrow cytology
Hypercellular marrow with 35% small lymphocytes and occasional intermediate sized lymphocytes. Slightly reduced myeloid and erythroid series, but maturation is complete. Megakaryocyte numbers appear mildly low.

Comment: The increased number of mature lymphocytes is consistent with chronic leukaemia.

Diagnosis
On the basis of flow cytometry, cell morphology and bone marrow evaluation, a diagnosis of **B cell chronic lymphocytic leukaemia** was made with infiltration of the spleen. The haematuria was attributed to a urinary tract infection with the lack of bacteria cultured being due to prolonged antibiotic therapy. The delayed response of the cystitis to routine therapy may have been due to the underlying leukaemia.

Treatment
Chemotherapy was started because of the extremely high lymphocytosis, moderate thrombocytopenia and the non-resolving cystitis. The leukaemia was treated with a combination of chlorambucil (4 mg/m^2 orally q48h) and prednisolone (20 mg/m^2 orally q24h for 7 days then q48h). Antibiotic therapy was continued with cefalexin (600 mg orally q12h) for 4 weeks.

Response to treatment
A good response to treatment was seen, with resolution of the haematuria and a dramatic reduction in the numbers of circulating lymphocytes over the first 3 weeks.

The dog continues to do well on a reduced treatment protocol 6 months later, with haematological values within the normal range.

Parameter	7 days	21 days	Reference range
Total RBC	6.06	5.80	5.5–8.5 x 10^{12}/l
Hct	0.41	0.39	0.37–0.55 l/l
Hb	14.6	13.5	12–18 g/dl
MCV	68	69	60–77 fl
MCH	24.1	23.3	19.5–24.5 pg
MCHC	35	34	32–37 g/dl
Platelets	324	337	175–500 x 10^9/l
Total WBC	52.82	19.9	6–17 x 10^9/l
Neutrophils	8.5	11.9	3–11.5 x 10^9/l
Lymphocytes	42.8	6.4	1–4.8 x 10^9/l
Monocytes	1.6	1.5	0.2–1.5 x 10^9/l
Eosinophils	0	0.1	0.1–1.3 x 10^9/l

References and further reading

Adam F, Villiers E, Watson S *et al.* (2009) Clinical pathological and epidemiological assessment of morphologically and immunologically confirmed canine leukaemia. *Veterinary and Comparative Oncology* **7**(3), 151–211

Avery AC and Avery PR (2007) Determining the significance of lymphocytosis. *Veterinary Clinics of North America: Small Animal Practice* **37**, 267–282

Breen M and Modiano JF (2008) Evolutionary conserved cytogenetic changes in hematological malignancies of dogs and humans – man and his best friend share more than companionship. *Chromosome Research* **16**, 145–154

Burnett RC, Vernau W, Modiano JF *et al.* (2003) Diagnosis of canine lymphoid neoplasia using clonal rearrangements of antigen receptor genes. *Veterinary Pathology* **40**, 32–41

Dunham SP and Graham E (2008) Retroviral infections of small animals. *Veterinary Clinics of North America: Small Animal Practice* **38**, 879–901

Kaneko N, Tanimoto T, Morimoto M *et al.* (2009) Use of formalin-fixed paraffin-embedded tissue and single-strand conformation polymorphism analysis for polymerase chain reaction of antigen receptor rearrangements in dogs. *Journal of Veterinary Medical Science* **71**(4), 535–538

Keller RL, Avery AC, Burnett RC *et al.* (2004) Detection of neoplastic lymphocytes in peripheral blood of dogs with lymphoma by polymerase chain reaction for antigen receptor gene rearrangement. *Veterinary Clinical Pathology* **33**(3), 145–149

Lana SE, Jackson TL, Burnett RC *et al.* (2006) Utility of polymerase chain reaction for analysis of antigen receptor rearrangement in staging and predicting prognosis in dogs with lymphoma. *Journal of Veterinary Internal Medicine* **20**(2), 329–334

McManus PM (2005) Classification of myeloid neoplasms: a comparative review. *Veterinary Clinical Pathology* **34**(3), 189–212

Pardanani A, Reeder T, Porrata LF *et al.* (2003) Imatinib therapy for hypereosinophilic syndrome and other eosinophilic disorders. *Blood* **101**(9), 3391–3397

Presley RH, Mackin A and Vernau W (2006) Lymphoid leukaemia in dogs. *Compendium on Continuing Education for the Practicing Veterinarian* **28**, 831–849

Tasca S, Carli E, Caldin M *et al.* (2009) Haematological abnormalities and flow cytometric immunophenotyping results in dogs with haemopoietic neoplasia: 210 cases (2002–2006). *Veterinary Clinical Pathology* **38**(1), 2–12

Usher SG, Radford AD, Villiers EJ *et al.* (2008) RAS, FLT3, and C-KIT mutations in immunophenotyped canine leukaemias. *Experimental Haematology* **37**(1), 65–77

Vail DM (2011) Tumours of the haemopoietic system. In: *BSAVA Manual of Oncology, 3rd edn*, ed. JM Dobson and BDX Lascelles, pp. 285—303. BSAVA Publications, Gloucester

Vardiman JW, Thiele T, Arber DA *et al.* (2009) The 2008 revision of the World Health Organization (WHO) classification of myeloid neoplasms and acute leukemia: rationale and important changes. *Blood* **114**(5), 937–951

Vernau W and Moore PF (1999) An immunophenotypic study of canine leukaemias and preliminary assessment of clonality by polymerase chain reaction. *Veterinary Immunology and Immunopathology* **69**, 145–164

Villiers W, Baines S, Law AM *et al.* (2006) Identification of acute myeloid leukemia in dogs using flow cytometry with myeloperoxidase, MAC387, and a canine neutrophil-specific antibody. *Veterinary Clinical Pathology* **35**(1), 55–71

Weiss D J (2005) Recognition and classification of dysmyelopoiesis in the dog: a review. *Journal of Veterinary Internal Medicine* **19**(2), 147–154

Weiss DJ (2006) Evaluation of dysmyelopoiesis in cats: 34 cases (1996-2005). *Journal of the American Veterinary Medical Association* **228**, 893–897

Wilkerson MJ, Dolce K, Koopmans T *et al.* (2005) Lineage differentiation of canine lymphoma/leukaemias and aberrant expression of CD molecules. *Veterinary Immunology and Immunopathology* **106**(3-4), 179–96

Willmann M, Milliner L, Schwendenwein I, *et al.* (2009) Chemotherapy in canine acute megakaryoblastic leukaemia: a case report and review of the literature. *In Vivo* **23**, 911–918

Workman HC and Vernau W (2003) Chronic lymphocytic leukaemia in dogs and cats; the veterinary perspective. *Veterinary Clinics of North America: Small Animal Practice* **33**, 1379–1399

17

Feline retrovirus infections

Andrew Sparkes and Kostas Papasouliotis

Introduction

There are three exogenous, contagious retroviruses transmitted between cats: feline syncytium-forming virus (FeSFV; spumavirus); feline leukaemia virus (FeLV; oncornavirus); and feline immunodeficiency virus (FIV; lentivirus). Of these viruses, FeSFV is generally considered to be non-pathogenic, whereas FeLV and FIV are important and common causes of disease. Infection with either FeLV or FIV can have a profound effect on haematological parameters, some of which may be diagnostically helpful in alerting the clinician to the possibility of these viruses as an underlying cause of the disease. Although there are many similarities in the diseases produced by these two viruses, there are also important differences in many aspects of their epidemiology, pathogenesis, diagnosis and control, and these aspects will therefore be briefly considered separately for each virus.

Feline leukaemia virus (FeLV)

Epidemiology

Cats persistently infected with FeLV excrete infectious virus in their saliva, nasal secretions, faeces and milk. Transmission of infection is mainly horizontal, and occurs primarily during prolonged direct social interaction between infected and susceptible cats where there is opportunity for exchange of virus (e.g. through mutual grooming, sharing of food and food bowls, sharing litter trays). Vertical transmission is also possible, but persistent FeLV infection usually results in infertility, abortion or resorption of fetuses in a pregnant queen. Environmental contamination is of minimal importance because the virus is very labile and is destroyed readily by disinfectants.

The outcome following exposure to FeLV depends on many factors including the dose of virus, the viral strain, and host resistance (which is strongly related to the age of the cat, its immunocompetence and probably also its genotype). In colonies of cats in which FeLV is endemic, typically around 30–40% will be persistently viraemic, around 30–40% will be transiently viraemic and mount an immune response that limits viral replication, and around 20–30% will seroconvert without having a detectable viraemic episode. Those cats that overcome viraemia develop latent infections (i.e. have proviral FeLV DNA integrated into certain host cells) for a variable period of time, and in a small proportion reactivation of infection may occur. Whether infected cats that mount a good immune response are ever able to eliminate infection completely, or whether proviral DNA remains incorporated in some host cells for the remainder of the cat's life, is unknown. It is likely that the proviral burden in most cats with an effective immune response declines over time, but provirus (latent infection) can be detected in a proportion of cats (up to around 10%) that do not test positive for virus by other methods (Lutz *et al.*, 2009).

Clinically and epidemiologically, it is the persistently viraemic cats that are most important, although a small proportion of latently or previously infected cats may also develop FeLV-related disease. However, because the life expectancy of FeLV-recovered cats is generally the same as that of FeLV naïve cats, the risk of significant FeLV-related disease in latently infected cats appears very low.

Worldwide it is estimated that 1–3% of the general healthy cat population is persistently infected with FeLV. However, the prevalence of infection varies according to the population of cats studied (their lifestyle and potential for exposure to FeLV), and there is also evidence of geographical and regional variations in the prevalence of FeLV. FeLV infection is most common in cats up to 5 years of age, with a declining prevalence thereafter (Hosie *et al.*, 1989).

Pathogenesis

If a cat infected with FeLV fails to eliminate the infection within the first 4–6 weeks, haemolymphoid infection is established that almost invariably results in persistent viraemia. FeLV replicates most effectively in rapidly dividing cells, and has a particular tropism for the haemopoietic stem cells in the bone marrow, the intestinal epithelial crypt cells, and the lymphocytes in the germinal centres of lymphoid follicles. Infection of bone marrow stem cells generally leads to very large quantities of virus being produced, which overwhelm the host's immune response, leading to persistent viraemia. Within the bone marrow, those cells of the myelomonocyte lineage develop an increasing virus burden as they mature, whereas among the erythrocyte precursors there is a greater viral burden in the early, undifferentiated cells. The persistent viraemia of bone marrow origin is partly cell-associated, with circulation of infected neutrophils, lymphocytes, monocytes and platelets, in addition to free virus being present in plasma.

Infection with FeLV can result in a variety of diseases (see below), and the outcome of infection is determined partly by the subgroup(s) or strain(s) of FeLV infecting that cat.

Individual cells are infected with FeLV when the major envelope glycoprotein (gp70) binds to specific cellular receptors, resulting in release of the viral RNA genome into the cell cytoplasm. Under the influence of the viral reverse transcriptase and the host cell's DNA polymerase, a double-stranded DNA copy (provirus) of the single-stranded RNA viral genome is produced. The provirus is integrated into the host cell genome during cellular division and can then lead to productive infection (cellular synthesis of viral proteins which are assembled into viral particles that bud from the cell surface). The pathogenesis of FeLV-related disease at a cellular level is not fully understood, but while infected cells are often able to function normally, in other cases the accumulation of certain viral proteins (e.g. p15E, gp70) within the cytoplasm may disrupt cellular function. In addition, the insertion of the proviral DNA into the host cell genome can disrupt or activate certain cellular proto-oncogenes, leading to insertional mutagenesis and neoplastic transformation of the cell. Another adverse effect seen with some FeLV strains is failure to integrate the proviral DNA into the genome, which leads to an accumulation of cytoplasmic viral DNA that can again disrupt cellular function and cause cytotoxicity.

According to the antigenic structure of the gp70 envelope glycoprotein, FeLV isolates are divided into four major subgroups: A, B, C and T. FeLV-A is invariably found in all FeLV-infected cats, whereas subgroup B is found in around 50% of infected cats, and subgroup C in just 1–2% of infected cats. Subgroup T has been described more recently and structural changes in this subgroup confer a particular tropism for T lymphocytes (Cheng *et al.*, 2007). Mixed infections with subgroups A and B are generally considered more pathogenic than infection with FeLV-A alone, and infections with subgroup C lead to the rapid development of erythroid aplasia, thymic atrophy and lymphoid depletion. Similarly, co-infection with FeLV-T is likely to be more pathogenic than infection with FeLV-A alone.

Rarely, FeLV DNA may recombine with certain cellular proto-oncogenes to form the acutely transforming feline sarcoma virus (FeSV). These viruses result in rapid neoplastic transformation of cells with the induction of multiple malignant sarcomas.

Diseases associated with FeLV infection

Uncommonly, but particularly if they are infected at a very young age, cats may develop FeLV-related disease and die within a few weeks of the onset of viraemia. More commonly, FeLV-related disease occurs after a prolonged period (months to years) of asymptomatic viraemia.

FeLV is a common cause of chronic disease in cats; the prevalence of viraemia in sick cats is typically 10–20% (Hosie *et al.*, 1989). Furthermore, FeLV-related disease commonly results in death of the infected cat – approximately 50% of infected cats die within 6 months of the diagnosis being made, and more than 80% die within 3.5 years. However, some infected cats remain healthy for many years, and occasionally cats with persistent infections appear to develop no significant FeLV-related disease.

Although FeLV is an oncogenic virus, the development of neoplasia accounts for only around 10–25% of FeLV-related deaths. Where neoplastic disease does develop, solid lymphomas are the most common type, with anterior mediastinal, alimentary, multicentric and atypical (miscellaneous) forms being described. Most FeLV-related lymphomas are T cell malignancies, and most are sub-leukaemic, although a proportion will be accompanied by lymphocytic leukaemia. In addition to lymphomas, FeLV infection may result in the development of a variety of leukaemias (predominantly of erythroid or myelomonocytic origin) or myeloproliferative disorders.

Cytosuppressive (degenerative) diseases account for 75% or more of FeLV-related deaths, and of the different syndromes recognized, FeLV-associated immunosuppression is the most important, probably accounting for around 50% of all FeLV-related diseases. The pathogenesis of the immunosuppression is complex and includes neutropenia and defective neutrophil function, dysfunction and numerical depletion of T lymphocytes, immune complex formation, complement depletion and thymic atrophy. The resulting immunosuppression leaves the infected cat susceptible to a wide variety of secondary and opportunistic infections.

Other manifestations of FeLV infection include anaemia (present in up to 30–50% of FeLV-infected cats and frequently non-regenerative), myelosuppression, enteropathy, reproductive failure, neurological disorders, fading kittens (thymic atrophy) and immune-complex related diseases (e.g. polyarthritis, glomerulonephropathies).

Specific haematological changes

Primary infection

Most FeLV strains will cause a relative or absolute lymphopenia in the first 2 months after infection, with a variable effect on lymphocyte subsets. Conversely, lymphocytosis is sometimes seen, but in most cases these leucocyte changes are reversed, and remain normal or near normal throughout the prolonged asymptomatic period. Occasionally, with infection by more virulent FeLV strains, a persistent decrease in lymphocyte numbers (including $CD4^+$ and $CD8^+$ T cells) is seen, which contributes to the early development of immunosuppression in these cats.

Anaemia

The development of anaemia is a common consequence of FeLV infection and may account for up to

25% of FeLV-related deaths. FeLV infection is also recognized as one of the most important causes of anaemia in the cat (Figure 17.1).

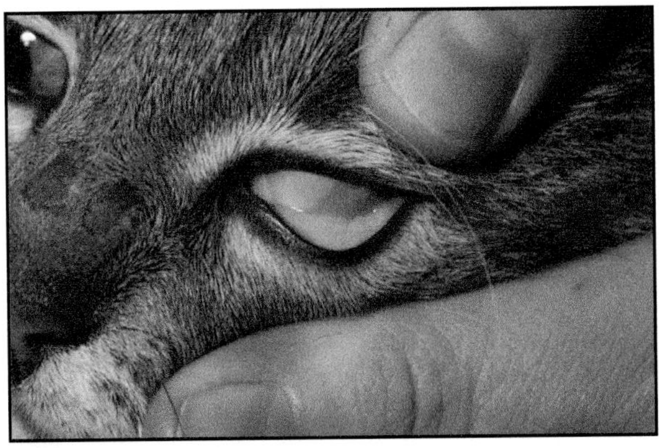

17.1 Pale mucous membranes in an anaemic cat.

The majority of FeLV-induced anaemias are non-regenerative, and they may be associated with myeloproliferative disorders (including myelofibrosis and osteosclerosis), dyserythropoiesis or erythroid aplasia (which can sometimes be a part of a pancytopenia). Anaemia of chronic disease (with abnormalities in iron usage and erythrocyte survival; Chapter 5) may also be involved in a number of cases of FeLV-associated anaemia, and co-infection with haemotropic mycoplasmas may also contribute to the non-regenerative anaemias seen in infected cats. Myeloproliferative diseases will sometimes lead to the appearance of leukaemic cells in blood smears, but more commonly the specific diagnosis of these cases requires examination of bone marrow aspirates. Some cases of dyserythropoietic anaemia exhibit high numbers of circulating nucleated red blood cells without concomitant reticulocytosis (Figure 17.2), and others demonstrate a marked megaloblastic anaemia (which is unrelated to vitamin B_{12} deficiency). Although generally classified as non-regenerative, some of these anaemias may in fact show evidence of partial (but inadequate) red cell regeneration.

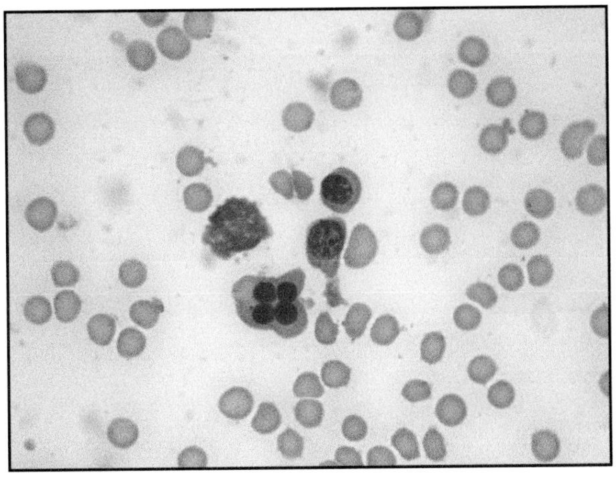

17.2 Blood dyserythropoiesis: peripheral blood smear (Modified Wright's stain; original magnification ×1000) from an FeLV-infected cat revealing anisocytosis, the presence of normochromic red blood cells and, in the centre, three dysplastic nucleated red blood cells.

In the past, 70% or more of non-regenerative anaemias in the cat have been attributed to FeLV infection. However, with the more widespread control of FeLV through testing and vaccination, this proportion may be lower now. Red cell aplasia (aplastic anaemia) is the most common cause of FeLV-associated anaemia, although in practice it may not be easy to distinguish this from certain myeloproliferative diseases and dyserythropoiesis, and these may occur concurrently in an infected cat.

Aplastic anaemia is characterized by normocytic normochromic (or sometimes macrocytic normochromic) anaemia with reticulocytopenia of both aggregate and punctate forms. Bone marrow aspirates reveal a marked increase in the myeloid:erythroid ratio caused by depletion of erythroid precursors. There is a strong association between the development of aplastic anaemia and infection with FeLV subgroup C, and the appearance of subgroup C in plasma immediately precedes the development of progressive aplastic anaemia during experimental FeLV infection. It appears that FeLV-C infects early erythroid precursors and interferes with a haem transport protein, leading to haem accumulation and death of the precursor cells. Despite progressive anaemia, serum erythropoietin levels are markedly elevated in these cats.

Between 10 and 20% of FeLV-related anaemias are regenerative. These are characterized by anisocytosis, polychromasia, reticulocytosis, macrocytosis and the appearance of nucleated red blood cells, which can be associated with extramedullary (splenic and hepatic) erythropoiesis. Most commonly, these anaemias are either immune-mediated or associated with concurrent infection with haemotropic mycoplasmas (e.g. *Mycoplasma haemofelis*; Chapter 7), although genuine autoimmune haemolytic anaemia has also been described in some FeLV-infected cats. Because of the established relationship between FeLV infection and haemotropic mycoplasmas (Bobade *et al.*, 1988), polymerase chain reaction (PCR) evaluation of blood for the presence of these organisms is advisable in all cases of FeLV-associated anaemia. However, the prognosis for these cats remains poor. Some may show temporary resolution of the anaemia – either spontaneously or in response to appropriate therapy – but recurrence of anaemia is common, and many will eventually progress to develop other FeLV-related disease. Thrombopathy or thrombocytopenia with secondary haemorrhage may also contribute occasionally to regenerative anaemia in cats with FeLV infection.

Lymphopenia and neutropenia

Although infection with FeLV can induce immunosuppression through functional disturbances of lymphocytes and neutrophils, many cats will also have numerical depletion of these cell lines. Up to 70% of infected cats will demonstrate lymphopenia and up to 35% may have absolute leucopenia. The lymphopenia appears to involve both B and T cells. However, while lymphopenia has been observed in many FeLV-infected cats, in a recent large study (Gleich and Hartmann, 2009) lymphocytosis was observed in 24% of FeLV-positive cats, a figure significantly higher than in a control population in which 10% of the cats had lymphocytosis. The cause of the lymphocytosis was not explored, but may relate to differences in viral pathogenicity, stage of the disease and perhaps different strains of the virus. Nevertheless, that study emphasized the variable haematological responses that can be seen with FeLV infection.

In addition to lymphopenia, neutropenia has also been reported frequently in FeLV-infected cats, and FeLV infection should be regarded as an important differential diagnosis for any neutropenic cat. In the study by Gleich and Hartmann (2009), 26% of nearly 100 FeLV-infected cats were neutropenic, compared with just 9% of the control population. Cyclic fluctuations in the numbers of neutrophils (cyclic neutropenia), lymphocytes and other circulating cells (cyclic haematopoiesis) have been reported in some FeLV-infected cats (Swenson *et al.*, 1987). Neutropenia is an important finding because it frequently leads to secondary infections that may overwhelm the cat. Although neutropenia and/or leucopenia may be a manifestation of the cytopathic effect of FeLV infection, these changes may also reflect underlying myeloproliferative diseases or preleukaemic syndromes.

FeLV myeloblastopenia

This consequence of FeLV infection is indistinguishable clinically from feline panleucopenia virus infection and is reported to occur relatively frequently in FeLV-infected cats. The syndrome is characterized by profound anaemia (frequently aplastic) in combination with severe leucopenia (i.e. pancytopenia), which is accompanied by dysentery, vomiting, anorexia and depression. Affected cats invariably die. The combination of signs in these cats presumably reflects the replication of FeLV in target cells of the intestinal epithelium and bone marrow, although the picture may be complicated by secondary bacterial infection in some cases.

'Normal' leucocyte responses

Although many if not all FeLV-viraemic cats are immunosuppressed to some degree, this does not necessarily prevent them mounting a response to secondary or opportunistic infections. Many infected cats will therefore exhibit neutrophilic leucocytosis, perhaps with a left shift, as an appropriate response to concurrent bacterial (or viral) infections.

Platelet abnormalities

Both megakaryocytes and platelets harbour FeLV infection. Macrothrombocytes with impaired function and decreased longevity are common in infected cats, and although thrombopathies and thrombocytopenias have been reported with FeLV infection, bleeding disorders have not commonly been described in FeLV-infected cats. In one study, FeLV infection was identified in 27% (11) of 41 thrombocytopenic cats, two of which had bleeding disorders (Jordan *et al.*, 1993), and in another study, 36% of FeLV-infected cats were thrombocytopenic (compared with 9% of the control population) (Gleich and Hartmann, 2009).

FeLV-induced leukaemias

Leukaemias are characterized by the presence of neoplastic cells in the peripheral circulation, and FeLV is responsible for most feline leukaemias (70–90%). Lymphoblastic or lymphocytic leukaemia may occur alone or in combination with solid lymphomas, and other FeLV-associated leukaemias include acute and chronic myelogenous leukaemia, and more rarely monocytic, myelomonocytic, erythro-, megakaryocytic, eosinophilic and also undifferentiated leukaemias (see Chapter 16).

Diagnosis

The diagnosis of FeLV is usually straightforward. The clinician will be alerted to the possibility of underlying FeLV as a cause of the disease by the clinical history (e.g. recurrent episodes of disease suggesting immunosuppression, presence of lymphoma), clinical findings and clinicopathological changes. Given that most cases of FeLV-related disease occur in persistently viraemic cats, detection of infection is readily achieved by assaying blood samples for the presence of p27, one of the core proteins of FeLV, which is almost invariably present in the plasma of persistently infected cats.

A variety of tests are available for detection of p27 in blood samples, including in-house diagnostic tests such as membrane-bound enzyme-linked immunosorbent assays (ELISAs; e.g. the SNAP test; Idexx) (Figure 17.3) and immunochromatographic (or rapid immunomigration; RIM) techniques (e.g. the Witness test; Synbiotics) (Figure 17.4). The simplicity of these tests (Figure 17.5) virtually eliminates the possibility of operator error, and they are therefore highly reliable.

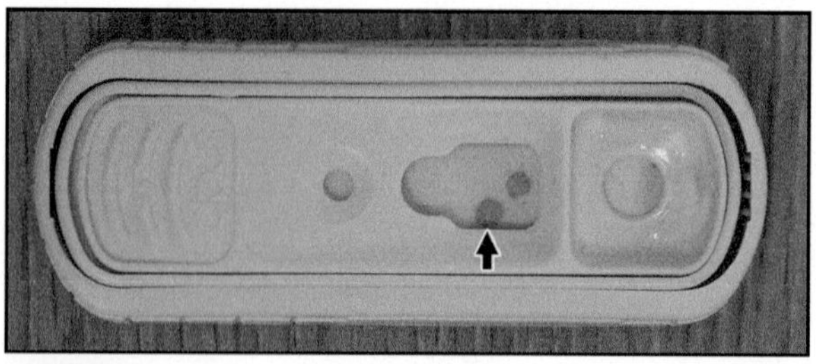

17.3 Positive FeLV test result (black arrow) in a SNAP test.

On rare occasions, as with any test, false positives and false negatives can occur, and if there is any reason to doubt the validity of a test result, repeating the test (ideally at a reference laboratory using a reference methodology) is recommended. Reference laboratories frequently use a plate ELISA for detection of p27 antigenaemia as an initial

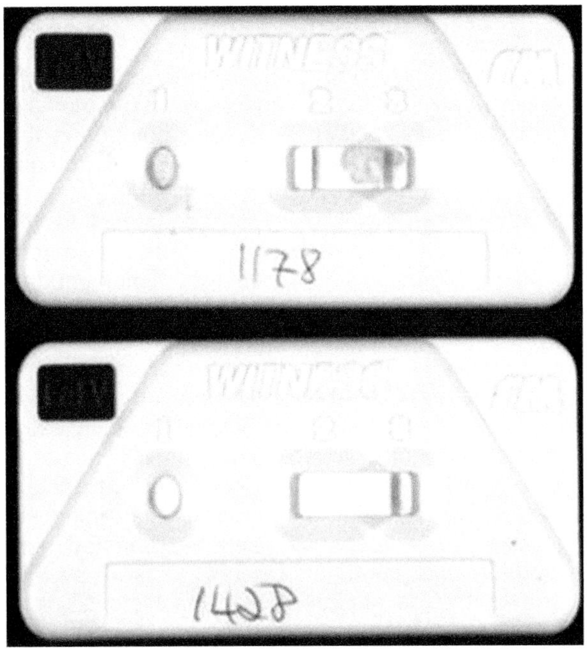

17.4 Witness test: FeLV-positive (sample 1178, above) and -negative (sample 1428, below) results.

Name of test	Company	Country of origin
Antigen Rapid	BioNote	Republic of Korea
DuoSpeed	BIO VETOTEST	France
FASTest	MegaCor	Germany
Mapic	Biotech	United States
One-Step	EVL	Netherlands
OnSite	Biotech	United States
SNAP	Idexx	United States
Witness	Synbiotics	United States

17.5 Some serological tests available for in-house detection of FIV antibody and FeLV antigen.

screening test, but may offer confirmation of test results with a variety of other methods such as virus isolation, PCR and immunofluorescence. Because these tests detect different aspects of infection, there is not complete agreement between them. Immunofluorescence detects cell-associated antigenaemia and as such is helpful in confirming the presence of viraemia. It usually correlates well with virus isolation, but may be more problematic with low viral burdens (low levels of fluorescence) or with autofluorescence causing false positive results. Virus isolation has long been held to be the 'gold standard' for detecting persistent viraemia, but this is a laborious test and is rapidly being replaced by PCR. However, PCR tests are not standardized across laboratories and care is needed to ensure that a reliable methodology and laboratory is chosen. Detection of viral RNA by reverse transcriptase PCR (RT-PCR) will detect and can quantify free viral loads, whereas conventional DNA PCR will detect proviral FeLV, and because this can be present in both viraemic and latently infected cats, the significance of a positive result may be more difficult to interpret.

It should also be remembered that not all cats with FeLV-related disease will be persistently viraemic, and it is estimated that 2–6% of cats that recover from FeLV infections (do not develop persistent viraemia) will go on to develop FeLV-related disease. The use of DNA PCR (peripheral blood/bone marrow) to detect proviral FeLV infection may be valuable in these rare situations.

Treatment

The decision on whether to treat an FeLV-infected cat must be made on an individual basis, but will be influenced by the clinical condition of the cat, the short- and long-term prognosis, the risk the infected individual poses to other cats, and the owners' wishes. However, the finding of FeLV infection *per se* in a pet cat is not a reason for euthanasia. Symptomatic and supportive therapy is most often provided for concurrent, secondary or opportunistic infections, and it is important that these infections are identified promptly and correctly to guide specific therapy (e.g. for *Mycoplasma haemofelis*). Regular 'wellness' examinations are important, and the cat should be confined appropriately to prevent infection of others (Levy *et al.*, 2008).

A wide variety of antiviral and/or biological response-modifying drugs have been used in an attempt to reverse the viraemia in FeLV-infected cats (reviewed by Rojko and Hardy, 1994). While some of these agents have apparently been of benefit in individual cases, overall the response is generally poor, including the response to interferons. Zidovudine (AZT) has both *in vitro* and *in vivo* antiviral effects against FeLV, and has been used clinically at doses of 5–10 mg/kg orally q12h, but the higher doses especially may contribute to anaemia in FeLV infection. Its use may reduce viral loads, improve immunological parameters and prolong life expectancy in some FeLV-infected cats (Levy *et al.*, 2008; Lutz *et al.*, 2009).

The use of corticosteroids may have some rationale in cases of immune-mediated or autoimmune haemolytic anaemia, and corticosteroids may also have a beneficial effect in cases of cyclic neutropenia (perhaps through release of the bone marrow pool of neutrophils). However, it is important that covering antibiotics are used at the same time because of the risk of severe immunosuppression.

FeLV-associated lymphoma and lymphoid leukaemia may respond to appropriate chemotherapy, but the longer-term prognosis is poorer in such cats because the underlying FeLV infection contributes to earlier recurrence of disease or development of other significant diseases.

Control

Traditionally, FeLV has been controlled in colonies of cats by the 'test and removal' policy, which has been demonstrated to work very well (Jarrett, 1994). The introduction of FeLV vaccination has meant that the general cat population has been afforded good protection against this disease, and this too has contributed to the decline in prevalence of this infectious agent. While it is important to appreciate that FeLV vaccination does not provide 100% protection, and therefore a vaccinated cat should not be exposed deliberately to the virus, vaccination is nevertheless a very valuable tool to help prevent infection in cats that could potentially encounter the virus (Lutz *et al.*, 2009).

Feline immunodeficiency virus (FIV)

Epidemiology

As with FeLV infection, the source of FIV is a cat persistently infected with this virus. Like FeLV, FIV is a labile virus and is secreted in the saliva of infected cats. However, in contrast to FeLV, the normal mucosal barrier provides a relatively strong defence against penetration by FIV, thus direct inoculation of the virus by biting is considered to be the major route of transmission. The risk of transmission by social contact is very much lower than with FeLV, and although vertical transmission and transmission via milk have been demonstrated with FIV, only a proportion of kittens will become infected, depending primarily on the viral load of the queen.

The fact that biting is the major route of transmission explains why FIV infection is much more common in male cats, free-roaming cats and in non-pedigree cats. The age distribution of FIV infection also differs from that of FeLV, infection being uncommon in young cats (less than 1 year of age), but increasing with age to reach a peak in the 6–10-year-old age group (Hosie *et al.*, 1989).

Importantly, once a cat has been infected with FIV it will remain permanently infected. The normal immune response is unable to eliminate the virus from the body.

FIV is endemic in cat populations throughout the world, although the prevalence varies considerably among different countries and regions, depending in part on the lifestyle of the cats studied and the density of the cat populations. Typically, in the general healthy cat population the prevalence of FIV in the UK and North America is 1–6%, but may be up to 14% in some regions (Hopper *et al.*, 1994; Hosie *et al.*, 2009). As with FeLV, the prevalence of infection is higher in sick cats, especially those with signs of chronic disease.

Pathogenesis

Following infection, FIV has been shown to have a tropism for both $CD4^+$ and $CD8^+$ T lymphocytes as well as macrophages and astrocytes, with cellular infection and integration of proviral DNA occurring in a similar way to FeLV infection. $CD4^+$ T lymphocytes (T helper cells) appear to be the major target for FIV (Hosie *et al.*, 2009). Marked viraemia is present during the first 2–4 weeks following infection, but coincidental with the development of an antibody response, the viraemia declines to very low levels for many months to years, until the terminal stages of disease.

Following initial exposure to the virus, most FIV-infected cats exhibit a prolonged asymptomatic period, typically lasting 2–5 years, but during this time there is progressive impairment of the immune system. Although replication of the virus occurs at only a low level during most stages of infection, FIV can nevertheless be recovered from many sources including circulating lymphocytes, lymph nodes, spleen, bone marrow, saliva, brain and cerebrospinal fluid. Many cells also become latently infected, with viral DNA incorporated into the cellular DNA.

Depletion of $CD4^+$ T lymphocytes and an inverted CD4:CD8 T cell ratio are characteristic early findings in FIV-infected cats, and these changes continue to progress with time (Novotney *et al.*, 1990; Barlough *et al.*, 1991). As early as 6 months post infection, impaired T cell responses can be detected, and eventually the immunodeficiency caused by FIV leads to the development of clinical signs, often related to recurrent secondary or opportunistic infections.

It is clear that there are many different strains of FIV (at least five subtypes or 'clades' have been described, labelled A–E), and this is one factor that may determine the clinical effect of infection, the rapidity with which lymphocyte subset changes occur, and the duration of the asymptomatic period. However, substantial genetic and antigenic differences occur within different clades as well as between them. Other factors may also be important to the development of disease, such as the age of the cat at the time of infection, exposure dose, route of infection and potential exposure to other pathogens.

Diseases associated with FIV infection

Infection with FIV is a significant cause of disease in cats, and it has been shown that the prevalence of infection among cats showing clinical signs compatible with an immunodeficiency syndrome (i.e. cats with chronic or recurrent disease) is typically 15–20%, but it may be up to 40% or more (Hopper *et al.*, 1992; Hosie *et al.*, 2009).

A distinct acute phase of infection is seen around 4 weeks post exposure, which is characterized by pyrexia lasting several days to weeks, neutropenia and generalized lymphadenopathy (lasting up to 9 months). The neutropenia may lead to the development of secondary infections, but fatalities at this stage are rare, and although changes are readily observed during experimental infections, it is likely that not all naturally infected cats will develop significant or detectable disease associated with the acute infection.

Following acute infection, cats enter an asymptomatic stage that usually lasts for several years, and some cats may never develop significant FIV-associated disease. The prognosis for an FIV-infected cat is generally better than for an FeLV-infected cat, with average survival times following diagnosis of around 5 and 2.5 years, respectively (Levy *et al.*, 2008). During the asymptomatic phase, the cat develops progressive impairment of the immune system, which in most cases ultimately leads to symptomatic FIV infection as a result of immunodeficiency or immune dysregulation and immunostimulation.

The signs that develop during the latter symptomatic phase of FIV infection are typically chronic or recurring signs of disease, with gingivostomatitis (Figure 17.6), chronic rhinitis, lymphadenopathy and malaise being particularly common findings. Weight loss, pyrexia and recurrent gastrointestinal, respiratory and dermatological problems are also commonly reported. Rarely, central nervous system (CNS) infection with FIV can develop, resulting in neurological signs that include altered sleep patterns, behavioural disorders and seizures. Many concurrent viral, bacterial, fungal and parasitic infections have been reported in FIV-infected cats, and the presence of an unusual infection or one that does not respond to appropriate therapy should alert the clinician to the possibility of underlying FIV infection. A variety of tumours have also been reported in FIV-infected cats; many may arise as a result of reduced immune surveillance in an infected cat, but occasionally the virus itself may be oncogenic and it may rarely cause direct development of lymphoma. Renal damage may also occur as a result of circulating immune complexes and the secondary damage they cause. As the disease progresses it is common to find multiple clinical signs in an infected individual.

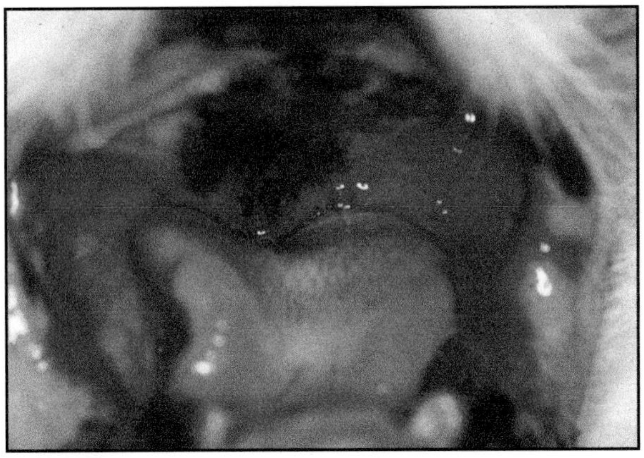

17.6 Severe stomatitis in an FIV-infected cat.

Specific haematological changes

Primary infection

Neutropenia with or without concomitant leucopenia is a common feature of the primary stage of FIV infection. Although many cats may pass through this stage with few or no overt clinical signs, a small proportion may develop significant disease, including secondary infections caused by the neutropenia. As with FeLV, testing for FIV is advisable in any cat that presents with neutropenia.

Haematological changes are commonly seen in association with the later stages of FIV infection, and these are comparable to the changes encountered in humans infected with the human immunodeficiency virus (HIV). However, even during the asymptomatic phase of FIV infection, haematological abnormalities (including anaemia, neutropenia and thrombocytopenia) have been reported in infected cats, as a result of bone marrow infection with the virus.

Anaemia

Anaemia is frequently found in the later (symptomatic) stages of FIV infection and studies of naturally occurring disease suggest a prevalence of between 15 and 40%. As with FeLV infection, FIV-induced immunosuppression will predispose cats to secondary infection with haemotropic mycoplasmas, and it is important to consider these organisms as a potential underlying cause of or contributory factor in the anaemia (consider appropriate PCR tests; Chapter 7). Both regenerative and non-regenerative anaemias are encountered in FIV-infected cats and with the latter, bone marrow aspirates are indicated to rule out myeloproliferative disorders or myelodysplasia. As with FeLV infection, anaemia of chronic disease may also be a contributory factor.

Thrombocytopenia is also occasionally seen in FIV-infected cats but this is rarely clinically significant.

Lymphopenia and neutropenia

Lymphopenia has been reported in 30–55% of FIV infected cats, and neutropenia in 5–35%. Both of these may contribute to leucopenia, which has been reported in 5–30% of infected cats. Along with FeLV, FIV should be considered a primary cause of neutropenia in the cat. The pathogenesis of this and other cytopenias in FIV infection is poorly understood, but undoubtedly involves multiple factors.

A reversible neutropenia has been reported in six of seven FIV-infected cats that were treated with griseofulvin, and this bears similarity to the observation of antibiotic-associated neutropenias in HIV-infected people, although again the precise pathogenesis of these changes is unclear.

The lymphopenia in advanced FIV infection is frequently profound, and while the stress of concurrent disease may be partly responsible for this change, the selective depletion of the $CD4^+$ T cells will also contribute to this finding. From studies of FIV-infected cats, and by analogy with HIV infection, other factors likely to be involved in the pathogenesis of the various cytopenias include FIV infection of bone marrow stem cells and accessory cells, viraemia and/or viral proteins inhibiting haemopoiesis, an imbalance of bone marrow T cells, the production of humoral inhibitory factors, an alteration in the profiles of T cell cytokine that affect haemopoiesis, and triggering of immune-mediated or autoimmune mechanisms.

'Normal' leucocyte responses

As with FeLV-induced immunosuppression, depending on the stage of disease many FIV-infected cats that have concurrent or secondary infections will still make an appropriate overt haematological response.

Studies have demonstrated leucocytosis and neutrophilia with a left shift as common findings in FIV-infected individuals, often in association with an obvious purulent or inflammatory disease process.

Haematological changes in terminal disease

Although it can be difficult to determine the clinical stage of FIV infection accurately, there is evidence that those cats with more advanced disease, and those that are entering the terminal stages of disease, are much more likely to have severe and multiple cytopenias present on haematological examination (Sparkes *et al.*, 1993). The results of routine haematology may therefore have some prognostic value for the individual, although it is important to interpret these findings in the light of the clinical picture. The ability to track $CD4^+$ cell numbers and the CD4:CD8 ratio in an infected cat over time may also provide significant prognostic information, although this is not incorporated as a routine part of the assessment of FIV-infected cats.

Lympho- and myeloproliferative disease

There is clear evidence that FIV infection predisposes cats to the development of lymphoproliferative and myeloproliferative disorders. It is generally thought that this occurs largely through reduced or ineffective immune surveillance as a consequence of the FIV infection, but on rare occasions it seems possible that it may result from insertional mutagenesis of the virus itself (similar to FeLV). Although much less common than FeLV as a cause of these disorders, a similar range of haematological changes can occur.

Diagnosis

Unlike the diagnosis of FeLV infection, there is too little FIV-derived antigen present in plasma and blood to be detected using currently available routine technologies. However, because FIV infections are persistent, the presence of circulating antibodies against the virus can be taken as indirect (and reliable) evidence of infection with the virus.

As with FeLV diagnosis, a number of 'in-house' diagnostic kits are available for the rapid detection of FIV antibodies, typically against the p24 and/or gp41 antigens. Again, the membrane ELISA kits (e.g. SNAP FIV; Idexx) and the immunochromatography techniques (e.g. 'Witness'; Synbiotics) have done much to minimize the danger of technical error when performing these tests and their results are generally very reliable.

However, both false positive and false negative results may be more of a concern with FIV testing than with FeLV testing, for a variety of different reasons. Some cats may experience delayed seroconversion after infection with FIV or simply fail to develop a good humoral immune response. Although such cases are likely to be uncommon, false negative results may be seen in such situations. Conversely, false positive results may occasionally be seen if cross-reacting antibodies are detected by the test (rare) or, more importantly, if a young cat is tested after receiving colostral antibodies from the queen or when a cat has been vaccinated against FIV. The commercially available FIV vaccine that is currently licensed in some countries unfortunately induces an antibody response that is indistinguishable from natural infection on routine serological tests.

As with routine FeLV testing, it is important to assess the results of routine 'in house' diagnostic tests carefully in the light of the clinical signs and the history of the cat being tested. If there is any doubt about the validity of the test result, again, confirmation of the result should be sought by submitting a sample to a reference laboratory with consideration also given to repeating the test at a later date if delayed seroconversion is suspected and/or if interference from maternally derived antibodies is suspected.

As with FeLV infection, laboratory-based diagnostics will often employ a plate ELISA test as an initial screening test for the presence of antibodies, but may also include western immunoblotting, virus isolation, immunofluorescence or PCR as a confirmatory test.

While virus isolation is perhaps the 'gold standard' for diagnosis of FIV, regrettably this is too laborious and expensive to be available as a routine diagnostic method. Western blotting allows detection of antibodies against individual viral proteins and can be a valuable confirmatory test (positive results should be reliable), but the sensitivity of western blotting may be poor and standardization among laboratories would be highly desirable. The use of PCR to detect integrated proviral DNA holds much promise for the detection of FIV infection, but is currently problematic. Studies of the PCR tests offered by different commercial laboratories show widely varying results, and for efficient detection of different FIV clades it is likely that multiplex PCRs will be needed with primers designed for different gene sequences. To develop a reliable PCR test will require wide cooperation between research and diagnostic laboratories, but caution is currently needed in the selection and interpretation of results. Nevertheless, PCR performed at a reputable laboratory using techniques to detect a wide range of FIV variants should be a valuable diagnostic tool.

Treatment

As with FeLV, treatment of FIV-infected cats is primarily symptomatic and supportive. Efforts should be made promptly to identify specific secondary or opportunistic infections and diseases that can be appropriately treated. Specific treatment for the haematological abnormalities is not feasible, but consideration of concurrent drug therapy and the possibility of drug-associated side effects should be considered when faced with a neutropenic FIV-infected cat.

The reverse transcriptase inhibitor zidovudine (AZT) used at a dose of 5–10 mg/kg orally q12h has shown some efficacy in the clinical management of FIV-infected cats, especially those with FIV-associated stomatitis. Reduced virus loads and enhanced clinical status may be seen in infected cats, but haematological monitoring is important to detect AZT-associated anaemia (seen more commonly with the higher doses), and resistant strains of FIV may emerge, so careful patient selection is warranted when considering therapy. Whether combined treatment with interferons would offer further benefits is unknown.

Control

A commercial FIV vaccine is available in some countries. This is a killed vaccine based on two strains of the virus and has been shown to provide some reasonable protection against infection in some studies. However, some of the challenge studies have failed to show substantial protection and it is likely therefore that the degree of protection afforded may vary considerably between strains and isolates. The biggest disadvantage with the vaccine is that it induces antibodies that are indistinguishable from those produced by natural infection in routine serological tests. Vaccine advisory panels have therefore recommended that the use of this vaccine should be restricted, and that it should be administered only where the benefit of vaccination can be clearly determined to outweigh the disadvantages. In addition, permanent identification (e.g. microchipping) of vaccinated cats is crucial.

Control of FIV relies greatly on the detection of infected cats, and on ensuring that they are managed in such a way that they are unlikely to transmit infection. This may involve the neutering of entire cats, and confining cats to prevent them from wandering and fighting.

References and further reading

Barlough JE, Ackley CD, George JW *et al.* (1991) Acquired immune dysfunction in cats with experimentally induced feline immunodeficiency virus infection: comparison of short-term and long-term infections. *Journal of Acquired Immune Deficiency Syndromes* **4**, 219–227

Bobade PA, Nash AS and Rogerson P (1988) Feline haemobartonellosis: clinical, haematological and pathological studies in natural infections and the relationship to infection with feline leukaemia virus. *Veterinary Record* **122**, 32–36

Cheng HH, Anderson MM and Overbaugh J (2007) Feline leukaemia virus T entry is dependent on both expression levels and specific interactions between cofactor and receptor. *Virology* **359**, 170–178

Day MJ, Horzinek MC, Schultz RD; WSAVA VGG (2010) Guidelines for the vaccination of dogs and cats. Compiled by the vaccination guidelines group (VGG) of the World Small Animal Veterinary Association (WSAVA). *Journal of Small Animal Practice* **51**, 1–32

Fujino Y, Horinchi H, Mizukoshi F *et al.* (2009) Prevalence of haematological abnormalities and detection of infected bone marrow cells in asymptomatic cats with feline immunodeficiency virus infection. *Veterinary Microbiology* **136**(3-4), 217–225

Gleich S and Hartmann K (2009) Hematology and serum biochemistry of feline immunodeficiency virus-infected and feline leukaemia virus-infected cats. *Journal of Veterinary Internal Medicine* **23**, 552–558

Hoover EA and Mullins JI (1991) Feline leukaemia virus infection and diseases. *Journal of the American Veterinary Medical Association* **199**, 1287–1297

Hopper CD, Sparkes AH and Harbour DA (1994) Feline immunodeficiency virus. In: *Feline Medicine and Therapeutics, 2nd edn*, ed. EA Chandler, CJ Gaskell and RM Gaskell, pp. 488–505. Blackwell Scientific Publications, Oxford

Horzinek MC, Addie D, Belak S *et al.* (2009) Infectious disease prevention and management. *Journal of Feline Medicine and Surgery* (special issue incorporating the ABCD guidelines) **7**, 527–618

Hosie MJ, Addie D, Belak S *et al.* (2009) Feline immunodeficiency: ABCD guidelines on prevention and management. *Journal of Feline Medicine and Surgery* **11**, 575–584

Hosie MJ, Robertson C and Jarrett O (1989) Prevalence of feline leukaemia virus and antibodies to feline immunodeficiency virus in cats in the United Kingdom. *Veterinary Record* **128**, 293–297

Jarrett O (1994) Feline leukaemia virus. In: *Feline Medicine and Therapeutics, 2nd edn*, ed. EA Chandler, CJ Gaskell and RM Gaskell, pp. 473–487. Blackwell Scientific Publications, Oxford

Jordan HL, Grindem CB and Brietschwerdt EB (1993) Thrombocytopenia in cats: a retrospective study of 41 cases. *Journal of Veterinary Internal Medicine* **7**, 261–265

Levy J, Crawford C, Hartmann K *et al.* (2008) 2008 American Association of Feline Practitioners' feline retrovirus management guidelines. *Journal of Feline Medicine and Surgery* **10**, 300–316

Lutz H, Addie D, Belak S *et al.* (2009) Feline leukaemia: ABCD guidelines on prevention and management. *Journal of Feline Medicine and Surgery* **11**, 565–574

Macy DW (1994) Feline immunodeficiency virus. In: Sherding RG (ed) In: *The Cat, Diseases and Clinical Management, 2nd edn,* ed. RG Sherding, pp.433–448. Churchill Livingstone, New York

Novotney C, English RV, Housman J *et al.* (1990) Lymphocyte population changes in cats naturally infected with feline immunodeficiency virus. *AIDS* **4**, 1213–1218

Pedersen NC and Barlough JE (1991) Clinical overview of feline immunodeficiency virus. *Journal of the American Veterinary Medical Association* **199**, 1298–1305

Richards JR, Elston TH, Ford RB *et al.* (2006) The 2006 American Association of Feline Practitioners Feline Vaccine Advisory Panel Report. *Journal of American Veterinary Medical Association* **229**, 1405–1441

Rojko JL and Hardy WD (1994) Feline leukaemia virus and other retroviruses. In: *The Cat, Diseases and Clinical Management, 2nd edn,* ed. RG Sherding, pp.263–432. Churchill Livingstone, New York

Shelton GH, Linenberger ML and Abkowitz JL (1991) Haematologic abnormalities in cats seropositive for feline immunodeficiency virus. *Journal of the American Veterinary Medical Association* **199**, 1353–1357

Sparkes AH, Hopper CD, Millard WG, Gruffydd-Jones TJ and Harbour DA (1993) Feline immunodeficiency virus infection – clinicopathological findings in 90 naturally occurring cases. *Journal of Veterinary Internal Medicine* **7**, 85–90

Swenson CL, Kociba GJ, O'Keefe DA *et al.* (1987) Cyclic haematopoiesis associated with feline leukaemia virus infection in two cats. *Journal of the American Veterinary Medical Association* **191**, 93–96

18

Ehrlichiosis

Mathios E. Mylonakis

Introduction

Canine ehrlichiosis (CE) is caused by Gram-negative, obligate intracellular, pleomorphic cocci of the genus *Ehrlichia* (order Rickettsiales, family Anaplasmataceae; Figure 18.1). *Ehrlichia canis* was the first species recognized to infect dogs and it is the principal causative agent of canine monocytic ehrlichiosis (CME; Neer *et al.*, 2002). *Ehrlichia chaffeensis*, the cause of human monocytic ehrlichiosis, has emerged recently as an infrequent cause of clinical disease in the dog, indistinguishable from that caused by *E. canis*. *Ehrlichia ewingii*, a species separate from, but closely related to *E. canis* and *E. chaffeensis*, is the cause of canine granulocytic ehrlichiosis. Given that the clinical importance and the bulk of information pertaining to *E. canis* infection far outweigh those for *E. chaffeensis* and *E. ewingii* infections in the dog, this review will emphasize the former, unless specified otherwise.

Life cycle and epidemiology

Ehrlichia canis is transmitted naturally by the brown dog tick, *Rhipicephalus sanguineus* (Figure 18.1). The mode of transmission is transstadial and intrastadial, but not transovarian; therefore, tick larvae and nymphs need to feed on rickettsaemic dogs to acquire the infection. Adult ticks may harbour the organism for at least 155 days post infection, which facilitates its wintering and transmission during the next tick season. The infection can also be transmitted by blood transfusion. Most dogs become infected and develop acute illness during the warm season of the year when ticks flourish; on the other hand, the extremely variable duration of the subclinical phase largely accounts for the lack of seasonality in the chronic phase of the disease. The lone star tick, *Amblyomma americanum*, has been incriminated in the transmission of *E. chaffeensis* and *E. ewingii*, although other tick species may also be suitable vectors (Figure 18.1). The global distribution of CE correlates, at least partially, with the density and geographical distribution of the tick vectors. *Ehrlichia* spp. infect primarily leucocytes, including monocytes, macrophages and lymphocytes (*E. canis* and *E. chaffeensis*) or neutrophils and eosinophils (*E. ewingii*), forming intracytoplasmic, membrane-bound bacterial aggregates called morulae.

Pathogenesis

During an incubation period of 8–20 days, *E. canis* enters the cells of the mononuclear phagocyte system, mainly in the spleen, liver and lymph nodes, where it replicates and spreads throughout the body. The course of the infection thereafter can be divided into the acute (non-myelosuppressive), subclinical and chronic (myelosuppressive) phases. Most untreated dogs recover spontaneously from the acute phase after 2–4 weeks, entering the subclinical phase, which may last several months to years, during which they show no clinical signs. Immunocompetent dogs may eliminate the infection during this period, but some will eventually develop the chronic phase of the disease, characterized by severe bone marrow (BM) aplasia, peripheral blood pancytopenia and high mortality due to septicaemia and/or severe bleeding. The conditions that may

Species	Geographical distribution	Vector [a]	Major mammalian host
Ehrlichia canis	Worldwide in tropical and temperate climates	*Rhipicephalus sanguineus, Dermacentor variabilis*	Dog
Ehrlichia chaffeensis	Southern United States, South Korea, Cameroon	*Amblyomma americanum, Dermacentor variabilis*	White-tailed deer
Ehrlichia ewingii	Southern and lower mid-eastern United States, Brazil, Cameroon	*Amblyomma americanum, Dermacentor variabilis, Rhipicephalus sanguineus*	White-tailed deer
Ehrlichia ruminantium [b]	Sub-Saharan Africa	*Amblyomma hebraeum*	Ruminants

18.1 Geographical distribution, vectors and major hosts of *Ehrlichia* spp. implicated in canine ehrlichiosis. [a] Known or strongly suspected; [b] Potential pathogen for dogs.

precipitate myelosuppression have yet to be elucidated. Breed-specific defective cell-mediated immunity (thought to occur in German Shepherd Dogs), co-infections with other vector-borne pathogens (e.g. *Leishmania infantum*, *Babesia* spp., *Rickettsia* spp., *Bartonella* spp.), strain virulence or inoculum size variation, and the cytokine profile induced within the host immune system following inoculation of *E. canis* (i.e. high levels of interferon (IFN)-γ have been associated with mild disease, as opposed to elevated interleukin (IL)-1β and IL-8, which are associated with more severe disease), may affect the clinicopathological diversity and the outcome of the disease.

Cellular immunity is pivotal for protection against *E. canis*; in contrast, the exuberant humoral immune response appears to confer no protection, and in fact may be detrimental to the host. A growing body of evidence indicates that several manifestations, including glomerulonephritis, uveitis, thrombocytopenia and anaemia, may be at least in part immune-mediated, as indicated by the presence of circulating immune complexes, plasmacytic infiltration of many parenchymal organs, polyclonal hypergammaglobulinaemia and the presence of anti-platelet and anti-erythrocyte antibodies. A bleeding tendency, the clinical hallmark of CME, is associated with impaired primary haemostasis resulting from thrombocytopenia, thrombocytopathy and/or mild vasculitis.

Thrombocytopenia appears to have a multifaceted pathogenesis. In the acute stage of CME, it is attributed to immune-mediated destruction, increased consumption secondary to mild vasculitis, splenic sequestration and possibly over-expression of platelet migration inhibition factor. The bone marrow failure in the myelosuppressive stage of CME accounts for the profound thrombocytopenia, bi- or pancytopenia that may be seen.

Characteristic	Acute CME (n = 50) [a]	Chronic CME (n = 19) [b]
	No. with finding/No. tested (%)	
Clinical manifestation		
Fever	47/50 (94)	10/19 (53)
Hypothermia	0	5/19 (26)
Depression	46/50 (92)	19/19 (100)
Anorexia	44/50 (88)	18/19 (95)
Weight loss	35/50 (70)	6/19 (32)
Lymphadenomegaly	32/50 (64)	9/19 (47)
Ocular discharge	23/50 (46)	2/19 (11)
Mucosal pallor	13/50 (26)	18/19 (95)
Splenomegaly	11/50 (22)	6/19 (32)
Bleeding diathesis	11/50 (22)	19/19 (100)
Respiratory distress	9/50 (18)	4/19 (21)
Uveitis	4/50 (8)	4/19 (21)
Tick infestation	22/50 (44)	3/19 (16)
Haematology		
Thrombocytopenia	49/50 (98)	19/19 (100)
Anaemia	41/50 (82)	19/19 (100)
Lymphopenia	21/50 (42)	18/19 (95)
Leucopenia	10/50 (20)	17/19 (89)
Neutropenia	1/50 (2)	17/19 (89)
Pancytopenia	8/50 (16)	17/19 (89)
Serum biochemistry		
Elevated ALT	29/44 (64)	13/18 (72)
Hypoproteinaemia	17/50 (34)	0
Hypoalbuminaemia	5/43 (12)	10/19 (53)
Hyperglobulinaemia	3/50 (6)	6/19 (32)
Elevated ALP	11/43 (26)	6/17 (35)

18.2 Frequency of clinical, haematological and biochemical abnormalities in 50 dogs with acute (non-myelosuppressive) and 19 dogs with chronic (myelosuppressive) naturally occurring canine monocytic ehrlichiosis (CME) caused by *Ehrlichia canis*. ALP, alkaline phosphatase; ALT, alanine aminotransferase. [a] Mylonakis *et al.*, 2003; [b] Mylonakis *et al.*, 2004.

Clinical presentation

E. canis infection causes a multisystemic disease ranging from mild (in the acute phase) to life-threatening (in the chronic phase) in severity (Figure 18.2). An unknown percentage of naturally infected dogs will never exhibit clinical signs; on the other hand, in dogs living in endemic areas, co-infections with other vector-borne pathogens may obfuscate the diagnosis. No gender or age predilection has been documented in CME; however, German Shepherd Dogs have higher morbidity and mortality compared with other breeds. Fever, depression, anorexia, lymphadenomegaly, splenomegaly, mucosal pallor, ocular abnormalities and bleeding tendency are common clinical manifestations in naturally occurring CME. Tick infestation may be noticed, especially in the acute phase of the disease, while ulcerative stomatitis and necrotic glossitis (Figure 18.3), hindlimb and/or scrotal oedema, bacterial pyoderma, icterus and central nervous system (CNS) signs have been more frequently reported in chronic CME.

Bleeding diathesis is also more common and severe in the chronic phase of CME, and in those dogs with concurrent conditions that predispose to bleeding (e.g. infection with *L. infantum*, von Willebrand's disease, drug-induced or uraemic thrombocytopathy). This feature of the disease is mainly expressed as cutaneous and mucosal petechiae and ecchymoses, hyphaema, epistaxis, microscopic or macroscopic haematuria, melaena and prolonged bleeding from venepuncture sites (Mylonakis *et al.*, 2004; Figures 18.4–18.8).

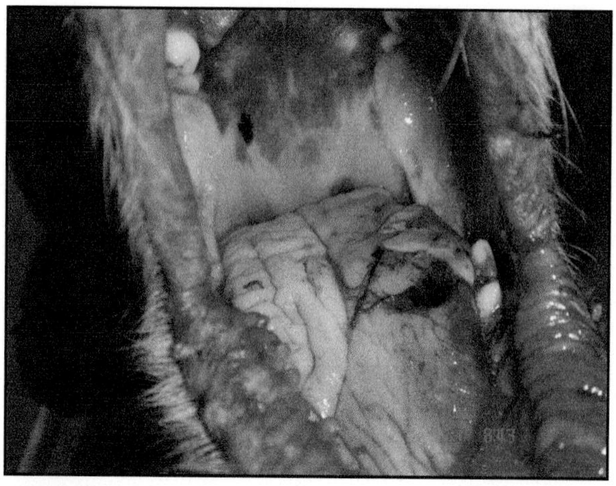

18.3 Severe necrotic glossitis in a dog with myelosuppressive *Ehrlichia canis* infection.

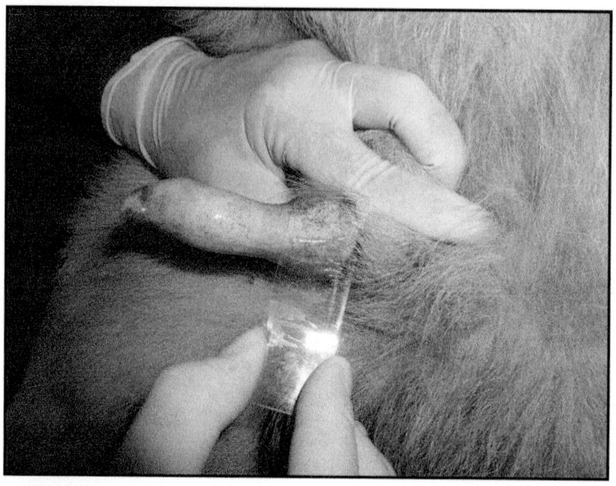

18.4 Numerous petechiae and ecchymoses in the penile mucosa of a dog with acute canine CME. The haemorrhagic lesions do not disappear on pressure (diascopy).

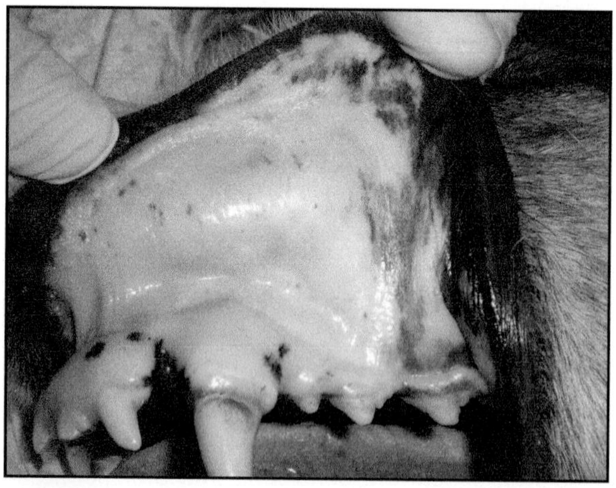

18.5 Mucosal pallor and petechiation in a dog with myelosuppressive CME.

Ocular lesions are commonly seen in CME, and may be the sole presenting complaint. Anterior or posterior uveitis is the most prevalent manifestation (Figure 18.9a). Ocular discharge, blepharitis,

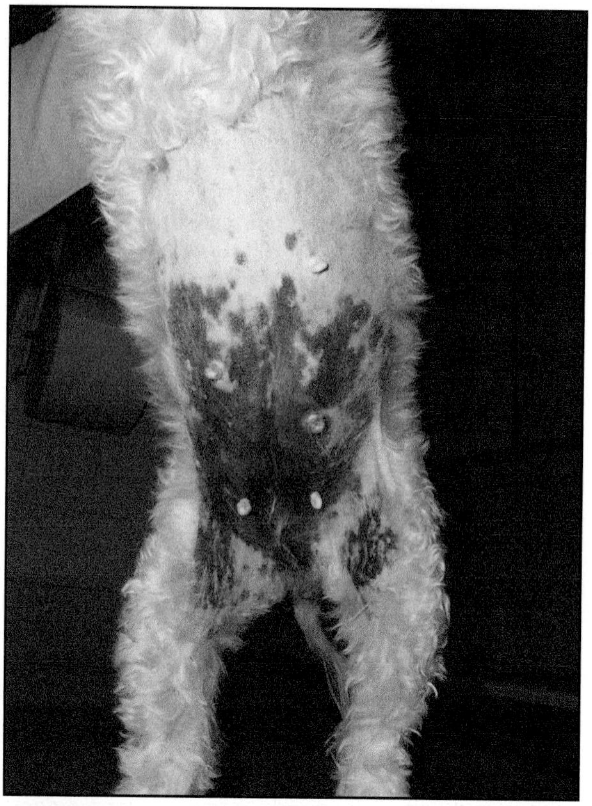

18.6 Extensive haemorrhagic lesions in a dog with concurrent CME and *L. infantum* infection.

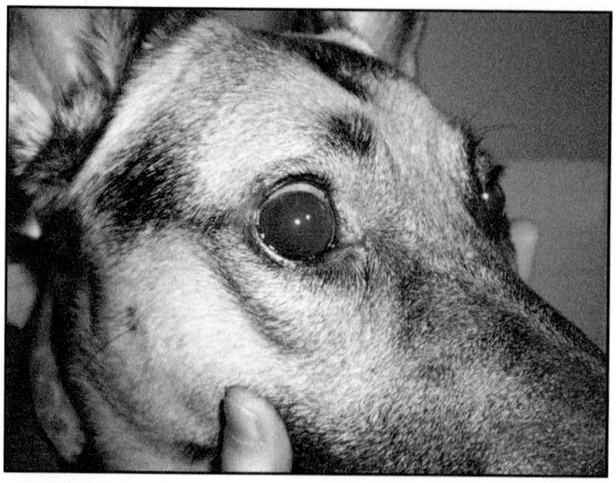

18.7 Anterior chamber bleeding (hyphaema) in a dog with CME. (Courtesy Dr A. Komnenou)

conjunctivitis, corneal ulceration, painful necrotic scleritis (Figure 18.9b), secondary glaucoma and retinal haemorrhage and/or detachment leading to blindness have also been reported.

The clinical manifestations of *E. chaffeensis* and *E. ewingii* infections in the dog overlap with those of *E. canis* infection, but their long-term clinical course and outcome are largely unknown. Notably, polyarthritis, manifesting as lameness, joint swelling and stiff gait, and CNS signs such as seizures, ataxia, vestibular dysfunction and cervical pain, are more frequent in granulocytic compared with monocytic ehrlichiosis.

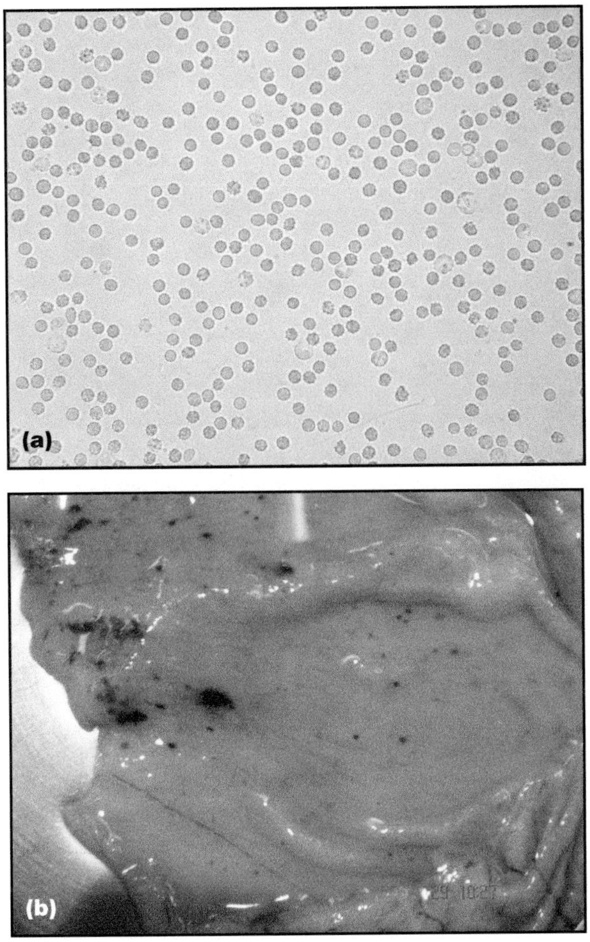

18.8 **(a)** Haematuria in a dog with chronic CME (urine sediment, objective × 40) and **(b)** same dog, post mortem: several petechiae and ecchymoses in the bladder mucosa. (Courtesy Dr V. Psychas)

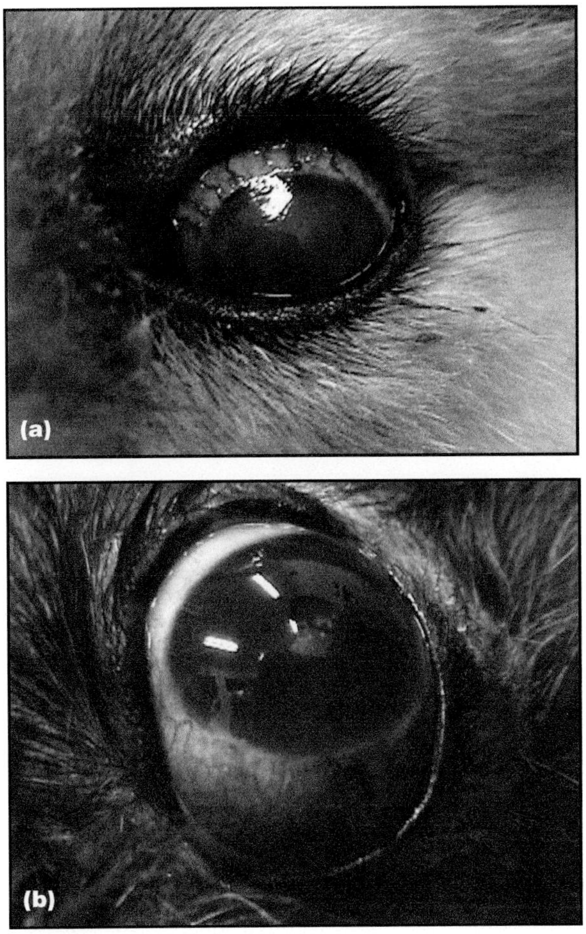

18.9 **(a)** Anterior uveitis and **(b)** necrotic scleritis in a dog with CME. (Courtesy Dr A. Komnenou)

Diagnosis

The diagnosis of CE is based on the historical (e.g. living in or travelling to endemic areas, evidence of tick infestation) and clinical compatibility, consistent clinicopathological abnormalities (see Figure 18.2) and *Ehrlichia*-specific testing.

Haematology

Thrombocytopenia is the most frequent haematological abnormality in CME, appearing in more than 80% of cases (see Figure 18.2). However, CME should not be ruled out solely on the basis of a normal platelet count. Megathrombocytosis (increased mean platelet volume and/or megathrombocyte percentage > 2% of the platelet count) is common in the acute phase of CME, and implies a regenerative thrombocytopenia. A non-regenerative anaemia, leucopenia and lymphopenia are additional abnormalities. Aplastic pancytopenia typifies the myelosuppressive form of the disease (Figure 18.10a); BM mast cell hyperplasia and plasmacytosis may be seen in these cases and should not be confused with systemic mastocytosis or multiple myeloma, respectively. Pancytopenia with normocellular BM (Figure 18.10b) may occur in acute CME, and is readily amenable to treatment. A mild-to-moderate thrombocytopenia is the most consistent haematological finding in subclinical CME. Granular lymphocytosis is a notable, although uncommon, feature of subclinical or chronic CME, and may imitate lymphocytic leukaemia. Thus, CME should be a differential for persistent lymphocytosis in the dog. Mild thrombocytopenia and non-regenerative anaemia predominate in *E. chaffeensis* and *E. ewingii* infections.

Biochemistry

Hypergammaglobulinaemia, hypoalbuminaemia and mildly elevated alkaline phosphatase and alanine aminotransferase activities are common biochemical abnormalities (see Figure 18.2) in *E. canis* infection. Hypergammaglobulinaemia does not correlate with the titre of anti-*E. canis* antibodies, and appears on serum electrophoresis to be polyclonal or, rarely, oligoclonal or monoclonal. Pancytopenic dogs tend to have lower gamma-globulin concentrations when compared with their non-pancytopenic counterparts. Proteinuria may be present, attributable to glomerulonephritis with or without immune complex deposition in the chronic and acute stages of CME, respectively.

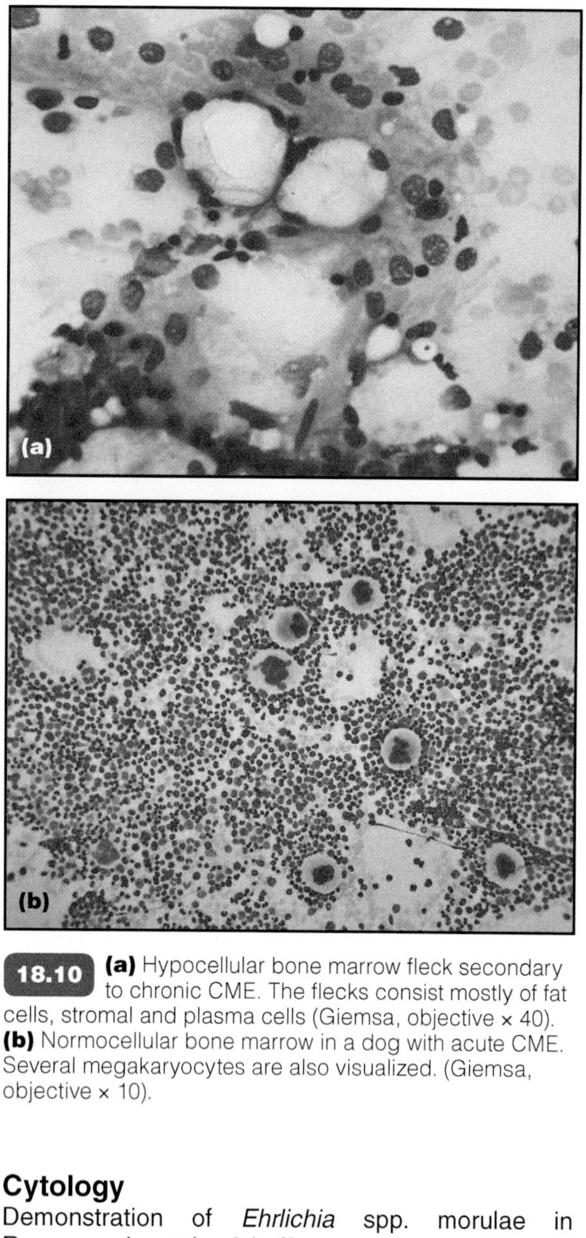

18.10 **(a)** Hypocellular bone marrow fleck secondary to chronic CME. The flecks consist mostly of fat cells, stromal and plasma cells (Giemsa, objective × 40). **(b)** Normocellular bone marrow in a dog with acute CME. Several megakaryocytes are also visualized. (Giemsa, objective × 10).

Cytology

Demonstration of *Ehrlichia* spp. morulae in Romanowsky-stained buffy coat smears, and less frequently in lymph node, BM, spleen, lung and cerebrospinal or joint fluid smears, is helpful in establishing a definitive diagnosis of acute CE. Morulae can be observed in monocytes (Figure 18.11), macrophages and lymphocytes (*E. canis*, *E. chaffeensis*) or in neutrophils and eosinophils (*E. ewingii*). In a study of dogs naturally infected by *E. canis*, the diagnostic sensitivity of buffy coat and lymph node cytology was 66% and 61%, respectively (Mylonakis *et al.*, 2003). As a rule, the visualization of morulae is easier in granulocytic (up to 25% infected granulocytes) compared with monocytic (< 1% infected mononuclear cells) ehrlichioses. Cytology is also valuable in documenting co-infections (e.g. *Babesia* spp., *Hepatozoon canis*, *L. infantum*), which may have therapeutic and prognostic implications. On the other hand, cytology is time consuming, notoriously insensitive in the diagnosis of subclinical and chronic CE, and its specificity is adversely affected by the inability to determine the species of ehrlichial organisms and

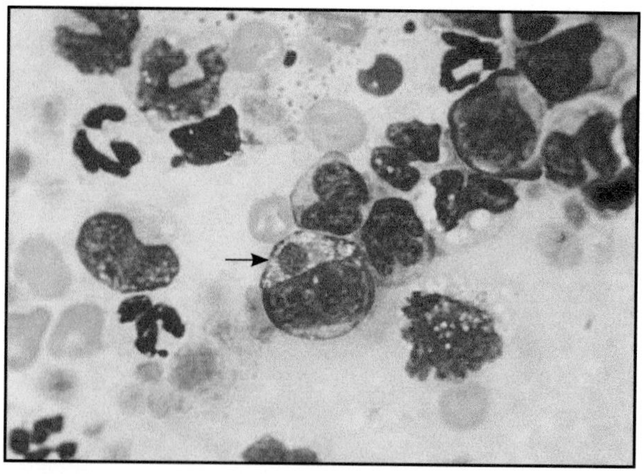

18.11 *Ehrlichia canis* morula in a monocyte of a dog with acute CME. (buffy coat, Giemsa, original magnification × 100)

the fact that extraneous material such as phagocytosed platelets or nuclear remnants and lymphocytic azurophilic granules can be confused with morulae.

Serological testing

Serology is the diagnostic modality employed most frequently for the confirmation of ehrlichial infections in the dog. Indirect fluorescent antibody (IFA) testing is considered the 'gold standard' for the detection and titration of anti-*Ehrlichia* antibodies, although enzyme-linked immunosorbent assays (ELISAs) are also used commonly. For most laboratories, an immunoglobulin (Ig)G titre equal to or greater than 80 is considered indicative of prior exposure to an *Ehrlichia* species. Antibodies develop 7–28 days post infection, but do not correlate reliably with the duration of infection, the current carrier status, or the presence and severity of clinical disease. In acutely infected dogs, clinical signs may occur before seroconversion, while myelosuppressed, moribund animals may on occasion demonstrate very low titres. Owing to the prolonged latent period and the persistent seropositivity following drug-mediated or self-eradication of the infection, clinicians should be aware that seroreactivity to *Ehrlichia* spp., especially in an endemic area, does not confirm that the clinical manifestations on presentation are attributable to an *Ehrlichia* spp. infection, unless a four-fold seroconversion is demonstrated in paired serum samples obtained 2–3 weeks apart.

The specificity of serology is also affected by the cross-reactivity that may occur among the same (i.e. *E. canis*, *E. chaffeensis* and *E. ewingii*) or, less likely, closely related (e.g. *Anaplasma phagocytophilum*) genogroup species. Although not available routinely, western immunoblotting may distinguish between infections with *Ehrlichia* spp. that display cross-reactivity, while the chronicity of *E. canis* infection may be inferred based on immunoblot patterns. Given that *in vitro* culture of *E. ewingii* has yet to be developed, no specific serological test is currently available for this organism. Numerous in-house ELISAs are available commercially for *E. canis* antibody testing. In general, these screening tests have been calibrated to be positive at an antibody level corresponding to an IFA titre of approximately 320 or higher; thus, a relatively low sensitivity may be anticipated, especially in acutely infected dogs.

Molecular testing

Polymerase chain reaction (PCR) is a highly sensitive method for the early detection (usually 4–10 days post inoculation), molecular characterization and quantification (real-time PCR) of ehrlichial organisms. Provided that the technique is subjected to stringent quality control, PCR may overcome several diagnostic limitations pertaining to serology and cytology. In addition, PCR is more useful than serology for the detection of concurrent ehrlichial infections and for post-treatment monitoring. Several PCR assays have been developed, targeting an array of genes, such as the 16S rRNA or the p30 genes, to specifically detect *E. canis*, *E. chaffeensis* or *E. ewingii* infections in the dog. Successful amplification of *Ehrlichia* DNA may be accomplished from several tissues, including whole blood, BM, spleen, liver, kidney, lung, lymph nodes and cerebrospinal fluid. In naturally-occurring CE, the sensitivity and the optimal tissue for PCR testing in the untreated dog have yet to be clarified; therefore, PCR should be used in conjunction with, rather than instead of, serology in the diagnosis of the disease (Neer *et al.*, 2002).

Treatment

In a dog with clinical and clinicopathological manifestations consistent with ehrlichiosis in conjunction with serological evidence of exposure, and/or molecular or cytological evidence of an ehrlichial infection, the decision for treatment is straightforward. The decision to treat a clinically healthy, seropositive dog may be particularly challenging, especially in endemic areas. A positive PCR result indicates active infection and warrants treatment, while a negative PCR (ideally performed on blood, BM or a splenic aspirate) does not justify initiation of treatment. However, if PCR is not available, the proper course of action should be decided on a case-by-case basis. The author inclines towards treating these dogs if they are thrombocytopenic and/or hypergammaglobulinaemic and no other potential causes of these abnormalities (e.g. iatrogenic thrombocytopenia and/or comorbid conditions) can be demonstrated.

Specific and supportive treatment

Tetracycline antibiotics

Historically, doxycycline, a semi-synthetic tetracycline, has been the first-line drug for the treatment of CE. In acute *E. canis* infection, several PCR-based studies have shown that doxycycline is very effective in eliminating the infection; however, in subclinical or chronic *E. canis* infection, this drug has been inconsistent in eradicating the infection. The consensus dosing recommendation for doxycycline in CE is 5 mg/kg orally q12h, for at least 28 days (Neer *et al.*, 2002). Importantly, in a recent study, the efficacy of the consensus doxycycline regimen was investigated during three different phases (namely acute, subclinical and chronic) following experimental *E. canis* infection in the dog. Despite the clinical and haematological recovery of the dogs and the negative blood PCR, *R. sanguineus* ticks that fed on the dogs after doxycycline treatment became PCR positive for *E. canis* DNA, regardless of the phase of disease in which treatment was initiated (McClure *et al.*, 2010). These results may imply that a very low level of rickettsiaemia, not detected by PCR, can persist even following prolonged doxycycline treatment, irrelevant of the clinical phase of the disease. Current evidence suggests that *E. chaffeensis* infection may be more refractory to doxycycline treatment compared with *E. canis*, and that granulocytic may be more responsive compared with monocytic ehrlichioses (Breitschwerdt *et al.*, 1998). Some dogs may experience nausea and vomiting with oral doxycycline, which may be mitigated by mixing the drug with food.

There is currently limited evidence-based justification for using other tetracyclines (e.g. minocycline, tetracycline, oxytetracycline), chloramphenicol or imidocarb dipropionate in the treatment of CE. The latter was recently found to be ineffective in eliminating natural and experimental *E. canis* infections (Eddlestone *et al.*, 2006); thus, it is no longer indicated except in dual infections with *Babesia canis*. In a recent report, rifampin at 15 mg/kg orally q12h, for 7 days, was as effective as doxycycline in completely eliminating experimental subclinical *E. canis* infection in two dogs (Schaefer *et al.*, 2008). Provided that a safe dose regime is established and further data on its efficacy are accumulated, rifampin might be a promising alternative to doxycycline in CE, as suggested by current clinical experience in human ehrlichiosis.

Glucocorticoids

Short-term glucocorticoid treatment (prednisolone 2 mg/kg q24h for 1 week) has been advocated in CE for attenuating the immune-mediated components of the disease. In the author's opinion, this is very rarely needed, because rapid improvement is noticed soon after the institution of doxycycline treatment in acutely infected dogs. On the other hand, the administration of glucococorticoids to a profoundly leucopenic dog may exacerbate the disease (Shipov *et al.*, 2008). Glucocorticoids may be considered, however, in dogs with severe thrombocytopenia-induced bleeding, when the differentiation of CE from the primary immune-mediated thrombocytopenia is not straightforward.

Supportive therapy

In the myelosuppressive form of CME, supportive treatment encompasses the administration of crystalloid solutions, periodic blood-typed and cross-matched whole blood transfusions, iron sulphate supplementation and the use of bactericidal antibiotics (e.g. enrofloxacin 10 mg/kg orally q24h) in dogs with moderate-to-severe neutropenia (neutrophil counts < 1×10^9/l).

Post-treatment monitoring

Post-treatment monitoring is particularly important in *E. canis* infections, which tend to become persistent. Unlike the myelosuppressive *E. canis* infection, which is refractory to treatment, acutely infected dogs experience a rapid clinical improvement within the first 24–48 hours, while resolution of haematological abnormalities takes 1–3 weeks. Failure of the dog to respond in that time period should prompt the clinician to reconsider the diagnosis. On the other hand, clinical and haematological recovery usually precedes the elimination of *E. canis*, thus treatment should not be terminated on the basis of clinicopathological normalization alone. Reappearance of thrombocytopenia 2–4 weeks after the cessation of doxycycline indicates treatment failure or re-infection. Hypergammaglobulinaemia tends to resolve 6–9 months after the initiation of treatment, and persistent hypergammaglobulinaemia indicates treatment failure or concurrent infectious or neoplastic conditions.

The antibody kinetics are unpredictable: frequently serum antibody persists for several months to years following eradication of the organism, which minimizes the value of serology as a post-treatment monitoring tool. In this respect, PCR applied to samples of blood, BM and more importantly splenic aspirates at least 2–4 weeks after completion of treatment is the most reliable method to prove the clearance of *E. canis* infection. Prognosis is good to excellent in granulocytic and acute monocytic ehrlichiosis; pancytopenia, severe leucopenia or neutropenia and severe anaemia herald a grave prognosis.

Prevention

Dogs treated successfully for CE do not acquire permanent immunity and may become re-infected. Therefore, tick control with careful manual removal or by application of appropriate acaricides on a year-round basis is the single most important measure for the prevention of CE. Tick control products such as those containing pyriprol, fipronil, permethrin, or amitraz-impregnated collars, have been shown to be very effective in reducing the incidence of *E. canis* infection and/or tick infestation, but owners should be aware that no product can prevent disease transmission completely in all dogs, under all circumstances. In highly endemic areas, when adequate tick control is hard to achieve, prophylactic daily use of low-dose doxycycline (3 mg/kg orally) during the tick season reduces the risk of infection, but this practice may induce drug resistance. Dogs entering a non-endemic area should be screened serologically and treated accordingly.

Feline ehrlichiosis

Feline ehrlichiosis is increasingly recognized worldwide, although cats seem to be less susceptible to the infections compared with dogs. Sero-epidemiological studies conducted in a number of countries indicate that cats are commonly exposed to *Ehrlichia* agents, although species have not been documented definitively. Experimentally, cats have been successfully infected with *A. phagocytophilum* and *Neorickettsia risticii.* Recent molecular studies in naturally exposed cats indicate that they can become infected by *A. phagocytophilum* (Chapter 19) and an *Ehrlichia canis*-like agent. In the latter cats, as well as in several others with morulae-like inclusions in the mononuclear cells, prominent clinical and clinicopathological manifestations included fever, anorexia, lethargy, joint pain, dyspnoea, mucosal pallor, splenomegaly, lymphadenomegaly, petechiation, thrombocytopenia, leucopenia or leucocytosis, non-regenerative anaemia, pancytopenia and hyperglobulinaemia (Lappin and Breitschwerdt, 2006). The diagnosis is based on clinicopathological compatibility and *Ehrlichia*-specific serological or PCR testing; however, some cats may have low or negative serum antibody titres in the presence of positive PCR. Doxycycline (5 mg/kg orally q12h, for at least 28 days) is the drug of choice for feline ehrlichiosis.

References and further reading

Breitschwerdt EB, Hegarty BC and Hancock SI (1998) Sequential evaluation of dogs naturally infected with *Ehrlichia canis, Ehrlichia chaffeensis, Ehrlichia equi, Ehrlichia ewingii,* or *Bartonella vinsonii. Journal of Clinical Microbiology* **36**, 2645–2651

Cohn LA (2003) Ehrlichiosis and related infections. *Veterinary Clinics of North America: Small Animal Practice* **33**, 863–884

Eddlestone SM, Neer TM, Gaunt SD *et al.* (2006) Failure of imidocarbe dipropionate to clear experimentally induced *Ehrlichia canis* infection in dogs. *Journal of Veterinary Internal Medicine* **20**, 840–844

Greig B, Breitschwerdt EB and Armstrong PJ (2006) Canine granulocytotropic ehrlichiosis (*E. ewingii* infection). In: *Infectious Diseases of the Dog and Cat, 3rd edn*, ed. CE Greene, pp. 217–219. Saunders Elsevier, St Louis

Harrus S, Kass PH, Klement E *et al.* (1997) Canine monocytic ehrlichiosis: a retrospective study of 100 cases, and an epidemiological investigation of prognostic indicators for the disease. *Veterinary Record* **141**, 360–363

Harrus S and Waner T (2010) Diagnosis of canine monocytic ehrlichiosis: An overview. *Veterinary Journal* **187**(3), 292–296

Komnenou A, Mylonakis ME, Kouti V *et al.* (2007) Ocular manifestations of canine monocytic ehrlichiosis (*Ehrlichia canis*): a retrospective study of 90 cases. *Veterinary Ophthalmology* **10**, 137–142

Lappin MR and Breitschwerdt EB (2006) Feline mononuclear ehrlichiosis. In: *Infectious Diseases of the Dog and Cat, 3rd edn*, ed. CE Greene, pp. 224–227. Saunders Elsevier, St Louis

Little SE (2010) Ehrlichiosis and anaplasmosis in dogs and cats. *Veterinary Clinics of North America: Small Animal Practice* **40**, 1121–1140

McClure JC, Crothers ML, Schaefer JJ *et al.* (2010) Efficacy of a doxycycline treatment regimen initiated during three different phases of experimental ehrlichiosis. *Antimicrobial Agents and Chemotherapy* **54**(12), 5012–5020

Mylonakis ME, Ceron JJ, Leontides L *et al.* (2011) Serum acute phase proteins as clinical phase indicators and outcome predictors in naturally-occurring canine monocytic ehrlichiosis. *Journal of Veterinary Internal Medicine* **25**, 811–817

Mylonakis ME, Koutinas AF, Billinis C *et al.* (2003) Evaluation of cytology in the diagnosis of acute canine monocytic ehrlichiosis (*Ehrlichia canis*): a comparison between five methods. *Veterinary Microbiology* **91**, 197–204

Mylonakis ME, Koutinas AF, Breitschwerdt EB *et al.* (2004) Chronic canine ehrlichiosis (*Ehrlichia canis*): a retrospective study of 19 natural cases. *Journal of the American Animal Hospital Association* **40**, 174–184

Neer TM, Breitschwerdt EB, Green RT *et al.* (2002) Consensus statement on ehrlichial diseases of small animals from the infectious disease study group of the ACVIM. *Journal of Veterinary Internal Medicine* **16**, 309–315

Neer TM and Harrus S (2006) Canine monocytotropic ehrlichiosis and neorickettsiosis (*E. canis, E. chaffeensis, E. ruminantium, N. sennetsu,* and *N. risticii* infections). In: *Infectious Diseases of the Dog and Cat, 3rd edn*, ed. CE Greene, pp. 203–216. Saunders Elsevier, St Louis

Schaefer JJ, Kahn J, Needham GR *et al.* (2008) Antibiotic clearance of *Ehrlichia canis* from dogs infected by intravenous inoculation of carrier blood. *Annals of the New York Academy of Science* **1149**, 263–269

Shipov A, Klement E, Reuveni-Tager L *et al.* (2008) Prognostic indicators for canine monocytic ehrlichiosis. *Veterinary Parasitology* **153**, 131–138

19

Anaplasmosis

Barbara Kohn

Introduction

Anaplasmosis is caused by several species of the bacterial genus *Anaplasma* that are implicated as emerging pathogens of dogs, cats, ruminants, horses and humans worldwide.

Anaplasma species infecting dogs and geographical distribution

Anaplasma spp. are closely related to members of the genus *Ehrlichia* and all of these organisms are transmitted by ticks. The *Anaplasma* species known to infect dogs are *A. phagocytophilum* and *A. platys*.

On the basis of analysis of 16S rRNA genes, *A. phagocytophilum* is the new name of the species formerly known as *Ehrlichia phagocytophila*, *E. equi* and the human granulocytic ehrlichiosis agent (Dumler *et al.,* 2001). These former *Ehrlichia* species are now considered to represent *A. phagocytophilum* strains in different geographical locations (Carrade *et al.,* 2009). It is not known whether genetic variation might be responsible for the differing pathogenicity of these strains. *A. phagocytophilum* is the cause of canine granulocytic anaplasmosis in Europe, America, Asia and Africa.

A. platys (formerly *E. platys*), the cause of canine cyclic thrombocytopenia, has been detected in the Mediterranean countries, the Middle East, regions of Asia, Africa, Australia, southern states of the USA and South America.

Granulocytic anaplasmosis

Anaplasma phagocytophilum is the causative agent of canine, feline, equine and human granulocytic anaplasmosis, and of tick-borne fever in ruminants.

Transmission, prevalence, life cycle and pathogenesis

A. phagocytophilum is an obligate, intracellular, coccoid bacterium (0.2–2.0 µm) with an outer cell wall structure that resembles that of Gram-negative bacteria.

Transmission occurs via ticks of the genus *Ixodes*: *I. ricinus* in Europe (Figure 19.1), *I. scapularis* and *I. pacificus* in the USA, and *I. persulcatus* and *Dermacentor silvarum* in Asia and Russia. Within Europe the prevalence of *A. phagocytophilum* in *I. ricinus*, as established by polymerase chain reaction (PCR), has been examined for various countries (range 0.1–14.1%). In the USA, the prevalence of ticks harbouring *A. phagocytophilum* ranges from 1.6% (in California, Florida and Georgia) to 13% (in New York State). In South America and Asia, *A. phagocytophilum* has also been identified in ticks (Kohn, 2010).

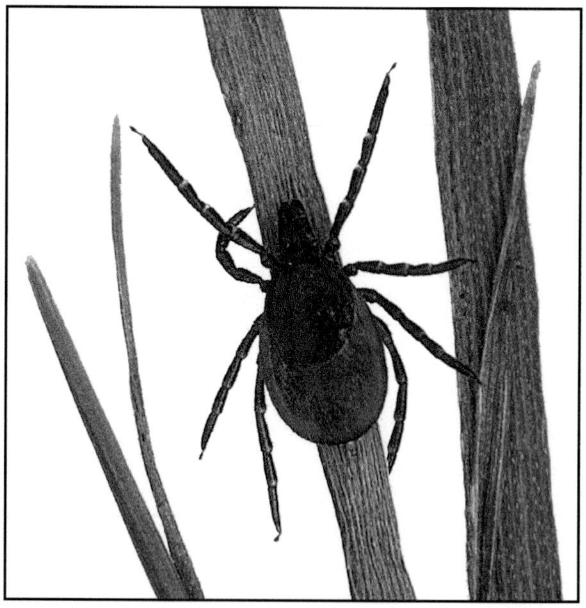

19.1 *Anaplasma phagocytophilum* is transmitted by ticks of the genus *Ixodes* (in Europe mainly *I. ricinus*).

Several mammalian species (e.g. small wild mammals, deer) and possibly birds may act as reservoir hosts. Dogs (and humans) are accidental hosts. Bacteraemia is probably short (< 28 days) and, therefore, dogs are not significant in transmission to other host species (Bakken and Dumler, 2008).

A further pathway for transmission in dogs is via infected blood, either experimentally or via blood transfusion (Egenvall *et al.*, 1998; Kohn, 2010). Single cases of nosocomial infection and perinatal transmission in humans and transplacental infection in cattle have been documented. In a postpartum bitch, a severe manifestation of infection was described with a lack of evidence of perinatal transmission to her puppies (Plier *et al.,* 2009).

Epidemiological studies evaluating the seroprevalence (rarely PCR prevalence) of *A. phagocytophilum* in dogs have been performed worldwide (Figures 19.2 and 19.3).

The seroprevalence in Europe ranges from 9 to 55%; PCR positive cases have to date not been described in the Mediterranean countries. These studies differ with regard to the dog population sampled (i.e. healthy or sick) and the test used (i.e. immunofluorescent antibody test (IFAT) or enzyme-linked immunosorbent assay (ELISA)). In addition, serological cross-reactivity with other *Anaplasma* species (e.g. *A. platys*) can potentially lead to overestimation of the true seroprevalence. In several studies, the seropositivity of dogs was correlated with increasing age, reflecting an increased likelihood of exposure over time (Kirtz *et al.,* 2007).

Two studies from Germany have reported that there was no difference in the percentage seropositivity between populations of healthy dogs and dogs suspected of having anaplasmosis. PCR-positive dogs can have haematological parameters within the reference range (Jensen *et al.,* 2007; Kohn *et al.,* 2011), which suggests that subclinical or mild disease and silent elimination might be common. Therefore, PCR screening of blood products is recommended in highly endemic areas to assure their safety.

A. phagocytophilum is transmitted transstadially within the tick. Transmission of *A. phagocytophilum* from the tick to mammals occurs 24–48 hours after the tick bite. *A. phagocytophilum* spreads within the mammalian host via blood or lymph and there is an incubation period of 1–2 weeks (Bjöersdorff, 2005).

After adhesion via P-selectin, which is abundant on the surface of the bacteria, *A. phagocytophilum* organisms enter the neutrophils (rarely eosinophils) via endocytosis (Greig and Armstrong, 2006) and are incorporated into phagosomes. Within the phagosome, the pathogens multiply by binary fission to form microcolonies (morulae) (Figure 19.4). Rupture of the phagosome and neutrophil membrane results in release of *A. phagocytophilum* with infection of other cells and multiple organs. *A. phagocytophilum* infects bone marrow stem cells, endothelial cells and megakaryocytes (Carrade *et al.,* 2009).

In order to survive and replicate, *A. phagocytophilum* inhibits key neutrophil bactericidal functions (e.g. neutrophil superoxide production, motility, neutrophil–endothelial cell interactions and phagolysosome fusion) and delays neutrophil apoptosis (Carrade *et al.,* 2009). Malfunction of infected phagocytes impairs immune defences and facilitates secondary infection. In addition, secondary immunopathology is suggested by severe pulmonary inflammation, alveolar damage and vasculitis of the extremities in the absence of bacterial organisms (Bjöersdorff, 2005).

Because of shared arthropod vectors and/or concurrent exposure to multiple vector ticks, co-infections may occur with other tick-borne pathogens (e.g. *Borrelia*, *Ehrlichia*, *Bartonella*, *Rickettsia*, *Babesia* spp. and arboviruses), thus complicating the clinical picture (Beall *et al.,* 2008).

Country	Number of tested dogs (*n*)	Prevalence (%)	Method	Reference
Germany	1124	50.1	IFAT	Barutzki *et al.*, 2006
	5881	21.5	SNAP 4Dx Test (ELISA)	Krupka *et al.*, 2008
	522	43.3 5.7	IFAT PCR	Kohn *et al.*, 2010
Italy	460	0	PCR	Solano-Gallego *et al.*, 2006
	5634	32.8	IFAT	Torina and Caracappa, 2006
Austria	1470	56.5	IFAT	Kirtz *et al.*, 2007
Sweden	246	20.7	IFAT	Jäderlund *et al.*, 2007
Spain	649	15.6	IFAT	Amusategui *et al.*, 2008
UK	120	0.8	PCR	Shaw *et al.*, 2005

19.2 Prevalence of infections with *A. phagocytophilum* in dogs from Europe. ELISA, enzyme-linked immunosorbent assay; IFAT, indirect immune fluorescent antibody test; PCR, polymerase chain reaction.

Region	Number of tested dogs (*n*)	Prevalence (%)	Method	Reference
Minnesota	731	55.4 10	ELISA (SNAP 4Dx) PCR	Beall *et al.*, 2008
USA: Northeast Midwest Southeast West	479,640 188,438 175,829 101,148 47,540	4.8 5.5 6.7 0.5 4.5	ELISA	Bowman *et al.*, 2009

19.3 Prevalence of infections with *A. phagocytophilum* in dogs from the USA. ELISA, enzyme-linked immunosorbent assay; IFAT, indirect immune fluorescent antibody test; PCR, polymerase chain reaction.

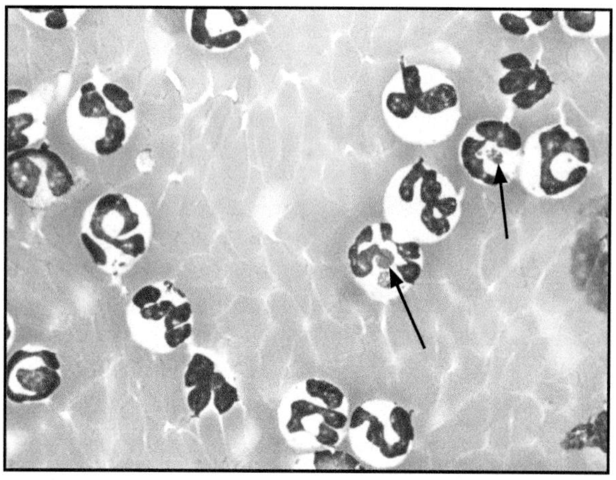

19.4 Morulae of *Anaplasma phagocytophilum* in neutrophils (arrowed) (original magnification x1000, Giemsa).

Clinical presentation

Most dogs naturally infected with *A. phagocytophilum* probably remain healthy, as indicated by the large number of seropositive dogs when compared with dogs with clinical disease. The infection appears to be self-limiting, because dogs with chronic disease have not been described.

Experimental infections with *A. phagocytophilum* have been performed in Sweden and the USA (Egenvall *et al.,* 1998; Alleman *et al.,* 2006). Natural infection was first identified in dogs in California in 1982 (Madewell and Gribble, 1982). Numerous case reports from Austria, Canada, Switzerland, the UK and the USA, and a few case series from Germany, Italy, Slovenia, Sweden and the USA, have been published (Kohn *et al.,* 2008; Carrade *et al.,* 2009).

Most dogs are diagnosed during the acute stage of disease. The duration of illness prior to diagnosis was > 7 days for 25% of the dogs in one study (Granick *et al.,* 2009). An age, sex or breed predisposition has not been described in most studies.

The most common clinical signs are non-specific and include lethargy, inappetance/anorexia and fever (Figure 19.5). Lameness may result from secondary immune-mediated (neutrophilic) polyarthritis. Rare signs are coughing, scleral injection, uveitis, limb oedema and polydipsia. Dogs may also exhibit central nervous system (CNS) signs, but in recent studies from Sweden and the USA there was no apparent association between neurological signs and infection (Jäderlund *et al.,* 2007; Barber *et al.,* 2010). Splenomegaly, diagnosed by radiography and ultrasonography, was present in all the dogs of one study (Kohn *et al.,* 2008; Figure 19.6).

The most consistent laboratory abnormality is thrombocytopenia, which can be severe (< 30 × 10^9/l; Figure 19.7). Thrombocytopenia may be attributed to increased platelet consumption resulting from disseminated intravascular coagulation (DIC), sequestration in an enlarged spleen, immune-mediated platelet destruction or the production of inhibitory factors.

Anaemia is described in approximately half of the patients. The anaemia is often mild, normocytic and normochromic, resembling the anaemia of chronic inflammation. Another pathomechanism might be (immune-mediated) haemolysis or blood loss (Kohn *et al.,* 2008). Abnormal findings in the leucocyte series include lymphopenia, neutrophilia, leucocytosis, leucopenia, monocytosis, lymphocytosis and neutropenia.

Reported abnormal serum biochemistry findings are listed in Figure 19.8. During an acute phase reaction, hepatic production of albumin is decreased and that of α- and β-globulins is increased, which may explain the presence of hypoalbuminaemia and hyperglobulinaemia. Increased liver enzymes and serum bilirubin may be due to reactive hepatitis or haemolysis, respectively.

Clinical signs	Dogs (*n* = 18) % [a]	Dogs (*n* = 34) % [b]
Lethargy	94	74
Anorexia	83	62
Fever	61	84
Pale mucous membranes	28	–
Tense abdomen	28	9
Diarrhoea	17	9
Vomiting	11	24
Lameness (polyarthritis)	11	32
Petechiae/melaena	11	–
Epistaxis	6	–
Tachypnoea	6	29
Collapse	11	–
Enlarged lymph nodes	–	32

19.5 Clinical findings in dogs with granulocytic anaplasmosis. [a]Kohn *et al.*, 2008; [b]Granick *et al.*, 2009.

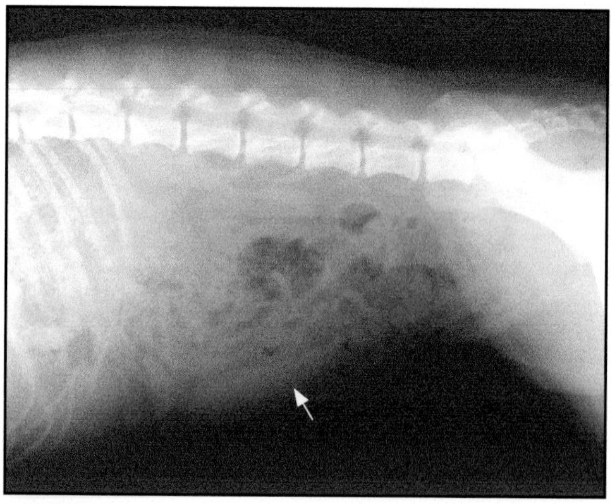

19.6 Lateral abdominal radiograph showing splenomegaly in a 2-year-old female Golden Retriever with granulocytic anaplasmosis. The position of the spleen is arrowed.

Parameter	Abnormal (n = 18) %[a]		Abnormal (n = 34) %[b]	
	↓	↑	↓	↑
Platelets	89	0	95	-
Haematocrit	61	6	47	-
Leucocytes	28	22	9	19
Band neutrophils	–	17	–	6
Segmented neutrophils	6	44	3	19
Eosinophils	72	6	–	–
Lymphocytes	50	11	65	–
Monocytes	0	39	–	–

19.7 Haematological abnormalities in dogs with granulocytic anaplasmosis. [a]Kohn *et al.*, 2008; [b]Granick *et al.*, 2009.

Parameter	Abnormal (*n* = 18) %[a]		Abnormal (*n* = 27) %[b]	
	↓	↑	↓	↑
Total protein	0	33	–	–
Albumin	67	0	44	–
Alanine aminotransferase	–	61	–	30
Aspartate aminotransferase	–	28	–	
Alkaline phosphatase	–	61	–	52
Bilirubin	–	22	–	37

19.8 Biochemical abnormalities in dogs with granulocytic anaplasmosis. [a]Kohn *et al.*, 2008; [b]Granick *et al.*, 2009.

Diagnosis

The diagnostic criteria for human granulocytic anaplasmosis are suggestive clinical signs and laboratory findings, together with:

- Detection of morulae within neutrophils (rarely eosinophils) on blood smears combined with a single positive antibody titre for *A. phagocytophilum* (or a positive PCR)
- A four-fold increase or decrease in the antibody titre within 4 weeks
- A positive PCR test using specific *A. phagocytophilum* primers
- Isolation of *A. phagocytophilum* from blood.

These criteria can also be applied to dogs and other species; however, isolation is not used routinely for diagnosis (Bjöersdorff, 2005; Bakken and Dumler, 2008).

In experimentally infected dogs, morulae appear as early as 4 days after inoculation and persist for 4-8 days. However, the morulae cannot be distinguished from those of *Ehrlichia* spp. (e.g. *Ehrlichia ewingii*), so it should be confirmed by PCR (or serology) that the organism is indeed *A. phagocytophilum*. Conventional or real-time PCR is a more sensitive diagnostic tool than identification of circulating morulae. Assays have been developed for the detection of *A. phagocytophilum* DNA in peripheral blood, buffy coat, bone marrow, and in cerebrospinal fluid, synovial fluid or splenic tissue. Assays based on the outer surface protein genes such as *msp2* are usually specific for *A. phagocytophilum*, whereas assays based on the 16S rRNA gene may detect other *Anaplasma* spp. or even other bacteria. In experimentally infected dogs, PCR tests on whole blood were positive for 6–8 days before and 3 days after morulae appeared on blood smears (Egenvall *et al.*, 2000).

Antibody testing can be performed by IFAT (Figure 19.9) or ELISA. Immunoglobulin (Ig) G antibodies are first detectable 8 days after initial exposure and 2–5 days after the appearance of morulae. Serological cross-reactivity between *A. phagocytophilum* and other related species (e.g. *A. platys*, *E. canis*, *E. ewingii* and *E. chaffeensis*) has been reported. Cross-reactivity with other non-ehrlichial species (e.g. *Coxiella burnettii*) might also occur (Greig and Armstrong, 2006; Santos *et al.*, 2009). During acute illness, antibodies may be inapparent. Given that the seroprevalence is high in endemic areas and that antibody titres may persist for several months or even years, a single positive titre is not diagnostic and may only reflect previous exposure. A fourfold or higher increase in antibody titres detected in paired serum samples taken at least 2–3 weeks apart is essential to confirm the diagnosis.

Therapy and outcome

The treatment of choice for granulocytic anaplasmosis in dogs is doxycycline (5 mg/kg orally q12h for 2 weeks), and most dogs show clinical improvement within 24–48 hours. *In vivo* effects against *A. phagocytophilum* have also been documented for rifampicin and chloramphenicol. In approximately half of dogs seropositive for *E. equi* with long-standing clinical signs, imidocarb diproprionate had a favourable effect (Bjöersdorff, 2005).

In dogs in which immune-mediated disease (e.g. reactive polyarthritis, secondary immune-mediated thrombocytopenia) is suspected, prednisolone can be administered in addition to doxycycline. However, the use of immunosuppressive glucocorticoids for treatment of secondary immune-mediated diseases must be considered very carefully when infection with a pathogen is likely.

It is not known whether natural infection provides long-term protection against the development of clinical anaplasmosis. Re-infection following the therapeutic elimination of the organism has not been reported in dogs; however, in human medicine one case has been documented.

The extent to which the pathogen induces chronic infection is also unknown. In one clinical study, all naturally infected dogs that were re-tested after 2–8 weeks had negative PCR test results using EDTA-anticoagulated blood and no morulae were

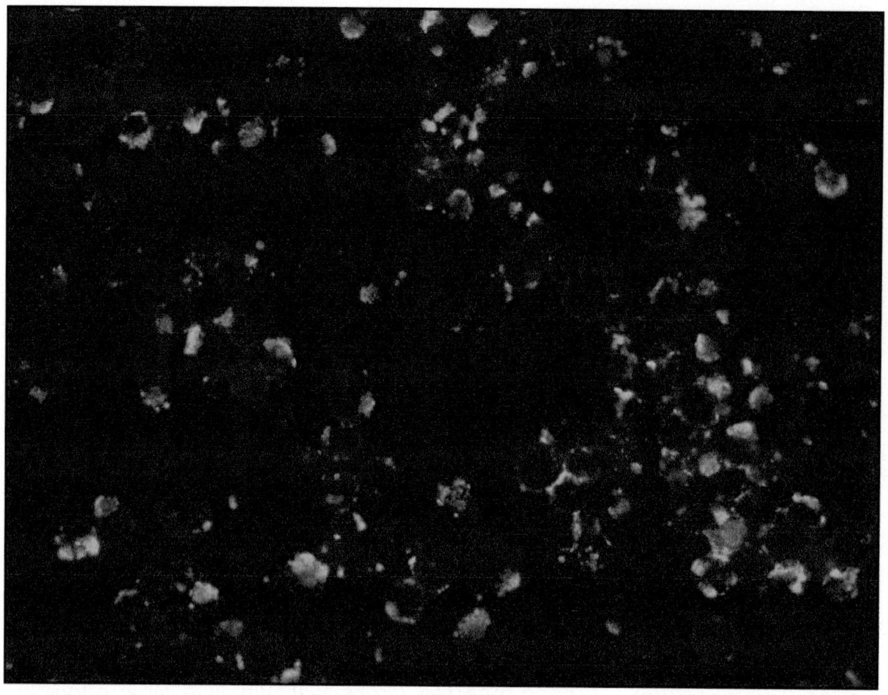

19.9 Positive *A. phagocytophilum* IFA test. In this test, serum from the patient is overlaid onto a monolayer of cells infected by the target organism. Binding of specific antibody is visualized by the use of a secondary antiserum conjugated to fluorescein and observation of the slide under light of an appropriate wavelength. (Kindly provided by Prof. K. Pfister).

detected in neutrophils (Kohn *et al.,* 2008). In an experimental study, glucocorticoid treatment of dogs that had been infected with *A. phagocytophilum* led to positive PCR results and re-appearance of morulae up to 6 months after infection (Egenvall *et al.,* 2000). In another study, persistent infections were established in two dogs using a human isolate of cultivated *A. phagocytophilum.* Both animals were positive on all PCR assays and doxycycline therapy did not eliminate the organism (Alleman *et al.,* 2006).

Prevention

No vaccine is available to prevent *A. phagocytophilum* infection. Prevention in endemic areas can be accomplished by maintaining strict tick control programmes. A thorough daily inspection for and removal of ticks is recommended, in combination with regular application of residual acaricidal products. Appropriate prophylactic administration of permethrin during the tick season protected 96% of dogs living in areas with high *Ixodes ricinus* populations from *A. phagocytophilum* infection.

Infectious canine cyclic thrombocytopenia

Anaplasma platys (formerly *Ehrlichia platys*) is an obligate, intracellular rickettsial organism that causes infectious cyclic thrombocytopenia in dogs.

Life cycle, transmission and pathogenesis

A. platys was first reported in the USA in 1978 and subsequently in Western Europe, Asia, South America, the Middle East, Australia and Africa (Harvey, 2006). Dogs are the primary reservoir host for *A. platys*, but the extent of the host spectrum has not been fully determined.

The organisms appear as round, oval or bean-shaped blue inclusions (0.35–1.25 µm in diameter) in platelets. *A. platys* multiplies by binary fission within membrane-bound vacuoles within the platelet, resulting in the formation of the typical morulae (Figure 19.10).

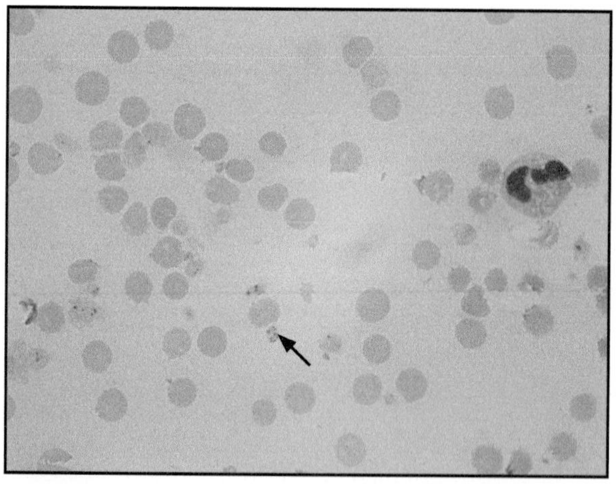

19.10 *Anaplasma platys* morulae in platelets from a dog (arrowed). (Kindly provided by Prof. K. Pfister).

The brown dog tick (*Rhipicephalus sanguineus*) is thought to transmit the pathogen, and *A. platys* has been detected in *Dermacentor* ticks collected from dogs in Thailand. Co-infection with other tick-transmitted pathogens has been reported and such co-infection may change the clinical course.

There is limited information available on the epidemiological aspects of *A. platys* infection. On the basis of serological studies, *A. platys* infection appears to be common in the southern states of the USA. One third of thrombocytopenic dogs had positive titres and over 50% of dogs that were seropositive for *E. canis* also had positive titres for *A. platys*. In subtropical areas of Japan 28% of free-roaming dogs were PCR-positive (Shaw, 2005; Harvey, 2006).

After an experimental inoculation of dogs with *A. platys*, parasitized platelets were detected in the peripheral blood after 8 to 15 days. The highest percentage of parasitized platelets occurred during the initial episode of parasitaemia. Within 3–5 days post inoculation, *A. platys* DNA could be amplified by PCR; by day 160 post inoculation all dogs were PCR negative, suggesting immunological clearance of *A. platys*. Experimentally infected dogs developed severe thrombocytopenia within 7 days of inoculation (Gaunt *et al.,* 2010). After a decrease in the circulating organisms, the platelet count increased within 3–4 days. These episodes of parasitaemia and severe thrombocytopenia occur at 1–2 week intervals. Thrombocytopenia might be due to direct platelet injury and/or immune-mediated destruction of platelets. Chronic infection is associated with low-level parasitaemia and mild, slowly resolving thrombocytopenia, which may reflect an adaptation of the host to *A. platys* infection (Harvey, 2006).

The differences in the severity of the illness that have been described may be due to differences in geographical origin of the *A. platys* strain and the presence of co-infections.

Clinical presentation

Experimentally infected dogs showed either no or only mild clinical signs, such as a slight increase in rectal temperature (Harvey, 2006; Gaunt *et al.,* 2010). Splenectomy before experimental infection does not alter the severity of disease.

More pathogenic strains of *A. platys* might occur outside the USA. Clinical signs in both experimental and natural studies of infected dogs in Greece, Portugal and Israel included fever, lethargy, anorexia, weight loss, pale mucous membranes, petechiae, nasal discharge and lymphadenomegaly (Kontos *et al.,* 1991; Harrus *et al.,* 1997; Santos *et al.,* 2009) . However, co-infections with other vector-transmitted diseases were not excluded by PCR in all dogs. Further findings described in single cases were bilateral uveitis and epistaxis. Thrombocytopenia is the major haematological finding. Cyclic thrombocytopenic episodes (with platelet counts $< 20 \times 10^9$/l) of 3–4 days' duration recur at 1- to 2-week intervals. A moderate non-regenerative anaemia may be present, probably as a result of inflammation. In rare cases with severe bleeding, the anaemia is regenerative. Moderate hyperglobulinaemia and occasional hypoalbuminaemia and hypocalcaemia have been reported. The occurrence of *A. platys* together with other infectious agents (e.g. *Ehrlichia canis*, *Babesia canis*) may potentiate the clinical disease and the laboratory abnormalities.

Diagnosis

Diagnosis of *A. platys* may be made by detecting organisms within platelets on stained blood smears. The sensitivity of this technique is greatly limited by the low levels of parasitaemia during severe thrombocytopenic episodes and in chronic infections (Shaw, 2005).

Species-specific PCR testing is the method of choice if appropriate primers are selected. Blood samples, but also bone marrow or spleen, can be used for testing. An IFAT for the detection of serum antibodies is available commercially, but cross-reactions may occur (e.g. with *A. phagocytophilum*; Santos *et al.,* 2009). After experimental infection with *A. platys*, antibodies were first detected by day 16. Antibody titres may persist for more than a year (Gaunt *et al.,* 2010).

Therapy and prevention

A. platys infection can be treated with tetracyclines (e.g. doxycycline 5–10 mg/kg q12h for 10 days or enrofloxacin 5 mg/kg q12h for 14–21 days; Harvey, 2006). Prevention is dependent on vector control using effective acaricides.

Feline granulocytic anaplasmosis

A. phagocytophilum may also infect cats, but less is known about tick-borne disease in cats than in dogs. The infrequent diagnosis of anaplasmosis might be due to a decreased pathogenicity of tick-borne pathogens in cats as compared with other species, or due to the more rapid removal of ticks by fastidious grooming, which results in decreased opportunity for disease transmission. In addition it is possible that there is general under-recognition of tick-borne diseases in cats.

Epidemiology

Susceptibility of cats to *A. phagocytophilum* infection was first documented in an experimental inoculation study with *E. equi*. Clinical abnormalities were not reported but two of five cats developed morulae in eosinophils. A cat naturally infected with *A. phagocytophilum* was first reported in Sweden (Bjöersdorff *et al.,* 1999). Since then positive PCR test results have been reported in several cats from the UK, Ireland, Denmark, North America, Italy, Spain, Austria, Switzerland and Germany.

Morulae-like structures in feline neutrophils have also been reported from cats in Brazil, Kenya and Italy; however, *A. phagocytophilum* infection was not confirmed by further testing (e.g. PCR tests).

Seroprevalence data for *A. phagocytophilum* infections in cats are available from several countries: the seroprevalence of *A. phagocytophilum* in Spain ranged from 1.8 to 7.7% (Ayllon *et al.,* 2009); it was 13% in Portugal (Alves *et al.,* 2009) and 9% in Germany (Morgenthal *et al.,* unpublished). Cross-reactions with other *Anaplasma* or *Ehrlichia* species must be considered in the interpretation of such data.

Clinical presentation

The clinical and laboratory findings in nine cats naturally infected with anaplasmosis were lethargy (in nine), anorexia (nine), fever (nine), lymphadenopathy (five), tachypnoea (two), a stiff gait (one), conjunctivitis (one), serous nasal discharge (one), cough (one), anaemia (six), thrombocytopenia (four), neutrophilia (two), eosinophilia (one), lymphopenia (one) and lymphocytosis (one). All the cats had outdoor access, and tick infestation had been noted in most of the cats (Bjöersdorff *et al.*, 1999; Lappin *et al.*, 2004; Kirtz *et al.*, 2005; Schaarschmidt-Kiener *et al.*, 2009).

Diagnosis

The diagnosis can be based on identification of morulae in granulocytes (e.g. three of the nine cats described above had detectable morulae). DNA was detected in eight of the nine cats described above, so PCR testing is the method of choice if the cat has not been pre-treated with anti-infective agents. If the PCR test is negative or not available both acute and convalescent serum samples should be examined for *A. phagocytophilum* antibody titres. The titre can be negative in an acutely infected cat; a fourfold increase of the titre is diagnostic. In naturally infected cats antibody persists for several months after treatment.

Therapy and prevention

Cats with anaplasmosis have been treated with doxycycline (5–10 mg/kg q24h for 20–30 days). Supportive care consisted of infusions with crystalloid solutions, non-steroidal anti-inflammatory drugs or antipyretic agents. Other treatment options are tetracyclines (22 mg/kg q8h for 21 days) or chloramphenicol (25 mg/kg q12h for 14 days; Lappin *et al.*, 2006). Clinical signs and laboratory abnormalities resolve quickly after tetracycline or doxycycline therapy in naturally infected cats and recurrence is not reported. Whether or not tetracycline treatment eliminates the organism is not known.

Given that *A. phagocytophilum* is transmitted by *Ixodes* spp., exposure of cats to arthropod vectors should be avoided or tick control should be maintained with acaricides. This is especially important for cats used as blood donors because *A. phagocytophilum* is likely to be transmitted by blood products (Lappin *et al.*, 2006).

References and further reading

Alleman AR, Chandrashaker R, Beall M *et al.* (2006) Experimental inoculation of dogs with a human isolate (Ny18) of *Anaplasma phagocytophilum* and demonstration of persistent infection following doxycycline therapy. *Proceedings 24th ACVIM Forum*, Louisville, Kentucky

Alves AS, Milhano N, Santos-Silva M, *et al.* (2009) Evidence of *Bartonella* spp., *Rickettsia* spp. and *Anaplasma phagocytophilum* in domestic, shelter and stray cat blood and fleas, Portugal. *Clinical Microbiology and Infection* **15**(Suppl. 2), 1–3

Amusategui I, Tesouro MA, Kakoma I *et al.* (2008) Serological reactivity to *Ehrlichia canis, Anaplasma phagocytophilum, Neorickettsia risticii, Borrelia burgdorferi* and *Rickettsia conorii* in dogs from Northwestern Spain. *Vector Borne Zoonotic Diseases* **8**, 797–803

Ayllon T, Villaescusa A, Tesouro MA *et al.* (2009) Serology, PCR and culture of *Ehrlichia/Anaplasma* species in asymptomatic and symptomatic cats from central Spain. *Clinical Microbiology and Infection* **15**(Suppl. 2), 4–5

Bakken JS and Dumler S (2008) Human granulocytic anaplasmosis. *Infectious Disease Clinics of North America* **22**, 443–448

Barber RM, Li Q, Diniz PP *et al.* (2010) Evaluation of brain tissue or cerebrospinal fluid with broadly reactive polymerase chain reaction for *Ehrlichia, Anaplasma*, Spotted Fever Group Rickettsia, *Bartonella*, and *Borrelia* species in canine neurological diseases (109 cases). *Journal of Veterinary Internal Medicine* **24**, 372–378

Barutzki D, De Nicola A, Zeziola M *et al.* (2006) Seroprevalence of *Anaplasma phagocytophilum* infection in dogs in Germany. *Berliner und Münchner Tierärztliche Wochenschrift* **119**, 342–347

Beall MJ, Chandrashekar R, Eberts MD *et al.* (2008) Serological and molecular prevalence of *Borrelia burgdorferi, Anaplasma phagocytophilum*, and *Ehrlichia* species in dogs from Minnesota. *Vector Borne Zoonotic Diseases* **8**, 455–464

Bjöersdorff A (2005) Granulocytic ehrlichiosis: *Anaplasma phagocytophilum* comb. nov (*E. phagocytophila* genogroup) infection. In: *Arthropod-borne Diseases of the Dog and Cat*, ed. SE Shaw and MJ Day, pp.127–132. Manson Publishing Ltd., London

Bjöersdorff A, Svendenius L, Owens JH *et al.* (1999) Feline granulocytic ehrlichiosis – a report of a new clinical entity and characterisation of the infectious agent. *Journal of Small Animal Practice* **40**, 20–24

Bowman D, Little SE, Lorentzen L *et al.* (2009) Prevalence and geographic distribution of *Dirofilaria immitis, Borrelia burgdorferi, Ehrlichia canis*, and *Anaplasma phagocytophilum* in dogs in the United States: Results of a national clinic-based serologic survey. *Veterinary Parasitology* **160**, 138–148

Carrade D, Foley JF, Borjesson DL *et al.* (2009) Canine granulocytic anaplasmosis: a review. *Journal of Veterinary Internal Medicine* **23**, 1129–1141

Dumler JS, Barbet AF, Bekker CP *et al.* (2001) Reorganization of genera in the families *Rickettsiaceae* and *Anaplasmataceae* in the order *Rickettsiales*: unification of some species of *Ehrlichia* with *Anaplasma, Cowdria* with *Ehrlichia* and *Ehrlichia* with *Neorickettsia*, descriptions of six new species combinations and designation of *Ehrlichia equi* and 'HGE agent' as subjective synonyms of *Ehrlichia phagocytophila. International Journal of Systematic and Evolutionary Microbiology* **51**, 2145–2165

Egenvall A, Bjöersdorff A, Lilliehöök I *et al.* (1998) Early manifestations of granulocytic ehrlichiosis in dogs inoculated experimentally with a Swedish *Ehrlichia* species isolate. *Veterinary Record* **143**, 412–417

Egenvall A, Lilliehöök I, Bjöersdorff A *et al.* (2000) Detection of granulocytic *Ehrlichia* species DNA by PCR in persistently infected dogs. *Veterinary Record* **146**, 186–190

Gaunt SD, Beall MJ, Stillman BA *et al.* (2010) Experimental infection and co-infection of dogs with *Anaplasma platys* and *Ehrlichia canis*: hematologic, serologic and molecular findings. *Parasites & Vectors* **3**, 33

Granick JL, Armstrong PJ and Bender JB (2009) *Anaplasma phagocytophilum* infection in dogs: 34 cases (2000–2007). *Journal of the American Veterinary Association* **234**(12), 1559–1565

Granick JL, Reneer DV, Carlyon JA *et al.* (2008) *Anaplasma phagocytophilum* infect cells of the megakaryocytic lineage through sialylated ligands but fails to alter platelet production. *Journal of Medical Microbiology* **57**, 416–423

Greig B and Armstrong PJ (2006) Canine granulocytotropic anaplasmosis (*A. phagocytophilum* infection). In: *Infectious Diseases of the Dog and Cat*, ed. CE Greene, pp.219–224. Elsevier Saunders, St. Louis

Harrus S, Aroch I, Lavy E *et al.* (1997) Clinical manifestations of infectious canine cyclic thrombocytopenia. *Veterinary Record* **141**, 247–250

Harvey JW (2006) Thrombocytopenic anaplasmosis (*A. platys* (*E. platys*) infection). In: *Infectious Diseases of the Dog and Cat*, ed. CE Greene, pp.229–231. Saunders Elsevier, St Louis.

Jäderlund KH, Egenvall A, Bergström K *et al.* (2007) Seroprevalence of *Borrelia burgdorferi sensu lato* and *Anaplasma phagocytophilum* in dogs with neurological signs. *Veterinary Record* **160**, 825–831

Jensen J, Simon D, Escobar HM *et al.* (2007) *Anaplasma phagocytophilum* in dogs in Germany. *Zoonoses and Public Health* **54**, 94–101

Kirtz B, Czettel B, Thum D *et al.* (2007) *Anaplasma phagozytophilum* in einer österreichischen Hundepopulation: eine Prävalenz-Studie (2001-2006). *Kleintierpraxis* **52**, 562–568

Kirtz G, Meli ML, Lutz H, *et al.* (2005) *Anaplasma phagocytophilum* Infektion bei 2 Katzen in Österreich. *Kleintierpraxis* **50** (8), 498–504

Kohn B (2010) *Anaplasma phagocytophilum* in the dog – update on epidemiology and clinical disease. *5th Canine Vector-borne Disease World Forum*, New York, 12–15 April, Proceedings pp.36–43

Kohn B, Galke D, Beelitz P *et al.* (2008) Clinical features of canine granulocytic anaplasmosis in 18 naturally infected dogs. *Journal of Veterinary Internal Medicine* **22**, 1289–1295

Kohn B, Silaghi C, Galke D *et al.* (2011) Infections with *Anaplasma phagocytophilum* in dogs in Germany. *Research in Veterinary Science* **91**, 71–76

Kontos VI, Papadopoulos O and French TW (1991) Natural and experimental canine infections with a Greek strain of *Ehrlichia platys*. *Veterinary Clinical Pathology* **20**, 101–105

Krupka I, Pantchev N, Lorentzen L *et al.* (2008) Prävalenz von Antikörpern gegen *Borrelia burgdorferi sensu lato*, *Anaplasma phagozytophilum* und *Ehrlichia canis* bei Hunden in Deutschland. 16. Jahrestagung der FG *Innere Medizin und klinische Labordiagnostik* der DVG, Gießen

Lappin MR, Bjöersdorff A and Breitschwerdt EB (2006) Feline granulocytic anaplasmosis. In: *Infectious Diseases of the Dog and Cat*, ed. CE Greene, pp.227–229. Saunders Elsevier, St Louis

Lappin MR, Breitschwerdt EB and Jensen WA (2004) Molecular and serological evidence of *Anaplasma phagocytophilum* infection of cats in North America. *Journal of the American Veterinary Medical Association* **225**, 893–896

Madewell B and Gribble D (1982) Infection in two dogs with an agent resembling *Ehrlichia equi*. *Journal of the American Veterinary Medical Association* **180**, 512–514

Plier ML, Breitschwerdt EB, Hegarty BC *et al.* (2009) Lack of evidence for perinatal transmission of canine granulocytic anaplasmosis from a bitch to her offspring. *Journal of the American Animal Hospital Association* **45**, 232–238

Santos AS, Alexandre N, Sousa R *et al.* (2009) Serological and molecular survey of *Anaplasma* species infection in dogs with suspected tickborne disease in Portugal. *Veterinary Record* **164**, 168–171

Schaarschmidt-Kiener D, Graf F, von Loewenich FD *et al.* (2009) *Anaplasma phagocytophilum* Infektion bei einer Katze in der Schweiz. *Schweizer Archiv für Tierheilkunde* **151**, 336–341

Shaw S (2005) Infectious canine cyclic thrombocytopenia: *Anaplasma platys* comb. nov infection. In: *Arthropod-borne Diseases of the Dog and Cat*, ed. SE Shaw and MJ Day, pp.132–133. Manson Publishing Ltd., London

Shaw SE, Binns SH, Birtles MJ *et al.* (2005) Molecular evidence of tick-transmitted infections in dogs and cats in the United Kingdom. *Veterinary Record* **157**, 645–648

Solano-Gallego L, Trotta M and Razia L (2006) Molecular survey of *Ehrlichia canis* and *Anaplasma phagocytophilum* from blood of dogs in Italy. *Annals of the* New York *Academy of Sciences* **1078**, 515–518

Torina A and Caracappa S (2006) Dog tick borne diseases in Sicily. *Parassitologia* **48,** 145–147

20

Canine leishmaniosis

Laia Solano-Gallego and Gad Baneth

Introduction

Canine leishmaniosis is one of the major zoonoses that cause severe fatal disease in humans and dogs globally. Infections caused by different *Leishmania* species are present in a variety of regions with different climatic conditions in the Old and New Worlds. On the basis of the clinical symptoms, the human disease has been divided into cutaneous, mucocutaneous and visceral forms. An estimated 12 million people suffer from leishmaniosis worldwide, with an estimated 1.5–2 million new cases occurring annually: 1–1.5 million cases of cutaneous leishmaniosis and 500,000 cases of visceral leishmaniosis (Desjeux, 2004). Epidemiologically, two different situations occur. The **zoonotic** form of visceral leishmaniosis is found in the Mediterranean basin and South America, with the dog as the main source of *L. infantum* infection for the female sandfly. The **anthroponotic** form is found in East Africa, Bangladesh, India and Nepal where *L. donovani* is passed from person to person through the sandfly vector without the need for a reservoir host (Desjeux, 2004). Anthroponotic visceral leishmaniosis caused by *L. donovani* is responsible for a large number of the fatalities associated with the visceral disease in humans (Alvar *et al.*, 2006).

Leishmania species that infect dogs and their geographical distribution

Domestic dogs are considered to be the main reservoirs for leishmaniosis in humans in the Mediterranean basin, Middle East and South America, where *L. infantum* (synonym *L. chagasi*) is the causative agent of infection (Baneth *et al.*, 2008). The seroprevalence in the Mediterranean basin ranges from 10 to 40%, depending on the region. Surveys employing other detection methods to calculate the prevalence of *Leishmania* infection by amplification of *Leishmania* DNA from different tissues (Solano-Gallego *et al.*, 2001) or by detection of specific anti-*Leishmania* cellular immunity (Cabral *et al.*, 1998) have revealed even higher infection rates, approaching 70% in some foci. Most dogs in these areas appear to have chronic infection that may be lifelong (Oliva *et al.*, 2006), but only a low proportion of dogs develop disease, with most being resistant to the development of clinical disease and maintaining a subclinical infection (Baneth *et al.*, 2008; Solano-Gallego *et al.*, 2009). It has been estimated, on the basis of seroprevalence studies from Italy, Spain, France and Portugal, that 2.5 million dogs in these countries are infected (Moreno and Alvar, 2002). The number of infected dogs in South America is also estimated in millions, with high infection rates in some areas of Brazil and Venezuela (Werneck *et al.*, 2007). Dogs can be infected by several other *Leishmania* species besides *L. infantum*. These species are responsible for cutaneous, mucocutaneous and visceral leishmanioses in humans, and include *L. braziliensis* in South America, *L. tropica* in North Africa and Asia, and *L. peruviana* and *L. panamanensis* in Latin America (Lemrani *et al.*, 2002; Dantas-Torres, 2007; Solano-Gallego *et al.*, 2009). For these species, dogs do not appear to be a significant reservoir of infection for humans (Dantas-Torres, 2007).

Canine leishmaniosis is also an important concern in non-endemic countries where imported disease constitutes a veterinary and public health problem (Petersen and Barr, 2009; Shaw *et al.*, 2009). In non-endemic countries, the disease can be diagnosed in dogs that have lived in or have travelled to endemic areas (Shaw *et al.*, 2009; Menn *et al.*, 2010). The increased numbers of dogs travelling to Southern Europe and imported as companion animals from endemic areas have raised serious concerns about the introduction of vector-borne diseases, such as leishmaniosis, into the non-endemic areas of Europe (Shaw *et al.*, 2009; Menn *et al.*, 2010). A study from the Netherlands found that about 58,000 dogs travel yearly from Holland to Southern Europe with their owners for vacations, and the risk of acquiring canine leishmaniosis is 0.027–0.23% (Teske *et al.*, 2002). Infected dogs in non-endemic areas may also contribute to the maintenance of the parasite within the canine population through non-vector transmission modes of infection (Solano-Gallego *et al.*, 2009). In addition, *L. infantum* infection is spreading northwards in Europe, having reached the foothills of the Alps in Northern Italy (Maroli *et al.*, 2008), the French Pyrenees (Dereure *et al.*, 2009), northern France (Chamaille *et al.*, 2010) and north-western Spain (Amusategui *et al.*, 2004). Transmission could occur in a new area if infected dogs are imported into the region and if the population of sandfly vectors is large enough. Changes in the dynamics of sandfly populations may lead to the creation of new permanent foci (Solano-Gallego *et al.*, 2009).

Life cycle and transmission of *L. infantum* in dogs

The natural life cycle of *Leishmania* infection involves a sandfly vector and a vertebrate host, in which two different forms of the parasite are found. Haemophagous female sandflies harbour the extracellular *Leishmania* promastigote (Figure 20.1) in their gut and transmit the parasite during a blood meal to a mammalian host, where the intracellular amastigote form develops (Figure 20.2). Dogs are infected by *Leishmania* promastigotes deposited in the skin when they are bitten by infected female sandfly vectors. The promastigotes invade host cells and replicate as intracellular amastigotes. Female sandflies from the genera *Phlebotomus* (Old World) or *Lutzomyia* (New World) are the principal agents of transmission of *Leishmania* in humans and dogs (Killick-Kendrick, 1999). The activity of the adult sandflies is crepuscular and nocturnal from early spring to late autumn in the Mediterranean basin and all year round in South America (Killick-Kendrick, 1999).

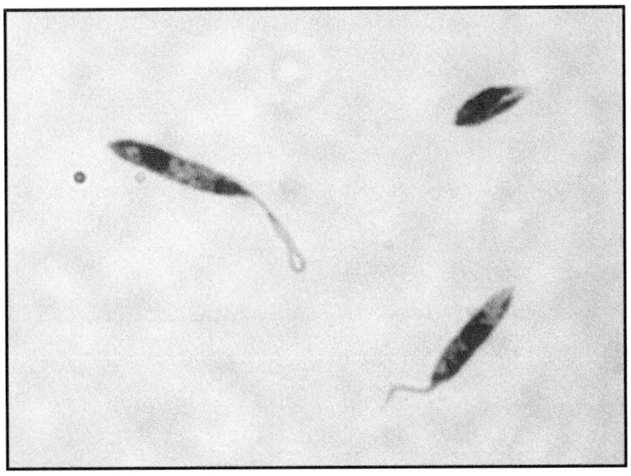

20.1 The promastigote form of *Leishmania infantum*.

Other less common routes of transmission have been reported in dogs. These could be more important in non-endemic areas where sandfly transmission does not appear to be established, such as the USA (Duprey *et al.*, 2006; Petersen, 2009), UK (Shaw *et al.*, 2009) and Germany (Menn *et al.*, 2010). Vertical transmission from a dam to its offspring has been documented in a few clinical reports (da Silva *et al.*, 2009) and during experimental (Rosypal *et al.*, 2005) and natural (Pangrazio *et al.*, 2009) infection. However, this mode of transmission has been disputed by other authors conducting studies of experimental infection (Andrade *et al.*, 2002). Venereal transmission of *L. infantum* from infected males to healthy bitches has

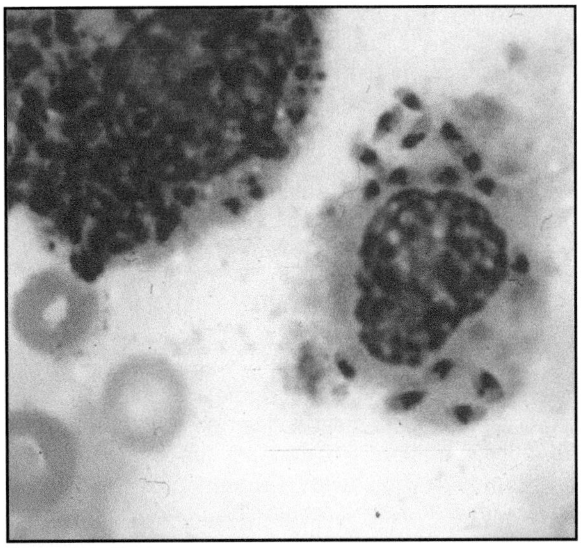

20.2 *Leishmania infantum* amastigotes in canine macrophages in a lymph node aspirate from a naturally infected dog.

also been described (Silva *et al.*, 2009). The transmission of *L. infantum* through blood products has been reported in dogs in North America (Owens *et al.*, 2001). This type of transmission is of special concern in endemic areas where blood donors are commonly infected subclinically (Tabar *et al.*, 2008). Therefore, it is important to test blood donors for *Leishmania* infection by serological and molecular tests and to exclude seropositive and/or polymerase chain reaction (PCR) positive dogs from donating blood (Solano-Gallego *et al.*, 2009). In addition, ticks and fleas have been proposed as alternative vectors of *Leishmania* (Coutinho *et al.*, 2005; Coutinho and Linardi, 2007; Dantas-Torres *et al.*, 2010a), but evidence of such transmission is sparse (Dantas-Torres *et al.*, 2010b) and controversial (Otranto and Dantas-Torres, 2010; Paz *et al.*, 2010). Sandflies are the only arthropod vector currently known to be adapted to the transmission of *Leishmania* (Killick-Kendrick, 1999). Direct dog-to-dog transmission has been suspected in non-endemic areas where sandfly vectors are apparently absent (e.g. the USA), but there is evidence of limited *L. infantum* infection in specific breeds such as Foxhounds and it has been suggested that direct transmission may occur in such breeds (Duprey *et al.*, 2006; Petersen and Barr, 2009).

Pathogenesis, clinical presentation and clinicopathological findings

A broad range of immune responses and clinical manifestations have been described in *L. infantum* infection in dogs. Infection may be subclinical, manifest as a self-limiting disease, or cause a non-self-limiting and severe illness (Solano-Gallego *et al.*, 2009). The two opposite extremes of this clinical spectrum are characterized in dogs by:

- 'Resistant' dogs with a protective $CD4^+$

T cell-mediated immune response characterized by release of Th1 cytokines such as interferon (IFN)-γ, interleukin (IL)-2 and tumour necrosis factor (TNF)-α, which induce anti-*Leishmania* activity in macrophages via nitric oxide production
- Sick dogs that characteristically have a marked humoral immune response, reduced cell-mediated immunity with a mixed Th1 and Th2 cytokine pattern, and a high parasite burden, which is detrimental to the animal (Baneth *et al.*, 2008).

Factors that may influence the progression from infection to clinical disease include age, breed, host genetics, nutrition, virulence of the parasite strain and concurrent diseases (Baneth *et al.*, 2008). In susceptible dogs, the incubation period prior to the appearance of clinical disease may last for months to years, during which time the parasite disseminates from the skin throughout the host's body, primarily to the haemolymphoid organs. Immune-mediated mechanisms are responsible for many of the pathological findings in canine leishmaniosis, in particular the deposition of immune complexes in the kidneys, blood vessels and joints. Renal pathology includes glomerulonephritis and interstitial nephritis (Poli *et al.*, 1991; Baneth *et al.*, 2008).

The main clinical and laboratory findings in canine leishmaniosis are listed in Figure 20.3. Skin lesions and lymphadenomegaly are the most frequent manifestations in affected dogs (Figures 20.4 and 20.5). About 25% of dogs with clinical leishmaniosis have ocular and periocular lesions, including keratoconjunctivitis and uveitis (Pena *et al.*, 2000). Atypical clinical signs are reviewed elsewhere (Solano-Gallego *et al.*, 2009) and include mucosal lesions, neurological, muscular, gastrointestinal and cardiovascular disorders. The main haematological abnormality in dogs with leishmaniosis is mild non-regenerative anaemia associated with chronic disease. Mild leucocytosis, leucopenia and pancytopenia are inconsistent findings (Petanides *et al.*, 2008); however, lymphopenia is reported frequently. Serum hyperviscosity, thrombocytopathy (Petanides *et al.*, 2008), secondary immune-mediated thrombocytopenia (Terrazzano *et al.*, 2006) and impaired secondary haemostasis and fibrinolysis (Ciaramella *et al.*, 2005) may also be detected. Antinuclear antibodies have been reported (Smith *et al.*, 2004). Parasites are rarely detected in peripheral blood smears and are more commonly found in aspirates from lymphoid organs. The main cause of death in dogs with leishmaniosis is immune-complex glomerulonephritis (Poli *et al.*, 1991).

General clinical signs	Local or generalized lymphadenomegaly, loss of body weight, exercise intolerance, decreased appetite, lethargy, splenomegaly, polyuria and polydypsia, epistaxis, onychogryphosis, lameness, vomiting and diarrhoea
Dermal lesions	Exfoliative dermatitis with alopecia, which can be generalized or localized over the face, ears and limbs, ulcerative dermatitis, nodular dermatitis, mucocutaneous proliferative dermatitis and papular dermatitis
Ocular lesions	Anterior uveitis, blepharitis (exfoliative, ulcerative or nodular) and keratoconjunctivitis, either common or sicca
Laboratory abnormalities	Hyperglobulinaemia (polyclonal gammaglobulinaemia), hypoalbuminaemia, decreased albumin:globulin ratio, mild to severe proteinuria, mild to moderate non-regenerative anaemia, renal azotaemia, elevated liver enzyme activities, thrombocytopenia and thrombocytopathy

20.3 Main clinical findings, including clinical signs and laboratory abnormalities, in classical canine leishmaniosis caused by *L. infantum*. (Source: Baneth *et al.*, 2008; Solano-Gallego *et al.*, 2009)

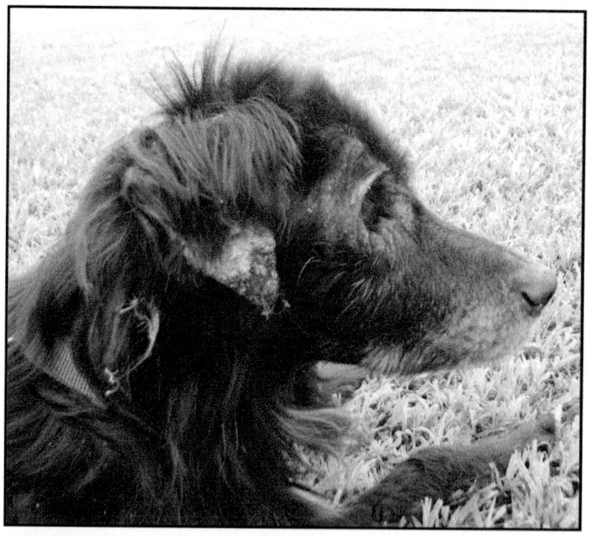

20.4 Dermal manifestations of canine leishmaniosis. Note the ulcerated pinnae, periocular alopecia and facial exfoliative dermatitis.

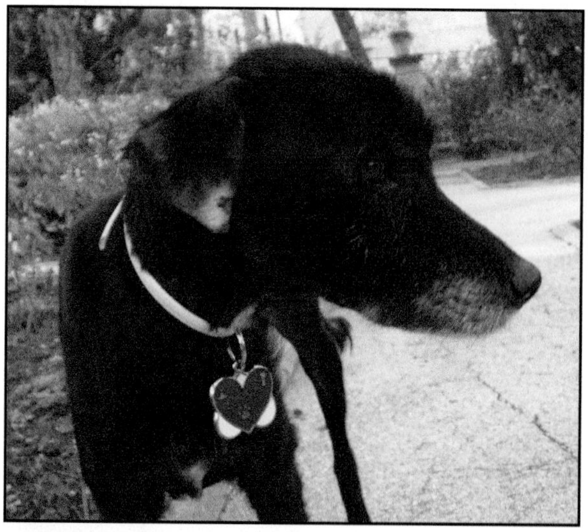

20.5 The dog in Figure 20.4 after 2 months of allopurinol treatment. Note the clinical improvement in the cutaneous lesions.

The variable and non-specific clinical signs make for an extensive list of differential diagnoses (Solano-Gallego *et al.*, 2009). In addition, the different degrees of disease severity require different treatments and carry different prognoses. A clinical staging system for canine leishmaniosis has been devised on the basis of the serological status, clinical signs and laboratory abnormalities. Four stages have been defined: mild, moderate, severe and very severe disease (Solano-Gallego *et al.*, 2009). Within this spectrum, clinical disease can range from mild (Stage I), such as a mild papular dermatitis associated with specific cellular immunity and low humoral responses (Ordeix *et al.*, 2005), to severe disease (Stage IV) characterized by end-stage renal disease with azotaemia and marked proteinuria caused by immune complex deposition in the renal glomeruli, associated with a massive humoral response and high parasite loads (Figure 20.6).

Diagnosis

Canine leishmaniosis has a high prevalence of subclinical infection. This makes the disease a diagnostic challenge for the veterinary practitioner, clinical pathologist and public health official in endemic countries, as well as in non-endemic regions where imported infection is a concern (Miró *et al.*, 2008).

Diagnostic investigation is usually performed for two main reasons:

- To confirm 'disease' (e.g. to find out whether a dog with clinical signs and/or clinicopathological abnormalities compatible with leishmaniosis indeed has the disease)
- To screen blood donors, to investigate the presence of 'infection' for epidemiological studies, to screen healthy dogs living in endemic regions, as often requested by the owners, to avoid importation of infected dogs to non-endemic countries, and to monitor the response to treatment (Miró *et al.*, 2008).

For these reasons, it is important to differentiate *Leishmania* infection from disease and to apply different diagnostic techniques accordingly (Solano-Gallego *et al.*, 2009).

Accurate diagnosis of canine leishmaniosis often requires an integrated approach combining clinicopathological assays and specific laboratory tests. This approach includes careful documentation of the clinical history, a thorough physical examination and several diagnostic tests such as complete blood count (CBC), serum biochemical profile, urinalysis, urine protein:creatinine ratio if proteinuria is detected, serum electrophoresis and a coagulation profile. Imaging of the abdomen by radiography and ultrasonography can assist in raising the index of suspicion for this disease. Several specific techniques have been developed to aid in the diagnosis of canine leishmaniosis (Figure 20.7). It is important to understand the basis of each diagnostic test, its limitations and the appropriate clinical interpretation (Solano-Gallego and Baneth, 2008).

Serology

The most useful diagnostic tools for the investigation of infection in sick and clinically healthy infected dogs include detection of serum anti-*Leishmania* antibodies by a quantitative assay and demonstration of parasite DNA in tissues by applying molecular techniques (Solano-Gallego *et al.*, 2009). In general, good sensitivities and specificities are gained with

Disease stage	Clinical signs	Laboratory abnormalities	Anti-*Leishmania* antibody levels
Stage I – mild disease	Mild, including peripheral lymphadenomegaly or papular dermatitis	Usually no clinicopathological abnormalities	Negative to low
Stage II – moderate disease	As for stage I. Plus diffuse or symmetrical cutaneous lesions (e.g. exfoliative dermatitis, onychogryphosis, ulceration), anorexia, weight loss, fever and epistaxis	Include mild non-regenerative anaemia, hyperglobulinaemia and hypoalbuminaemia, and serum hyperviscosity syndrome. Two sub-stages. Stage IIa: renal profile normal, with creatinine < 1.4 mg/dl, the dog is not proteinuric and the urine protein:creatinine ratio (UPC) is < 0.5. Stage IIb: creatinine < 1.4 mg/dl and UPC 0.5–1	Low to high
Stage III – severe disease	As for stages I and II. Plus dogs may present with signs caused by immune-complex deposition – lesions associated with vasculitis, arthritis, uveitis and glomerulonephritis.	As for stage II except for chronic kidney disease (CKD) International Renal Interest Society (IRIS) stage I with UPC > 1 or stage II with creatinine of 1.4–2 mg/dl	Moderate to high
Stage IV – very severe disease	As for stage III. Plus pulmonary thromboembolism, or nephrotic syndrome, or end stage renal disease	As for stage II plus CKD IRIS stage III (creatinine 2–5 mg/dl) or stage IV (creatinine > 5 mg/dl). The nephrotic syndrome includes a marked proteinuria with UPC > 5	Moderate to high

20.6 Clinical signs, laboratory abnormalities and serological status in the different stages of canine leishmaniosis. (Source: Solano-Gallego *et al.*, 2009)

Methods	Diagnostic technique/samples
Serology	Indirect fluorescent antibody test (IFAT) Enzyme-linked immunosorbent assay (ELISA) Direct antiglobulin test (DAT) Antigen-specific rK39 serology In-house immunochromatographic devices Western blot
Cytology	Skin touch preparation Fine-needle aspirates from lymph nodes, bone marrow, spleen, other tissues and body fluids
Histopathology	Formalin-fixed tissues stained with haematoxylin & eosin *Leishmania* immunohistochemistry
Detection of *Leishmania* DNA by PCR targeting the kinetoplast DNA or genomic ribosomal RNA genes	Conventional PCR Nested PCR Quantitative real-time PCR
Parasite culture	Samples from the bone marrow, buffy coat, spleen, lymph node, cutaneous lesions and other tissues in a specialized medium for the culture of *Leishmania*

20.7 Diagnostic techniques used for canine leishmaniosis.

quantitative serological methods for the diagnosis of clinical leishmaniosis (Miró *et al.*, 2008). High antibody levels are usually associated with disease and a high parasite density (Reis *et al.*, 2006) and, for this reason, they provide a conclusive diagnosis of leishmaniosis. However, the presence of lower antibody levels is not necessarily indicative of patent disease and needs to be confirmed by another diagnostic method such as PCR, cytology or histology (Miró *et al.*, 2008; Solano-Gallego *et al.*, 2009). Serological cross-reactivity with different pathogens is possible with some serological tests, especially those based on whole parasite antigen. Cross-reactivity has been reported with other species of *Leishmania* and *Trypanosoma cruzi* (Barbosa-De-Deus *et al.*, 2002).

Cytology and histology

Microscopic detection of amastigotes by cytology is frequently unrewarding owing to a low to moderate number of detectable parasites present even in dogs with full-blown clinical disease (Moreira *et al.*, 2007). *Leishmania* parasites may also be seen in histopathological formalin-fixed, paraffin wax-embedded biopsy sections of skin or other infected organs. *Leishmania* parasites should be suspected in granulomatous, pyogranulomatous or lymphoplasmacytic inflammation in different tissues (Solano-Gallego *et al.*, 2004; Pena *et al.*, 2008) or in lymphoid organ reactive hyperplasia (Mylonakis *et al.*, 2005) detected by cytology or histopathology. Definite identification of parasites within tissue macrophages may be difficult and an immunohistochemical method can be employed to detect or verify the presence of *Leishmania* in the tissue (Ferrer *et al.*, 1988).

PCR

PCR assays with various target sequences using genomic or kinetoplast DNA (kDNA) have been developed. Assays based on kDNA appear to be the most sensitive for direct detection in infected tissue (Francino *et al.*, 2006; Gomes *et al.*, 2008; Miró *et al.*, 2008). The PCR can be performed on DNA extracted from tissue, blood, body fluids or even from histopathological specimens (Solano-Gallego *et al.*, 2009). PCR of bone marrow, lymph node or skin is most sensitive and specific for the diagnosis of canine leishmaniosis (Mathis and Deplazes, 1995; Reale *et al.*, 1999; Solano-Gallego *et al.*, 2001). PCR of whole blood, buffy coat and urine samples is less sensitive than on the aforementioned tissues (Mathis and Deplazes, 1995; Reale *et al.*, 1999; Solano-Gallego *et al.*, 2007). PCR carried out on aspirates of lymph node and bone marrow has been shown to be more sensitive than microscopy of stained smears or parasite culture (Moreira *et al.*, 2007). PCR of conjunctival swabs has been shown to be helpful in the non-invasive diagnosis of canine infection (Strauss-Ayali *et al.*, 2004).

PCR is not the first confirmatory assay recommended for dogs with clinical signs that are suspected of leishmaniosis because, in endemic areas, a large portion of the dog population is likely to harbour *Leishmania* without clinical disease, or while suffering from a different medical condition. Given that high serological titres are closely associated with clinical disease and less frequent among clinically healthy carriers of *Leishmania*, quantitative serology would be the assay first recommended for diagnosis of disease (Solano-Gallego *et al.*, 2009). The presence of *Leishmania* DNA in the blood or other tissues of clinically healthy dogs living in endemic areas indicates that these dogs harbour infection (Solano-Gallego *et al.*, 2001), but they may never develop clinical disease (Oliva *et al.*, 2006).

Therapy, prevention and public health considerations

The main drugs used in the treatment of canine leishmaniosis include: the pentavalent antimonial meglumine antimonate, which selectively inhibits leishmanial glycolysis and fatty acid oxidation; miltefosine, which is an alkylphospholipid that has a direct toxic effect against *Leishmania*; and allopurinol, which acts by inhibiting protein translation through interfering with RNA synthesis. The main anti-leishmanial drugs, with dosages and side effects are listed in Figure 20.8.

Anti-leishmanials

The combination of meglumine antimonate and allopurinol is the most common treatment used for canine leishmaniosis in Europe (Baneth and Shaw, 2002; Noli and Auxilia, 2005). Miltefosine has recently been shown to be effective against the

Generic name	Dosage, route, interval and duration	Side effects	References
Meglumine antimonate	75 mg/kg s.c. q12h or 100 mg/kg s.c. q24h for 4–8 weeks	Cutaneous abscesses/cellulitis, gastrointestinal signs, potential nephrotoxicity	Noli and Auxilia, 2005; Bianciardi *et al.*, 2009
Allopurinol	10 mg/kg orally q12h, for 6–12 months or longer if needed	Xanthine urolithiasis	Ling *et al.*, 1991
Miltefosine	2 mg/kg orally q24h, for 4 weeks	Gastrointestinal signs	Miró *et al.*, 2009; Woerly *et al.*, 2009

20.8 The main anti-leishmanial drugs for the treatment of canine leishmaniosis. Combinations of meglumine antimonate and allopurinol, or miltefosine and allopurinol can be used.

canine disease and it is recommended as an alternative to meglumine antimonate in combination with long-term allopurinol treatment (Manna *et al.*, 2009; Miró *et al.*, 2009; Woerly *et al.*, 2009). Amphotericin B, which acts by binding to ergosterol in the parasite cell membrane and altering its permeability, is also used (Cortadellas, 2003), but it is highly nephrotoxic. New drugs (Miró *et al.*, 2008) and immunotherapy (Borja-Cabrera *et al.*, 2004) are currently under investigation in dogs. Anti-*Leishmania* treatment often achieves only clinical improvement in dogs with leishmaniosis and it is frequently not associated with the elimination of the parasite (Noli and Auxilia, 2005).

Preventive measures

Insecticides

The use of topical insecticides (Alexander and Maroli, 2003) in collars (Maroli *et al.*, 2001) or spot-on formulations has been shown to be effective in reducing *Leishmania* transmission (Otranto *et al.*, 2007). Deltamethrin-impregnated collars reduce the number of dog sandfly bites significantly under experimental conditions (Killick-Kendrick *et al.*, 1997) and decrease infection transmission in field studies (Maroli *et al.*, 2001). In a study supported by the World Health Organization in Iran, application of collars to dogs in intervention and control villages reduced the seroconversion rate in dogs and in children living in the intervention villages significantly (Gavgani *et al.*, 2002a).

Vaccination

A commercial vaccine against canine leishmaniosis has been approved in Brazil (Borja-Cabrera *et al.*, 2002; Dantas-Torres, 2006) and another vaccine has been approved in Europe. Several vaccine candidates are under experimental (Ramos *et al.*, 2008) or field evaluation in Europe (Lemesre *et al.*, 2007).

Public health

Human visceral leishmaniosis caused by *L. infantum* is a serious public health problem. It is mostly a disease of young children, and malnutrition has been recognized as a risk factor for infantile leishmaniosis. This may explain why this disease is more prevalent among children in poor countries despite high prevalence rates in the dog populations of both affluent and developing countries (Alvar *et al.*, 2006). Human disease is also prevalent in immunosuppressed individuals, and patients with human immunodeficiency virus infection are now the predominant risk group for the human visceral disease in southern Europe (Alvar *et al.*, 2008). Several studies have investigated the association between canine and human leishmaniosis in the same region and examined to what degree the infection in dogs poses a risk for the human population (Miró *et al.*, 2008). Increased prevalence of infection in the canine population has been found to be associated with an increased incidence of human leishmaniosis (Werneck *et al.*, 2007). Poor socioeconomic conditions are risk factors for the association between canine and human infections (Werneck *et al.*, 2007), and dog density and ownership of infected dogs are risk factors for infantile human leishmaniosis (Gavgani *et al.*, 2002b). The relationship between canine and human infections probably differs from one region to another and could depend on several factors, including human nutrition, lifestyle, time spent outdoors, the density of dogs, and the behaviour of sandfly vectors. Infected pets may remain carriers of disease despite treatment, and it is recommended that appropriate topical insecticides are applied to them in order to prevent further transmission.

Feline leishmaniosis

The *Leishmania* species shown to cause feline leishmaniosis are: *L. infantum* in southern Europe (Ozon *et al.*, 1998; Poli *et al.*, 2002; Pennisi *et al.*, 2004), Brazil (Savani *et al.*, 2004) and Iran (Hatam *et al.*, 2010); *L. mexicana* in Texas (Craig *et al.*, 1986); and *L. amazonensis* (de Souza *et al.*, 2005) and *L. braziliensis* (Simoes-Mattos *et al.*, 2005) in Brazil. Despite the high prevalence of *L. infantum* in dogs in the Mediterranean Basin, with common manifestations of clinical disease (Solano-Gallego *et al.*, 2001), far fewer cases of clinical feline *Leishmania* infection have been described in this region. The lesions described most frequently in feline leishmaniosis due to *L. infantum* are ulcerocrusting and nodular dermatitis, alopecia and scaling (Ozon *et al.*, 1998; Poli *et al.*, 2002; Pennisi *et al.*, 2004), with the visceral form of the disease involving the spleen, liver, lymph nodes and kidney being described less commonly (Ozon *et al.*, 1998; Leiva *et al.*, 2005).

Although clinical cases of leishmaniosis have been reported in cats with co-infection of feline leukaemia virus (FeLV) or feline immunodeficiency virus (FIV; Poli *et al.*, 2002), the true association between *Leishmania* and retroviral infections in cats remains unclear. Diagnosis is made in the majority of cases by serology, cytology, histology or PCR assays. The most common treatment of feline leishmaniosis is with allopurinol at the same dosage as used for dogs. The recent description of a high prevalence of subclinical *Leishmania* infection in cats in the Mediterranean Basin countries shown by PCR of blood (Martin-Sanchez *et al.*, 2007), and the demonstration of transmission from a cat to sandfly vectors (Maroli *et al.*, 2007), raise the possibility that cats may have a role as a reservoir host for *L. infantum*.

References and further reading

Alexander B and Maroli M (2003) Control of phlebotomine sandflies. *Medical and Veterinary Entomology* **17**, 1–18

Alvar J, Aparicio P, Aseffa A *et al.* (2008) The relationship between leishmaniasis and AIDS: the second 10 years. *Clinical Microbiology Reviews* **21**, 334–359

Alvar J, Yactayo S and Bern C (2006) Leishmaniasis and poverty. *Trends in Parasitology* **22**, 552–557

Amusategui I, Sainz A, Aguirre E *et al.* (2004) Seroprevalence of *Leishmania infantum* in northwestern Spain, an area traditionally considered free of leishmaniasis. *Annals of the New York Academy of Sciences* **1026**, 154–157

Andrade HM, de Toledo Vde P, Marques MJ *et al.* (2002) *Leishmania* (*Leishmania*) *chagasi* is not vertically transmitted in dogs. *Veterinary Parasitology* **103**, 71–81

Baneth G, Koutinas AF, Solano-Gallego L *et al.* (2008) Canine leishmaniosis – new concepts and insights on an expanding zoonosis: part one. *Trends in Parasitology* **24**, 324–330

Baneth G and Shaw SE (2002) Chemotherapy of canine leishmaniosis. *Veterinary Parasitology* **106**, 315–324

Barbosa-De-Deus R, Dos Mares-Guia ML, Nunes AZ *et al.* (2002) *Leishmania major*-like antigen for specific and sensitive serodiagnosis of human and canine visceral leishmaniasis. *Clinical and Diagnostic Laboratory Immunology* **9**, 1361–1366

Bianciardi P, Brovida C, Valente M *et al.* (2009) Administration of miltefosine and meglumine antimoniate in healthy dogs: clinicopathological evaluation of the impact on the kidneys. *Toxicological Pathology* **37**, 770–775

Borja-Cabrera GP, Correia Pontes NN, da Silva VO *et al.* (2002) Long lasting protection against canine kala-azar using the FML-QuilA saponin vaccine in an endemic area of Brazil (Sao Goncalo do Amarante, RN). *Vaccine* **20**, 3277–3284

Borja-Cabrera GP, Cruz Mendes A, Paraguai de Souza E *et al.* (2004) Effective immunotherapy against canine visceral leishmaniasis with the FML-vaccine. *Vaccine* **22**, 2234–2243

Cabral M, O'Grady JE, Gomes S *et al.* (1998) The immunology of canine leishmaniosis: strong evidence for a developing disease spectrum from asymptomatic dogs. *Veterinary Parasitology* **76**, 173–180

Chamaille L, Tran A, Meunier A *et al.* (2010) Environmental risk mapping of canine leishmaniasis in France. *Parasites and Vectors* **3**, 31

Ciaramella P, Pelagalli A, Cortese L *et al.* (2005) Altered platelet aggregation and coagulation disorders related to clinical findings in 30 dogs naturally infected by *Leishmania infantum*. *Veterinary Journal* **169**, 465–467

Cortadellas O (2003) Initial and long-term efficacy of a lipid emulsion of amphotericin B desoxycholate in the management of canine leishmaniasis. *Journal of Veterinary Internal Medicine* **17**, 808–812

Coutinho MT, Bueno LL, Sterzik A *et al.* (2005) Participation of *Rhipicephalus sanguineus* (Acari: Ixodidae) in the epidemiology of canine visceral leishmaniasis. *Veterinary Parasitology* **128**, 149–155

Coutinho MT and Linardi PM (2007) Can fleas from dogs infected with canine visceral leishmaniasis transfer the infection to other mammals? *Veterinary Parasitology* **147**, 320–325

Craig TM, Barton CL, Mercer SH *et al.* (1986) Dermal leishmaniasis in a Texas cat. *American Journal of Tropical Medicine and Hygiene* **35**, 1100–1102

da Silva SM, Ribeiro VM, Ribeiro RR *et al.* (2009) First report of vertical transmission of *Leishmania* (*Leishmania*) *infantum* in a naturally infected bitch from Brazil. *Veterinary Parasitology* **166**, 159–162

Dantas-Torres F (2006) Leishmune vaccine: the newest tool for prevention and control of canine visceral leishmaniosis and its potential as a transmission-blocking vaccine. *Veterinary Parasitology* **141**, 1–8

Dantas-Torres F (2007) The role of dogs as reservoirs of *Leishmania* parasites, with emphasis on *Leishmania* (*Leishmania*) *infantum* and *Leishmania* (*Viannia*) *braziliensis*. *Veterinary Parasitology* **149**, 139–146

Dantas-Torres F, Lorusso V, Testini G *et al.* (2010a) Detection of *Leishmania infantum* in *Rhipicephalus sanguineus* ticks from Brazil and Italy. *Parasitology Research* **106**, 857–860

Dantas-Torres F, Martins TF, de Paiva-Cavalcanti M *et al.* (2010b) Transovarial passage of *Leishmania infantum* kDNA in artificially infected *Rhipicephalus sanguineus*. *Experimental Parasitology* **125**, 184–185

Dereure J, Vanwambeke SO, Male P *et al.* (2009) The potential effects of global warming on changes in canine leishmaniasis in a focus outside the classical area of the disease in southern France. *Vector Borne Zoonotic Disease* **9**, 687–694

Desjeux P (2004) Leishmaniasis: current situation and new perspectives. *Comparative Immunology and Microbiology of Infectious Disease* **27**, 305–318

de Souza AI, Barros EM, Ishikawa E *et al.* (2005) Feline leishmaniasis due to *Leishmania* (*Leishmania*) *amazonensis* in Mato Grosso do Sul State, Brazil. *Veterinary Parasitology* **128**, 41–45

Duprey ZH, Steurer FJ, Rooney JA *et al.* (2006) Canine visceral leishmaniasis, United States and Canada, 2000-2003. *Emerging Infectious Diseases* **12**, 440–446

Ferrer L, Rabanal RM, Domingo M *et al.* (1988) Identification of *Leishmania donovani* amastigotes in canine tissues by immunoperoxidase staining. *Research in Veterinary Science* **44**, 194–196

Francino O, Altet L, Sanchez-Robert E *et al.* (2006) Advantages of real-time PCR assay for diagnosis and monitoring of canine leishmaniosis. *Veterinary Parasitology* **137**, 214–221

Gavgani AS, Hodjati MH, Mohite H *et al.* (2002a) Effect of insecticide-impregnated dog collars on incidence of zoonotic visceral leishmaniasis in Iranian children: a matched-cluster randomised trial. *Lancet* **360**, 374–379

Gavgani AS, Mohite H, Edrissian GH *et al.* (2002b) Domestic dog ownership in Iran is a risk factor for human infection with *Leishmania infantum*. *American Journal of Tropical Medicine and Hygiene* **67**, 511–515

Gomes YM, Paiva Cavalcanti M, Lira RA *et al.* (2008) Diagnosis of canine visceral leishmaniasis: biotechnological advances. *Veterinary Journal* **175**, 45–52

Hatam GR, Adnani SJ, Asgari Q *et al.* (2010) First report of natural infection in cats with *Leishmania infantum* in Iran. *Vector Borne Zoonotic Diseases* **10**, 313–316

Killick-Kendrick R (1999) The biology and control of phlebotomine sand flies. *Clinical Dermatology* **17**, 279–289

Killick-Kendrick R, Killick-Kendrick M, Focheux C *et al.* (1997) Protection of dogs from bites of phlebotomine sandflies by deltamethrin collars for control of canine leishmaniasis. *Medical and Veterinary Entomology* **11**, 105–111

Leiva M, Lloret A, Pena T *et al.* (2005) Therapy of ocular and visceral leishmaniasis in a cat. *Veterinary Ophthalmology* **8**, 71–75

Lemesre JL, Holzmuller P, Goncalves RB *et al.* (2007) Long-lasting protection against canine visceral leishmaniasis using the LiESAp-MDP vaccine in endemic areas of France: double-blind randomised efficacy field trial. *Vaccine* **25**, 4223–4234

Lemrani M, Nejjar R and Pratlong F (2002) A new *Leishmania tropica* zymodeme -- causative agent of canine visceral leishmaniasis in northern Morocco. *Annals of Tropical Medicine and Parasitology* **96**, 637–638

Ling GV, Ruby AL, Harrold DR *et al.* (1991) Xanthine-containing urinary calculi in dogs given allopurinol. *Journal of the American Veterinary Medical Association* **198**, 1935–1940

Manna L, Vitale F, Reale S *et al.* (2009) Study of efficacy of miltefosine and allopurinol in dogs with leishmaniosis. *Veterinary Journal* **182**, 441–445

Maroli M, Mizzon V, Siragusa C *et al.* (2001) Evidence for an impact on the incidence of canine leishmaniasis by the mass use of deltamethrin-impregnated dog collars in southern Italy. *Medical and Veterinary Entomology* **15**, 358–363

Maroli M, Pennisi MG, Di Muccio T *et al.* (2007) Infection of sandflies by a cat naturally infected with *Leishmania infantum*. *Veterinary Parasitology* **145**, 357–360

Maroli M, Rossi L, Baldelli R *et al.* (2008) The northward spread of leishmaniasis in Italy: evidence from retrospective and ongoing studies on the canine reservoir and phlebotomine vectors. *Tropical Medicine and International Health* **13**, 256–264

Martin-Sanchez J, Acedo C, Munoz-Perez M *et al.* (2007) Infection by *Leishmania infantum* in cats: epidemiological study in Spain.

Veterinary Parasitology **145**, 267–273
Mathis A and Deplazes P (1995) PCR and in vitro cultivation for detection of *Leishmania* spp. in diagnostic samples from humans and dogs. *Journal of Clinical Microbiology* **33**, 1145–1149
Menn B, Lorentz S and Naucke TJ (2010) Imported and travelling dogs as carriers of canine vector-borne pathogens in Germany. *Parasites and Vectors* **3**, 34
Miró G, Cardoso L, Pennisi MG *et al.* (2008) Canine leishmaniosis -- new concepts and insights on an expanding zoonosis: part two. *Trends in Parasitology* **24**, 371–377
Miró G, Oliva G, Cruz I *et al.* (2009) Multicentric, controlled clinical study to evaluate effectiveness and safety of miltefosine and allopurinol for canine leishmaniosis. *Veterinary Dermatology* **20**, 397–404
Moreira MA, Luvizotto MC, Garcia JF *et al.* (2007) Comparison of parasitological, immunological and molecular methods for the diagnosis of leishmaniasis in dogs with different clinical signs. *Veterinary Parasitology* **145**, 245–252
Moreno J and Alvar J (2002) Canine leishmaniasis: epidemiological risk and the experimental model. *Trends in Parasitology* **18**, 399–405
Mylonakis ME, Papaioannou N, Saridomichelakis MN *et al.* (2005) Cytologic patterns of lymphadenopathy in dogs infected with *Leishmania infantum. Veterinary Clinical Pathology* **34**, 243–247
Noli C and Auxilia ST (2005) Treatment of canine Old World visceral leishmaniasis: a systematic review. *Veterinary Dermatology* **16**, 213–232
Oliva G, Scalone A, Foglia Manzillo V *et al.* (2006) Incidence and time course of *Leishmania infantum* infections examined by parasitological, serologic, and nested-PCR techniques in a cohort of naive dogs exposed to three consecutive transmission seasons. *Journal of Clinical Microbiology* **44**, 1318–1322
Ordeix L, Solano-Gallego L, Fondevila D *et al.* (2005) Papular dermatitis due to *Leishmania* spp. infection in dogs with parasite-specific cellular immune responses. *Veterinary Dermatology* **16**, 187–191
Otranto D and Dantas-Torres F (2010) Fleas and ticks as vectors of *Leishmania* spp. to dogs: caution is needed. *Veterinary Parasitology* **168**, 173–174
Otranto D, Paradies P, Lia RP *et al.* (2007) Efficacy of a combination of 10% imidacloprid/50% permethrin for the prevention of leishmaniasis in kennelled dogs in an endemic area. *Veterinary Parasitology* **144**, 270–278
Owens SD, Oakley DA, Marryott K *et al.* (2001) Transmission of visceral leishmaniasis through blood transfusions from infected English foxhounds to anemic dogs. *Journal of the American Veterinary Medical Association* **219**, 1076–1083
Ozon C, Marty P, Pratlong F *et al.* (1998) Disseminated feline leishmaniosis due to *Leishmania infantum* in Southern France. *Veterinary Parasitology* **75**, 273–277
Pangrazio KK, Costa EA, Amarilla SP *et al.* (2009) Tissue distribution of *Leishmania chagasi* and lesions in transplacentally infected fetuses from symptomatic and asymptomatic naturally infected bitches. *Veterinary Parasitology* **165**, 327–331
Paz GF, Ribeiro MF, Michalsky EM *et al.* (2010) Evaluation of the vectorial capacity of *Rhipicephalus sanguineus* (Acari: Ixodidae) in the transmission of canine visceral leishmaniasis. *Parasitology Research* **106**, 523–528
Pena MT, Naranjo C, Klauss G *et al.* (2008) Histopathological features of ocular leishmaniosis in the dog. *Journal of Comparative Pathology* **138**, 32–39
Pena MT, Roura X, Davidson MG (2000) Ocular and periocular manifestations of leishmaniasis in dogs: 105 cases (1993-1998). *Veterinary Ophthalmology* **3**, 35–41
Pennisi MG, Venza M, Reale S *et al.* (2004) Case report of feline leishmaniasis in four cats. *Veterinary Research Communications* **28**, 363–366
Petanides TA, Koutinas AF, Mylonakis ME *et al.* (2008) Factors associated with the occurrence of epistaxis in natural canine leishmaniasis (*Leishmania infantum*). *Journal of Veterinary Internal Medicine* **22**, 866–872
Petersen CA (2009) New means of canine leishmaniasis transmission in North America: the possibility of transmission to humans still unknown. Interdisciplinary Perspectives on Infectious Diseases **2009**, 802712.
Petersen CA and Barr SC (2009) Canine leishmaniasis in North America: emerging or newly recognized? *Veterinary Clinics of North America: Small Animal Practice* **39**, 1065–1074, vi
Poli A, Abramo F, Barsotti P *et al.* (2002) Feline leishmaniosis due to *Leishmania infantum* in Italy. *Veterinary Parasitology* **106**, 181–191
Poli A, Abramo F, Mancianti F *et al.* (1991) Renal involvement in canine leishmaniasis. A light-microscopic, immunohistochemical and electron-microscopic study. *Nephron* **57**, 444–452
Ramos I, Alonso A, Marcen JM *et al.* (2008) Heterologous prime-boost vaccination with a non-replicative vaccinia recombinant vector expressing LACK confers protection against canine visceral leishmaniasis with a predominant Th1-specific immune response. *Vaccine* **26**, 333–344
Reale S, Maxia L, Vitale F *et al.* (1999) Detection of *Leishmania infantum* in dogs by PCR with lymph node aspirates and blood. *Journal of Clinical Microbiology* **37**, 2931–2935
Reis AB, Teixeira-Carvalho A, Vale AM *et al.* (2006) Isotype patterns of immunoglobulins: hallmarks for clinical status and tissue parasite density in Brazilian dogs naturally infected by *Leishmania (Leishmania) chagasi. Veterinary Immunology and Immunopathology* **112**, 102–116
Rosypal AC, Troy GC, Zajac AM *et al.* (2005) Transplacental transmission of a North American isolate of *Leishmania infantum* in an experimentally infected beagle. *Journal of Parasitology* **91**, 970–972
Savani ES, de Oliveira Camargo MC, de Carvalho MR *et al.* (2004) The first record in the Americas of an autochthonous case of *Leishmania (Leishmania) infantum chagasi* in a domestic cat (*Felix catus*) from Cotia County, Sao Paulo State, Brazil. *Veterinary Parasitology* **120**, 229–233
Shaw SE, Langton DA and Hillman TJ (2009) Canine leishmaniosis in the United Kingdom: a zoonotic disease waiting for a vector? *Veterinary Parasitology* **163**, 281–285
Silva FL, Oliveira RG, Silva TM *et al.* (2009) Venereal transmission of canine visceral leishmaniasis. *Veterinary Parasitology* **160**, 55–59
Simoes-Mattos L, Mattos MR, Teixeira MJ *et al.* (2005) The susceptibility of domestic cats (*Felis catus*) to experimental infection with *Leishmania braziliensis. Veterinary Parasitology* **127**, 199–208
Smith BE, Tompkins MB and Breitschwerdt EB (2004) Antinuclear antibodies can be detected in dog sera reactive to *Bartonella vinsonii* subsp. *berkhoffii, Ehrlichia canis*, or *Leishmania infantum* antigens. *Journal of Veterinary Internal Medicine* **18**, 47–51
Solano-Gallego L and Baneth G (2008) Canine leishmaniosis – a challenging zoonosis. *European Journal of Companion Animal Practice* **18**, 232–241
Solano-Gallego L, Fernandez-Bellon H, Morell P *et al.* (2004) Histological and immunohistochemical study of clinically normal skin of *Leishmania infantum*-infected dogs. *Journal of Comparative Pathology* **130**, 7–12
Solano-Gallego L, Koutinas A, Miró G *et al.* (2009) Directions for the diagnosis, clinical staging, treatment and prevention of canine leishmaniosis. *Veterinary Parasitology* **165**, 1–18
Solano-Gallego L, Morell P, Arboix M *et al.* (2001) Prevalence of *Leishmania infantum* infection in dogs living in an area of canine leishmaniasis endemicity using PCR on several tissues and serology. *Journal of Clinical Microbiology* **39**, 560–563
Solano-Gallego L, Rodriguez-Cortes A, Trotta M *et al.* (2007) Detection of *Leishmania infantum* DNA by fret-based real-time PCR in urine from dogs with natural clinical leishmaniosis. *Veterinary Parasitology* **147**, 315–319
Strauss-Ayali D, Jaffe CL, Burshtain O *et al.* (2004) Polymerase chain reaction using noninvasively obtained samples, for the detection of *Leishmania infantum* DNA in dogs. *Journal of Infectious Disease* **189**, 1729–1733
Tabar MD, Roura X, Francino O *et al.* (2008) Detection of *Leishmania infantum* by real-time PCR in a canine blood bank. *Journal of Small Animal Practice* **49**, 325–328
Terrazzano G, Cortese L, Piantedosi D *et al.* (2006) Presence of anti-platelet IgM and IgG antibodies in dogs naturally infected by *Leishmania infantum. Veterinary Immunology and Immunopathology* **110**, 331–337
Teske E, van Knapen F, Beijer EG *et al.* (2002) Risk of infection with *Leishmania* spp. in the canine population in the Netherlands. *Acta Veterinaria Scandinavica* **43**, 195–201
Werneck GL, Costa CH, Walker AM *et al.* (2007) Multilevel modelling of the incidence of visceral leishmaniasis in Teresina, Brazil. *Epidemiology and Infection* **135**, 195–201
Woerly V, Maynard L, Sanquer A *et al.* (2009) Clinical efficacy and tolerance of miltefosine in the treatment of canine leishmaniosis. *Parasitol Research* **105**, 463–469

21

Overview of haemostasis

Reinhard Mischke

Introduction

The haemostatic system is a vital mechanism, the main functions of which are:

- To guarantee maintenance of vascular integrity, i.e. to minimize blood loss, if injuries to the vessel wall occur
- To maintain blood fluidity under physiological conditions, i.e. in an intact vascular system.

According to the classical understanding of haemostasis, primary (platelet function) and secondary (coagulation system) haemostasis mechanisms are distinct (Figure 21.1). This classical model of blood coagulation is helpful in explaining the main reactions and clinical manifestations of different haemostatic disorders and is an excellent basis for an understanding of the haemostatic tests. Nevertheless, these processes take place simultaneously rather than consecutively. In addition, there are important relationships between the coagulation proteins and platelets as well as other cell types. Our current understanding is summarized in the 'cell-based model of haemostasis/blood coagulation'.

Mechanisms for the regulation and control of blood coagulation include inhibitors and the fibrinolytic system. The delicate balance between clot formation and clot dissolution (fibrinolysis) may be disturbed in either direction in a variety of pathological conditions. Fibrinolysis is also important in the final steps of haemostasis, where the clot dissolves once the blood vessel has been repaired, re-establishing normal blood flow.

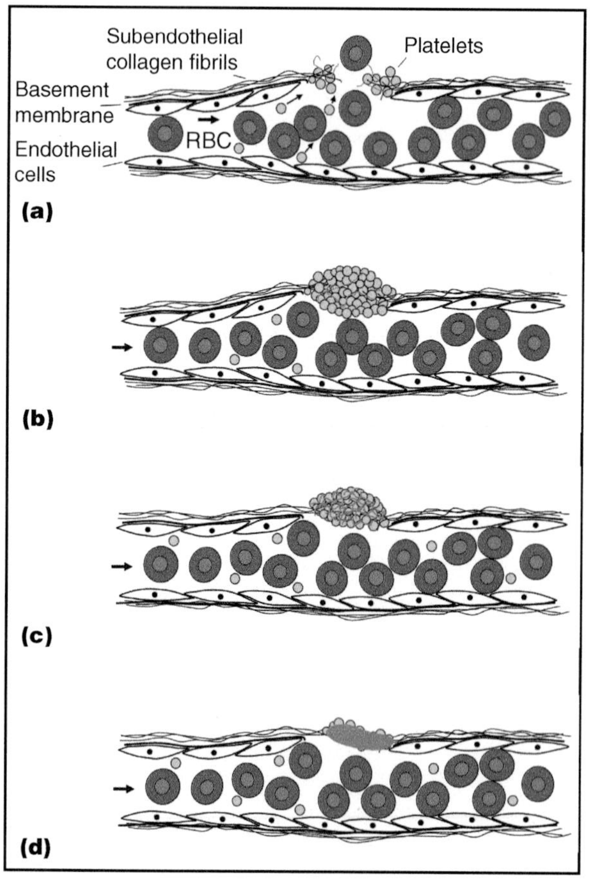

21.1 Schematic diagram of haemostasis. **(a)** Vasoconstriction results in deceleration of blood flow (red blood cells; RBC), which supports adhesion and aggregation of platelets. **(b)** Further platelets are attracted, leading to complete occlusion by a primary platelet plug. **(c)** Stabilization by fibrin and cross-linkage of fibrin prevent loss of the clot by increasing blood pressure following decreased vasoconstriction. There is dissolution of boundaries between platelets. **(d)** Reduction of the size of the clot is caused by retraction of platelets and fibrin strands with near normalization of blood flow.

Primary haemostasis

Primary haemostasis describes the processes of the primary closure of an injured blood vessel by the rapid formation of the labile 'primary platelet plug' (Figure 21.1). This is based mainly on an adequate platelet count and function, and the interaction between platelets and damaged vascular endothelium (Hawiger, 1990). In combination with vasoconstriction, this initial platelet plug may provide adequate haemostasis in capillaries and venules. In vessels in which flow and pressure are greater, it is essential to stabilize this plug with an overlying mesh of insoluble fibrin formed by the blood coagulation system (secondary haemostasis).

Platelet activation is initiated by exposure of the platelets to subendothelial substances such as collagen, which promotes platelet adhesion (Figure 21.2), whereas the normal endothelium inhibits platelet adhesion by means of prostacycline and endothelium-derived relaxing factor. Platelets adhere

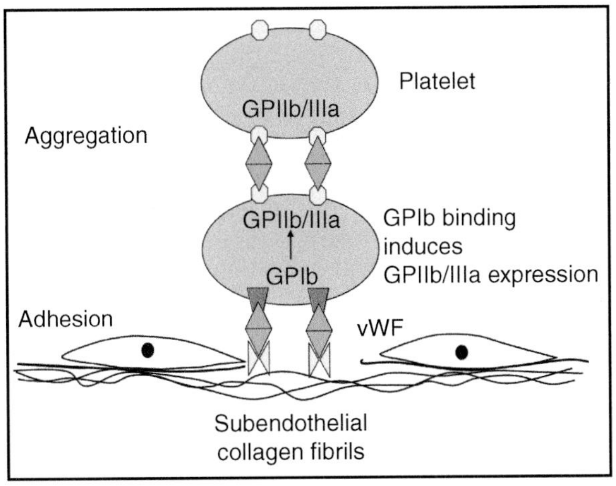

21.2 Schematic diagram of the mechanisms underlying platelet adhesion and aggregation.

to the subendothelial collagen via a specific plasma membrane receptor. Under conditions of high shear rates (i.e. in arterioles and in the microcirculation), binding of platelets to the subendothelial matrix is inadequate and interaction of von Willebrand factor (vWf) with its platelet receptor glycoprotein (GP) 1b/V/IX is necessary.

Formation of the platelet plug is supported by simultaneous local vasoconstriction that reduces the rate of blood flow. This vasoconstriction is induced by the release of vasoactive substances such as thromboxane A_2, serotonin and adrenaline by the platelets and endothelium.

Binding of collagen to the platelet receptor signals a message to the platelets that initiates a series of events. With their contractile proteins, activated platelets perform a shape change from smooth and discoid to round with numerous projecting pseudopods, which greatly increase the platelet surface area. Activation exposes fibrinogen and vWf receptors on the platelet membrane and allows fibrinogen- or vWf-mediated platelet aggregation. The contents of the platelet dense granules (cations, nucleotides and amines) and α-granules (numerous proteins, including fibrinogen, vWf and factors that promote vascular repair) are released locally and help to recruit further platelets to the site of injury. They also provide material for clotting reactions and agonists to induce further platelet activation. The exposure of the subendothelial tissues also results in a conformational change in vWf that allows platelets to recognize and bind vWf, resulting in further adherence of platelets to the subendothelium as well as promoting further platelet activation. The primary haemostatic platelet plug over the site of vessel injury is formed by the combination of platelets adherent to the subendothelium and platelets aggregated to each other. Finally, the membranes of the aggregated platelets dissolve and they merge together.

vWf is a large protein synthesized by endothelial cells. It consists of multiple subunits, with both smaller and larger multiple-subunit molecules, with the latter being the most effective at binding to platelets. vWf is synthesized mainly in the vascular endothelial cells and is released into the plasma and the subendothelial tissues. A small amount of vWf is synthesized by megakaryocytes and stored within platelet granules (Ruggeri and Ware, 1992). Apart from its important role in platelet adhesion at sites of vascular damage (and aggregation), vWf functions as a carrier molecule for factor (F) VIII in the circulation.

Secondary haemostasis (blood coagulation)

Traditional blood coagulation system

The blood coagulation system results in the generation of thrombin. Thrombin converts soluble fibrinogen to insoluble fibrin ('secondary haemostasis'), which stabilizes the platelet clot in a meshwork of fibrin strands. Secondary haemostasis comprises different coagulation factors, which are synthesized by the liver in their inactive forms (precursors, proenzymes). After completion of protein synthesis, F II (prothrombin), FVII, FIX and FX require vitamin-K-dependent γ-carboxylation, which enables them to bind via ionized calcium (Ca^{2+}) to the negatively charged phospholipid surface of activated platelets. Under conditions of vitamin K deficiency or the ingestion of vitamin K antagonists, this γ-carboxylation does not take place. Consequently, haemostatically incompetent proteins will be stored in the liver, and when the blood level of the functional factors decreases below a certain level, they are released into the circulation as 'proteins induced by vitamin K absence' (PIVKA). Most of the coagulation factors are proteases (often serine proteases with a reactive serine at the active site) and they activate another coagulation protein in the sequence directly.

Most of the clotting process occurs on the phospholipid membrane of activated platelets at the site of vascular injury and requires Ca^{2+}, especially the two major enzyme–cofactor complexes (tenase and prothrombinase) that are formed during coagulation (Zwaal and Schroit, 1997). When platelets are activated, these negatively charged phospholipids translocate from the inner leaflet of the lipid bilayer of the plasma membrane to the outer surface of the platelet membrane, where they are exposed to the circulating coagulation factors. The anchoring of the tenase and prothrombinase complexes to the platelets in the platelet plug also leads to localization of the coagulation cascade and thrombin generation at the site of injury (Walsh, 2004).

The coagulation cascade

Since the 1960s, the blood coagulation system has been described mainly as a cascade involving a sequence of stages in which activated coagulation factors, mostly acting as enzymes, convert the subsequent coagulation factor (proenzyme) to its active form. Based on this theory, the amplification of the initial signal at different steps results finally in the formation of adequate amounts of thrombin and subsequently formation of sufficient fibrin. Factor V and FVIII, which are non-enzymatic protein cofactors, serve as catalysts in coagulation. Thrombin itself further activates inactive factors (e.g. FV and FVIII), significantly increasing the reaction rates of the tenase (FVIIIa) and prothrombinase (FVa) complexes, and thus amplifies the coagulation process (Figure 21.3).

Traditionally, the coagulation cascade has been divided into the extrinsic, intrinsic and common pathways, although the intrinsic and extrinsic pathways are interactive *in vivo*. The intrinsic system is initiated (within the blood) by contact activation of FXII on negatively charged surfaces (subsequently activating other contact components), and the extrinsic system is initiated by the interaction of tissue factor (TF, released by tissue trauma) and activated FVII. Both pathways result finally in FX activation to FXa. At that point the two paths converge into the common pathway (Figure 21.3).

This classical model has limitations in describing the situation *in vivo*, because it is now generally accepted that:

- *In vivo* the extrinsic pathway (i.e. via TF and FVIIa) is the primary pathway in the initiation of blood coagulation, whereas the intrinsic system seems to be more important in sustaining the coagulation process (Mann, 1999)
- The contact activation of blood coagulation *in vivo* does not play a major role as a starting reaction of the intrinsic system
- There are inter-relationships between coagulation factors of the extrinsic and intrinsic systems (i.e. the borderlines between the extrinsic and intrinsic pathways have blurred)
- The blood coagulation system functions in a close relationship with cells.

Nevertheless, the classical schedule with the separation of the intrinsic and extrinsic systems still has validity. The widely used group and global tests prothrombin time (PT) and activated partial thromboplastin time (aPTT) mimic activation via the extrinsic or intrinsic system, respectively (see Chapter 22). Therefore, the classical depiction of secondary coagulation provides an excellent basis for the understanding and interpretation of *in vitro* blood coagulation analyses and is helpful in the classification of clotting disorders.

Extrinsic pathway

The extrinsic pathway comprises the activation of FVII by association with TF. In comparison to other clotting factors, FVIIa is less inhibited by the major natural anticoagulant, antithrombin (AT). Of the total amount of FVII, 1–2% circulates under physiological conditions in its active form as FVIIa (Morrisey *et al.*, 1993). This FVIIa is available to initiate coagulation in response to endothelial damage and release of TF, a transmembrane glycoprotein of various cell and tissue types including endothelial cells and subendothelial fibroblasts. TF is not normally present in the circulation or expressed on cell surfaces, but when endothelial or subendothelial cells are damaged or activated, TF is expressed and exposed to the circulating coagulation factors. Activated FVII and TF with calcium ions (Ca^{2+}) comprise the 'tissue factor complex', which activates FX, but also FIX (the so called 'Josso loop'). In a positive feedback mechanism, further FVII molecules are activated by FVIIa–TF complexes and FXa. TF acts as a regulatory protein and increases (> 10^7 times) the rate at which FX, FIX and FVII are activated, which amplifies the process. The FVIIa–TF complex delivers only a small amount of FXa (by direct activation), and the additional activation of FX via FIXa as part of the tenase complex is therefore essential for the generation of an adequate amount of thrombin and subsequently fibrin.

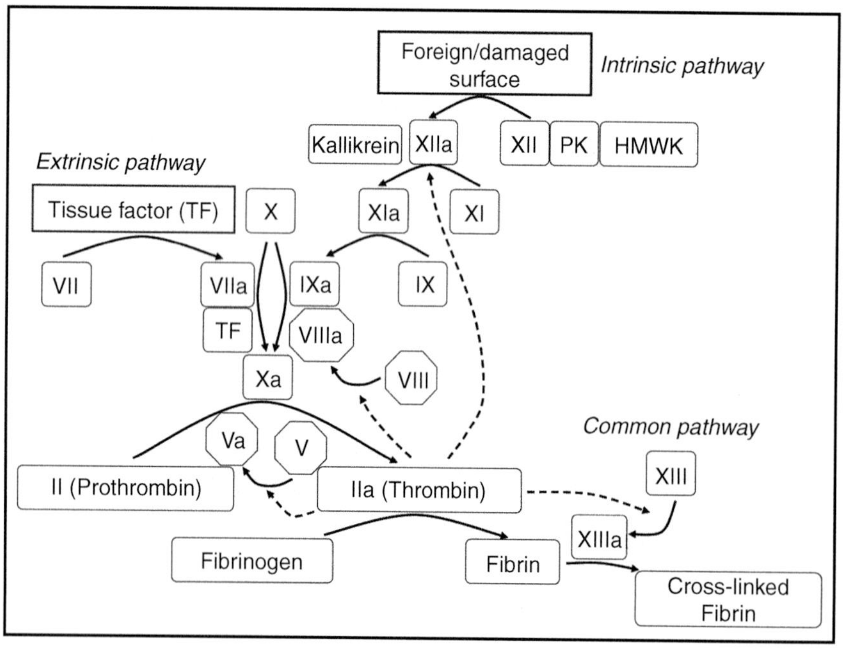

21.3 Schematic diagram of the classical cascade model of blood coagulation. HMWK, high molecular weight kininogen; PK, prekallikrein.

Intrinsic system, contact activation

Based on *in vitro* observations (e.g. the clotting of blood in glass tubes), the interaction of contact activation factors (FXII, prekallikrein and high molecular weight kininogen (HMWK)) was traditionally thought to initiate the intrinsic branch of the coagulation pathway. The essential initial autoactivation of FXII to FXIIa (which is associated with a change in its confirmation) is triggered by binding to a negatively charged surface such as (*in vitro*) glass, kaolin, ellagic acid and other contact activators that are used for the measurement of aPTT and activated clotting time. Surfaces that induce autoactivation of FXII under pathophysiological conditions *in vivo* include exposed subendothelial collagen, released platelet polysomes, aggregated proteins and tissue RNA (Schmair and LaRusch, 2010). In a positive feedback mechanism, FXIIa converts prekallikrein to kallikrein, which activates further FXII molecules. In addition, kallikrein also converts HMWK to the inflammatory mediator bradykinin. HMWK also acts as a non-enzymatic cofactor in the interaction between prekallikrein and FXII and the activation of FXI. FXIIa is able to initiate the intrinsic coagulation pathway by converting FXI to FXIa, which then activates FIX to FIXa. The contact activation culminates in the production of the 'tenase' complex, which consists of FIXa, FVIIIa, phospholipid and Ca^{2+} and effectively activates FX.

However, although the contact factors FXII, prekallikrein and HMWK are important for *in vitro* clotting tests, their significance for coagulation *in vivo* is doubtful, because deficiencies in these three contact factors are not associated with clinical bleeding disorders (see Chapter 25). *In vivo*, these three factors trigger a range of responses and are more important in the initiation of inflammation and fibrinolysis. In contrast, deficiencies in FXI, FIX and FVIII lead to bleeding disorders, which underlines the importance of these factors for normal coagulation. *In vivo* activation of these factors takes place efficiently in several steps by proteolytic action of the initially small amounts of thrombin generated during the initial activation of the extrinsic system (FXI, FVIII) and by FVII and TF (FIX; see above). *In vivo*, the intrinsic system seems to be more important in sustaining rather than initiating the coagulation cascade.

Common pathway, fibrin formation

The common pathway comprises activation of prothrombin by the prothrombinase complex (FXa, FVa, phospholipid and Ca^{2+}) as the final and central step in a cascade of enzymatic reactions and the subsequent rapid conversion of soluble fibrinogen to insoluble fibrin/fibrin monomers. Owing to the thrombin-mediated feedback activation of FV, FVIII and FXI, even minute amounts of thrombin result in a marked amplification of the coagulation cascade.

Fibrinogen is a large plasma protein that consists of two identical halves, each of which has three polypeptide chains (Aα, Bβ and γ) wound around each other to form a linear molecule. The so-called fibrinopeptides A and B represent the amino ends of the Aα and Bβ chains. These fibrinopeptides are highly negatively charged and this keeps the fibrinogen molecules apart from each other. Thrombin cleaves the negatively charged fibrinopeptides A and B from the fibrinogen molecule to form fibrin monomers. The amount and speed of thrombin generation determines whether a critical mass of fibrin monomers is achieved to induce polymerization of the soluble fibrin molecules into fibrin strands, which then aggregate spontaneously and precipitate as an insoluble fibrin matrix.

Further actions of thrombin are the activation of the fibrin stabilizing FXIII, which then cross-links the fibrin molecules, resulting in increased mechanical strength of the clot and increased resistance to fibrinolysis, and activation of thrombin activatable fibrinolysis inhibitor (TAFI). Therefore, fibrin structure depends on the amount of thrombin generated and the rate of thrombin generation. Only after generation of a large amount of thrombin does a tight, stable fibrin haemostatic plug form, which is resistant to fibrinolysis and is required for full and sustained haemostasis.

The firm cross-linked fibrin mesh (within the platelet plug) is less vulnerable to proteolysis by the fibrinolytic enzyme plasmin and results in a much stronger occlusion than the primary platelet plug. In addition, thrombin is a potent platelet agonist and guarantees continued formation of the platelet plug in primary haemostasis.

The cell-based model of blood coagulation

The classical model of haemostasis, which describes mostly separate functions for platelets (primary haemostasis) and coagulation factors (secondary haemostasis), and the blood coagulation system as a 'coagulation cascade', with enhancement of the signal from one step to the next step, has now been replaced by a new, cell-based model of coagulation (Figure 21.4) (Hoffman and Monroe, 2001; Smith, 2009). This understanding of *in vivo* haemostasis accentuates the role of the interaction of coagulation proteins with cell surfaces. In this model, the coagulation process is described in overlapping phases and with participation of two different cell types: TF-bearing cells and platelets.

Initiation

According to current knowledge, the main mechanism that initiates haemostasis is the formation of a complex between TF and pre-existing traces of FVIIa that are present in the circulating blood under physiological conditions (see above). Functionally active TF is expressed by cells localized outside the vasculature and, like collagen, it is present in the subendothelial matrix. In contrast, circulating cells such as monocytes and tumour cells, as well as microparticles, may express TF on their surfaces; this is normally encrypted and inactive. Thus, TF is exposed to blood after a vessel wall injury and FVIIa leaving the vasculature will bind to TF and

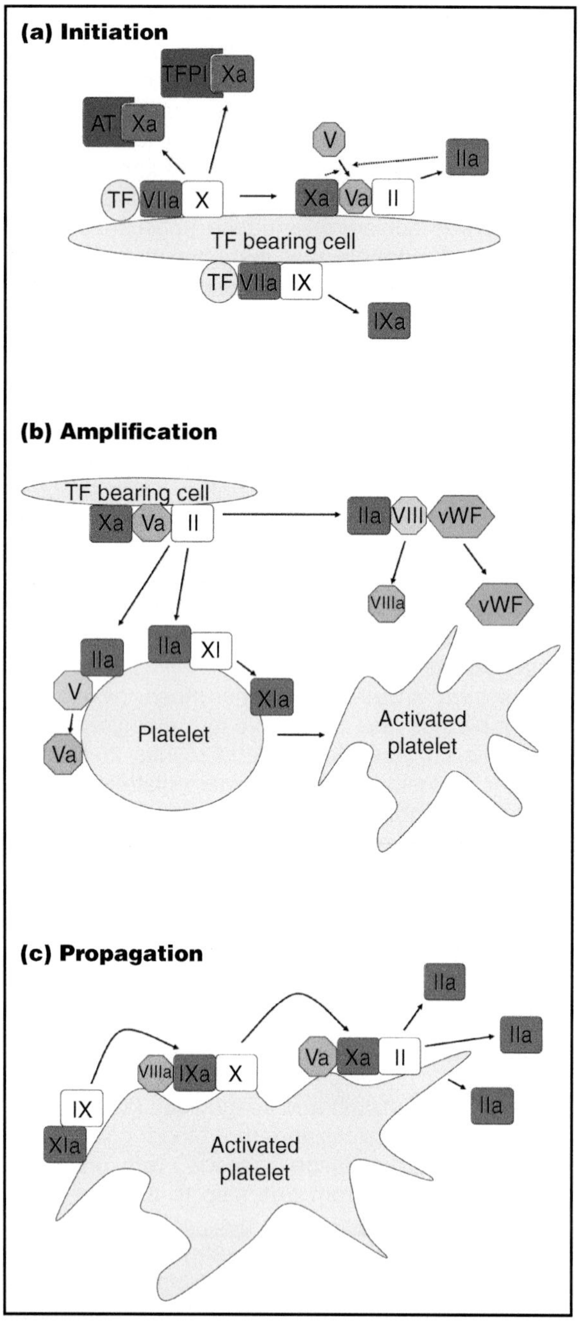

21.4 The cell-based model of fibrin formation accentuates the role of different cell types in fibrin generation in overlapping phases. **(a)** The initiation phase on the tissue factor (TF)-bearing cell after exposure of blood to TF-bearing cells at the site of injury results in generation of small amounts of factor (F)IXa and thrombin, which both diffuse away from the TF-bearing cell towards the platelet. **(b)** Amplification phase. A small amount of thrombin generated on the TF-bearing cell activates platelets, releases von Willebrand factor (vWF) and activates FV, FVIII and FXI. **(c)** Propagation phase. Activated clotting factors (in phases a and b) assemble on the procoagulant membrane surface of the activated platelet to form intrinsic tenase, which results in FXa generation on the platelet surface. A prothrombinase complex forms and results in the generation of large amounts of thrombin directly on platelets.

potentially initiate coagulation. Under physiological conditions (intact endothelium) initiation of coagulation is prevented.

Exposure of the blood to a TF-bearing cell at the site of vascular injury results in immediate binding of FVIIa to the exposed TF. In a positive feedback mechanism the TF–FVIIa complex activates additional FVII to FVIIa, resulting in an even larger amount of TF–FVIIa complexes. The TF–FVIIa complexes are activators of FX (into FXa) on the TF-bearing cell and also activate FIX. Initially, only small amounts of these two coagulation proteins are generated. The FXa binds to a small number of available active molecules of its cofactor FVa (FX is able to activate FV directly, but this occurs more slowly) to form a prothrombinase complex, which subsequently cleaves small amounts of prothrombin to generate thrombin. The activity of FXa is limited to the surface of the TF-bearing cell, because FXa molecules, which dissociate from the activated membrane surface, are inactivated immediately by AT or tissue factor pathway inhibitor (TFPI). In contrast, the FIXa generated can dissociate from the membrane and move to the surface of platelets or other nearby cells, because FIXa is much more slowly inhibited by AT than FXa and is not inhibited at all by TFPI.

Amplification

The small amount of thrombin that is generated initially on a TF-bearing cell diffuses into the flowing blood and promotes significant activation of blood coagulation, i.e. positive feedback, via different mechanisms:

- Thrombin-induced activation of FV and FVIII is important, because FVa and FVIIIa enhance blood coagulation and, thereby, result in marked amplification of the further generation of thrombin. In addition, FXI is activated; this, like activation of FV, takes place on the platelet surface
- Furthermore, before FVIII can be activated, it must be cleaved from vWF by thrombin. vWF circulates together with FVIII and, thereby, stabilizes FVIII and increases its half-life. The isolated vWF mediates platelet adhesion and aggregation
- Thrombin (released from the TF-bearing cell) binds to surface receptors of platelets that have leaked from the vasculature at the site of injury and is a potent platelet activator. Thrombin-activated platelets show a shape change that results in the exposure of negatively charged phospholipids (especially expression of phosphatidylserine) to create a procoagulant membrane surface that is the ideal template for the generation of larger amounts of FX and thrombin. In addition, activated platelets release granule contents that enhance haemostasis (see Primary haemostasis).

Propagation

The release of granule contents by the first small number of activated platelets (in the amplification phase) results in recruitment of a larger number of platelets to the site of injury. Their surface provides the location for the propagation phase. The platelets express ligands on their surface as the basis for platelet aggregation. FVIIIa (generated in the amplification phase) binds with FIXa on the platelet surface. Small amounts of FIXa are initially (initiation phase) generated by TF–FVIIa complexes and additional amounts are generated by cleavage of FIX by the FXIa that was generated on the platelet surface in the amplification phase.

The intrinsic tenase complex (FIXa, FVIIIa, Ca^{2+}) rapidly starts to generate large amounts of FXa on the (activated) platelet surface. The smaller amounts of FXa that have already been generated on the TF-bearing cell during the initiation phase are rapidly inhibited in the blood stream (after leaving the TF-bearing cell surface; Figure 21.5). The FXa that is generated on the platelet surface rapidly binds FVa (which is generated by thrombin in the amplification phase), and this prothrombinase complex effectively activates prothrombin, resulting in marked generation of thrombin. Thrombin cleaves fibrinopeptides from fibrinogen, resulting in fibrin formation (see Common pathway).

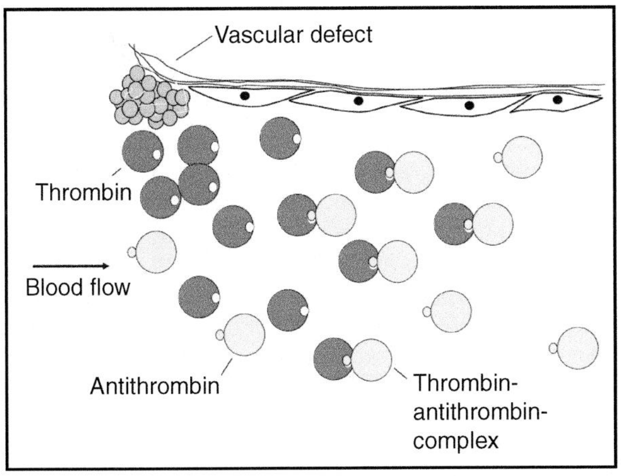

21.5 Schematic diagram illustrating the importance of blood flow in the inactivation of thrombin by antithrombin.

Inhibitors of coagulation

Natural inhibitors of blood coagulation are an essential regulatory mechanism for blood coagulation. The most important are AT, the protein C pathway and TFPI. They are located primarily on intact endothelial cells (e.g. in the periphery of the vessel wall defect), and control inappropriate activation, limit it to the essential site and terminate the clotting process. In addition, activated clotting factors that enter the flowing blood are diluted rapidly when the blood flows away from the site of injury, resulting in a decrease in the concentration of activated factors to levels below the inhibitory capacity of the inhibitors (Figure 21.5).

Antithrombin

AT is a glycoprotein (molecular mass 58 kDa) and is the most important plasma inhibitor of activated coagulation factors of the serine protease type. Its most important target is thrombin, followed by FXa, FIXa and FXIa, but it is probably a poor inhibitor of FVIIa. The anticoagulant activity of circulating AT is enhanced greatly by binding to the heparan sulphate polymers. Small amounts of heparin sulphate proteoglycans are normally present on endothelial cell surfaces and participate in controlling the coagulation process at the margin of the site of vascular injury. In addition, the catalytic effect on the induction of inhibitory interactions between activated factors and AT is the main anticoagulant effect of therapeutically administered heparin.

Protein C pathway (protein C, thrombomodulin, protein S)

The protein C pathway comprises thrombin, thrombomodulin, the endothelial cell protein C receptor (EPCR), protein C and protein S (Figure 21.6). Proteins C and S are vitamin K-dependent anticoagulant plasma proteins that circulate in the plasma as inactive precursors. The protein C pathway is one of the most important systems controlling thrombosis.

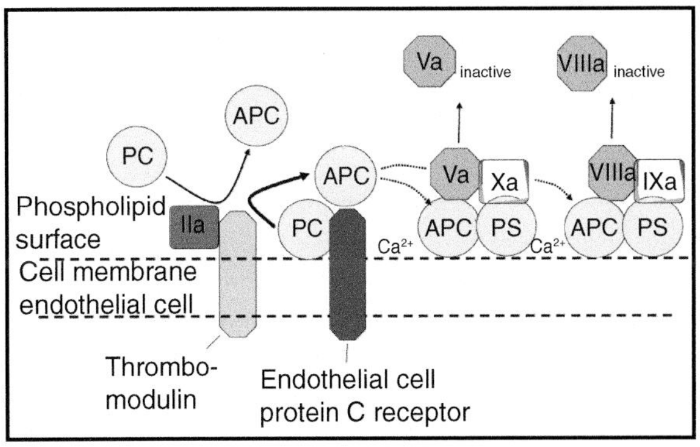

21.6 The protein C system. APC, activated protein C; PC, protein C; PS, protein S.

The pathway starts with the binding of thrombin to thrombomodulin on the surface of intact endothelial cells in the area surrounding the vascular defect, which limits the clot formation to this site (Esmon, 2003). By binding to thrombomodulin, the procoagulant potential of thrombin is inhibited directly. In addition, thrombin bound to thrombomodulin is inactivated by plasma protease inhibitors faster than free thrombin, and it then dissociates rapidly from thrombomodulin, resulting in enhanced clearance from the circulation. Proportional to the amount of thrombin present, i.e. the extent of the coagulation response, the complex activates protein C to its active form (APC), i.e. the potent procoagulant thrombin is not only activated but converted to an anticoagulant. The complex also activates TAFI. By binding to EPCR, *in vivo* activation of protein C is augmented approximately 20-fold and presented to the thrombin–thrombomodulin complex. After dissociation from EPCR, APC binds to its cofactor protein S via Ca^{2+} on appropriate negatively charged phospholipid cell surfaces. The activated protein C–protein S complex inactivates FVa and FVIIIa, resulting in inhibition of the tenase and prothrombinase complexes and limiting further thrombin generation. The activated protein C–protein S complex also initiates fibrinolysis.

In addition, thrombomodulin has direct anti-inflammatory activity, which reduces cytokine formation by the endothelium and decreases leucocyte–endothelial cell adhesion. APC–EPCR complexes appear to play a role in the cellular signalling mechanisms that down-regulate formation of inflammatory cytokines such as tumour necrosis factor and interleukin-6.

Tissue factor pathway inhibitor

TFPI (also called extrinsic pathway inhibitor) is bound to endothelial cell surfaces and is also released in small amounts from activated platelets. It inhibits FXa and then the FVIIa–TF complex (but not free FVIIa). TFPI is the most important inhibitor of the extrinsic pathway. The system acts as a further negative feedback mechanism, because after formation of a certain amount of FXa, this is partly bound to TFPI and inhibits FVIIa–TF. The concentration of TFPI is increased during heparin therapy, owing to its release from the vasculature as an important side-effect of this therapy, and contributes to prolongation of aPTT.

Fibrinolysis

The final stage in haemostasis is the repair of the damaged vessel wall and dissolution of the fibrin clot to re-establish vascular patency and restore normal blood flow (Narayanan, 1998) (Figure 21.7). Fibrinolysis is mediated by the proteolytic enzyme plasmin. This is derived from an inactive precursor (plasminogen), which is synthesized by the liver. Plasmin degrades fibrinogen and fibrin, including cross-linked fibrin, within a clot to release fibrin degradation products, including the cross-linked fragment D-dimer.

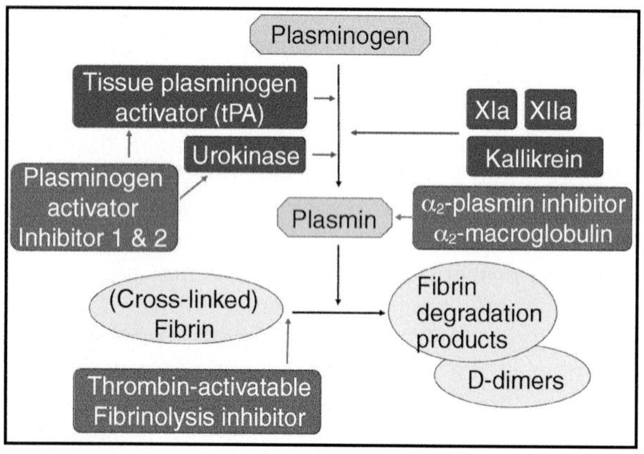

21.7 The fibrinolytic system. Activators are indicated in blue boxes; inhibitors of fibrinolysis are indicated in red boxes.

The most potent activators of plasminogen to plasmin are tissue-type plasminogen activator (tPA) and urokinase-type plasminogen activator (uPA). The tPA is synthesized and released by vascular endothelial cells in response to a wide range of stimuli, including bradykinin from contact activation and catecholamines. The released tPA binds initially to fibrin and only then is able to bind plasminogen and activate it to plasmin, whereas circulating tPA is rapidly removed by the liver resulting in a short half-life of about 5 minutes. Therefore, tPA activity is localized to the site of clot formation.

The uPA is secreted primarily by the kidneys as an inactive precursor. It is activated by the contact factors kallikrein, HMWK and FXII as well as by plasmin, and appears to function primarily within urine and tissues. FXIIa also activates plasminogen, either directly or via activation of FXI and prekallikrein. Kallikrein then activates HMWK, which also converts plasminogen to plasmin.

Similar to blood coagulation, fibrinolysis is controlled by specific plasma inhibitors that inactivate plasmin and the plasminogen activators. Plasmin is inhibited by α_2 plasmin inhibitor and α_2 macroglobulin. Plasminogen-activator inhibitor I (PAI-1), secreted by endothelial cells, hepatocytes and platelets, is the most important inhibitor of tPA and uPA. Almost all circulating tPA is bound to PAI-1, and only the tPA attached to fibrin is able to activate plasminogen. TAFI partly degrades the carboxyterminal binding sites for plasminogen in fibrin, which are a prerequisite for binding and interaction with tPA.

Fibrin(ogen) degradation products, which are released by fibrinogen(olysis), have anticoagulant effects, mainly by interfering with fibrin polymerization. In addition, plasmin degrades FVa and FVIIIa. These are further important negative feedback mechanisms that control excessive coagulation.

References and further reading

Esmon CT (2003) The protein C pathway. *Chest* **124**(Suppl.3), 26S–32S
Hawiger J (1990) Platelet-vessel wall interactions. Platelet adhesion and aggregation. *Atherosclerosis Reviews* **21**, 165–186
Hoffman M and Monroe DM 3rd (2001) A cell-based model of hemostasis. *Thrombosis and Hemostasis* **85**, 958–965.
Mann KG (1999) Blood coagulation. *Alcoholism: Clinical and Experimental Research* **23**, 1111–1113
Morrisey JH, Macik BG, Neuenschwander PF and Comp PC (1993) Quantitation of activation factor VII levels in plasma using a tissue factor mutant selectively deficient in promoting factor VII activation. *Blood* **81**, 734–744
Narayanan S (1998) Current concepts of coagulation and fibrinolysis. *Advances in Clinical Chemistry* **33**, 133–168
Ruggeri ZM and Ware J (1992) The structure and function of von Willebrand factor. *Thrombosis and Haemostasis* **67**, 594–599
Schmair AH and LaRusch G (2010) Factor XII: New life for an old protein. *Thrombosis and Haemostasis* **104**, 915–918
Smith SA (2009) The cell-based model of coagulation. *Journal of Veterinary Emergency and Critical Care* **19**, 3–10
Walsh PN (2004) Platelet coagulation-protein interactions. *Seminars in Thrombosis and Hemostasis* **30**, 461–471
Zwaal RFA and Schroit AJ (1997) Pathophysiologic implications of membrane phospholipid asymmetry in blood cells. *Blood* **89**, 1121–1132

22

Haemostasis: diagnostic techniques

Reinhard Mischke

Introduction

Adequate haemostasis depends on normal structure and function of the blood vascular system, the number and functional integrity of platelets, and an adequate coagulation system, including stability of the fibrin clot. The vascular component is rarely diagnosed as the cause of haemostatic disorders, because standardized tests for vascular haemostatic dysfunctions do not exist in veterinary medicine. In contrast, haemostatic disorders caused by quantitative or qualitative platelet defects or coagulation system disorders can be defined.

A detailed history and a thorough clinical examination can suggest an underlying haemostatic disorder and the nature of the disorder. The pattern of bleeding can indicate the cause of a haemorrhagic diathesis. Mucosal and cutaneous petechiae, purpura and ecchymoses are characteristic findings in disorders of primary haemostasis (i.e. thrombocytopenia, thrombocytopathia). In contrast, blood coagulation disorders such as haemophilia are associated with larger areas of haemorrhage (e.g. subcutaneous or intramuscular haematomas, body cavity and joint haemorrhages). Bleeding from mucosal surfaces (e.g. epistaxis, oral cavity haemorrhage, haematemesis, haematuria, haematochezia and melaena) can be associated with disorders of primary or secondary haemostasis.

Laboratory tests are required to establish the presence or absence of most haemostatic disorders. A basic haemostasis profile can be performed in a practice laboratory. This enables a rational assessment of haemostatic function and, in case of a disorder, in many cases allows definition of the haemostatic disorder or indicates which specific tests should be chosen to make a final diagnosis. The performance of these specific tests (e.g. factor (F) VIII and IX measurements for the diagnosis of haemophilia) is usually restricted to a specialist veterinary diagnostic laboratory.

Indications for haemostasis testing

Spontaneous bleeding (without detectable cause), bleeding disproportionate to the degree of trauma and bleeding from multiple sites are indicative of a haemostatic disorder and, therefore, these clinical findings should prompt laboratory tests of haemostasis (Figure 22.1). These may also be indicated in animals without actual or historical bleeding, for example as preoperative screening or as part of breeding programmes.

- Haemorrhages, swellings and body cavity effusions of uncertain origin
- Underlying diseases that are frequently associated with haemostatic disorders (e.g. liver diseases, haemangiosarcoma)
- Monitoring of known haemostatic disorders
- Control of anticoagulant and fibrinolytic therapy
- Preoperative screening
- Breeding programmes

22.1 Indications for laboratory evaluation of haemostasis in small animals.

Sample collection and handling

Haemostasis tests rely more on blood sampling techniques than most other laboratory diagnostic procedures. Blood anticoagulated with potassium–ethylenediamine tetra-acetic acid (EDTA) is the standard sample required for platelet counts. Citrated blood can also be used, and may be better for cats because formation of platelet clumps is reduced. It may also be used in rare cases of suspected pseudothrombocytopenia (i.e. artificially low platelet counts caused by EDTA-induced aggregates). Platelet counts from citrated blood must be multiplied by 1.11 to correct the dilution caused by the citrate solution.

Coagulation tests are performed with plasma prepared from blood anticoagulated with sodium citrate or citrate buffer. For platelet aggregation studies (e.g. with the Multiplate analyser) hirudin-anticoagulated blood provides the best results (Kalbantner *et al.*, 2010).

Sample tubes for citrated blood

Sample containers are available from various manufacturers. These are prefilled with 0.11 mol/l sodium citrate or citrate buffer solution to guarantee a ratio of 9 parts blood to 1 part anticoagulant when the tubes are filled appropriately. Alternatively, graduated plastic tubes or syringes can be filled with an adequate amount of anticoagulant. In cases of remarkably increased or decreased haematocrit (Hct), controlled over- or underfilling, respectively, of the tubes with blood is recommended to achieve an adequate ratio between the plasma and citrate solution (Figure 22.2).

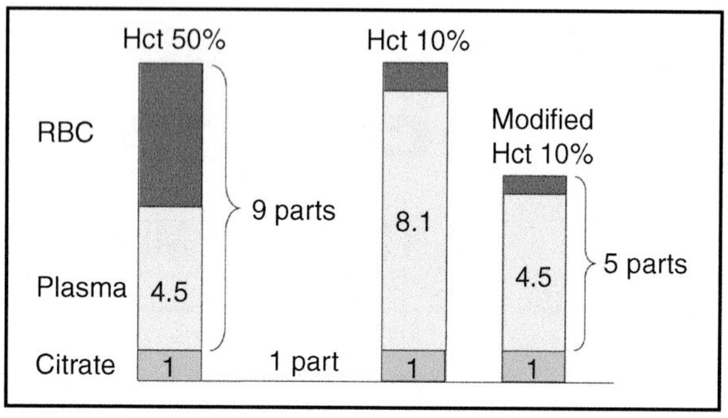

22.2 Influence of haematocrit (Hct) on the ratio of blood to anticoagulant in citrated blood. In a sample with normal haematocrit (50%), the ratio between plasma and citrate is approximately 4.5:1 (left-hand column), whereas the ratio is approximately 8:1 in a sample with a haematocrit of 10% (middle column). Deliberate underfilling of the tube to approximately 60% results in an adequate ratio (right-hand column).

Blood collection

Blood collection should be carried out without raising the vein if possible, or by raising the vein only slightly and briefly (< 30 seconds), to avoid significant activation of the haemostatic and fibrinolytic system. A sharp disposable needle with an adequate lumen (e.g. 20 gauge/1.1 mm (dogs), 18 gauge/0.9 mm (cats)) should be used. The first drops of blood should be discarded or used for other sample tubes to avoid contamination of the samples with tissue thromboplastin, because this may result in misleading results caused by activation of clotting factors and/or platelets. The blood should flow gently from the needle along the wall of the tube. If citrated blood is obtained with a syringe, aspiration should be performed carefully, because a high vacuum can lead to activation of the coagulation system. Therefore, the vacutainer system is not ideal for coagulation tests. To guarantee correct mixing of the collected blood with the anticoagulant (sodium citrate), tubes should be swayed gently while the blood is being collected, and after the blood collection is finished the tube (or syringe) must be gently agitated or revolved several times.

Citrated plasma preparation

Centrifugation of the sample (for 10 minutes at 1500–2000 × *g*) and subsequent removal by pipette of the (platelet-poor) citrated plasma supernatant should be performed as quickly as possible, at the latest within 2 hours of blood collection. Immediately before centrifugation, the sample should be checked for possible clots and partially or completely coagulated samples should be discarded.

Storage stability and sample transport

For many years the storage stability of blood coagulation factors in unfrozen samples was underestimated. Only minimal changes in the results of routine coagulation tests (i.e. prothrombin time (PT) and activated partial thromboplastin time (aPTT)) occur after storage at room temperature for up to 48 hours (Furlanello *et al.*, 2006). Therefore, transport of samples of citrated plasma or blood to specialized laboratories via overnight express is possible and the sample does not require freezing or special cooling. The exact requirements may differ among laboratories, and it is advisable to discuss these with the laboratory beforehand.

Global testing

Global tests assess the overall haemostatic function of a blood sample, including the interaction between the platelets and the coagulation system. These include simple tests, such as the whole blood clotting time or the activated clotting time (ACT), as well as automatic viscoelastic point-of-care haemostatic assays. These methods are easy to perform and can be used as patient-side tests. Generally, these methods have limited sensitivity with respect to the detection of decreased individual haemostatic components.

Activated clotting time

Test principle

The ACT is a simple screening test that measures the clotting time of fresh whole blood after contact activation and, thereby, the intrinsic and common coagulation pathways. A normal result also requires an adequate platelet count (Bateman *et al.*, 1999). It is important to avoid contamination of the blood sample with tissue factor (TF) at the time of collection because this will activate the extrinsic pathway.

Method

An ACT tube containing diatomaceous earth is prewarmed to 37°C and venepuncture performed. To minimize contamination with tissue factor, 0.25–0.5 ml of blood is drawn into the syringe and discarded, and 2 ml of blood is then drawn and added to the ACT tube. Alternatively, if collected directly into a vacutainer tube, the first 0.25–0.5 ml can be collected into one tube, which may be discarded, and the ACT tube can then be attached and filled. The timer is started as soon as the blood enters the ACT tube. The sample is mixed gently by inversion, then placed in a 37°C heating block or water bath (60 seconds for dogs and 45 seconds for cats) or incubated in the closed hand of the investigator. It is then tilted at 10-second intervals until the first clot is observed; this may precede coagulation of the entire sample.

Interpretation

The ACT ranges from 60–110 seconds in normal dogs and from 50–75 seconds in normal cats. Prolongation of the ACT indicates a severe abnormality of the intrinsic and/or common pathways (e.g. hypofibrinogenaemia). The ACT will also be prolonged in severe thrombocytopenia (< 10×10^9 platelets/l).

Thromboelastography/thromboelastometry

The current leading point-of-care systems for the investigation of haemostasis are thromboelastography (TEG) and rotation thromboelastometry (ROTEM).

Test principle and indication

The method assesses the viscoelastic properties of clotting whole blood, including fibrinolysis, under low shear conditions. It gives an overview of the whole function of haemostasis. The method is particularly useful for the detection of hypercoagulable states (Wiinberg *et al.*, 2008).

Method

Blood is collected in a purpose-designed cup that is heated to 37°C. Either native blood or recalcified citrated blood can serve as the sample, in each case with or without addition of activating agents (i.e. tissue factor or kaolin). A pin is suspended within the cup and connected to a detector system (a torsion wire in TEG and an optical detector in ROTEM). The cup and pin are oscillated relative to each other through an angle of 4 degrees for 45 minutes. The movement is initiated from either the cup (TEG) or the pin (ROTEM). When fibrin forms between the cup and pin, the rotation transmitted from the cup to the pin (TEG) or the impedance of the rotation of the pin (ROTEM) are detected at the pin and registered on a graph. The different parts of the graph reflect different stages of the haemostatic process (clotting time, kinetics of fibrin formation, strength of the clot, and fibrinolysis) (Figure 22.3a). The nomenclature is slightly different between TEG and ROTEM.

Interpretation

Different haemostatic disorders are indicated by characteristic tracings (Figure 22.3b), whereas the automated numerical analysis of the graph is less important. The evaluation of the haemostatic system in whole blood allows investigation of the combined influence of cellular (i.e. platelets, erythrocytes and leucocytes) and plasma elements on clot formation. Therefore, viscoelastic tests give an impression of the total haemostatic potential of a sample. In contrast to clotting tests, the method provides information about the strength/stability of the clot and possible hyperfibrinolysis.

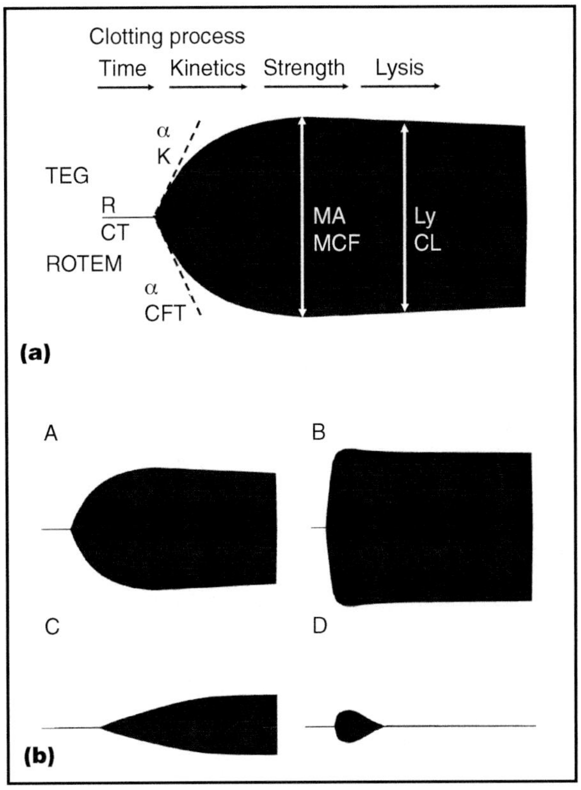

22.3 Schematic TEG/ROTEM traces indicating: **(a)** the commonly reported variables: reaction time (R)/clotting time (CT), clot formation time (K/CFT), alpha angle (α), maximum amplitude (MA)/maximum clot firmness (MCF), and lysis (Ly)/clot lysis (CL), and **(b)** different characteristic patterns: A normal, B hypercoagulability, C hypocoagulability (e.g. thrombocytopenia/thrombocytopathia), D primary hyperfibrinolysis.

Basic haemostasis profile

A basic profile for haemostasis usually includes platelet count, PT (one-stage PT, thromboplastin time) and aPTT. It may be expanded by measurement of thrombin time and/or fibrinogen concentration when PT and aPTT are prolonged, in order to differentiate further whether the final stage of blood coagulation (thrombin–fibrinogen interaction, fibrin formation) is affected. Additional measurement of capillary bleeding time is indicated in cases where platelet dysfunction or von Willebrand's disease (vWD) are suspected.

Platelet count

Estimation in blood smear

The semiquantitative estimation of the platelet count in a peripheral blood smear can be used to verify the thrombocytopenia measured by an automated blood cell counter. In addition, platelet morphology (size, activation status, aggregates) can be evaluated. Normal platelets appear as small (2–4 µm diameter, quarter to half the diameter of an erythrocyte (in dogs)) anucleate round to oval cells that stain faintly basophilic. Small reddish granules may be visible in the centre, especially in feline platelets, which are usually larger and more visible than those from dogs.

Method: A blood smear from a sample collected in EDTA is stained with a Romanowsky stain such as Wright, Giemsa, Diff-Quik or RapiDiff and scanned under low power to determine the presence of any platelet clumps. If present, these are usually found in the feathered edge and along the sides of the smear and will result in falsely decreased platelet counts. The presence of platelet clumps does not necessarily mean that the platelet count is adequate (Grindem *et al.*, 1991). Inwards from the feathered edge, a good blood smear should have a monolayer area with evenly distributed cells, which is ideal for detailed assessment of platelets and other cells. In this area, each platelet in an oil immersion field (×1000 total magnification) represents approximately 15 × 10^9 platelets/l.

Interpretation: More than 10 platelets/oil immersion field (as a median of several fields assessed) is equivalent to an approximate platelet count of ≥ 150 × 10^9/l. Large platelets (shift platelets or megathrombocytes) may be seen when there is excessive platelet destruction and a regenerative platelet response, with the exception of primary immune-mediated thrombocytopenia (Dircks *et al.*, 2009). Shift platelets may also be seen in infiltrative diseases of the bone marrow and as a breed variant in Cavalier King Charles Spaniels and Norfolk Terriers (Gelain *et al.*, 2010). Small platelets (microthrombocytosis) may be seen in iron-deficiency anaemia.

Manual (visual) platelet count

Method: Manual platelet counts are simple to perform, but have an inherent coefficient of variation of 20–25%, even when performed by experienced personnel. Commercial kits that include a diluent system (e.g. Unopette Microcollection System for WBC/Platelet Determination, Becton-Dickinson, Oxford, UK; ThromboPlus, Sarstedt, Nümbrecht, Germany) simplify visual platelet counting in EDTA blood by use of a counting chamber. EDTA-blood is added to commercial tubes containing 2 ml of a medium that dilutes the sample appropriately and causes haemolysis of red cells. Addition of the blood to these tubes can be achieved using the EDTA-coated capillary tubes provided in the kits or by pipetting the same volume of EDTA-blood (20 µl, or 100 µl in cases of thrombocytopenia) into the tube (Figure 22.4a). After complete haemolysis (about 10 minutes), a Neubauer haemocytometer is loaded by capillary action, taking care not to overfill the counting chamber. The haemocytometer is placed in a humid chamber (a small container with a lid, such as a Petri dish, containing a layer of wet filter paper) for 5–10 minutes while the platelets settle. The platelets in five group quadrants are counted in the central part of the haemocytometer by using the high-dry (40×) objective and a lowered condenser (Figure 22.4b). This count is performed for both sides of the chamber and an average is calculated. If 100 µl of EDTA-blood is used, the average is the platelet count (× 10^9/l), and if 20 µl is used, the result must be multiplied by 5.

Interpretation: Healthy dogs have platelet counts of 150–500 × 10^9/l and healthy cats 180–550 × 10^9/l. Platelet numbers must decrease below 60 × 10^9/l to cause a significantly increased risk of bleeding.

Automated platelet count

Numerous cell counters optimized for veterinary medicine with integrated software packages for animals, and which have been validated for different animal species, are currently available for veterinary practice. Automated platelet counts are more precise and, in dogs, more accurate than manual counts because many thousands of cells are evaluated in each sample. In contrast, cell counters often provide inaccurate platelet counts in cats because of the small size of red blood cells in cats and the tendency of feline platelets to form aggregates. Spurious thrombocytopenia occurs in Cavalier King Charles Spaniels, partly caused by the presence of large platelets as a breed variant. False counting can also occur if small or large platelets are not detected by the machine because of inappropriate machine settings or calibration.

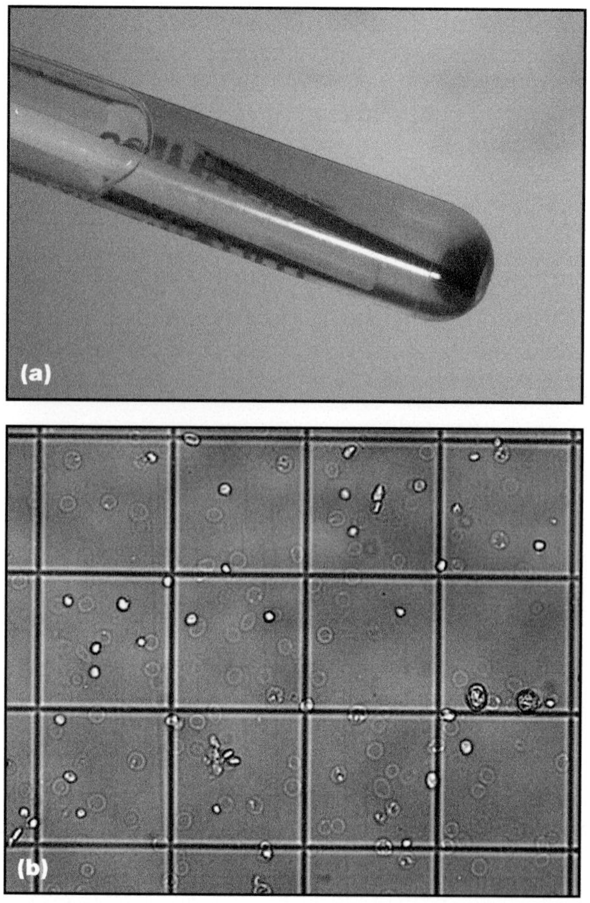

22.4 Visual platelet count. **(a)** The contents of a capillary tube containing EDTA blood are emptied into a sample tube containing a haemolytic and dilution medium (Thrombo Plus system). The figure also demonstrates the sample applicator stick (within the tube), which is attached to the lid of the sample tube and can be used to load the haemocytometer by capillary action. **(b)** In the counting chamber, platelets are detected as small dots with a light centre and must be differentiated from the larger white blood cells (in the middle of the right-hand side, two white blood cells can be seen; cell shadows in the background represent lysed red blood cells).

Bleeding time

The (capillary) bleeding time is defined as the time until a standardized episode of capillary bleeding ceases; it is a useful *in vivo* screening test for the function of primary haemostasis. It is indicated in patients with suspected platelet function disorders or vWD, i.e. in patients with haemorrhagic diathesis with normal platelet counts and clotting test results. Furthermore, it is a useful pre-surgical screening test to rule out defective primary haemostasis in an animal with no current clinical evidence of bleeding.

Capillary bleeding time in dogs is measured preferably in the non-anaesthetized dog held in lateral recumbency (Nolte *et al.*, 1997). This method is, in the experience of the author, superior to the widely used buccal mucosal bleeding time (BMBT) with regard to feasibility, possibility of standardization, and safety (i.e. the ability to stop bleeding with a bandage in cases with severe haemostatic disorders). Some experience with either of these techniques in healthy animals is essential if meaningful and reproducible bleeding times are to be obtained.

A technique for measuring the cuticle bleeding time has been described (Giles *et al.*, 1982). This is sensitive to coagulation defects as well as primary haemostatic defects, but anaesthesia is recommended and the endpoint may be more difficult to determine than with the capillary bleeding times.

Bleeding time at the toe

Technique: Non-anaesthetized dogs are held in lateral recumbency (Nolte *et al.*, 1997) (Figure 22.5).

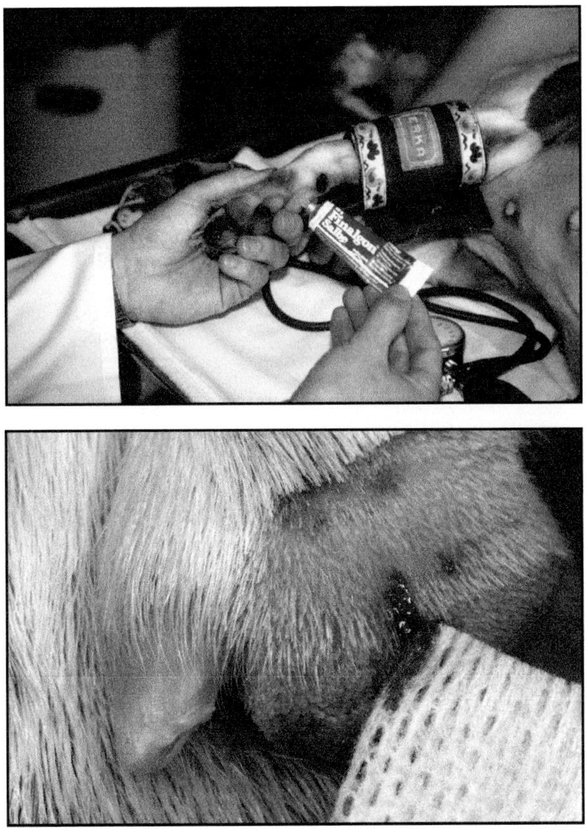

22.5 Capillary bleeding time. A non-anaesthetized dog is held in lateral recumbency and a hyperaemic agent is applied to the shaved lateral side of a front toe. A blood lancet is used to make two punctures close to the edge of the keratinized skin of the footpad. The bleeding time is detected by carefully dabbing the blood from these two sites with a swab every 15 seconds until the bleeding stops.

The skin of the lateral side of a front toe is shaved and a hyperaemic agent (Finalgone Creme, Boehringer Ingelhelm, Germany) is applied to the shaved area for 1 minute and wiped off. Subsequently, a sphygmomanometer cuff, which was previously placed above the antebrachium, is inflated to apply a pressure of 60 mmHg. This is performed to increase and standardize blood flow in the puncture area. One minute after applying this pressure, the skin is punctured twice, 5 mm apart, with a sterile manual or semi-automatic blood lancet, close to the edge of the keratinized skin of the footpad. The blood is dabbed off carefully every 15 seconds with a swab until the bleeding stops (i.e. until there are no traces of blood noticeable on the swab). The average time from making the two punctures is calculated as the capillary bleeding time. The reference value in the dog is 1–2.5 minutes.

Interpretation: Prolonged capillary bleeding times can be associated with severe thrombocytopenia, platelet function disorders or vWD. In patients with normal platelet counts, capillary bleeding time serves as a screening test for platelet function disorders and vWD. Severe vWD can be associated with extremely prolonged haemorrhage from puncture sites that may require application of a bandage.

Buccal mucosal bleeding time (BMBT)

Method: The BMBT test is performed with the animal held in lateral recumbency, with minimal physical restraint or light sedation. The upper lip is folded back and held in place by a gauze bandage; this must be tied tightly enough to impede the venous return from the lip and cause congestion (Figure 22.6). An incision is made in a non-vascular area of the mucosa with a spring-loaded cutting device (e.g. Simplate II, Organon Teknika, Cambridge, UK; Surgicutt, Ortho Diagnostic Systems, High Wycombe, UK). The edge of a piece of filter (blotting) paper is used to absorb the blood (the paper must be held away from the edges of the incision so as not to disturb the developing clot). The time from making the incision to the cessation of bleeding is recorded. If the animal has signs of defective primary haemostasis, caution is needed because it can be difficult to stop the bleeding in this location.

Interpretation: The bleeding time ranges from 1.7 to 4.2 minutes for healthy dogs (Jergens *et al.*, 1987) and from 1.0 to 2.4 minutes for healthy cats (Parker *et al.*, 1988). These values may differ slightly depending on technique, and each clinician should test the method on healthy animals before using the BMBT on animals with suspected bleeding disorders.

Blood coagulation tests (global tests, group tests)

In order to test the plasma coagulation system, the screening tests PT and aPTT are widely used. These tests evaluate the whole plasma coagulation system with the exception of the FXIII-dependent fibrin cross-linking (Figure 22.7). Each of these 'group tests' evaluates several coagulation factors of

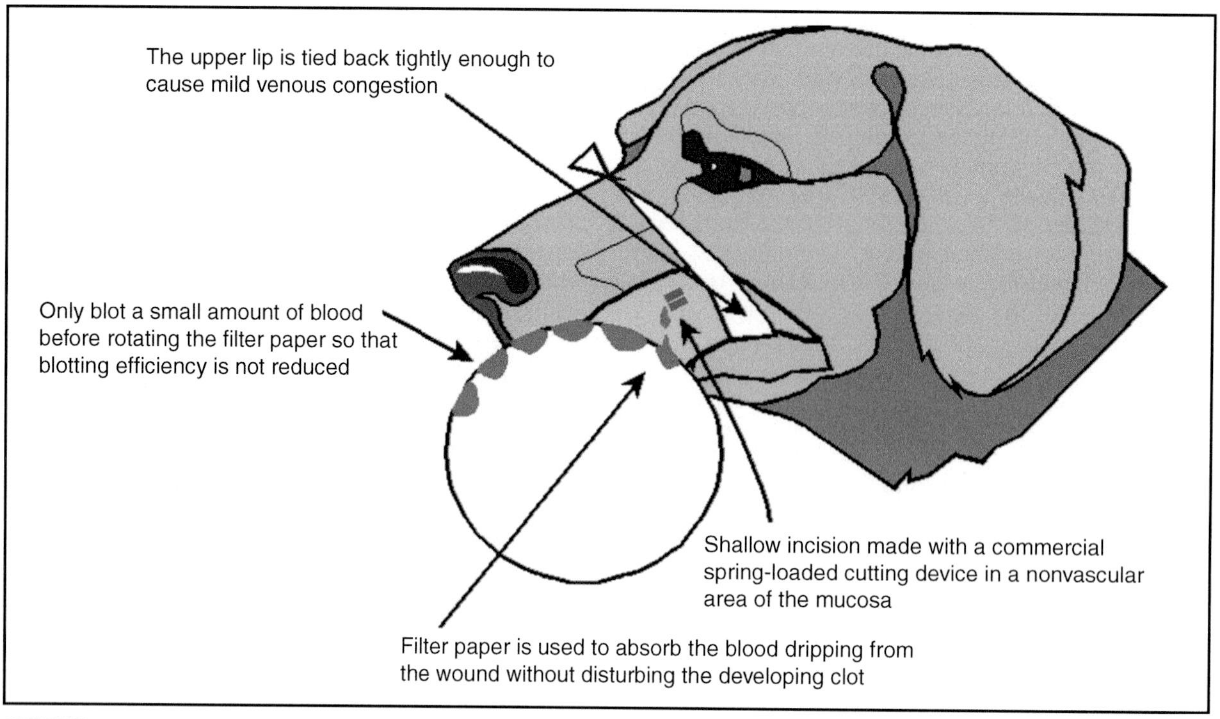

The upper lip is tied back tightly enough to cause mild venous congestion
Only blot a small amount of blood before rotating the filter paper so that blotting efficiency is not reduced
Shallow incision made with a commercial spring-loaded cutting device in a nonvascular area of the mucosa
Filter paper is used to absorb the blood dripping from the wound without disturbing the developing clot

22.6 Technique for the measurement of buccal mucosal bleeding time (BMBT) in the dog.

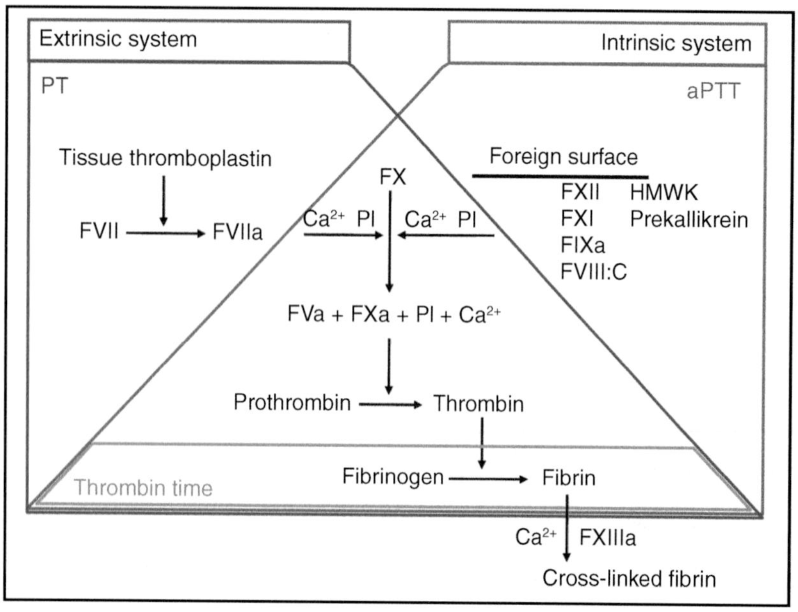

22.7 Classical schedule of the haemostasis system, indicating areas examined by the three group tests: prothrombin time (PT), activated partial thromboplastin time (aPTT) and thrombin time. Ca, calcium ions; F, (coagulation) factor; HMWK, high molecular weight kininogen; PL, phospholipid.

the extrinsic and common or intrinsic and common pathways, respectively. Both screening tests may miss mild reductions in individual factors, especially when measurements are performed with tests optimized for the determination of human plasma and/or with insensitive reagents. On the other hand, deficiency of selected clotting factors (e.g. prekallikrein, FXII) may produce abnormal screening test results although the animal does not show an increased bleeding tendency. When both tests are prolonged, the complementary measurement of thrombin time, the third group test, is indicated.

Coagulation tests measure the time taken for citrated platelet-poor plasma to clot when coagulation is initiated by the addition of calcium and activating agents. Blood coagulation tests are usually performed with coagulometric methods, but can also be performed with chromogenic assays. Coagulation times can be measured by manual techniques (tilt tube, hook technique) with visual detection of the time point of clot formation, but these techniques require considerable practice to obtain reliable results. Preferably, semi-automated or automated coagulometers are used, which are based on different electromechanical principles (e.g. Schnitger and Gross coagulometer based on the hook technique, ball coagulometer) or photo-optical techniques that detect a change in the intensity of light transmission when clot formation occurs. In addition, point-of-care analysers with test cartridges for PT and aPTT in animals are available (e.g. VetScan VSpro Coagulation Analyzer).

Prothrombin time

Test principle: The PT imitates the activation of coagulation via the extrinsic pathway and measures the coagulation factors of the extrinsic (FVII) and common pathways (FX, FV, FII and fibrinogen). Clotting is initiated by adding calcium and tissue thromboplastin, which provides tissue factor and substitutes for the negatively charged phospholipid surface provided by platelets *in vivo*.

Method: The PT measured in canine or feline plasma following the manufacturer's test instructions ('PT standard test') is significantly shorter than in humans; the test is not sufficiently sensitive to detect decreased coagulation factor activity. In specialized laboratories, the use of an optimized test (e.g. 100 µl 1:20 diluted sample, 100 µl fibrinogen solution (to guarantee adequate fibrin clot formation), incubation for 2 minutes, 100 µl Ca-thromboplastin reagent) is preferable to the standard test for use in dogs and cats (Mischke and Nolte, 1997). Apart from the modified test, commercial PT test modifications such as Hepato Quick (Roche Diagnostics GmbH, Mannheim, Germany) or Normotest (Technoclone GmbH, Vienna, Austria) are suitable screening tests of the extrinsic system in dogs and cats. In general, reagents based on animal-derived thromboplastins appear to be better activators of animal coagulation than synthetic or recombinant human thromboplastins.

Standardization: Commercial reagents have a low batch-to-batch variability, indicating that the preparation of lot-specific reference values is not required. Calculation of prothrombin (time) ratios or percentage activity values (derived from a reference curve prepared with pooled canine/feline plasma) may minimize differences between different lots of one defined reagent, if an adequate and consistent standard material is available. However, even after calculating a prothrombin ratio or converting the result to the percentage of normal activity, it is impossible to get a reagent-independent result (Mischke, 2011).

Reference values: The use of reference values specific for the animal species, reagent, method and instrumentation is important for the interpretation of the results of group tests and also of other haemostasis test procedures. Therefore, these reference values are best established in the laboratory itself and should be based on a sufficient number of healthy animals of the respective species (at least 40). Alternatively, as a rough guide, one or preferably two controls from healthy individuals from the relevant animal species can be used, especially if samples are submitted to a human laboratory that does not have much experience in the measurement of animal samples.

Interpretation: Prolongation of the PT standard test indicates a significant deficiency in coagulation, because clotting factors must be decreased to < 30% of normal to cause prolongation of PT, whereas the optimized test can also detect milder factor deficiencies. The PT is frequently prolonged in acquired vitamin K deficiency, liver disease, specific factor deficiencies and disseminated intravascular coagulation (DIC). Deficiency of FVII causes prolongation of the PT with no change in aPTT and thrombin time. Owing to the short half-life of FVII, the PT is selectively prolonged in the early stages of acquired vitamin K deficiency.

Activated partial thromboplastin time

Test principle: aPTT imitates coagulation via contact activation and identifies coagulation abnormalities in the intrinsic (high-molecular weight kininogen, prekallikrein, FXII, FXI, FIX and FVIII) and common pathways (FX, FV, FII and fibrinogen).

Method: Clotting is initiated by the addition of a surface activator (e.g. ellagic acid, silica or kaolin), phospholipid (which substitutes for the negatively charged phospholipid surface provided by platelets *in vivo*) and excess calcium. The reagents used in the aPTT vary greatly in composition and therefore in sensitivity and specificity. Dilution of the plasma does not increase the sensitivity of this test when using electro-optical detection of fibrin formation (Johnstone, 1984). For reference values see under PT.

Interpretation: With sensitive aPTT reagents (e.g. Hemos IL SynthAFAX, Instrumentation Laboratory Warrington, UK), aPTT tests optimized for human plasma can detect mild individual coagulation factor deficiencies in canine and feline plasma (Mischke, 2000). Haemophiliacs have usually prolonged aPTT; in dogs with haemophilia A this will be approximately 1.5–2.5 times normal. With less sensitive reagents even significant factor deficiencies to values < 30% may result in false negative (normal) results. Haemophilic heterozygous carriers with residual activities of 40–60% of FVIII or FIX cannot be detected with sufficient certainty. The optimal aPTT ratio for heparin treatment (i.e. corresponding to 0.3–0.7 IU/ml) must be assessed by calibration specific for the aPTT reagent and heparin preparation used.

Thrombin time (thrombin clot time)

Indication: Thrombin time measurements are indicated in cases of combined prolongation of PT and aPTT to assess whether the final generation of fibrin is involved in the haemostatic disorder. In addition, the thrombin time is used to monitor heparin therapy.

Test principle: Thrombin time measures the clotting time of citrated plasma after the addition of exogenous thrombin. Therefore, this test depends only on the availability of an adequate concentration of fibrinogen, and possible inhibitors of the thrombin–fibrinogen interaction (heparin) and of fibrin polymerization (fibrin(ogen) degradation products (FDPs), abnormal serum proteins).

Method: Commercial test kits (e.g. Test Thrombin Reagent, Siemens Healthcare Diagnostics GmbH, Eschborn, Germany; STA Thrombin Reagent, Roche Diagnostics GmbH) are used to measure the thrombin time in dogs and cats. High thrombin concentrations are required to monitor animals receiving therapeutic doses of unfractionated heparin.

Interpretation: The thrombin time in dogs and cats gives very similar results to tests performed in human patients, but reference values must be established specifically for each species and method. The thrombin time will be prolonged if there is either hypofibrinogenaemia (< 0.7 g/l) or dysfibrinogenaemia. In samples with a normal fibrinogen concentration, FDPs cause prolongation at concentrations of ≥ 0.1 mg/ml (Mischke and Wolling, 2000).

Interpretation of test results for the basic programme: Combined interpretation of results from platelet count and group tests and, if necessary, capillary bleeding time, often allows a tentative diagnosis to be made, which may then require confirmation or differentiation by further tests, especially individual clotting factor analyses (Figure 22.8).

Further and specific tests

In individual cases, additional specific tests, which can usually only be measured in specialist laboratories, are necessary to confirm diagnosis or to accompany therapy.

Individual clotting factors

Indication

Determination of plasma activities of individual clotting factors is important for the diagnosis and monitoring of haemostatic disorders, particularly hereditary individual clotting factor deficiencies such as haemophilia A and B.

Test principle

Levels of FII, FV, FVII, and FX are measured with a modified PT test; FVIII, FIX, FXI and FXII are measured with a modified aPTT test. The tests are performed with a diluted sample and the addition of a sample of plasma that is known to lack a single individual factor. Therefore, the coagulation time of the test depends on the residual activity of the coagulation factor under test.

Method

Coagulometric tests that incorporate human factor-deficient plasma are typically used for the determination of clotting factor activities in dogs and cats. Owing to the fact that FV and FVIII:C activities in canine and feline plasma are several times higher than in human plasma, accurate measurement of coagulation factor activities in canine or feline plasma, using human deficient plasma, requires higher sample dilution (i.e. 1: > 20) than typically

Platelet count	↓–↓↓↓	→	→/↓	↓↓	→	→
Bleeding time	↑–↑↑/→	↑–↑↑↑	→	→	→	→
PT	→	→	↑↑↑	↑↑	↑	→
aPTT	→	→	↑↑	↑↑↑	↑	↑–↑↑
Thrombin time	→/⇣	→	⇣/→	↑↑	→/⇣	→/⇣
Diagnosis/ differential diagnosis	Thrombocytopenia	vWD Platelet dysfunction	Anticoagulant rodenticide intoxication	DIC (final stage)/ hyperfibrinolysis	DIC Liver induced Vitamin K-dependent	Haemophilia Contact factor deficiencies DIC, etc.
Further recommended tests to confirm diagnosis	—	vWf Collagen binding activity Platelet function tests	Control of therapeutic effect after vitamin K_1	—	Individual coagulation factors (Activation markers)	Individual coagulation factors

PT – prothrombin time; aPTT – activated partial thromboplastin time; vWD – von Willebrand's disease; vWf – von Willebrand factor; DIC – disseminated Intravascular coagulation

↓–↓↓↓ Mild to severe decrease/shortening; ↑–↑↑↑ Mild to severe prolongation; → Normal finding; ⇣ Reactive shortening; / or (alternative finding)

22.8 Combined interpretation of test results from routine tests of haemostatic function and further tests recommended to differentiate between haemostatic disorders.

used for human plasma. Differences in activities between human and canine or feline plasma and non-parallelism of the standard curves emphasize the necessity to use species-specific standard curves prepared with a sample of pooled plasma for the accurate determination of clotting factor activity.

Interpretation

Factor activities of 30% are usually sufficient for physiological haemostasis. Haemophilic patients have usually < 10% of normal levels of FVIII or FIX, respectively.

Fibrinogen

Indication

Fibrinogen is determined in an extended coagulation profile and also with regard to its role as an acute phase reactant.

Test principle and method

Fibrinogen concentration is usually determined using the functional clotting method, as described by Clauss (1957). This method is a modified thrombin time measurement, and is based on the principle that at low fibrinogen concentrations the clotting time is proportional to the fibrinogen concentration. Commercially available standard curves for human fibrinogen or human standard material can be used for calibration, because calibration curves prepared with canine or feline specific fibrinogen standards show very similar results.

Interpretation

The fibrinogen concentration ranges from 1.0 to 3.0 g/l in normal dogs and cats. Hyperfibrinogenaemia occurs frequently, and also occurs in cases of DIC. Hypofibrinogenaemia occurs primarily because of increased fibrinolysis in DIC with dominant hyperfibrinolysis.

Antithrombin (AT)

Together with protein C, AT is the most important physiological inhibitor of the blood clotting system and the main inhibitor of thrombin.

Indication

Measurement of AT is particularly important in cases of DIC that are receiving therapeutic (high dose) heparin treatment, to guarantee an adequate AT level. Heparin functions mainly by enhancing the inhibition of thrombin by AT and, therefore, increases AT consumption. Assessment of AT activity is also useful in animals suspected of having a hypercoagulable state.

Test principle and method

Common assays for AT activity are based on synthetic FXa- or thrombin-dependent chromogenic substrates and are well suited for measurement of AT activity in animals (Mandell *et al.*, 1991). Canine and feline pooled plasma are ideal standards.

Interpretation

Subnormal AT levels (< 75%) are associated with decreased effectiveness of heparin therapy. In DIC the concentration of AT is decreased. In one study, 85% of dogs (35 of 41) with confirmed DIC had decreased AT concentrations (Feldman *et al.*, 1981). AT also decreases in hepatic disease owing to decreased synthesis. AT is similar in size to albumin and is lost in protein-losing nephropathies and protein-losing enteropathies.

D-dimer, activation markers

Plasma markers that are useful to detect activation of the clotting system in small animals (e.g. thrombosis, DIC) include D-dimers, soluble fibrin and thrombin–antithrombin complex concentrations.

Indication

D-dimers are used primarily as markers of coagulation activation, and their measurement is indicated in cases of suspected DIC or thrombosis.

Test principle and method

Given that antibodies against human D-dimers cross-react with canine and feline D-dimers, human tests are suitable. Immunoturbidimetric methods are useful reference methods. In addition, semiquantitative latex agglutination test kits (e.g. Minutex, formerly Accuclot, D-dimer, Tcoag Ireland Ltd, Bray, Ireland) can be used to detect increased D-dimers in dogs (Boutet *et al.*, 2009).

Interpretation

Healthy dogs have D-dimer concentrations of < 0.25 µg/ml. Generation of D-dimers requires the action of thrombin and plasmin, so increased D-dimers are markers of intravascular clotting (DIC, or thrombosis). A negative result more or less rules out thrombosis, but a positive result is relatively nonspecific. Many DIC diagnostic scoring systems include increased D-dimer levels.

von Willebrand factor (vWf)

vWf plays a major role in the adherence of platelets to the subendothelial collagen at the site of vascular injury and platelet aggregation. In most cases, it is sufficient to measure the concentration of plasma vWf. Specific assays that detect selective loss of the functionally active large multimers (collagen binding assays, electrophoretic multimeric analysis) to characterize a type II vWD have limited availability. Genetic tests are available for different mutations in various dog breeds (see Chapter 27).

Indication

Measurement of vWf concentration is indicated in cases with a suspected haemorrhagic disorder in which results of platelet count and of clotting tests have not revealed corresponding changes, and/or in cases of otherwise unexplained prolonged bleeding time.

Test principle and method

vWf in plasma stored at either 4°C or 22°C (and even in blood when stored at 22°C) is relatively stable for up to 48 hours (Johnstone *et al.*, 1991). Measurement of the concentration of canine vWf in citrated plasma can be performed with human test kits based on latex agglutination or enzyme-linked immunosorbent assay (ELISA) test principles, owing to cross-reactivity of the antibodies. Canine pooled plasma should serve as the standard (activity usually defined as 100%).

Interpretation

vWf has a wide reference range (50–180%). It is an acute phase reactant and may be increased in conditions such as strenuous exercise, age, azotaemia, liver disease, parturition and after application of the vasopressin analogue 1-desamino-8-D-arginine vasopressin (DDAVP).

Platelet function tests

Special functional assays of primary haemostasis are indicated in cases suspected of having platelet function disorders. This is particularly important in cases with haemorrhagic diathesis that show prolonged capillary bleeding time despite normal platelet count and in which vWD has been ruled out. Further indications exist in patients suffering from primary diseases that are frequently associated with platelet functional disorders (e.g. liver disease), or for the monitoring and evaluation of anti-platelet drug treatment.

Global tests of primary haemostasis such as capillary bleeding time and automated platelet function analyses are also indicated for the estimation of the overall function of primary haemostasis in thrombocytopenic dogs that require surgery. There are numerous tests that may be used to characterize platelet function disorders, including flow cytometric platelet function tests, evaluation of platelet adhesion, viscoelastic whole blood tests, and detection of platelet microparticles.

Inherited (congenital) functional abnormalities of platelets are rare in domestic animals and in humans, but acquired platelet dysfunction is more frequent and may occur in association with many diseases and after administration of a number of drugs, including anti-platelet agents. Therefore, it is essential to obtain an accurate history of all drugs the animal has received in the past 10 days to rule out their effects, especially aspirin and non-steroidal anti-inflammatory agents.

Functional platelet tests such as platelet aggregation tests should be completed within 4 hours after blood collection and they require specialized and expensive equipment. For these reasons, specific testing of platelet function is usually only available at veterinary teaching hospitals.

Platelet function analyser

Instrument: The platelet function analyser PFA-100 (Siemens Healthcare Diagnostics GmbH) has been evaluated and is suitable for use in dogs (Callan and Giger, 2001; Mischke and Keidel, 2003). The system comprises a microprocessor-controlled instrument and disposable test cartridges that contain a biologically active membrane (Figure 22.9). The instrument aspirates a blood volume under constant vacuum from a sample reservoir in the test cartridge through a capillary and a microscopic aperture cut into the membrane at the end of the capillary. The membrane is coated with collagen and adenosine diphosphate (ADP) (collagen/ADP cartridge) or collagen and adrenaline (epinephrine) (collagen/adrenaline cartridge). The presence of these biochemical stimuli, and the high shear rates developed under standardized flow conditions, result in platelet attachment, activation, aggregation, and slow formation of a stable platelet plug at the aperture. The 'closure time' is reported by the analyser.

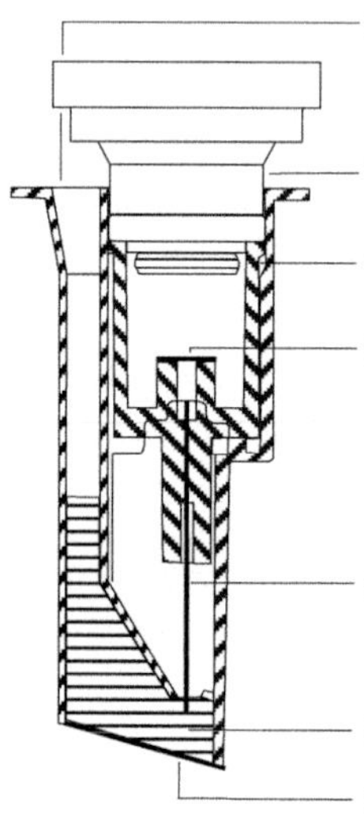

22.9 Schematic diagram of the cross-sectional view of the functional unit of the platelet function analyser PFA-100.

Technical aspects: The cartridges, which are stored at refrigerator temperature, should be pre-warmed at room temperature for at least 15 minutes before inserting them into the analyser and starting the measurement. The analysis should be performed between 30 minutes and 2 hours after collection of the citrate buffer-anticoagulated blood, which is the standard sample (Mischke and Keidel, 2002). It is advisable to use only one position (e.g. position A) of the two alternative measuring positions of the analyser, because spontaneous sedimentation can lead to artificial results in the second cartridge inserted in parallel into position B.

Reference values:

- Collagen/ADP cartridge: 52–86 seconds (Callan and Giger, 2001), 53–98 seconds (Mischke and Keidel, 2003).
- Collagen/adrenaline cartridge: 97–225 seconds (Callan and Giger, 2001), 92–> 300 seconds (Mischke and Keidel, 2003).

Interpretation: The method can be regarded as a global screening test of primary haemostasis. Apart from platelet function, the result is significantly influenced by platelet count and Hct (Callan and Giger, 2001; Mischke and Keidel, 2003). Even slightly subnormal Hct values are associated with prolongation of the closure time, which limits the clinical applicability of the analyser. Because measurements using the collagen/adrenaline cartridge exceed the upper limit of the measuring range in a small percentage of healthy dogs (Mischke and Keidel, 2003), this cartridge type is less suitable for tests of primary platelet function in dogs.

Platelet aggregation

The measurement of platelet aggregation following the addition of agonists is one of the most important *in vitro* methods of assessing platelet function.

Test principle: The turbidimetric method measures the increase of light transmission in platelet-rich plasma during aggregation, while impedance aggregometry measures the increase in the electrical resistance in blood that results from the accumulation of platelet aggregates on sensor wires (Dyszkiewicz-Korpanty *et al.*, 2005). The advantage of the turbidimetric method is that the platelet count can be adjusted to a defined value, but the preparation of the platelet-rich plasma requires additional equipment and time, large sample volumes, and experienced personnel. This preparation procedure can also alter the quality of the sample through loss of large platelets with increased or decreased reactivity. In contrast, impedance aggregometry does not require cell separation, which means that shorter preparation times and smaller sample volumes can be used. Furthermore, lipaemic samples may be evaluated. Impedance aggregometry on whole blood may also better reflect *in vivo* platelet function, given that platelets can interact with other blood cells in this system. The electrical probes of the impedance method create an artificial surface and therefore may better mimic *in vivo* platelet aggregation, which occurs typically on injured or inflamed vascular surfaces, while the platelets aggregate in the liquid phase in the turbidimetric method.

Multiplate analyser: The novel Multiplate impedance aggregometer (Dynabyte Medical GmbH, Munich, Germany) is well suited for use in dogs (Kalbantner *et al.*, 2010). The device has five parallel test channels. The single-use test cells have a pipette-intake, a cup portion with a dual sensor unit protruding into the blood, which is stirred by a Teflon-coated stirring magnet, and a jack portion which connects the test cell to the device and records the electrical resistance between the sensor wires. The change in impedance determined by each sensor is recorded independently and provides an internal control. The test can be performed as recommended by the manufacturer for human samples (300 µl isotonic sodium chloride solution, 300 µl of hirudin-anticoagulated blood, 3 minutes incubation and stirring at 37°C, addition of 20 µl agonist solution; Kalbantner *et al.*, 2010). The change in impedance caused by the adhesion and aggregation of platelets on the electrodes is detected continuously for 6 minutes (standard setting) to 12 minutes (the setting used in our laboratory, which allows the aggregation curve to almost reach plateau).

Agonist concentrations: With regard to optimal sensitivity, minimum effective (threshold) concentrations of agonists should be used (i.e. agonist concentrations that induce constant high maximum aggregation values in healthy animals). In a canine study using the Born method, the following threshold concentrations (final test concentrations) were established: 25 µmol/l ADP, 10 µg/ml collagen and 1 IU/ml thrombin (Mischke and Schulze, 2004). In an actual study using the Multiplate instrument, the following optimal agonist concentrations (sourced from Dynabyte Medical GmbH) were defined for dogs: 10 µmol/l ADP, 5 µg/ml of collagen, and 1 mmol/l arachidonic acid (Kalbantner *et al.*, 2010).

Reference values: These should be established for the particular reagents, instrument and laboratory performing the test.

Interpretation: Platelet aggregation is particularly useful for the detection of decreased platelet function. Because low agonist concentrations are associated with a wide range of results, it is almost impossible to detect hyperaggregability in individual patients. Platelet counts influence the result, especially when measurements are performed with the turbidimetric method.

References and further reading

Bateman SW, Mathews KA, Abrams-Ogg ACG *et al.* (1999) Evaluation of point-of-care tests for diagnosis of disseminated intravascular coagulation in dogs admitted to an intensive care unit. *Journal of the American Veterinary Medical Association* **215**, 805–810

Boutet P, Heath F, Archer J and Villiers E (2009) Comparison of quantitative immunoturbidimetric and semiquantitative latex-agglutination assays for D-dimer measurement in canine plasma. *Veterinary Clinical Pathology* **38**, 78–82

Callan MB and Giger U (2001) Assessment of a point-of-care instrument for identification of primary hemostatic disorders in dogs. *American Journal of Veterinary Research* **62**, 652–658

Clauss A (1957) Rapid physiological coagulation method in determination of fibrinogen. *Acta Haematologica* **17**, 237–246

Dircks BH, Schuberth HJ and Mischke R (2009) Underlying diseases and clinicopathologic variables of thrombocytopenic dogs with and without platelet-bound antibodies detected by use of a flow cytometric assay: 83 cases (2004-2006). *Journal of the American Veterinary Medical Association* **235**, 960–966

Dyszkiewicz-Korpanty AM, Frenkel EP and Sarode R (2005) Approach to the assessment of platelet function: Comparison between optical-based platelet-rich plasma and impedance-based whole blood platelet aggregation methods. *Clinical and Applied Thrombosis/Hemostasis* **11**, 25–35

Feldman BF, Madewell BR and O'Neill S (1981) Disseminated intravascular coagulation: antithrombin, plasminogen, and coagulation abnormalities in 41 dogs. *Journal of the American Veterinary Medical Association* **179**, 151–154

Furlanello T, Caldin M, Stocco A *et al.* (2006) Stability of stored canine plasma for hemostasis testing. *Veterinary Clinical Pathology* **35**, 204–207

Gelain ME, Tutino GF, Pogliani E and Bertazzolo W (2010) Macrothrombocytopenia in a group of related Norfolk terriers. *Veterinary Record* **167**, 493–494

Giles AR, Tinlin S and Greenwood R (1982) A canine model of hemophilic (factor VIII:C deficiency) bleeding. *Blood* **60**, 727–730

Grindem CB, Breitschwerdt EB, Corbett WT and Jans HE (1991) Epidemiologic survey of thrombocytopenia in dogs: a report on 987 cases. *Veterinary Clinical Pathology* **20**, 38–43

Jergens AE, Turrentine MA, Kraus KH and Johnson GS (1987) Buccal mucosal bleeding time of healthy dogs and of dogs in various pathological states, including thrombocytopenia, uremia and von Willebrand's disease. *American Journal of Veterinary Research* **48**, 1337–1342

Johnstone IB (1984) The activated partial thromboplastin time of diluted plasma: variability due to method of fibrin detection. *Canadian Journal of Comparative Medicine* **48**, 198–201

Johnstone IB, Keen J, Halbert A and Crane S (1991) Stability of factor VIII and von Willebrand factor in canine blood samples during storage. *Canadian Veterinary Journal* **32**, 173–175

Kalbantner K, Baumgarten A and Mischke R (2010) Measurement of platelet function in dogs using a novel impedance aggregometer. *The Veterinary Journal* **185**, 144–151

Mandell CP, O'Neill SL and Feldman BF (1991) Antithrombin III concentrations associated with L-asparaginase administration. *Veterinary Clinical Pathology* **21**, 68–70

Mischke R (2000) Activated partial thromboplastin time as a screening test of minor or moderate coagulation factor deficiencies for canine plasma: sensitivity of different commercial reagents. *Journal of Veterinary Diagnostic Investigation* **12**, 433–437

Mischke R (2011) Prothrombin time standardisation in canine samples with regard to inter-batch and inter-reagent variability. *The Veterinary Journal* **188**, 301–306

Mischke R and Keidel A (2002) Preclinical studies for the use of the platelet function analyser PFA-100 with the collagen/ADP cartridge in dogs. *Deutsche Tieraerztliche Wochenschrift* **109**, 235–238

Mischke R and Keidel A (2003) Influence of platelet count, acetylsalicylic acid, von Willebrand's disease, coagulopathies, and haematocrit on results obtained using a platelet function analyser in dogs. *The Veterinary Journal* **165**, 43–52

Mischke R and Nolte I (1997) Optimization of prothrombin time measurements in canine plasma. *American Journal of Veterinary Research* **58**, 236–241

Mischke R and Schulze U (2004) Studies on platelet aggregation using the Born method in normal and uraemic dogs. *The Veterinary Journal* **168**, 270–275

Mischke R and Wolling H (2000) Influence of fibrinogen degradation products on thrombin time, activated partial thromboplastin time and prothrombin time of canine plasma. *Haemostasis* **30**, 123–130

Nolte I, Niemann C, Bowry SK, Failing K and Müller-Berghaus G (1997) A method for measuring capillary bleeding time in non-anaesthetized dogs. Prolongation of the bleeding time by acetylsalicylic acid. *Journal of Veterinary Medicine (Zentralblatt Veterinaermedizin) Series A* **44**, 625–628

Parker MT, Collier LL, Kier AB and Johnson GS (1988) Oral mucosal bleeding times of normal cats and cats with Chediak-Higashi syndrome or Hageman trait (factor XII deficiency). *Veterinary Clinical Pathology* **17**, 9–12

Wiinberg B, Jensen AL, Johansson PI *et al.* (2008) Thrombelastographic evaluation of hemostatatic function in dogs with disseminated intravascular coagulation. *Journal of Veterinary Internal Medicine.* **22**, 357–365

23

Disorders of platelet number

Ann Hohenhaus and Carrie White

Introduction

Platelets adhere to injured vascular endothelium in the primary step of haemostasis. Following adherence, platelets are activated and release granules, which recruit additional platelets to the area of injury. Activated platelets aggregate to form a temporary platelet plug. Quantitative disorders of platelets include thrombocytopenia and thrombocytosis. Most quantitative platelet disorders result from underlying diseases; however, primary disorders of platelet number do occur. Any of these disorders can disturb the normal platelet response and result in either haemorrhage or thrombosis.

Quantitative disorders of platelets are among the most common haematological disorders diagnosed in veterinary medicine. Dogs are more likely to be diagnosed with a quantitative platelet disorder than cats. In a large population of cats seen at a veterinary teaching hospital in the UK, reactive thrombocytosis was diagnosed in 4.6% of the feline population, while thrombocytosis was diagnosed in approximately 8.5% of dogs in the USA (Hammer, 1991; Rizzo *et al.*, 2007). Thrombocytopenia has been reported in 1.3% of cats seen at a veterinary teaching hospital in the UK. Similar numbers have been reported for the occurrence of thrombocytopenia in cats from the USA (Jordan *et al.*, 1993). The occurrence of thrombocytopenia in two large canine populations, one in the USA and one in Germany, was between 5 and 7% (Grindem *et al.*, 1991; Botsch *et al.*, 2009).

Thrombocytopenia is defined as an absolute decrease in the number of circulating platelets. Typical laboratory reference ranges for platelet counts are wide (200–400 $\times$ 10^9/l), and less than approximately 150 $\times$ 10^9/l would be considered to represent thrombocytopenia. Unless platelet function is abnormal or other coagulation defects are present, haemorrhage does not occur typically until the platelet count is less than approximately 30 $\times$ 10^9/l. Clinical impression suggests that cats, but not dogs, may have profoundly low platelet counts without overt haemorrhage (Jordan *et al.*, 1993; Putsche and Kohn, 2008; Wondratschek *et al.*, 2010). Haemorrhage due to thrombocytopenia is characterized by surface bleeding: petechiae, ecchymosis and bleeding from mucosal surfaces such as epistaxis, melaena and haemoptysis (Putsche and Kohn, 2008) (Figures 23.1 and 23.2).

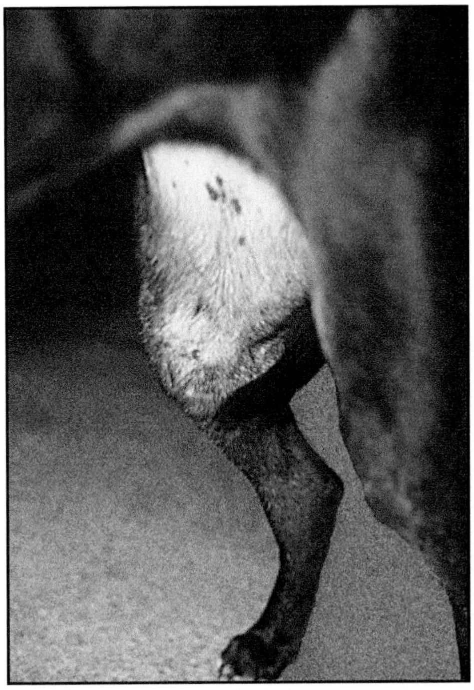

23.1 Petechiae on the medial thigh of a dog.

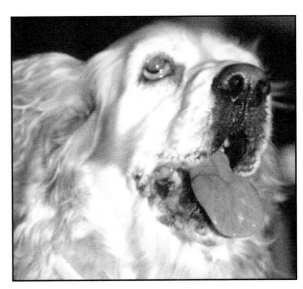

23.2 Epistaxis in a Cocker Spaniel with thrombocytopenia secondary to administration of levamisole as an immunomodulatory agent.

Thrombocytosis is defined as an absolute increase in the number of circulating platelets. In veterinary medicine, convention defines thrombocytosis as a platelet count > 700 × 10^9/l (Chisholm-Chait, 1999). Typically, thrombocytosis is an incidental finding when a complete blood count is performed for an unrelated purpose. Clinical signs, related to either the underlying disease or the elevated platelet count, are not always present in thrombocytosis. Reactive thrombocytosis has no clinical signs referable to the elevation in platelet count. Both thrombosis and haemorrhage have been associated with myelodysplastic thrombocytosis.

Thrombocytopenia

Thrombocytopenia can be a primary disorder of decreased platelet production by the bone marrow or increased platelet destruction in the periphery. Thrombocytopenia can also develop secondary to a wide variety of conditions such as infectious, inflammatory and neoplastic diseases. Classification of thrombocytopenia by mechanism into four categories helps to guide the diagnostic evaluation. These groups are: increased destruction, decreased production, excessive consumption and platelet sequestration (Figure 23.3). There is considerable

Mechanism and causes		Associated factors	
		Dogs	*Cats*
Increased destruction	Primary immune-mediated	Thrombocytopenia, Evans' syndrome, systemic lupus erythematosus, immune-mediated thrombocytopenia and neutropenia	Thrombocytopenia, Evans' syndrome, systemic lupus erythematosus
	Secondary immune-mediated	Gold salts, sulphonamide antibiotics, post-transfusion purpura, inflammatory bowel disease, infectious diseases (*see text for details*)	Methimazole
Decreased production	Myelophthisis	Lymphoma, leukaemia, plasma cell disorders	
	Myelotoxicity	Chemotherapeutic agents, radiation therapy, phenylbutazone, oestrogens, griseofulvin	Chemotherapy agents, radiation therapy, griseofulvin
	Infectious agents	*Ehrlichia*, *Anaplasma*, *Neorickettsia*, parvovirus	Feline leukaemia virus, feline immunodeficiency virus, feline panleucopenia, *Ehrlichia canis*- like infection
	Myelodysplasia	Idiopathic	
	Genetic	Cavalier King Charles Spaniel (β-tubulin defect), cyclic haemopoiesis	
Increased consumption	Severe haemorrhage	Anticoagulant rodenticide intoxication	
	Overwhelming infection	Histoplasmosis, sepsis	
		Snake envenomation	
	Disseminated intravascular coagulation	Infection: canine infectious hepatitis, leptospirosis, babesiosis, histoplasmosis. Neoplasia: haemangiosarcoma, lymphoma. Inflammation	Infection: feline infectious peritonitis. Neoplasia: lymphoma
	Microangiopathic	Dirofilariasis, incompatible transfusions, heatstroke, haemolytic–uraemic syndrome, transvenous coil	Incompatible transfusions, haemolytic–uraemic syndrome
Sequestration		Hypersplenism, liver disease, neoplasia	
Unknown or multifactorial mechanism	Infective endocarditis	Gram +ve or –ve bacteria, *Bartonella*	
	Miscellaneous infections	Hepatozoonosis, babesiosis, leptospirosis	*Cytauxzoon felis*
		Acute pancreatitis	
	Neoplasia	Carcinoma, sarcoma, lymphoid	
	Other	Heatstroke	

23.3 Classification of thrombocytopenia in dogs and cats. In addition, clinically insignificant thrombocytopenia is found as a breed variation in Greyhounds and Shiba Inus. Pseudothrombocytopenia is also found in dogs and cats.

overlap between the mechanisms of thrombocytopenia and the categorization is not rigid.

Clinically insignificant thrombocytopenia

Pseudothrombocytopenia occurs in 1 in 1000 people and has been reported rarely in dogs. The diagnosis of pseudothrombocytopenia should be considered in a dog or cat with a severely low platelet count (platelets < 30 × 10^9/l) without clinical signs of thrombocytopenia-related haemorrhage. Anticoagulants such as EDTA induce pseudothrombocytopenia by causing platelet aggregation following traumatic venepuncture, which causes automated haematology analysers to report falsely low platelet counts. Differentiation between actual and pseudothrombocytopenia prevents unnecessary treatment.

Several reports suggest that platelet counts in Greyhounds are lower than established reference ranges, and a reference range of 64–292 × 10^9/l should be used for this breed (Steiss *et al.*, 2000). The cause of Greyhound thrombocytopenia may be a breed variation because anti-platelet antibodies have not been detected. Other studies suggest that a platelet count < 100 × 10^9/l is abnormal in Greyhounds and should be investigated. The Shiba Inu dog may also have a breed variation in platelet count. A small number of clinically normal Shiba Inus with microcytic red blood cells also had a platelet count ranging from 110–196 × 10^9/l.

Causes of excessive platelet destruction

Loss of self-tolerance and induction of an anti-platelet antibody response are mechanisms responsible for premature destruction of platelets. Primary immune-mediated destruction is mediated by an antibody response possibly directed against glycoproteins IIb and IIIa on the platelet surface. Production of the antibody is due to a loss of self-tolerance; consequently this process is occasionally termed autoimmune thrombocytopenia. Binding of this antibody to an epitope on the platelet surface results in accelerated destruction of platelets by macrophages in the reticuloendothelial system. The mechanism of platelet destruction in secondary immune-mediated thrombocytopenia (IMTP) is similar to that of primary IMTP; however, underlying neoplastic, infectious or inflammatory disease, or a drug, vaccine or transfusion of a blood product may induce the anti-platelet antibody.

Primary immune-mediated thrombocytopenia

By definition, primary IMTP has no inciting cause. In both dogs and cats, primary IMTP may occur as the sole haematological disorder or as a component of multi-lineage disorders, including: Evans' syndrome (concurrent immune-mediated haemolytic anaemia (IMHA) and IMTP); immune-mediated neutropenia (IMNP) and IMTP; or systemic lupus erythematosus (SLE). One quarter of dogs diagnosed with SLE have thrombocytopenia. The diagnosis of primary IMTP is one of exclusion. Diagnostic testing aims to identify possible inciting causes of secondary IMTP (Figure 23.4) and if none are found, primary IMTP is diagnosed.

Primary IMTP is the most common acquired disorder of haemostasis in the dog. Approximately 5% of all dogs with thrombocytopenia have primary immune-mediated platelet destruction (Grindem *et al.*, 1991; Botsch *et al.*, 2009). Dogs with severe thrombocytopenia and surface haemorrhage raise the clinical suspicion of primary IMTP (Botsch *et al.*, 2009). Laboratory findings of a normal to decreased mean platelet volume and demonstration of platelet-bound antibodies are supportive of this diagnosis.

Primary IMTP is rare in cats. In a series of 41 cats diagnosed with thrombocytopenia, only one was believed to have IMTP (Jordan *et al.*, 1993). Most other reports of primary IMTP in cats are single cases or small case series. Review of the sparse literature on feline thrombocytopenia suggests that petechiation and ecchymoses can occur anywhere on the body, but there may be a propensity for haemorrhage in the head and neck region (Wondratschek *et al.*, 2010). Platelet counts of cats with IMTP ranges from 1–46 x 10^9/l.

Secondary immune-mediated thrombocytopenia

Unlike primary IMTP where the cause of anti-platelet antibody production is unknown, secondary IMTP has an identifiable cause possibly responsible for induction of anti-platelet antibodies. Causes include infections, medications, and incompatible transfusions (see Figure 23.2).

Infectious causes: Infectious diseases are the underlying cause of IMTP in 20–60% of dogs. Multiple infectious agents have been reported as an underlying cause and more will probably be described. When considering an infectious agent as the cause of thrombocytopenia in a dog or cat, the simultaneous contribution of multiple infectious agents should be considered, because co-infection is common. Not all infectious agents that cause thrombocytopenia cause immune destruction of platelets and additional infectious agents are listed in Figure 23.3 under multiple categories of thrombocytopenia.

Rocky Mountain spotted fever (RMSF), caused by *Rickettsia rickettsii*, is an acute, fulminant, febrile illness. Canine cases are seen typically during the warmer months. The most common findings are anorexia, lethargy, fever, thrombocytopenia, leucocytosis and hypoproteinaemia (Gasser *et al.*, 2001). Thrombocytopenia can be severe (< 75 × 10^9/l). Although RMSF is a tick-borne illness, owners are infrequently aware of tick infestation in dogs diagnosed with RMSF. RMSF is poorly named and is typically found east of the Rocky Mountains; however, it is reported in nearly all of the continental United States.

Angiostrongylus vasorum is a metastrongyloid nematode parasite of dogs, which is an increasingly significant cause of disease in Europe. Infection is acquired from ingestion of larvae-infected slugs or snails. Clinical signs range from none to subcutaneous swelling and lower respiratory signs.

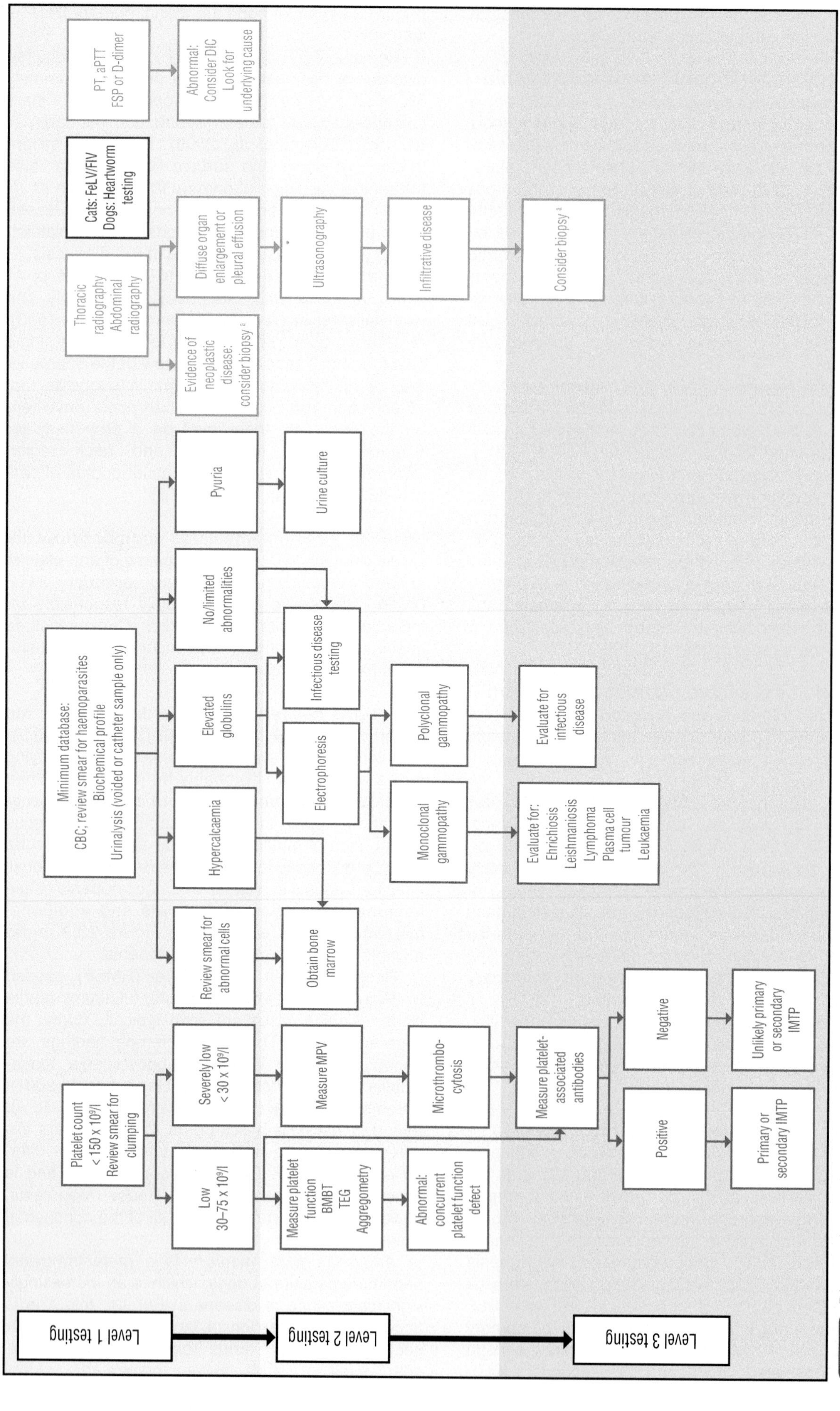

23.4 Diagnostic algorithm for a dog or cat with thrombocytopenia and surface bleeding. aPTT, activated partial thromboplastin time; BMBT, buccal mucosal bleeding time; DIC, disseminated intravascular coagulation; FeLV, feline leukemia virus; FIV, feline immunodeficiency virus; FSP, fibrin split products; IMTP, immune-mediated thrombocytopenia; MPV, mean platelet volume; PT, prothrombin time; TEG, thromboelastography. [a] High risk of bleeding; platelet products should be available.

Haemorrhage related to thrombocytopenia is an important clinical presentation in affected dogs. The diagnosis is based on the demonstration fo larvae in samples of bronchoalveolar lavage fluid or faeces.

Leishmaniosis is a common protozoal disease of dogs found in particular geographical areas throughout the world. Among infected dogs, 25–50% are believed to develop secondary IMTP. Hyperglobulinaemia is also common; it may be either mono- or polyclonal and results in thrombocytopathia.

Hyperthyroidism drug therapy: Treatment of feline hyperthyroidism with methimazole has been associated with development of thrombocytopenia. Slightly less than 3% of treated cats develop thrombocytopenia within the first 3 months of treatment. Thrombocytopenia can be severe (platelet count < 75 × 10^9/l) and can result in clinical haemorrhage. Cessation of methimazole treatment results in resolution and re-administration of the drug leads to recrudescence. Immunological destruction of platelets is considered the likely mechanism because cats treated with methimazole also develop positive direct antiglobulin tests and positive antinuclear antibody tests.

Antibiotics: Administration of sulphonamide antibiotics may be associated with a systemic hypersensitivity reaction. Hydroxylamine metabolites, formed from oxidation of the para-amino group of the sulphonamide molecule, have been implicated. Dobermanns are susceptible to this systemic disorder (Figure 23.5), probably because many of these dogs have decreased ability to detoxify hydroxylamine metabolites of sulphonamides, but many other breeds may be affected. One component of this systemic disorder is thrombocytopenia. In addition to thrombocytopenia, fever and hepatopathy are the most common clinical signs (Trepanier *et al*., 2003). Neutered bitches, Samoyeds and Miniature Schnauzers were over-represented in one study. Discontinuation of drug therapy results in resolution of clinical signs in most dogs; although dogs with thrombocytopenia recover less often than dogs without thrombocytopenia (63% vs. 90%; Trepanier *et al*., 2003).

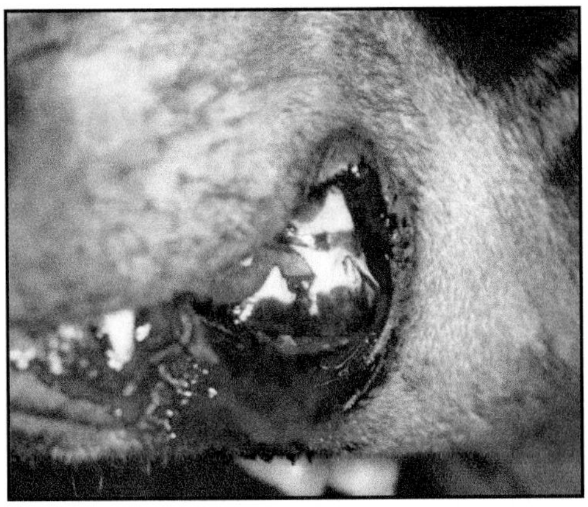

23.5 Surface bleeding in a Dobermann with thrombocytopenia secondary to administration of sulphonamide antibiotic.

Post-transfusion purpura: Post-transfusion purpura is a rare disorder caused by antibodies induced by previous transfusion and directed at platelets. Post-transfusion purpura is a form of delayed immunological transfusion reaction that occurs 1–2 weeks after a transfusion because of the time required for memory cells to initiate antibody production. The transfusion recipient lacks a particular platelet antigen, and exposure to that antigen in the transfused blood induces antibody production. Thrombocytopenia can be severe (platelet count < 10 × 10^9/l) and result in clinically significant haemorrhage. Post-transfusion purpura has been reported in a dog with haemophilia A after multiple blood transfusions. Anti-platelet antibodies were identified (Wardrop *et al*., 1997).

Causes of decreased platelet production

Genetic causes

The Cavalier King Charles Spaniel (CKCS) suffers from an inherited disorder of platelet production. This autosomal recessive disorder is the consequence of a mutation in the β1-tubulin gene (Davis *et al*., 2008). CKCSs homozygous for the mutation have a platelet count < 100 × 10^9/l, heterozygous dogs have a platelet count approximately 200 × 10^9/l and dogs with two wild type alleles have a platelet count > 250 × 10^9/l. The single nucleotide mutation renders platelet microtubule protofilaments unstable, resulting in abnormal proplatelet formation. Clinically, macrothrombocytosis is apparent on blood smears (Figure 23.6) and, despite a low platelet count, haemorrhage does not occur. The diagnosis can be confirmed using molecular testing.

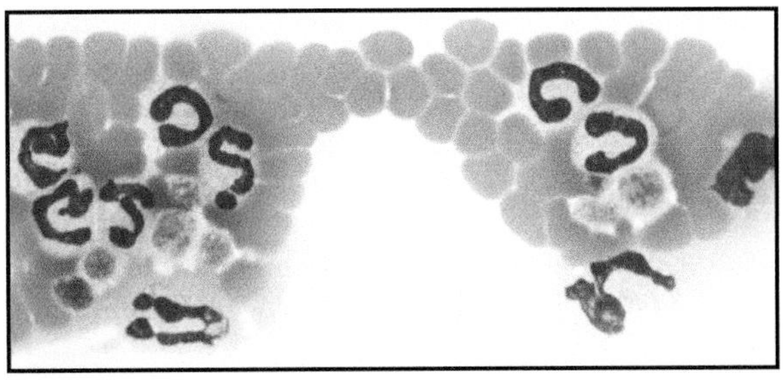

23.6 Photomicrograph (original magnification × 1000) of a blood smear from a Cavalier King Charles Spaniel with macrothrombocytosis. Note that the platelets are nearly as large as the red blood cells.

Drug-related causes: Multiple therapeutic agents may damage bone marrow haemopoietic cells and result in thrombocytopenia as well as other cytopenias. Griseofulvin, phenylbutazone and chemotherapeutic agents can all cause bone marrow suppression and thrombocytopenia. Any chemotherapeutic agent can cause thrombocytopenia; however, carboplatin, melphalan and lomustine (CCNU) are commonly associated with thrombocytopenia. Radiation therapy rarely causes thrombocytopenia, but if the radiation field involves a large portion of bone marrow, thrombocytopenia can occur.

Oestrogen is unique among the agents that cause bone marrow suppression and thrombocytopenia. In dogs, oestrogen causes pancytopenia when administered as a therapeutic agent or when produced by a Sertoli cell tumour. If the source of oestrogen is removed, bone marrow recovery begins in about 30 days, but not all dogs recover.

Infectious causes: Infectious diseases can suppress bone marrow production of one or more cell lines. Infection with feline panleucopenia virus or canine parvovirus causes pancytopenia. Other infections associated with bone marrow suppression include ehrlichiosis (*Ehrlichia canis*), feline leukaemia virus (FeLV) and feline immunodeficiency virus (FIV). FeLV causes bone marrow suppression by infecting progenitor cells and induces aplastic anaemia, myelodysplasia or neoplasia. Examination of bone marrow cells from cats infected with FIV using polymerase chain reaction and immunohistochemistry demonstrates megakaryocytes infected with FIV and dysplastic megakaryocytes. Over 30% of cats infected with FeLV have thrombocytopenia, while this is reported in only 11% of cats infected with FIV. In one study, the mean platelet count was statistically different between FeLV- and FIV-infected cats; the mean platelet count was 260 × 10^9/l and 325 × 10^9/l, respectively, although the range was similar, 8–750 × 10^9/l *versus* 35–755 × 10^9/l (Gleich and Hartmann, 2009).

Bone marrow disorders: Primary (idiopathic) disorders of the bone marrow can result in thrombocytopenia; however, multiple cell lines are normally affected. Aplastic anaemia is characterized by a decrease in all cell lines. Myelophthisis, infiltration of the bone marrow by cancer cells, occurs with lymphoproliferative disorders such as lymphoma, lymphoid leukaemia and plasma cell tumours. The infiltrating cells crowd out normal marrow cells. Myelodysplasia, a non-neoplastic dysregulation of normal haemopoietic cell production, results in decreased production of platelets and red and white blood cells. Another bone marrow disorder that results in abnormalities of multiple cell lines is canine cyclic haemopoiesis (see Chapter 13).

Causes of excessive platelet consumption

Rodenticide poisoning

Anticoagulant rodenticide intoxication is a reported cause of thrombocytopenia in dogs and cats. While the exact mechanism is unknown, consumption of platelets during haemorrhage probably contributes to thrombocytopenia. Approximately half of the dogs and cats diagnosed presumptively with anticoagulant rodenticide intoxication have a moderate thrombocytopenia (platelet count 50–150 × 10^9/l); although severe thrombocytopenia has been seen (platelet count < 50 × 10^9/l). The combination of haemorrhage, elevated prothrombin (PT) and activated partial thromboplastin times (aPTT) and thrombocytopenia can lead to a misdiagnosis of disseminated intravascular coagulation (DIC). Thrombin time (TT) can often help to differentiate anticoagulant rodenticide intoxication (TT within normal range) and severe DIC (TT prolonged). To differentiate further between the two diseases, a search for an underlying cause is essential.

Disseminated intravascular coagulation

DIC is always associated with an underlying cause such as infection, inflammation or neoplasia. The trigger for DIC is systemic activation of coagulation, typically by the systemic release of tissue factor and the generation of proinflammatory cytokines (see Chapter 30). Clotting factors and platelets are consumed and replaced until consumption surpasses the ability of the body to replace them. When this occurs, disseminated coagulation becomes evident clinically and organ dysfunction ensues. Thrombocytopenia can be severe in dogs with DIC, with a mean platelet count of 55 × 10^9/l in one study (Botsch *et al.*, 2009). In addition to thrombocytopenia, laboratory analysis demonstrates prolonged PT and aPTT, and elevated fibrin split products or D-dimers. Schistocytes are seen on the blood smear if intravascular haemolysis occurs. In cats, neoplasia, pancreatitis and sepsis are the most common causes of DIC. In dogs, haemangiosarcoma of all anatomical locations, liver disease and sepsis are the most common causes. DIC carries a poor prognosis, especially in cats. Fewer than 10% of cats diagnosed with DIC were discharged from hospital in one study, compared with approximately 50% of dogs.

Histoplasmosis

Histoplasma capsulatum is a saphrophytic fungus found in soil, and is capable of causing disseminated infection. Histoplasmosis is found throughout the USA, especially in the Ohio and Mississippi river valleys. Histoplasmosis occurs sporadically in Europe. Clinical signs in dogs include chronic diarrhoea, intestinal blood loss, weight loss and anaemia. Thrombocytopenia is found in approximately half of the infected dogs, and can be mild or severe. DIC is the major cause of thrombocytopenia in dogs with disseminated histoplasmosis, but consumption and splenic sequestration may also play a role.

Microangiopathic disease

Microangiopathic disease results from the induction of platelet aggregation by a lesion in the endothelium of small blood vessels. Thrombi form in the arteries, causing erythrocyte fragmentation and haemolysis. Haemolytic–uraemic syndrome, dirofilariasis and intravascular coils have been associated with microangiopathic disease in dogs and cats. Haemolytic–uraemic syndrome (HUS) is a microangiopathic disorder that has been reported in both dogs and cats. In dogs, HUS is characterized by prodromal haemorrhagic gastroenteritis, severe thrombocytopenia and anuric renal failure. The mean platelet count has been reported to be < 20 × 10^9/l. Supportive care and treatment of anuria with dopamine and furosemide has been used to induce urine production. Post-mortem examination confirms the presence of arterial thrombi (Holloway *et al.*, 1993). HUS has also been reported in cats that were administered ciclosporin as part of a protocol for renal transplantation. Renal allograft rejection, in the presence of low ciclosporin levels, decreases renal allograft function and initiates a microangiopathic process. The result is haemolytic anaemia and thrombocytopenia. Ciclosporin-associated HUS is associated with elevated concentrations of the drug, microangiopathic haemolysis, thrombocytopenia and renal failure.

Heartworm: Another microangiopathic process seen in both dogs and cats occurs in dirofilariasis. *Dirofilaria immitis* is a widely distributed parasite, found most commonly in the southern United States, but with populations also found in southern Europe, as well as throughout other continents. Heartworm disease is inaptly named, because the nematode *Dirofilaria immitis* resides in the pulmonary arterial vasculature. The presence of the adult nematodes in the pulmonary arteries induces villous myointimal proliferation and activates platelets, causing thrombocytopenia. Thrombocytopenia is found in the severe, fulminate systemic forms of dirofilariasis, caval syndrome and DIC. Although the worm burden is lower in cats with heartworm disease, the pulmonary vascular lesions are more severe. Platelet counts have not been reported in heartworm-infected cats, but thrombocytopenia would be expected given the degree of pulmonary artery disease.

Transvenous or transarterial coils: Transvenous or transarterial coils used to correct vascular anomalies can serve as an inciting cause for a microangiopathic process. Haemolytic anaemia, schistocytes and thrombocytopenia have been seen following coil embolization of patent ductus arteriosus in dogs.

Envenomation

Snake venom contains multiple factors that affect coagulation. The component of snake venom with thrombin-like activity activates platelets and consumes fibrinogen, resulting in thrombocytopenia. In addition to surface bleeding, envenomation causes tissue necrosis at the site of the bite, cardiac arrhythmias and neurological signs.

Causes of increased platelet sequestration

At any one time, a normal spleen contains 30–40% of the total platelet pool. Enlargement of the spleen or perturbation of the splenic blood flow can result in sequestration of an increased number of platelets in the spleen. Enlargement of the spleen may be caused by infiltrative neoplasia or portal hypertension, which limits blood flow out of the spleen. Hypersplenism is characterized by splenomegaly, peripheral cytopenias and bone marrow hyperplasia. Hypersplenism rarely occurs. Platelets may not be the only cell line affected, and the bone marrow shows hyperplastic cell production corresponding to the cytopenias. Enlargement of the spleen occurs for an unknown reason and splenectomy is the treatment of choice.

Multifactorial or unknown causes of thrombocytopenia

Neoplasia

Thrombocytopenia is commonly associated with neoplasia. Studies of platelet counts in dogs with cancer identify 10–30% with thrombocytopenia (Botsch *et al.*, 2009). Approximately 16–37% of dogs with lymphoid tumours, carcinomas and sarcomas had thrombocytopenia. In the majority of these dogs, the aetiology of thrombocytopenia could not be determined. None of the dogs in this study was diagnosed with IMTP. In one study of immune diseases, dogs diagnosed with IMTP had an increased risk of developing lymphoma.

One of the most common tumours associated with thrombocytopenia is haemangiosarcoma. Over 75% of dogs and 10–30% of cats have thrombocytopenia concurrent with a diagnosis of haemangiosarcoma. Thrombocytopenia has been attributed to microangiopathic disease and to DIC. The mean platelet count in dogs with haemangiosarcoma is 138×10^9/l; therefore, the haemorrhage is not a consequence of thrombocytopenia, but is multifactorial.

Heatstroke

Heatstroke-induced thrombocytopenia is another disease with multiple aetiologies. Traditionally, DIC has been thought to be the most common cause. Recently, an immune-mediated aetiology has been proposed based on the identification of anti-platelet antibodies and response to immunomodulatory drugs in a small group of dogs with heatstroke.

Infectious causes

Infection with members of the genera *Rickettsia*, *Ehrlichia*, *Anaplasma* and *Neorickettsia* is commonly associated with thrombocytopenia caused by a variety of mechanisms. *Ehrlichia canis* and *Anaplasma phagocytophilum* are both associated with IMTP. Of dogs infected with *A. phagocytophilum*, 80% have thrombocytopenia, and a majority of these dogs have platelet-bound antibodies, indicating secondary immune platelet destruction (see Chapter 19). Although thrombocytopenia is common with *A. phagocytophilum* infection, surface bleeding is not. *A. phagocytophilum* is endemic in the UK. *Ehrlichia chaffeensis*, the agent of human monocytic ehrlichiosis, is associated with thrombocytopenia, but infection is typically subclinical in dogs. *Anaplasma platys* causes a cyclic thrombocytopenia in dogs, with a periodicity of 1–2 weeks. Morulae can be identified in platelets via light microscopy and thrombocytopenia may be caused by a secondary immune reaction (see Chapter 19). *Neorickettsia helminthoeca,* the causative agent of salmon poisoning, and *N. risticii* (formerly *E. risticii*), the causative agent of Potomac horse fever, both infect dogs and cause thrombocytopenia. In dogs with salmon poisoning the prevalence of thrombocytopenia is as high as 80%. *E. canis*-like infection and *A. phagocytophilum* infection have been reported in a limited number of cats with haematological abnormalities such as thrombocytopenia. In cats with *E. canis*-like infection, haematological abnormalities were accompanied by bone marrow hypoplasia (see Chapter 18).

Babesiosis is an important protozoal tick-borne disease of the dog. Although infection with *Babesia canis* and *B. gibsoni* primarily causes haemolytic anaemia, thrombocytopenia is common in dogs with babesiosis and is likely to be multifactorial. Platelets undergo immune destruction owing to the formation of anti-platelet antibody, sequestration in an enlarged spleen or consumption by DIC in complicated cases of babesiosis. A wide range of platelet counts has been reported with *Babesia* spp. infections (platelet count 32–147 $\times$ 10^9/l). Surface bleeding is uncommon in uncomplicated cases of babesiosis, and if surface bleeding is identified, the finding suggests a form of babesiosis complicated by DIC (see Chapter 8).

Thrombocytopenia occurs in approximately half of the dogs infected with *Leptospira* spp. *Leptospira* organisms cause endothelial damage and platelet activation. Dogs infected with the Pomona serogroup are five times more likely to be thrombocytopenic. According to one study, dogs infected with *L. pomona* had a lower rate of hospital discharge than dogs infected with other serogroups. Other laboratory findings in dogs infected with any serogroup include azotaemia, anaemia, leucocytosis and elevated liver enzymes. In severe cases, elevations of PT and aPTT occur, consistent with a diagnosis of DIC.

Thrombocytopenia occurs in cases of infective endocarditis. The infecting organism is not related to the type of disease because thrombocytopenia is reported with Gram-positive and Gram-negative organisms, as well as *Bartonella* spp. The mechanism of thrombocytopenia in this condition has not been investigated.

Pancreatitis is a common diagnosis in dogs. In one study, 59% of dogs diagnosed with acute pancreatitis had concurrent thrombocytopenia. Most of the dogs had coexisting coagulation disorders. Laboratory findings of thrombocytopenia coupled with gastrointestinal signs should provoke further investigation for possible pancreatitis.

Clinical presentation

The patient history will often suggest possible aetiologies for thrombocytopenia. Dogs and cats with infectious diseases may have a history of flea or tick infestation. Drugs administered to treat medical conditions are known causes of thrombocytopenia. Historical information is diagnostic for thrombocytopenia associated with heatstroke and snake envenomation. Dogs and cats with a history of travel may have contracted an infection not endemic to their normal geographical location (e.g. leishmaniosis or histoplasmosis). Pets allowed to roam freely outdoors are exposed to organisms such as retroviruses or *Leptospira* spp., known causes of thrombocytopenia.

Signalment appears to be strongly associated with the development of primary IMTP. Bitches develop the disorder twice as often as male dogs. Several breeds of dog also develop primary IMTP more commonly, including the Cocker Spaniel, German Shepherd Dog, Rottweiler, Golden Retriever, Old English Sheepdog, and the Miniature and Toy Poodle. Age does not seem to be a predictor of primary IMTP. The reported age range is < 1–14 years; however, the majority of dogs are between 4 and 6 years of age. Because primary IMTP is rare in cats, age, breed and gender predilections have not been reported.

Every tissue in the body requires platelets to maintain haemostatic balance; consequently, thrombocytopenia results in clinical signs referable to multiple body systems. The major clinical sign of thrombocytopenia, regardless of the cause, is surface bleeding. In dogs with thrombocytopenia surface bleeding manifests as petechial and ecchymotic haemorrhage, epistaxis, haematuria, melaena, hyphaema, haemoptysis and prolonged bleeding after trauma or surgery (see Figures 23.1, 23.2 and 23.5). The clinical presentation of cats with thrombocytopenia appears to be similar to that of dogs, although cats seem to be less likely to show signs of haemorrhage even when the platelet count is very low (Jordan *et al.*, 1993).

In addition to clinical signs of haemorrhage, there may be clinical signs specific to an underlying disorder. Fever is common with infection and also with primary immune diseases. Masses, either external or discovered by diagnostic imaging, suggest cancer as the underlying cause. Body cavity haemorrhage, haemothorax or haemoabdomen, would be unlikely with thrombocytopenia as the primary haemostatic disorder and these findings suggest a global coagulation disorder such as anticoagulant rodenticide intoxication or DIC.

Diagnostic evaluation

The goal of the diagnostic investigation of thrombocytopenia is to differentiate between primary immune-mediated disease and thrombocytopenia secondary to an underlying cause. In primary IMTP, the only laboratory abnormality may be thrombocytopenia. An approach to the diagnostic evaluation is outlined in Figure 23.4.

Complete blood count

A complete blood count can elucidate potential underlying causes of thrombocytopenia. Certain automated haematology analysers give a visual depiction of platelet count in addition to that of reticulocytes and erythrocytes (Figure 23.7). Anaemia is common and is often secondary to blood loss. The presence of schistocytes suggests DIC or a microangiopathic process. Leucocytosis is often seen with infection; although leucopenia can occur with infections such as parvovirus or feline retrovirus infections. Aggregation of platelets occurs commonly during sampling and artefactually lowers the platelet

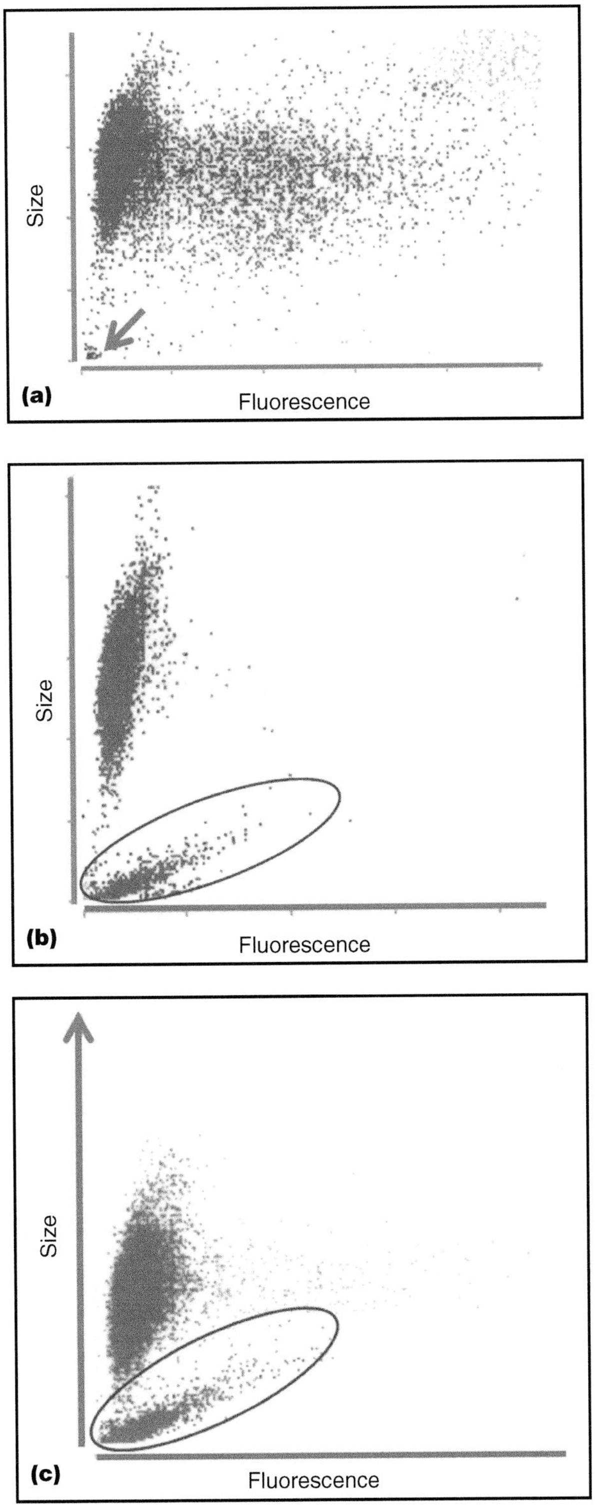

23.7 Plateletgrams from an automated haematology analyser demonstrating various platelet counts. Each blue dot represents one platelet. The red dots are red blood cells, **(a)** Canine platelet count = 2 x 10^9/l. **(b)** Canine platelet count = 268 x 10^9/l. **(c)** Feline platelet count = 765 x 10^9/l.

count. Review of the blood smear can determine the degree of clumping.

Biochemical profile

Clues to an underlying disease can be obtained from the biochemical profile. A decreased albumin to globulin ratio (< 0.7) should be followed up with serum protein electrophoresis. Monoclonal gammopathy will be seen with lymphoproliferative neoplasia, and sometimes in chronic infectious diseases (e.g. ehrlichiosis, anaplasmosis or leishmaniosis). Polyclonal gammopathy is a non-specific finding. Azotaemia suggests HUS as a potential cause of thrombocytopenia and if liver enzymes are elevated as well, leptospirosis should be considered.

Urinalysis

In dogs and cats with bleeding and thrombocytopenia, urine for analysis should not be obtained via cystocentesis owing to the risk of serious haemorrhage. Urinalysis results should be reviewed carefully for evidence of infection or proteinuria.

Faecal analysis

In dogs with thrombocytopenia and pulmonary infiltrates, a diagnosis of *Angiostrongylus vasorum* should be considered. Faecal analysis or evaluation of bronchoalveolar lavage fluid will detect larvae.

Platelet count and mean platelet volume

The platelet count can be estimated by counting platelets per oil immersion field as described in Chapter 22.

Blood samples intended for assessment of platelet parameters should be collected in EDTA. This anticoagulant causes less platelet aggregation and gives more accurate values for platelet count and mean platelet volume than citrate. When compared with EDTA, samples anticoagulated in citrate demonstrate increased aggregation. Increased aggregation and loss of the discoid shape of platelets account for the increase in mean platelet volume when citrate is used as the anticoagulant (Stokol and Erb, 2007).

Thrombocytopenia identified by an automated platelet count should be confirmed by a manual count. Platelets are prone to aggregation and in the cat are of similar size to red blood cells (RBCs). Automated methods cannot always distinguish between platelets, platelet clumps and feline RBCs. Automated platelet counts are not reliable in CKCSs with macrothrombocytosis. In addition to a manual platelet count, a blood smear should be reviewed for platelet aggregation as an artefactual cause of thrombocytopenia. Artefactual thrombocytopenia may occur in as many as 10–20% of dogs diagnosed with thrombocytopenia using an automated impedance analyser.

Repeated blood sampling with atraumatic venepuncture may be sufficient to identify pseudothrombocytopenia secondary to platelet clumping. Pseudothrombocytopenia from the use of EDTA anticoagulant has been reported in a dog. If the platelet count is still low when performed on a sample obtained via atraumatic venepuncture, collection of blood in citrate should be performed and the platelet count repeated on the citrated sample to determine whether EDTA pseudothrombocytopenia exists.

The mean platelet volume, as measured by automated haematology analysers, can be used in the diagnosis of IMTP. The combination of severe thrombocytopenia and microcytic platelets strongly suggests that the disorder is immune mediated. Increased mean platelet volume appears to be associated with active thrombopoiesis, although it is not specific for primary IMTP.

Coagulation testing

Thrombocytopenia may occur alone, or as a component of DIC. A coagulation profile can be used to differentiate the two disorders. Dogs with DIC will have elevations in at least two of the following tests in addition to thrombocytopenia: PT, aPTT, fibrin degradation products or D-dimers. Identification of an underlying disease known to be associated with DIC is also necessary.

Diagnostic imaging

When the cause of thrombocytopenia is not obvious from the history and physical examination or the minimum database, diagnostic imaging should be performed. Images should be reviewed carefully for abnormalities related to neoplastic, inflammatory and infectious diseases. A mass lesion or organ enlargement suggests a neoplastic disorder. Pleural effusion or alveolar infiltration is a non-specific finding potentially caused by haemorrhage from thrombocytopenia, or an underlying cause such as anticoagulant rodenticide intoxication or infection.

Abnormal findings on routine radiography of the thorax and abdomen may warrant follow-up with ultrasonography. Ultrasonography of the abdomen allows evaluation of the organ parenchyma for infiltrative neoplastic or inflammatory disease and can identify small mass lesions not recognized with radiography. An enlarged cardiac silhouette found with radiography should prompt echocardiography to evaluate the patient for cardiac diseases. Ultrasound examination of the thoracic cavity can identify intrathoracic masses obscured by pleural effusion, especially when thoracocentesis is contraindicated in the face of severe thrombocytopenia.

Platelet function testing

Haemorrhage from thrombocytopenia due to a platelet count between 30 and 150 × 10^9/l suggests a concurrent thrombopathia, because haemorrhage is uncommon with this degree of thrombocytopenia as a solitary abnormality. If thrombocytopenia and haemorrhage occur with a platelet count between 30 and 150 × 10^9/l, platelet function testing is indicated. Several tests have been used to evaluate global haemostasis in thrombocytopenic dogs: buccal mucosal bleeding time (BMBT), platelet aggregometry and thromboelastography (Boudreaux, 2008). Of these, only BMBT can be performed in routine clinical practice. The other tests are available at large referral centres. Additional tests of platelet function are available, but are not typically used in dogs with thrombocytopenia.

BMBT is a global assay of platelet function (see Chapter 22). Thrombocytopenia, thrombocytopathia vasculitis and von Willebrand's disease can all result in an abnormal BMBT. The BMBT is normal in CKCS with macrothrombocytopenia.

Thromboelastography is a global assay of coagulation that uses whole blood and measures the interaction between the cellular and plasma components of haemostasis during clot formation and dissolution (see Chapter 22).

Platelet aggregometry is considered the gold standard test for platelet function (see Chapter 22). Platelet aggregometry can be a direct assay, evaluating the patient's platelets, or it can be indirect, evaluating the patient's plasma for platelet inhibiting factors. Indirect platelet aggregometry has been used to identify a concurrent platelet function defect in dogs with primary IMTP (Kristensen *et al.*, 1994). Conversely, normal platelet function has been found using direct platelet aggregometry in CKCS with macrothrombocytosis.

Infectious disease testing

Multiple test methodologies are available to determine whether an infectious disease is the cause of thrombocytopenia; however, not all methodologies are available for every infectious agent. Diagnostic tests include light microscopy, culture, histology, serum antigen testing, serum antibody testing and polymerase chain reaction (PCR). The gold standard test depends on the disease being investigated. Of these tests, serum antibody testing is generally the least specific. It documents exposure to an infective agent, but does not confirm current infection. Serum antibody tests are rapid and readily available and, depending on sensitivity and specificity, may be useful in the diagnosis of a disease. Antibody tests include enzyme-linked immunosorbent assay (ELISA), western blot, immunofluorescence, agar gel immunodiffusion and agglutination assays. Antibody testing is used in the diagnosis of FIV, leishmaniosis, histoplasmosis and in leptospirosis where paired rising titres are considered diagnostic of infection. Culture of an infectious agent confirms the diagnosis, and is useful clinically in bacterial and fungal diseases; however, culture is insensitive, time-consuming and is not practical for many infectious diseases. Histopathology can confirm the presence of an infectious agent such as *Hepatozoon canis*, and blood smear cytology is useful for the diagnosis of large and small *Babesia* spp. as well as *Anaplasma phagocytophilum* and, rarely, *Ehrlichia canis* morulae. Antigen testing is considered the gold standard for diseases such as FeLV and dirofilariasis. PCR testing is very sensitive and specific. This methodology determines the presence or absence of minute quantities of DNA derived from an infectious agent. PCR testing is available for many infectious agents such as *Ehrlichia*, *Anaplasma*, *Leishmania* and *Babesia*.

Bone marrow evaluation

Bone marrow examination is not warranted in every patient with thrombocytopenia, and in dogs with severe (< 20 × 10^9/l) thrombocytopenia it does not appear to provide specific diagnostic or prognostic information (Miller and Lunn, 2007). Bone marrow examination is warranted when thrombocytopenia persists despite treatment and there is a suspicion of myelophthisis, based on the finding of abnormal cells on the haemogram, or bicytopenia/pancytopenia occurs. Expected findings for bone marrow aspiration in cases of thrombocytopenia are listed in Figure 23.8.

Megakaryocyte hypoplasia
• Drug toxicity • Toxic agents • Infection: chronic ehrlichiosis/anaplasmosis • Amegakaryocytic thrombocytopenia • Radiation • Cyclic haemopoiesis
Megakarocyte hyperplasia
• Immune-mediated thrombocytopenia • Disseminated intravascular coagulation • Platelet sequestration
Abnormal cells; variable megakaryocyte numbers
• Myelofibrosis • Myeloproliferative disorders • Lymphoproliferative diseases • Myelodysplastic syndrome • Myelophthisis • Infection: histoplasmosis

23.8 Bone marrow findings in thrombocytopenia and associated orders.

Antiplatelet and antimegakaryocyte antibodies

Demonstration of antibodies bound to the surface of platelets or megakaryocytes would be a useful test for the diagnosis of primary IMTP. Several methods of detecting these antibodies have been developed, including ELISA and flow cytometry to measure directly or indirectly the presence of platelet antibodies in both the dog and cat. However, these tests are not specific for the diagnosis of primary IMTP. When an anti-platelet antibody test is positive, the thrombocytopenia can be assumed to have an immunological component. Demonstration of anti-megakaryocyte antibodies has similar difficulties to the demonstration of anti-platelet antibodies. In addition, the demonstration of anti-megakaryocyte antibodies requires an adequate bone marrow sample.

Treatment

The treatment of thrombocytopenia is dictated by the aetiology. Frequently, the aetiology is unknown until the results of infectious disease testing become available. One rational approach to the treatment of a dog or cat with thrombocytopenia is to obtain the results of the tests listed as Level 1 tests in the algorithm in Figure 23.4. If initial testing eliminates neoplasia, DIC, heartworm disease and severe infection as the cause of thrombocytopenia, doxycycline therapy should be initiated (10 mg/kg orally q24h or divided q12h). At this time, prednisone or prednisolone therapy could be started if haemorrhage is severe, but if haemorrhage is mild, prednisone or prednisolone therapy should be delayed to allow assessment of the response to doxycycline therapy in 24–48 hours. Improvement with doxycycline therapy suggests that prednisone or prednisolone will not be required. Lack of improvement 24–48 hours following initiation of doxycycline therapy signifies that a doxycycline-responsive disease, such as Rocky Mountain spotted fever, is not likely and glucocorticoid treatment should be considered. If infectious disease testing confirms a doxycycline-responsive disease, therapy should continue as appropriate for the disease. The concern when initiating glucocorticoid therapy in cases of thrombocytopenia without a definitive diagnosis is the possibility that treatment will mask an underlying lymphoproliferative disorder. Given that IMTP has been associated with an increased risk of the development of lymphoma, bone marrow aspiration should be considered prior to initiation of glucocorticoid therapy to eliminate occult lymphoproliferative disease from the differential list.

Drug therapy

Multiple drugs have been used in the management of platelet disorders. Prednisone and prednisolone are considered the first line drugs for dogs and cats, respectively, in treatment of IMTP, although some clinicians favour dexamethasone or methylprednisolone (Wondratschek *et al.*, 2010). Glucocorticoids inhibit macrophage clearance of antibody-bound platelets by the spleen. The optimal dosage has not been determined, but a general recommendation of 1.5–2 mg/kg prednisolone daily is often made. Once a normal platelet count has been attained, the glucocorticoid dose is tapered by 25% per week until a dosage of 0.5 mg/kg every other day is reached. A normal platelet count is typically reached in 7–10 days. After approximately 6 months passes without relapse, glucocorticoids can be discontinued.

Vincristine belongs to a group of cytotoxic drugs known as the vinca alkaloids. Most commonly used for the treatment of lymphoproliferative neoplasia, vincristine binds platelet cytoskeletal tubulin avidly. Administration of vincristine and prednisone to dogs with IMTP results in a more rapid increase in platelet numbers and shortened hospitalization time when compared with treatment with prednisone alone (see Chapter 26). The mechanism of platelet increase is unknown and is speculated to be either an increase in platelet production or a decrease in platelet destruction. The dose of vincristine typically used in dogs to increase platelet count is 0.02 mg/kg i.v. once; most dogs respond in 3–7 days. The dose can be repeated in 7 days if the platelet count has not improved.

A rapid improvement in platelet count has been seen in cases of canine IMTP treated with a single dose of intravenously administered human immunoglobulin G (IVIG). Strong evidence supports the use of this product for short-term management of severe IMTP. A randomized, double blind placebo controlled clinical trial demonstrated superior results when dogs were treated with glucocorticoids and IVIG compared with treatment with glucocorticoids alone (Bianco *et al.*, 2009). All dogs treated with IVIG responded and had platelet counts > 40 × 10^9/l within 7 days of treatment. The median time to response was 3.5 days. The use of IVIG is limited because of the risk of anaphylaxis associated with antibody formation following repeated administrations, its cost, and the concern that a single administration of the drug does not result in long-term immunosuppressive effects. The dosage of IVIG is 0.5 g/kg administered as an i.v. infusion over 6–12 hours.

Ciclosporin and azathioprine are adjunct immunosuppressive agents that may be used to treat IMTP when glucocorticoid and vincristine therapy failure to resolve the thrombocytopenia. Neither has been studied in a randomized clinical trial. Ciclosporin is a polypeptide macrolide that modulates cell-mediated immunity by blocking production of cytokines by activated T cells. The dose of ciclosporin is adjusted on the basis of trough levels. The target trough concentration is not universally agreed. Some recommend a trough concentration of 400–600 ng/ml and a starting dose of 15–30 mg/kg q24h, others use 250–400 ng/ml with a starting dose of 10 mg/kg q24h. Azathioprine is a cytotoxic analogue of adenine that is used primarily for immunosuppression. It is converted to its active form though a series of metabolic steps in the liver. Azathioprine interferes with DNA and RNA synthesis, inhibits coenzyme formation and modifies T cell function. Administration of azathioprine is typically at a dose rate of 2 mg/kg orally q24h in dogs, tapering to 1 mg/kg every other day when a response is seen. Cats are very sensitive to the toxic effects of azathioprine and its use is not recommended in this species. Profound myelosuppression occurs in cats and some dogs and is believed to be caused by a deficiency in the enzymes required to inactivate azathioprine. Hepatotoxicity and pancreatitis have also been reported.

Successful use of danazol, an anabolic steroid, has been reported anecdotally in dogs with IMTP. Danazol is thought to improve the platelet count by reducing Fc receptors on macrophages and decreasing anti-platelet IgG antibodies. A dosage of 5–10 mg/kg q12h has been recommended. A response may not be seen until the therapy has been given for 1–3 months.

Vitamin K_1 is the antidote for anticoagulant rodenticide toxicity. Vitamin K_1 anticoagulant factors (II, VII, IX, X) are produced by the liver in an inactive form and require vitamin K_1 for activation. Anticoagulant rodenticides inhibit vitamin K_1 activation of these coagulation factors, resulting in coagulation factor depletion and clinical haemorrhage. The route of administration varies depending on the formulation of vitamin K_1 administered. Review of the product insert before administration is necessary because some products may cause anaphylaxis if administered intravenously. The recommended dosage is 2.2 mg/kg divided q8h or q6h. The duration of administration depends on the type of poisoning being treated. For short-acting anticoagulant rodenticides 2 weeks of therapy might be adequate, but for long-acting anticoagulant rodenticides 6 weeks of therapy is required; however, the dose can be tapered over the 6-week treatment period. The PT should be measured 48 hours after discontinuation of vitamin K_1.

Transfusion support

Transfusion of a variety of blood products is an important supportive therapy during the treatment of thrombocytopenia. Packed red blood cell transfusions should be administered to control the clinical signs associated with anaemia, regardless of the cause of anaemia. Red blood cell transfusion should be considered when the following occur: weakness, tachycardia, hypotension unresponsive to volume expansion, and hypoxaemia unresponsive to oxygen supplementation. Dogs with gastrointestinal bleeding secondary to thrombocytopenia have high transfusion requirements compared with dogs with surface bleeding. Plasma transfusion has a limited role in the management of thrombocytopenia, unless the thrombocytopenia is attributable to coagulation factor deficiencies such as occur in anticoagulant rodenticide toxicity or DIC. Platelet transfusion is reserved typically for treatment of life-threatening haemorrhage because of the short lifespan of the transfused platelets and because platelets require specialized conditions for collection and storage. The need for platelet transfusion is met most often by the transfusion of fresh whole blood. Platelets stored in CPDA-1 (citrate phosphate dextrose adenine anticoagulant) on a continuous rocker for up to 8 hours following collection at 20–24°C maintain adequate function and post-transfusion survival. The ability of this product to increase the platelet count and control haemorrhage has not been evaluated in clinical cases of thrombocytopenia.

Surgery

Splenectomy has been used in primary IMTP when the dose of immunosuppressive agents required to maintain an adequate platelet count results in unacceptable side effects, or when immunosuppressive agents fail to control relapses of thrombocytopenia. Based on limited reports of dogs with thrombocytopenia, the use of all immunosuppressive agents can be discontinued in approximately 50–75% of dogs treated with splenectomy (Feldman *et al.*, 1985; Jans *et al.*, 1990).

Prognosis

The prognosis of dogs and cats with thrombocytopenia depends on the inciting cause and the response to treatment. Of 13 cats diagnosed presumptively with feline primary IMTP, 11 responded to immunosuppressive treatment and supportive measures such as blood transfusion and were released from the hospital (Wondratschek *et al.*, 2010; Bianco *et al.*, 2008). The prognosis for dogs with primary IMTP is considered good to guarded, with mortality rates ranging from 3–30%. The prognosis reported for concurrent IMTP and IMHA varies among reports. European dogs with concurrent IMTP and IMHA have a similar prognosis to those with ITP, and dogs from North America have a less favourable prognosis, with many dogs dying or being euthanized within a month of diagnosis. Relapse is common in dogs treated for primary IMTP. Estimates of relapse suggest that 25–50% of dogs will relapse and require long-term intermittent immunosuppression (Jans *et al.*, 1990; Putsche and Kohn, 2008).

Thrombocytosis

Thrombocytosis has been defined in veterinary medicine as a platelet count > 700 × 10^9/l. Three forms of thrombocytosis have been described: primary, also known as myeloproliferative thrombocytosis; secondary or reactive thrombocytosis; and physiological thrombocytosis (Chisholm-Chait, 1999). Myeloproliferative thrombocytosis occurs in disorders such as essential thrombocythaemia, polycythaemia vera and leukaemias arising from the various white blood cell lines. Reactive thrombocytosis is the most common disorder, and occurs as a sequel to an underlying condition. The elevated platelet count in reactive thrombocytosis does not result in clinical signs related to the elevated platelet count. Physiological thrombocytosis is the result of platelet mobilization in response to excitement or exercise.

Mechanism and causes

Myeloproliferative thrombocytosis is a component of several different myeloproliferative disorders. Myeloproliferative disorders result from clonal proliferation of haematopoietic stem cells, and when the proliferating cell is the megakaryocyte or a megakaryocyte progenitor cell, myeloproliferative thrombocytosis ensues. Morphological and functional abnormalities of megakaryocytes and platelets are also components of myeloproliferative thrombocytosis. Essential thrombocythaemia is a specific myeloproliferative disorder of platelets. In humans, polycythaemia vera is a myeloproliferative disorder with clonal proliferation of red blood cells and platelets. Canine and feline polycythaemia vera generally lack thrombocytosis as a laboratory feature of the disease, but not uniformly (see Chapter 4).

Secondary (reactive) thrombocytosis results from a physiological stimulation of the bone marrow by cytokines in response to an underlying condition. The cytokines responsible for this condition are unknown in dogs and cats, but in humans they include thrombopoietin, interleukin 6 and catecholamines. Conditions that may underlie secondary thrombocytosis in dogs and cats are outlined in Figure 23.9. Gastrointestinal and endocrine diseases predominate among cats diagnosed with reactive thrombocytosis.

A transient elevation of platelet count resulting from splenic contraction and lasting 15–30 minutes is the hallmark of physiological thrombocytosis. No clinical signs have been attributed to physiological thrombocytosis and treatment is unnecessary.

- Blood loss
- Chemotherapy rebound:
  - Doxorubicin in cats
- Haemolysis
- Infection:
  - *Hepatozoon canis*
- Inflammation:
  - Steroid-responsive meningitis/arteritis
  - Reactive amyloidosis
- Endocrine disease:
  - Glucocorticoid excess
  - Hyperthyroidism
- Iron deficiency
- Neoplasia:
  - Renal adenocarcinoma
  - Lymphoma
  - Myeloproliferative disorders
- Splenectomy
- Surgery
- Vincristine administration

23.9 Conditions associated with secondary (reactive) thrombocytosis.

Clinical presentation

A complete history and physical examination will be critical to differentiate between myelodysplastic and reactive thrombocytosis. Specific associations between breed and sex have not been made in cases of thrombocytosis. Young cats (< 1 year of age) appear to be affected commonly with thrombocytosis (Rizzo *et al.*, 2007). A history of prior administration of chemotherapeutic agents, especially vincristine in dogs or doxorubicin in cats, has been associated with thrombocytosis. Recent surgery or splenectomy explains an elevated platelet count, and a cat with a poor body condition and a thyroid nodule suggests reactive thrombocytosis associated with hyperthyroidism.

As is typical for patients with haematological disorders, dogs and cats with thrombocytosis may present with minimal or vague clinical signs (Hammer, 1991; Rizzo *et al.*, 2007). In the few reported cases of essential thrombocythaemia, lethargy, anorexia and weight loss were seen. Physical examination may reveal splenomegaly and pale or hyperaemic mucous membranes if anaemia or polycythaemia are concurrent. Dogs and cats with thrombocytosis should be examined carefully for signs of haemorrhage or thrombosis because both have been reported in cases of essential thrombocythaemia. Surprisingly, thrombocytosis is not a hallmark of aortic thromboembolism in either the dog or the cat.

Diagnostic evaluation

The diagnostic criteria for essential thrombocythaemia in humans cannot be adapted easily to veterinary patients because genetic testing is considered pathognomonic for the diagnosis of essential thrombocythaemia in human patients (Beer and Green, 2009). Mutations in the tyrosine kinase gene, *JAK2V617F*, or the gene for the thrombopoietin receptor, MPL, are found in human patients with essential thrombocythaemia and have not been evaluated in dogs and cats believed to have the same disorder. In addition, essential thrombocythaemia shares features of chronic myeloproliferative syndromes, and cytogenetic testing is performed to identify the Philadelphia chromosome. Consequently, the diagnosis of essential thrombocythaemia will be made in animals with persistent thrombocytosis when causes of reactive thrombocytosis and other myeloproliferative disorders have been excluded and abnormalities in platelet/megakaryocyte morphology and function have been identified.

The diagnostic plan for a dog or cat with a platelet count above 700 × 10^9/l should be developed to differentiate myelodysplastic thrombocytosis from reactive thrombocytosis (Chisholm-Chait, 1999). Typically, a complete blood count will already have been analysed when the thrombocytosis was identified initially. Platelet counts should be repeated once or twice to determine whether thrombocytosis is persistent. The complete blood count should be reviewed for characteristic features of iron deficiency, such as a non-regenerative anaemia with microcytosis and hypochromia, and for morphological abnormalities in additional cell lines that may suggest a myeloproliferative disorder. Serum iron levels should be obtained if indicated. Biochemical profiling may also support a diagnosis of iron deficiency or blood loss if the total protein is decreased or the blood urea nitrogen increased in the absence of other indicators of kidney disease. Biochemical profiling will also suggest a diagnosis such as hyperadrenocorticism as the cause of reactive thrombocytosis. Because of the high intra-platelet concentration of potassium, factitious hyperkalaemia is associated with thrombocytosis. Elevated serum potassium levels should be confirmed by measuring the plasma concentration of potassium in blood collected in lithium heparin tubes. Routine urinalysis assists in the diagnosis of kidney disease as the underlying cause of thrombocytosis, or blood loss due to urinary tract haemorrhage. Diagnostic imaging of both the thoracic and abdominal cavities is critical to eliminate neoplastic causes of reactive thrombocytosis. If no potential causes for reactive thrombocytosis are identified during the diagnostic evaluation, a diagnosis of essential thrombocythaemia should be considered and additional platelet testing performed.

Both functional and morphological abnormalities of platelets and megakaryocytes have been reported in cases with essential thrombocythaemia. Evaluation of a fresh blood smear may demonstrate megaplatelets, hypogranular platelets or platelets with serpentine shape. Evaluation of a bone marrow aspirate allows quantification and morphological assessment of megakaryocytes. The bone marrow aspirate of a dog or cat with essential thrombocytosis will show a marked increase in the number of megakaryocytes. These megakaryocytes can be dimorphic, have abnormal or absent alpha granules, giant platelet granules and increased cytoplasmic vacuolation. Platelet function, as assessed by *in vitro* aggregometry, reflects decreased responsiveness to adenosine diphosphate (ADP) and arachidonic acid. Thromboelastography has not been used to study the platelets of dogs and cats with thrombocytosis; however, human patients with thrombocytosis have a hypercoagulable state as determined by thromboelastography.

Treatment and prognosis

The optimal treatment of essential thrombocytosis in animals is unknown and is typically based on treatment of human patients. Low dose aspirin is prescribed to prevent thrombosis in human patients. A dosage of 0.5 mg/kg orally q24h has been recommended as the antithrombotic dose in dogs. The dosage for cats is 10–20 mg/kg orally every 2–3 days. The first-line treatment for essential thrombocythaemia in humans is hydroxycarbamide (hydroxyurea), which has been used with variable success in veterinary patients. One reported dosing scheme is 25 mg/kg q12h for 7 days followed by a maintenance dosage of 16.25 mg/kg q24h. A few reports indicate that radioactive phosphorus, ^{32}P, affects remission in essential thrombocythaemia, but limited availability restricts its usage. Specific treatment of reactive thrombocytosis is not required. The treatment should focus on the underlying disorder.

The prognosis for dogs and cats with thrombocytosis is variable. The underlying disorder determines the prognosis in reactive thrombocytosis. Dogs and cats with essential thrombocytosis may have rapidly progressive haemopoietic failure, slowly progressive disease, or succumb to the toxic effects of therapeutic agents.

References and further reading

Beer PA and Green AR (2009) Pathogenesis and management of essential thrombocythemia. *Hematology: American Society of Hematology Education Program*, pp.621–628

Bianco D, Armstrong PJ and Washabau RJ (2008) Presumed primary immune-mediated thrombocytopenia in 4 cats. *Journal of Feline Medicine and Surgery* **10**, 495–500

Bianco D, Armstrong PJ and Washabau RJ (2009) A prospective, randomized, double-blinded, placebo-controlled study of human intravenous immunoglobulin for the acute management of presumptive primary immune-mediate d thrombocytopenia in dogs. *Journal of Veterinary Internal Medicine* **23**, 1071–1078

Botsch V, Küchenhoff H, Hartmann K *et al.* (2009) Retrospective study of 871 dogs with thrombocytopenia. *Veterinary Record* **21**, 647–651

Boudreaux MK (2008) Characteristics, diagnosis and treatment of inherited platelet disorders in mammals. *Journal of the American Veterinary Medical Association* **233**, 1251–1259

Chisholm-Chait A (1999) Essential thrombocythemia in dogs and cats. Part I and Part II. *Compendium on Continuing Education for the Practicing Veterinarian* **21**, 158–167 and 218–229

Davis B, Toivio-Kinnucan M, Schuller S *et al.* (2008) Mutation in β-1 tubulin correlated with macrothrombocytopenia in Cavalier King Charles Spaniels. *Journal of Veterinary Internal Medicine* **22**, 540–545

Feldman BF, Handagama P and Lubberink AAME (1985) Splenectomy as an adjunctive therapy for immune-mediated thrombocytopenia and haemolytic anemia in the dog. *Journal of the American Veterianry Medical Association* **187**, 617–629

Gasser AM, Birkenheuer AJ and Breitschwerdt EB (2001) Canine Rocky Mountain spotted fever: a retrospective study of 30 cases. *Journal of the American Animal Hospital Association* **37**, 41–48

Gleich S and Hartmann K (2009) Hematology and serum biochemistry of feline immunodeficiency virus infected and feline leukemia infected cats. *Journal of Veterinary Internal Medicine*

23, 552–558
Grindem CB, Breitschwerdt EB, Corbett WT *et al.* (1991) Epidemiologic survey of thrombocytopenia in dogs: a report on 987 cases. *Veterinary Clinical Pathology* **20**, 38–43
Hammer AS (1991) Thrombocytosis in dogs and cats: a retrospective study. *Comparative Haematology International* **1**, 181–186
Holloway S, Senior D, Roth L *et al.* (1993) Hemolytic uremic syndrome in dogs. *Journal of Veterinary Internal Medicine* **7**, 220–227
Jans HE, Armstong PJ and Price GS (1990) Therapy of immune mediated thrombocytopenia. *Journal of Veterinary Internal Medicine* **4**, 4–7
Jordan HL, Grindem CB and Breitschwerdt EB (1993) Thrombocytopenia in cats: a retrospective study of 41 cases. *Journal of Veterinary Internal Medicine* **7**, 261–265
Kristensen AT, Weiss DJ and Klausner JS (1994) Platelet dysfunction associated with immune-mediated thrombocytopenia in dogs. *Journal of Veterinary Internal Medicine* **8**, 323–327
Miller MD and Lunn KF (2007) Diagnostic use of cytologic examination of bone marrow from dogs with thrombocytopenia: 58 cases (1994–2004). *Journal of the American Veterinary Medical Association* **213**, 1540–1544
Putsche JC and Kohn B (2008) Primary immune-mediated thrombocytopenia in 30 dogs (1997–2003). *Journal of the American Animal Hospital Association* **44**, 250–257
Rizzo F, Tappin SW and Tasker S (2007) Thrombocytosis in cats: a retrospective study of 51 cases (2000–2005). *Journal of Feline Medicine and Surgery* **9**, 319–325
Steiss JE, Brewer WG, Welles E *et al.* (2000) hematologic and serum biochemical reference values in retired greyhounds. *Compendium on Continuing Education for the Practicing Veterinarian* **22**, 243–248
Stokol T and Erb HN (2007) A comparison of platelet parameters in EDTA- and citrate-anticoagulated blood in dogs. *Veterinary Clinical Pathology* **36**, 48–154
Trepanier LA, Danhof R, Toll J *et al.* (2003) Clinical findings in 40 dogs with hypersensitivity associated with administration of potentiated sulfonamides. *Journal of Veterinary Internal Medicine* **17**, 647–652
Wardrop KJ, Lewis D, Mark S *et al.* (1997) Posttransfusion purpura in a dog with hemophilia A. *Journal of Veterinary Internal Medicine* **11**, 261–263
Wondratschek C, Weingart C and Kohn B (2010) Primary immune-mediated thrombocytopenia in cats. *Journal of the American Animal Hospital Association* **46**, 12–19

24

Disorders of platelet function

Tracy Stokol and James Catalfamo

Introduction

The platelet disorders encountered most commonly in veterinary practice are quantitative abnormalities, particularly thrombocytopenia. Defects in platelet function, i.e. thrombopathias (thrombocytopathies), are much less common and are difficult to diagnose because they require specialized tests, most of which are not readily available to the general practitioner. However, the practitioner may have the ability to utilize recently developed molecular diagnostic tests that simply require collection and submission of a blood sample for genetic analysis. Abnormalities in platelet function have been documented in domestic animals and result in abnormal bleeding in affected individuals. Thrombopathias should always be suspected if an animal is bleeding excessively, but has a normal platelet count and coagulation profile. Knowledge of normal platelet physiology and function is helpful in understanding the different forms of disturbed platelet function.

Platelet structure

Platelets are small anucleate cells produced by megakaryocytes in the bone marrow and pulmonary vasculature. In the absence of vessel injury, platelets circulate as discoid cells and have minimal interaction with other blood components, including the vessel wall. When stimulated, platelets function as the primary defence mechanism against bleeding. Despite its small size, the platelet is a complex cell. The platelet is enclosed by a plasma membrane, which is invaginated at multiple points to increase the extracellular surface area and encloses a cytoplasm rich in organelles, membranous structures, specialized secretory granules and structural contractile proteins (Figure 24.1). The platelet can be divided into several compartments, each having distinctive roles in platelet function. These include the plasma membrane, the dense tubular system, secretory granules and the structural proteins that comprise the platelet cytoskeleton.

Plasma membrane

The platelet is surrounded by a plasma membrane that extends through a system of channels to form the open canalicular system (Figure 24.1). This membrane structure maintains cytoplasmic integrity and is the surface that sustains the external interactions among vascular and plasma proteins, platelets and other blood cells and the network of

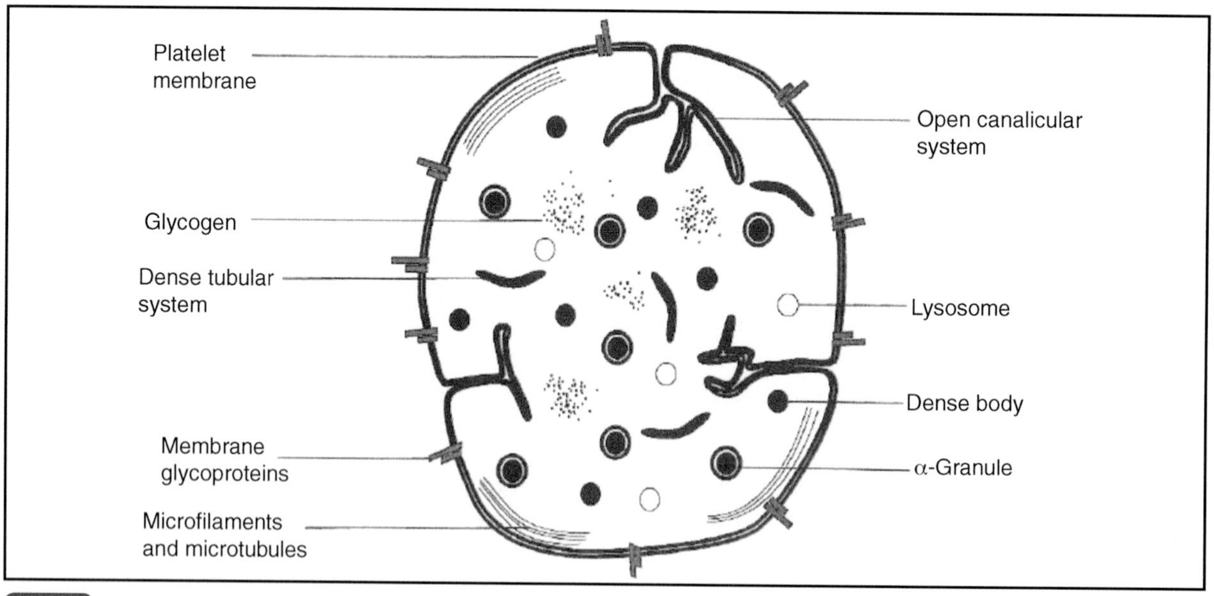

24.1 Schematic illustration of platelet ultrastructure.

structural proteins that make up the platelet cytoskeleton. It is selectively permeable and controls the movement of substances in and out of the cell. It is pivotal to platelet adhesion, aggregation, secretion, contraction and procoagulant activity.

The plasma membrane consists primarily of a phospholipid bilayer containing integral membrane proteins and cholesterol. Variations in cholesterol:phospholipid ratios modulate membrane fluidity. Phospholipids within the membrane are distributed asymmetrically; the asymmetry is maintained by phospholipid-specific transporter proteins. In the resting platelet, the outer layer is rich in phosphatidylcholine and sphingomyelin, whereas the inner layer is rich in phosphatidylserine and phosphatidylethanolamine. This asymmetry is essential for proper platelet function, because the alterations in the distribution of the phospholipids (specifically, the preferential movement of phosphatidylserine to the outer layer of the membrane) that occur on platelet activation convert the platelet into a procoagulant surface. Numerous glycoproteins (GPs) are embedded within the lipid bilayer. These proteins span the membrane and have extracellular and cytoplasmic domains. GPs often function as receptor molecules for platelet activation, adhesion and aggregation, allowing the platelet to interact with other cells and the subendothelial matrix. The glycoproteins are labelled consecutively with Roman numerals and belong to several different gene families, including integrins, leucine-rich glycoproteins, selectins, the immunoglobulin superfamily and quadraspanins. Figure 24.2 lists the major cell surface proteins with known roles in platelet function.

The different plasma membrane components have specific roles in platelet function. The translocation of phosphatidylserine to the outer membrane provides a binding surface for activated coagulation factors (especially those associated with the activation of factor (F) X and prothrombin) and promotes their catalytic activity (Figure 24.3). This is essential for the amplification and propagation of thrombin generation and fibrin clot formation. The

Platelet membrane receptor	Ligand	Role in platelet function
Integrins		
GPIIb-IIIa ($\alpha_{IIb}\beta_3$)	Fibrinogen, von Willebrand factor (vWF), fibronectin, vitronectin	Aggregation and spreading, outside–in and inside–out signalling
Vitronectin receptor ($\alpha_v\beta_3$)	Vitronectin, fibrinogen, fibronectin, thrombospondin	Adhesion (low shear)
GPIa-IIa ($\alpha_2\beta_1$)	Collagen	Adhesion (low shear)
GPIc-IIa ($\alpha_5\beta_1$)	Fibronectin	Adhesion (low shear)
GPIc-IIa region ($\alpha_6\beta_1$)	Laminin	Adhesion (low shear)
Leucine-rich glycoproteins		
GPIb-IX	vWF	Adhesion (high shear) and shape change
GPV	Forms a complex with GPIb-IX	Binding site for α-thrombin and binds vWF
GPVI	Collagen	Major signalling receptor for collagen, required for aggregation and secretion
Nucleotide receptors		
$P2Y_{12}$	ADP	Aggregation, inhibition of adenylyl cyclase
$P2Y_1$	ADP	Aggregation, shape change, mobilizes ionized calcium, stimulates IP3 formation
$P2X_1$	ATP	Rapid calcium influx, shape change
Thrombin-cleaved receptors		
PAR1 and PAR3 (human)	Primary thrombin receptors	Aggregation, shape change, ionized calcium mobilization, IP3 formation and granule secretion
PAR3 and PAR4 (mice)	Primary thrombin receptors	Aggregation, shape change, ionized calcium mobilization, IP3 formation and granule secretion
Selectins		
P-selectin (α-granule)	Lectins	Leucocyte–platelet interactions

24.2 Platelet cell surface receptors and their role in platelet function. ADP, adenosine diphosphate; ATP, adenosine triphosphate; IP3, inositol 1, 4, 5-triphosphate; PAR, protease-activated receptor.

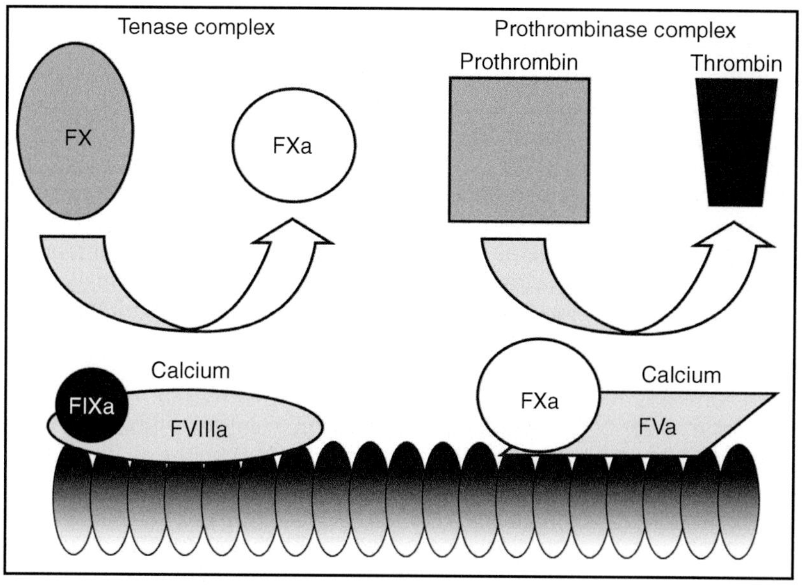

24.3 Schematic illustration of assembly of the tenase and prothrombinase complexes on the platelet surface. During platelet activation, phosphatidylserine is enriched in the outer leaflet of the platelet membrane. The tenase complex consists of the platelet membrane-associated assembly of activated factor IX (FIXa), activated factor VIII (FVIIIa), phosphatidylserine and ionized calcium (calcium) and is responsible for the activation of factor X. Similarly, the prothrombinase complex consists of a complex of activated factor X (FXa), activated factor V (FVa), phosphatidylserine and ionized calcium and is responsible for the activation of prothrombin to thrombin.

exposure of phosphatidylserine and the release of platelet membrane derived microparticles are essential for platelet procoagulant activity. This activity was previously called platelet factor 3 (PF3) activity. Arachidonic acid is produced by the action of phospholipase A_2 on membrane phospholipids (particularly phosphatidylcholine). Arachidonic acid is the initial substrate in a series of reactions that result in eicosanoid (prostaglandin) synthesis (Figure 24.4). The most important platelet eicosanoid is thromboxane A_2, a potent mediator of platelet aggregation and recruitment. The surface glycoproteins, especially the complexes of GPIb-IX and GPIIb-IIIa, act as receptors for both soluble (e.g. fibrinogen) and insoluble platelet-anchoring ligands (e.g. collagen) and are essential for platelet aggregation and platelet adhesion to the vascular subendothelium. A qualitative or quantitative defect in these receptors results in abnormal platelet function.

The open canalicular system, produced by invaginations of the plasma membrane, maintains direct contact with the plasma and is the likely site of endocytosis of plasma proteins into the platelet (see Figure 24.1). The contents of both α-granules and dense bodies are exocytosed into the open canalicular system during the release reaction.

Dense tubular system

The dense tubular system (composed of residual smooth endoplasmic reticulum) actively sequesters calcium by means of a calcium pump, the activity of which is enhanced by cyclic adenosine monophosphate (cAMP). The concentration of cyclic AMP is regulated by two enzymes: adenylate cyclase, which increases cAMP concentrations, and phosphodiesterase, which destroys cAMP. The release of ionized calcium from the dense tubular system is essential for platelet activation, including platelet granule secretion and aggregation. Therefore, agents that stimulate adenylate cyclase, such as prostacyclin, increase cAMP concentrations. This in turn promotes calcium sequestration in the dense tubular system and inhibits aggregation and release. The dense tubular system also contains a platelet-specific peroxidase and enzymes involved in prostaglandin synthesis.

Secretory organelles

Blood platelets are rich in cell organelles including two platelet-specific granules, α-granules and δ-granules (dense bodies), as well as organelles common to other cell types including mitochondria, peroxisomes and lysosomes. Figure 24.5 lists the contents of the platelet-specific granules. The α-granule localized proteins (von Willebrand factor (vWf) and fibrinogen) are secreted during the release reaction and support platelet adhesion and aggregation. α-Granule localized fibrinogen, FXI, FVIII and FV, when secreted during platelet activation, support thrombin generation and subsequent fibrin formation. The dense bodies are the storage sites for the non-metabolic pool of adenosine triphosphate (ATP), adenosine diphosphate (ADP), serotonin and calcium. Two thirds of the platelet's adenine nucleotides are in this storage pool, with an ATP:ADP ratio of 2:3. The metabolic pool has an ATP:ADP ratio of 8:1. Deficiency within the storage pool, resulting from reduced or absent dense bodies, is characterized by an increased ATP:ADP ratio in the storage pool, approaching that of the metabolic pool.

Cytoskeleton

Platelets have a membrane skeleton that consists of two-dimensional assemblies of spectrin strands that interconnect at their ends by binding actin filaments. The cytoskeletal system defines the discoid shape of the resting platelet and maintains cell integrity as the platelets encounter high fluid shear forces generated by blood flow over the vascular endothelium. When platelets are activated the internal actin cytoskeleton is remodelled. These changes contribute to platelet shape change, spreading along exposed subendothelial surfaces, granule release and clot retraction.

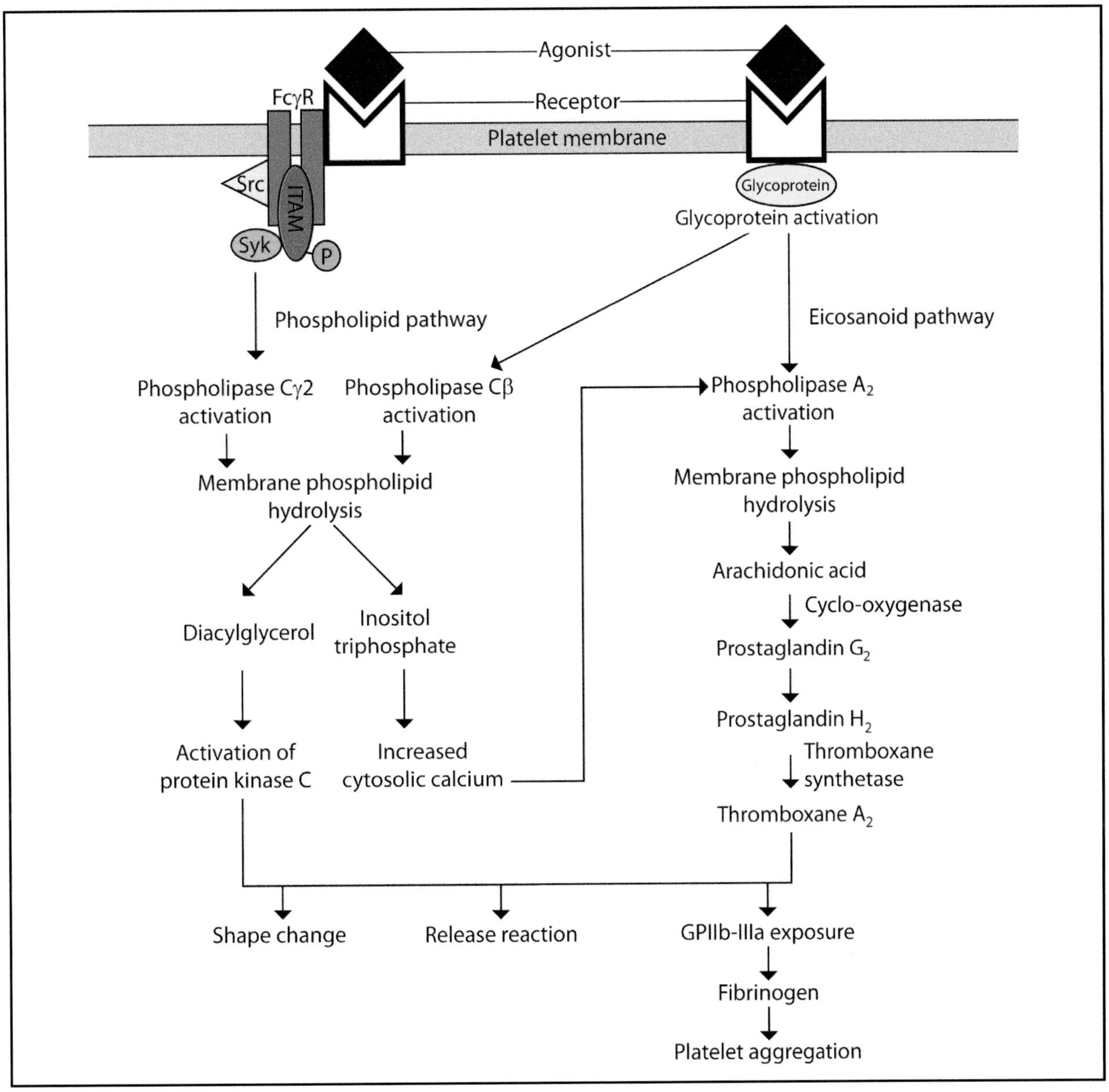

24.4 Basic platelet reaction. This is the sequence of signalling events that occurs during platelet activation. The reaction is initiated when an agonist binds to its specific receptor on the platelet plasma membrane. Receptors for ADP, thromboxane A_2, thrombin, adrenaline (epinephrine), serotonin and prostaglandins E_2 and I_2 are coupled to messengers called glycoproteins (GPs); receptors for IgG, the collagen receptor GPVI and C-type lectin-like receptor 2 are FcγR-linked. Upon activation, GPs trigger activation of phospholipase A_2 (eicosanoid or arachidonate pathway) or phospholipase Cβ (phospholipid pathway). In the eicosanoid pathway, phospholipase A_2 catalyses the release of arachidonic acid from phospholipids (especially phosphatidylcholine) in the platelet membrane; leading to the synthesis of prostaglandin endoperoxides and thromboxane A_2. Thromboxane A_2 plays a critical role in platelet recruitment and granule secretion. The phospholipid pathway is activated by both GP- and FcγR-coupled receptors. The FcγR-linked platelet receptors contain an immunoreceptor tyrosine-based activation motif (ITAM) similar to the primary signalling domain of classical immunoreceptors. Following agonist binding, the ITAM domain is phosphorylated; Syk (a tyrosine kinase) binds to the phosphorylated ITAM domain of the FcγR chain and triggers phospholipase Cγ activation. Activated phospholipase C (γ or β) in turn hydrolyses phosphatidylinositol 4, 5-bisphosphate to diacylglycerol and inositol 1, 4, 5-triphosphate (IP). Diacylglycerol activates protein kinase C, which, through secondary messengers, leads to platelet aggregation, shape change, and secretion. Inositol triphosphate increases cytosolic calcium concentrations by promoting calcium release from the dense tubular system and entry of extracellular ionized calcium. The increased intracellular calcium has several effects, including shape change, granule secretion and activation of the fibrinogen receptor, GPIIb-IIIa. Although these two pathways of platelet activation are illustrated as relatively distinct from one another, they do interact with, and amplify, each other. For example the inositol triphosphate-mediated increase in intracellular calcium concentration also leads to activation of phospholipase A_2 (eicosanoid pathway). Platelets contain the enzyme adenylate cyclase (AC), which regulates intraplatelet levels of cyclic AMP (cAMP). Activation of GP-coupled receptors signals either activation or inhibition of AC (pathway not shown). When adrenaline, for example, binds to its GP-coupled receptor, it leads to inhibition of AC and decreased platelet cAMP, which in turn promotes calcium release from the dense tubular system and leads to increased platelet reactivity. When prostacyclin (PGI_2) released by vascular endothelial cells binds to its GP-linked receptor it signals activation of AC and increased levels of cAMP, which act to inhibit platelet reactivity. This is an important non-thrombotic effect of normal vascular endothelium.

α-Granules
• Adhesive proteins – promote platelet aggregation and adhesion to subendothelium and leucocytes: – von Willebrand factor[a], fibronectin[a] – Fibrinogen[b] – Thrombospondin, vitronectin, P-selectin • Growth modulators – stimulate the growth and proliferation of smooth muscle cells and fibroblasts and the deposition of extracellular matrix material (roles in inflammation, wound repair and atherosclerosis): – Platelet-derived growth factor, transforming growth factor β – Platelet factor 4, connective tissue activating peptide III, thrombospondin – C1-inhibitor, high molecular weight kininogen • Coagulation factors – participate in fibrin formation and fibrinolysis: – Fibrinogen – FV[a], FXI[a], FVa, FVIIIa, FXIa – High molecular weight kininogen – Plasminogen activator inhibitor I, Protein S
δ-Granules (dense bodies)
• Adenosine triphosphate • Guanine triphosphate • Adenosine diphosphate • Guanine diphosphate • Calcium • Serotonin • Pyrophosphate

24.5 Contents of platelet-specific granules. [a]Substances produced by megakaryocytes. [b]Along with albumin and immunoglobulin G, fibrinogen is endocytosed by platelets and packaged into α-granules.

Platelet function

Platelets contribute to both primary and secondary haemostasis (see Chapter 21). They are the first line of defence in maintaining vascular integrity and rapid arrest of bleeding. They plug sites of vascular injury by adhering to, and aggregating around, breaches in vessel walls. When formation of an initial platelet plug is insufficient to stop bleeding, activated adherent platelets recruit additional platelets to the site where they serve to localize, amplify and sustain the coagulant response. Activated platelets release stored coagulation factors and provide an anchoring surface for the assembly of plasma derived coagulation factors that form reaction complexes (tenase and prothrombinase complexes) to amplify and propagate thrombin formation and fibrin generation (Colman *et al.*, 2006).

It is becoming increasingly clear that platelets contribute significantly to pathological vascular events, including inflammation, thrombosis, and atherosclerosis and cancer metastasis. Defects in platelet function are, however, recognized clinically by the abnormal bleeding that results from failure of platelets to form an adequate platelet plug or sustain platelet procoagulant reactions. Therefore, only the role of platelets in haemostasis will be discussed here.

Platelet function in haemostasis can be separated into several steps: adhesion, aggregation, the release reaction and platelet procoagulant activity (Figure 24.6). Although these processes are discussed separately, these events occur simultaneously in the vasculature, and this distinction is an artificial one.

Adhesion

Under normal circumstances, the endothelium prevents interaction of platelets with the vessel wall by acting as a physical barrier and secreting the platelet inhibitors prostacyclin and nitric oxide. Vessel injury disrupts the endothelium and exposes the thrombogenic subendothelium to circulating cells. Immediately, platelets adhere to the damaged vessel wall through the interaction of platelet membrane activation and anchoring receptors with ligands in the vascular subendothelial matrix. The type of receptors and ligands differs, depending on the site of vessel damage and, more specifically, on the shear rate of blood flow in that area. Studies performed *in vitro* indicate that under conditions of low shear, as found in the venous circulation or areas of blood stasis, platelets adhere to collagen, laminin and fibronectin through integrin receptors. Under conditions of high shear, as found in the arterioles and microcirculation, adhesion is accomplished by vWf and GPIb-IX (see Figure 24.2). Humans, dogs, horses and mice with abnormalities in vWf (von Willebrand's disease (vWD)) or human patients with defects in GPIb-IX (Bernard–Soulier syndrome) exhibit defective platelet adhesion under conditions of high shear, illustrating the importance of this interaction and providing a physiological basis for the haemorrhage observed in these two conditions. vWD has been diagnosed in several breeds of dog (vWD types 1, 2 and 3), horses and mice; however, an animal model of Bernard–Soulier syndrome has not been identified. The interaction of vWf with GPIb-IX triggers platelet activation and subsequent aggregation through a complex series of intracellular signal transduction events termed the basic platelet reaction. In contrast to most platelet agonists, vWf–collagen induced platelet activation is not GP coupled. It proceeds through an immunoreceptor tyrosine-based activation motif (ITAM) similar to the primary signalling domain of classical immunoreceptors. The signalling events stimulated by collagen interaction with its platelet receptors parallel events initiated following stimulation of antigen receptors on B and T lymphocytes. The cytoplasmic domain of platelet FcRγ is non-covalently complexed with platelet GPVI and contains the ITAM motif. GPVI-induced platelet activation is initiated by tyrosine phosphorylation of ITAM; this signal is then transduced to other signalling partners. The activation pathways for GP-coupled and FcRγ-linked platelet signalling then converge to follow two separate but interacting pathways, one involving phospholipid hydrolysis (the phospholipid pathway) and the other, arachidonic acid metabolism (the arachidonate or eicosanoid pathway) (see Figure 24.4). An important consequence of triggering both pathways is the activation (by conformational change) of the

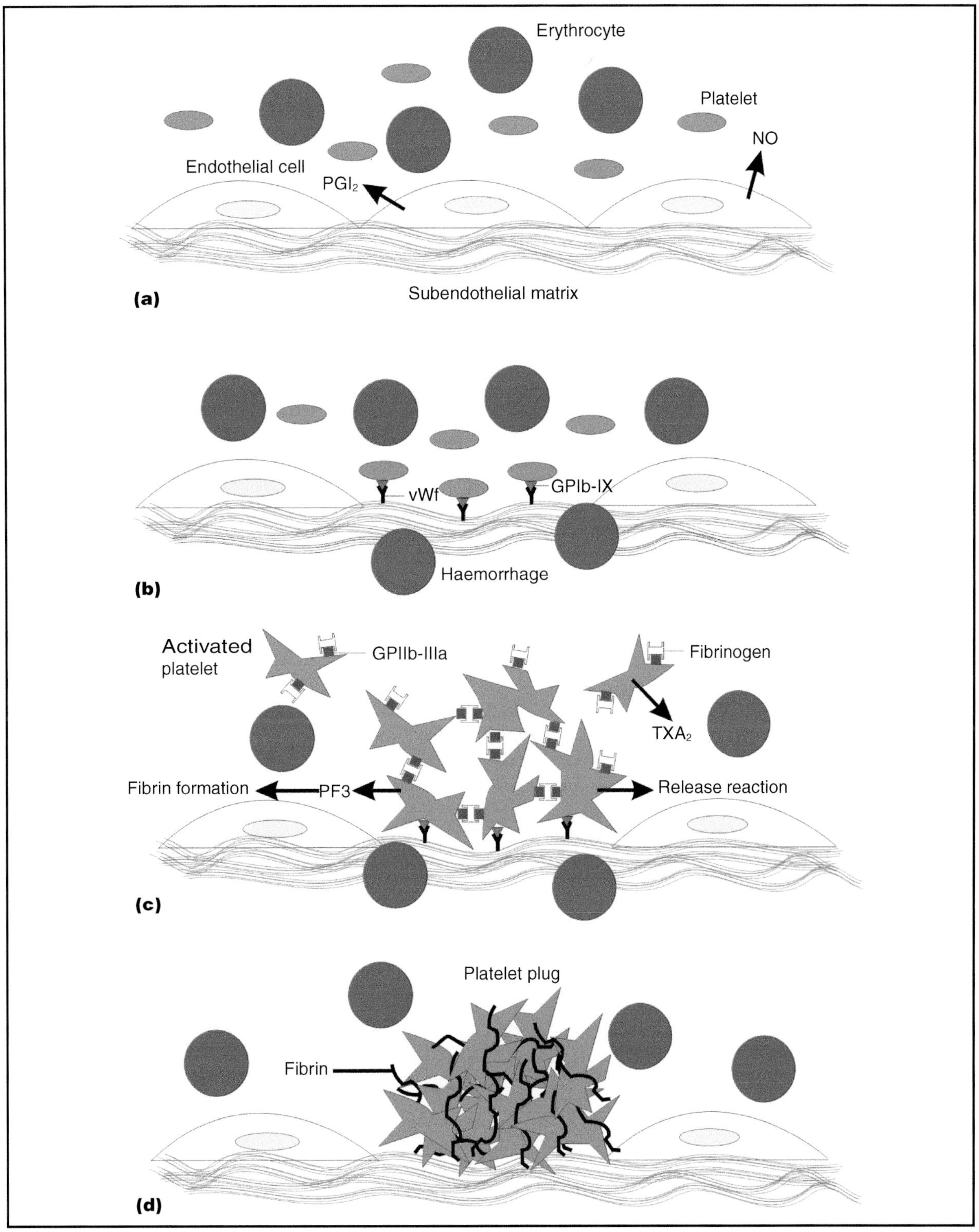

24.6 Schematic illustration of primary haemostasis. **(a)** The intact endothelium prevents platelet adherence by acting as a physical barrier and releasing inhibitors of platelet function, including prostacyclin (PGI_2) and nitric oxide (NO). These substances inhibit platelet function by increasing platelet concentrations of cyclic adenosine monophosphate and cyclic guanosine monophosphate, respectively. **(b)** When the endothelium is disrupted, platelets adhere to the exposed subendothelium. Under conditions of high shear, platelets adhere through an interaction between GPIb-IX and von Willebrand factor (vWF). **(c)** Under conditions of low shear, platelets adhere, through integrin receptors, to collagen, laminin and fibronectin in the subendothelial matrix. Adhesion activates platelets through the basic platelet reaction, resulting in shape change, the release reaction and thromboxane A_2 (TXA_2) generation. This culminates in platelet recruitment, further platelet activation and aggregation. Platelet aggregation occurs when fibrinogen binds to its receptor, GPIIb-IIIa, on the platelet membrane. Consequently, the primary platelet plug is produced by a fused mass of platelets. Platelet procoagulant activity (PF3) becomes available (through translocation of phosphatidylserine to the outer leaflet of the platelet membrane) upon platelet activation and promotes secondary haemostasis, resulting in the formation of fibrin. **(d)** Fibrin solidifies the primary platelet plug, forming a stable thrombus.

fibrinogen receptor, GPIIb-IIIa, which culminates in platelet aggregation.

Aggregation

Under physiological conditions, platelet aggregation occurs after platelets have attached and spread along the subendothelium or have interacted with agonists, such as collagen, thrombin or ADP. These interactions initiate the basic platelet reaction, resulting in activation of GPIIb-IIIa. Platelet aggregation is mediated by the binding of soluble plasma proteins, particularly fibrinogen, to GPIIb-IIIa (in the presence of divalent cations) on the same or adjacent platelets, thus effectively cross-linking the platelets. Plasma and platelet vWF (released from α-granules) may contribute to this aggregation in healthy humans. Aggregation is potentiated by other mediators, including thrombin, ADP (released from dense bodies, damaged endothelial cells or erythrocytes), serotonin, platelet-activating factor and thromboxane A_2. Irreversible platelet aggregation requires both platelet metabolism and stimulation by one or more specific agonists.

Platelet aggregation can be measured *in vitro* using light transmission or impedance aggregometry (see Chapter 22). Aggregation is initiated when one or more agonists bind to specific receptors in the platelet membrane and trigger outside–in and inside–out cell signalling events that result in a conformational change in the platelet integrin receptor for fibrinogen to generate fibrinogen cross-linked platelets. Figure 24.7 lists the various types of platelet agonist. Strong agonists, such as collagen and thrombin, induce aggregation through both the phospholipase C (hydrolysis of phospholipid) and eicosanoid pathways (generation of thromboxane A_2). They can trigger granule secretion even when aggregation is inhibited. Weak agonists, such as ADP, activate the eicosanoid pathway and rely on thromboxane A_2 for irreversible aggregation. The irreversible phase of platelet aggregation triggered by high concentrations of these weaker agonists is inhibited by drugs that interfere with eicosanoid synthesis, such as aspirin.

Agonist	Aggregation inhibited by aspirin
Weak agonists	
Adenosine diphosphate	Yes
Adrenaline	Yes
Platelet-activating factor	Partial
Arachidonic acid	Yes
Vasopressin (antidiuretic hormone)	Partial
Thromboxane A_2	No
Strong agonists	
Collagen	At low concentrations of agonist
Thrombin	At low concentrations of agonist
Calcium ionophores	No

24.7 Platelet agonists.

Granule secretion

The release reaction involves the secretion of the constituents of the α-granule and dense body into the open canalicular system. The released constituents can then participate in platelet aggregation and fibrin formation. The release reaction can be measured by detecting the amount of ^{14}C-serotonin or ATP released during aggregation.

Procoagulant activity

The generation of platelet procoagulant activity requires an influx of calcium and is associated with the redistribution of phosphatidylserine to the outer platelet membrane leaflet and the shedding of membrane vesicles from the platelet surface. The translocation of phosphatidylserine provides a binding site for activated coagulation factors and is essential for the generation of activated FX and thrombin. Platelets also secrete enzymes and cofactors during the release reaction, all of which participate in thrombin generation. Similarly, FXIII is released from the platelet cytoplasm and cross-links fibrin.

Diagnosis of thrombopathias

Thrombopathias should be suspected in an animal with excessive haemorrhage typical of primary haemostatic disorders (Figure 24.8) and a normal platelet count and coagulation profile. In many thrombopathias, minor bleeding episodes often go undetected and major spontaneous bleeding is uncommon; however, bleeding complications associated with abnormal platelet function frequently present following trauma or surgery.

- Petechiae and purpura
- Mild to moderate bleeding from mucosal surfaces:
  - Gastrointestinal
  - Genitourinary
  - Nasal
  - Gingival
- History of easy bruising and haematoma formation
- Excessive bleeding after trauma, surgery and venepuncture

24.8 Clinical findings in thrombopathias.

The minimal database in patients with excessive haemorrhage includes a complete history (including sex, age and breed of dog, family history, details of previous bouts of haemorrhage, possible access to anticoagulant rodenticides or drugs), a thorough physical examination (noting the type and distribution of haemorrhage and the presence of underlying disease), a platelet count, a blood smear examination for platelet morphology, and a coagulation profile (i.e. activated partial thrombo-plastin time, prothrombin time and fibrinogen and vWf concentrations). If all these tests are within reference intervals, the animal should be evaluated for a thrombopathia (Figure 24.9). Unfortunately, many of the tests for thrombopathias are performed only at referral institutions and are not readily available to the general practitioner. Some of these tests will be mentioned briefly here (see also Chapter 22).

- Buccal mucosal bleeding time [a]
- PFA-100 closure time [a]
- von Willebrand factor testing
- Glass bead retention test
- Platelet aggregation
- Platelet secretion (serotonin or ATP)
- Platelet procoagulant activity (prothrombin consumption index (PCI) test)
- Platelet ATP:ADP ratio
- Platelet activation and glycoprotein analysis using flow cytometry or immunoblot analysis
- Molecular diagnostic testing

24.9 Tests for diagnosis of thrombopathias. [a] Can be performed in private practice.

Buccal mucosal bleeding time

The buccal mucosal bleeding time (BMBT) is a relatively simple *in vivo* test of primary haemostasis. The BMBT is the length of time needed for haemorrhage to cease from a small standardized cut in the buccal mucosa made with a special disposable device (e.g. Simplate II, Organon Teknika, Jessup, MD, USA or Surgicutt, International Technidyne Corporation, Edison, NJ, USA). The technique has been well described in the veterinary literature.

In human medicine the BMBT has been replaced by the platelet function analyser (PFA)-100 assay system as a screening tool for disorders of primary haemostasis, owing to the increased reproducibility and sensitivity of the PFA-100 assay (Harrison *et al.,* 2009). The Multiplate impedance aggregometer (Dynabate GmbH) has been used to monitor antiplatelet therapies (Paniccia *et al.,* 2009) and may have utility as a screening tool for disorders of primary haemostasis. These are discussed in Chapter 22.

von Willebrand factor

Evaluation of von Willebrand factor (vWf) is discussed in Chapter 27.

Clot retraction

Clot retraction is a crude and subjective test of platelet number and function. Abnormal retraction may be caused by hypofibrinogenaemia, thrombocytopenia or thrombopathia.

Glass bead retention

In the glass bead retention test, platelet numbers are determined before and after a standard volume of venous blood is passed at a standard rate through a plastic column packed with glass beads. Retention is dependent on vWF, ADP release from haemolysed erythrocytes, normal platelet function and coagulation. Platelet retention is decreased in thrombopathias and vWD (Brassard and Meyers, 1991). This test is, however, difficult to standardize and is not recommended because there are more specific tests for the diagnosis of these disorders. The PFA-100 closure time can be used to screen for vWD (see below).

Platelet aggregometry

Platelet aggregation is induced *in vitro* in response to agonists. The assay is performed in an instrument called a 'platelet aggregometer', of which there are two types: optical and impedance. The optical aggregometer is sensitive to changes in light transmission, whereas the impedance method is sensitive to changes in electrical resistance generated across two electrodes when platelet aggregates accumulate on the electrode. Special optical aggregometers, lumiaggregometers, measure ATP release simultaneously with aggregation. The impedance method, which also measures whole blood platelet aggregation, is thought to be a more accurate indicator of the physiological processes that occur *in vivo* than the optical method, which uses platelet-rich plasma. Whole blood impedance lumiaggregometers are now available to monitor platelet aggregation and secretion simultaneously.

Platelet release and ATP:ADP ratio

The release reaction can be assessed by determination of total platelet ATP and ADP content and by the release of ATP or ^{14}C-serotonin from dense bodies during aggregation. In storage pool defects, dense bodies and their associated nucleotides are reduced or absent; therefore the ATP:ADP ratio of the storage pool increases.

Platelet function analyser (PFA-100)

New instruments have been developed that assess platelet function by simulation of vessel injury *in vivo*. Citrate anticoagulated blood is passed through a tiny aperture punched into a collagen-coated membrane impregnated with ADP or adrenaline. These instruments measure the time taken (closure time) for platelets to adhere to the membrane and aggregate to produce a platelet plug, thus closing the aperture. In human and canine patients this process depends on vWF and normal platelet function. Preliminary testing in dogs has shown that, with the ADP channel, the closure time is abnormally long in dogs with vWD (Callan and Giger, 2001) and Glanzmann's thrombasthenia, and in Basset Hound thrombopathia (MB Brooks, personal communication) (see also Chapter 22).

Platelet procoagulant activity

In the past, the procoagulant activity of platelets was measured by the PF3 test, an obsolete assay that was used primarily for the detection of anti-platelet antibodies. Currently, the procoagulant activity of platelets can be determined in human patients using a prothrombinase assay or flow cytometry.

Platelet glycoproteins

Platelet membrane glycoproteins can be purified using gel filtration chromatography and labelled. With advances in immunological techniques, the presence or absence of these glycoproteins, as well as their state of activation, can be assessed with monoclonal antibodies in procedures such as flow cytometry and immunoblotting (Welles *et al.*, 1994; Boudreaux *et al.*, 1996).

Defects in platelet function

Thrombopathias can be inherited or acquired. Acquired disorders are far more common, especially those induced by drug treatment or disease. Thrombopathias typically are associated with haemorrhage and a decrease in platelet function. However, there are many disorders (e.g. diabetes mellitus, immune-mediated haemolytic anaemia, pancreatitis, nephrotic syndrome and hyperadrenocorticism) that are associated with thrombosis. Although thrombosis is usually caused by endothelial injury, deficient or abnormal coagulation inhibitors and abnormalities of fibrinolysis, there is no doubt that platelet hyperaggregability is a contributing factor in thrombus formation. Thrombotic disorders will not be discussed further because hyperfunctional platelets have been implicated in thrombosis in only a few animal diseases (Figure 24.10).

Thrombopathias are recognized more readily in dogs than in cats. In general, cats do not often exhibit excessive haemorrhage, which may be attributed to their small size and lifestyle. Inherited disorders should be suspected in a young animal, especially if family members display similar bleeding tendencies and there is no history of drug treatment. Thrombopathias can affect any component of platelet function from adhesion to aggregation. The defects can involve quantitative or qualitative abnormalities in membrane proteins needed for platelet adhesion and interplatelet interactions, aberrant cAMP metabolism, abnormalities in cell signalling pathways, impaired synthesis of proaggregatory prostaglandin metabolites, decreased or absent granule pools, and low concentrations or abnormal function of essential cofactors such as vWF and fibrinogen.

Inherited platelet disorders (thrombopathias)

Many inherited thrombopathias have been characterized in human medicine, however only a

Disease	Proposed mechanism of platelet dysfunction
Decreased platelet function	
Neoplasia: Acute megakaryoblastic leukaemia Essential thrombocythaemia Polycythaemia vera	 Defective adhesion and aggregation Defective adhesion and aggregation Defective adhesion and aggregation
Dysproteinaemias (lymphoma, multiple myeloma)	Paraprotein (IgG, IgM, IgA) coats platelets causing defective adhesion, aggregation and procoagulant activity
Infectious agents: *Ehrlichia canis* *Anaplasma (Ehrlichia) platys*	 Decreased adhesion, procoagulant activity, ? antibody-mediated dysfunction Decreased aggregation (secondary to platelet activation with subsequent exhaustion)
Hepatic disease	Decreased aggregation attributed to a variety of causes
Renal disease	Decreased adhesion
Pancreatitis	Decreased aggregation (secondary to platelet exhaustion after initial hyperresponsiveness and DIC)
Disseminated intravascular coagulation (DIC)	Fibrinogen degradation products coat platelets interfering with function
Immune-mediated thrombocytopenia	Decreased aggregation
Increased platelet function	
Nephrotic syndrome	Enhanced arachidonic acid availability
Neoplasia	?
Feline hypertropic cardiomyopathy	?
Infectious agents: *Rickettsia rickettsi* *Dirofilaria immitis*	 ? Due to larger more functional platelets ? Parasite liberates biogenic amines, which interact with platelet surface
Feline infectious peritonitis virus	Unknown: ? Direct viral interaction with platelets, and DIC

24.10 Animal diseases associated with acquired thrombopathias.

few have been diagnosed in companion animals (Figure 24.11). Some of these will be discussed in detail.

von Willebrand's disease

Although vWD does not affect platelets directly, vWF is essential for platelet adhesion to the subendothelium and, to a lesser extent, platelet aggregation. The clinical signs in this disorder are therefore similar to thrombopathias (see Chapter 27).

Glanzmann's thrombasthenia

Glanzmann's thrombasthenia has been diagnosed in Otterhounds and a Great Pyrenees dog (Boudreaux *et al.*, 1996). The defect appears to be inherited in an autosomal recessive fashion, and affected dogs have excessive mucosal haemorrhage (Figure 24.12). Haemostatic testing shows a normal to mildly decreased platelet count, normal to increased mean platelet volume and prolonged BMBT. Characteristic features include decreased platelet retention, absent platelet aggregation to collagen, ADP, platelet-activating factor and thrombin, and decreased granule secretion. Change in platelet shape does occur. Clot retraction is abnormal, which helps to differentiate this disorder from Basset Hound thrombopathia. Flow cytometric studies have shown a noticeable reduction in GPIIb-IIIa on the platelet surface in both Otterhounds and Great Pyrenees dogs. In the Otterhound, there is a single nucleotide change in exon 12 of the GPIIb gene, which disrupts a calcium-binding domain and forms an unstable GPIIb-IIIa complex, preventing its expression on the platelet surface (Boudreaux and Catalfamo, 2001). An mRNA splicing defect in exon 13 of the GPIIb gene has been identified in the Great Pyrenees dog. This defect also disrupts a calcium-binding domain and results in a truncated protein, which destabilizes the GPIIb-IIIa complex (Lipscomb *et al.*, 2000). Molecular diagnostic testing is available by contacting Dr Boudreaux's laboratory, University of Auburn, USA.

Platelet signalling disorders

An inherited platelet signalling defect has been described in the Basset Hound, Eskimo Spitz dog and in some cattle, but has not been reported in humans. The clinical signs in affected dogs consist of petechiae, aural haematomas and prolonged haemorrhage with shedding of deciduous teeth. Severe bleeding complications are often reported

Disorder	Breeds affected	Defects/characteristics
Glanzmann's thrombasthenia	Otterhound Great Pyrenees	Mutation in *GPIIb* gene; decreased GPIIb-IIIa expression; absent or reduced platelet fibrinogen binding; absent platelet aggregation to multiple platelet agonists; abnormal clot retraction and PFA-100 closure times
Signal transduction defect	Basset Hound (thrombopathia) Eskimo Spitz dog (thrombopathia) Landseer ECT (thrombopathia)	Various mutations in *CalDAG-GEF1* gene; abnormal activation of GPIIb-IIIa with impaired platelet aggregation and secretion; abnormal Rap1b GTP loading; normal clot retraction; abnormal PFA-closure time
Storage pool deficiency	American Cocker Spaniel	Affected gene unknown; platelets deficient in storage pools of adenine nucleotides; exhibit impaired platelet aggregation and secretion; uptake and release of serotonin normal
Chédiak–Higashi syndrome	Blue Smoke Persian cat	Absent dense bodies; platelets deficient in storage pools of ATP, ADP, serotonin and divalent cations; platelet aggregation and secretion abnormal
von Willebrand's disease	Multiple dog breeds (vWD types 1, 2 and 3)	Qualitative or quantitative abnormalities in von Willebrand factor; impaired vWf-mediated platelet adhesion and anchoring
Macrothrombocytopenia	Cavalier King Charles Spaniel	Mutation in gene for beta-1 tubulin; platelet aggregation and release normal; large platelets with platelet numbers decreased due to altered megakaryocyte proplatelet release
Cyclic haemopoiesis	Grey collies	Mutation in *AP3B1* gene; characterized by cyclic fluctuations in the number of circulating neutrophils, reticulocytes and platelets; platelet reactivity to collagen reduced; platelet content of serotonin, ATP and ADP reduced; impaired clot retraction
Canine procoagulant deficiency (canine Scott syndrome)	German Shepherd Dog	Affected gene unknown; abnormal platelet procoagulant activity; abnormal prothrombin consumption index; abnormal externalization of platelet membrane phosphatidylserine and release of platelet microparticles; normal platelet aggregation, secretion and clot retraction

24.11 Inherited platelet function disorders in animals. ECT, European Continental Type.

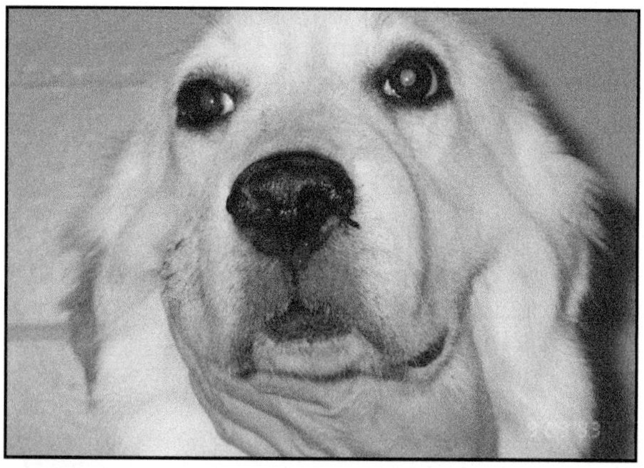

24.12 Spontaneous epistaxis in a Great Pyrenees dog with Glanzmann's thrombasthenia. (Courtesy of Dr M Boudreaux)

following surgical procedures or trauma. An autosomal recessive condition, this form of thrombopathia is characterized by decreased platelet retention and absent platelet aggregation in response to all agonists, except thrombin, to which there is a delayed onset and reduced rate of aggregation. Platelet ^{14}C-serotonin release is decreased in response to collagen, but normal to thrombin. Change in shape does occur and clot retraction is normal. Results of flow cytometric assays confirm the existence of glycoprotein IIb-IIIa complexes on the platelet surface. Platelets from affected Basset Hounds have slightly increased basal cAMP concentrations, which have been attributed to impaired phosphodiesterase activity. Increased cAMP inhibits intracellular calcium release, agonist–receptor binding and agonist-induced phospholipid hydrolysis. Cyclic AMP metabolism has not been evaluated in the Eskimo Spitz dog.

The molecular basis for these disorders involves distinct mutations in the gene encoding a guanine nucleotide exchange factor (GEF), which is essential for normal platelet signal transduction. The GEF that is mutated in thrombopathic Basset Hounds and Eskimo Spitz dogs is calcium diacylglycerol guanine nucleotide exchange factor 1 (CalDAG-GEF1). The activity of this GEF requires the generation of ionized calcium and diacylglycerol (see Figure 24.4). Normal function of this calcium- and diacylglycerol- sensitive GEF is critical to the GPIIb/GPIIIa conformational changes required to support normal platelet aggregate formation (Boudreaux *et al.*, 2007). A murine CalDAG-GEF1 knock-out model has been developed, and it exhibits a platelet function and bleeding phenotype similar to affected dogs. Molecular diagnostic tests are available from Dr Boudreaux's laboratory, University of Auburn, USA.

Storage pool deficiency in American Cocker Spaniels

American Cocker Spaniels with storage pool deficiency have moderate to severe haemorrhage after trauma, venepuncture or surgery. They have normal platelet counts, a prolonged BMBT, decreased platelet aggregation and ^{14}C-serotonin release in response to collagen, and an increased platelet ATP:ADP ratio. Dense bodies are visible on electron microscopy. The disorder has been attributed to a selective defect in ADP transport in dense granules. Haemorrhage is often severe enough to require fresh platelet transfusions (Callan *et al.*, 1995).

Inherited macrothrombocytopenia

Cavalier King Charles Spaniels (CKCS) can inherit macrothrombocytopenia as an autosomal recessive trait. Affected dogs have large platelets with numbers ranging from 50–100 $\times$ 10^9/l blood. The molecular basis for the defect is a mutation in the gene encoding β1-tubulin (Davis *et al.*, 2008). It has been postulated that the mutation results in microtubule instability, which alters megakaryocyte proplatelet release. Dogs with the mutation are not at risk for expression of a bleeding tendency. Some CKCSs have a reported bleeding tendency associated with mitral valve disease. A molecular diagnostic test is available from Dr Boudreaux's laboratory, University of Auburn, USA.

Canine procoagulant deficiency (canine Scott syndrome)

A canine hereditary bleeding disorder with the characteristic features of human Scott syndrome has been reported in German Shepherd Dogs (Brooks *et al.*, 2002). The affected animals were from a single, inbred colony and experienced clinical signs of epistaxis, hyphaema, intramuscular haematoma and prolonged bleeding with cutaneous bruising after surgery. The haemostatic abnormalities identified were restricted to tests of platelet procoagulant activity, whereas platelet count, bleeding time, clot retraction, and platelet aggregation and secretion in response to thrombin, collagen, and ADP stimulation were normal. While the platelet phospholipid content was normal, flow cytometric analyses revealed diminished phosphatidylserine exposure and a failure of microvesiculation in response to calcium ionophore, thrombin and collagen stimulation. Pedigree studies indicated a homozygous recessive inheritance pattern of the defect.

Acquired thrombopathias

Acquired thrombopathias should be suspected in animals with specific diseases known to be associated with platelet dysfunction (see Figure 24.10) and in animals that have been treated with certain drugs (Figure 24.13). The risk of bleeding is unpredictable and typically less severe and consistent than in animals with inherited disorders. Although abnormal platelet function occurs in these diseases, there may be other causes for the excessive haemorrhage seen in these conditions (e.g. thrombocytopenia). However, it should be recognized that platelets potentially do not function normally in these situations, and drugs that may exacerbate platelet dysfunction should therefore be avoided.

Inhibitors of prostaglandin synthesis
• Cyclo-oxygenase inhibitors: – Aspirin – Non-steroidal anti-inflammatory drugs (phenylbutazone, indomethacin, ibuprofen) • Thromboxane synthetase inhibitors (diazoxiben)
Drugs that increase concentrations of cyclic adenosine monophosphate (cAMP) or cyclic guanosine monophosphate (cGMP)
• Adenylate cyclise or guanylate cyclise activators: – Prostaglandin I_2, E_1 and D_2 (cAMP) – Nitric oxide, nitroglycerin, nitroprusside (cGMP) • Phosphodiesterase inhibitors: – Dipyridamole – Methylxanthines (caffeine, theophylline, aminophyline)
Calcium antagonists
• Diltiazem, nifepidine, verapamil • Barbiturates (? interfere with agonist-receptor binding and prevent increase in cytosolic calcium concentration)
Membrane-active drugs (interfere with platelet receptors)
• Antibiotics (penicillin, ampicillin, ticarcillin, gentamicin, sulphonamides, cephalothrin, cefmetazole, moxalactum) • Antihistamines (phenothiazines) • Plasma expanders (dextran, hetastarch, pentastarch) • Propanolol, isoproterenol • Anaesthetic agents (procaine, lidocaine, halothane, glycerol guiacolate)
Unknown
• Heparin • Ticlopidine (? interfere with fibrinogen-receptor exposure) • Oestrogens, chondroitin sulphate, carbenicillin

24.13 Drugs that can interfere with platelet function. Most cases have been reported in humans and not in domestic animals.

Drug-associated thrombopathias

An enormous variety of drugs can interfere with platelet function (Rao, 2006). The most commonly used of these is aspirin, which in some situations is prescribed precisely for its antiplatelet effects, such as in the prevention of thromboembolism in feline cardiomyopathy and canine heartworm disease. Aspirin inhibits platelet function by irreversibly acetylating platelet cyclo-oxygenase, thus preventing generation of thromboxane A_2, which is needed for secretion and aggregation. Other non-steroidal anti-inflammatory agents (e.g. phenylbutazone) inhibit cyclo-oxygenase activity reversibly. Aspirin is unique, however, as its effect lasts for the lifespan of the platelet (7–10 days in the dog). Inhibitory effects can persist for 7 days after treatment ceases. Aspirin should be avoided as an analgesic in dogs with inherited platelet function defects and haemostatic disorders such as vWD and haemophilia A.

Disseminated intravascular coagulation

DIC is caused by the systemic generation of thrombin resulting in widespread coagulation, with resultant microcirculatory thromboembolism and multiorgan failure. DIC is not a primary disorder; it is initiated by an underlying disease process, typically septicaemia, pancreatitis, heat stroke, surgery, viral infections, neoplasia, transfusion reactions or tissue necrosis. DIC is initiated by increased tissue factor expression by monocytes and possibly endothelial cells, mediated by cytokines or exposure of subendothelial tissue factor by massive endothelial cell injury. Some tumours (e.g. mucinous adenocarcinoma) and snake venoms can initiate DIC by activating coagulation factors such as FX directly. As a result, there is widespread activation of coagulation, with fibrin deposition and thrombus formation. Consequently, there is consumption of platelets, fibrinogen and coagulation factors with secondary fibrinolysis and generation of fibrin degradation products (FDPs) and D-dimers. Erythrocytes shear as they traverse damaged blood vessels, producing a microangiopathic haemolytic anaemia. The clinical signs may be related to tissue hypoxia, infarction or haemorrhage. Typically, haemorrhage is attributed to depletion of platelets and coagulation factors and abnormal fibrin polymerization, but there is often concurrent platelet dysfunction. Platelet dysfunction is mediated by high concentrations of FDPs (especially fragments D and E), which have a high affinity for platelet membranes and compete with fibrinogen for platelet receptors, thus impairing aggregation.

Immune-mediated thrombocytopenia

Some dogs with immune-mediated thrombocytopenia (IMTP) have abnormal platelet aggregation, which is mediated by IgG antibodies (Kristensen *et al.*, 1994). In chronic IMTP in humans, most antibodies are directed against GPIIb-IIIa and GPIb-IX (McMillan *et al.*, 1987), and studies in dogs by Lewis and Meyers (1996) indicate that, in some dogs with IMTP, there is an autoantibody against GPIIb-IIIa. Given that this glycoprotein has an essential role in platelet aggregation, it is not surprising that dogs with IMTP have concurrent platelet dysfunction. For unknown reasons, in IMTP the clinical signs of haemorrhage do not always correlate with the platelet count. It may be that the clinical signs of IMTP depend on the extent of platelet dysfunction as well as the severity of the thrombocytopenia. Further studies need to be performed in this area.

Renal disease

Mucosal bleeding, reduced platelet retention and a prolonged BMBT are features of natural and experimentally induced uraemia in dogs. These abnormalities correlate with the extent of azotaemia. Platelet aggregation is either normal or mildly decreased, which implicates defective adhesion as the main haemostatic abnormality (Brassard *et al.*, 1994). The amount and multimeric composition of vWF are normal, indicating that the adhesion defects are not caused by vWF abnormalities (Brassard and Meyers, 1994).

Hepatic disease

Hepatic disease is often associated with prolonged haemorrhage, which is attributable to a combination of reduced synthesis of coagulation factors, DIC and platelet dysfunction. Dogs with various types of hepatic disease have defective platelet aggregation in whole blood, and display excessive haemorrhage related to platelet dysfunction (Willis *et al.*, 1989). This dysfunction is thought to be caused by circulating FDPs, increased bile acids, altered platelet phospholipids, enhanced nitric oxide production (a result of hyperammonaemia) and increased proportions of older, less active platelets (Bowen *et al.*, 1988; Willis *et al.*, 1989).

Management

Assessment of the risk of bleeding in thrombopathias is difficult, because none of the platelet function tests predicts the likelihood of haemorrhage accurately. The BMBT is considered by some to be the best indicator of '*in vivo*' haemostatic competence in patients with thrombopathias. The PFA-100 closure time may also be useful as a global screening assay for platelet function. The BMBT and the PFA-100 closure times can be used as screening tests before invasive surgery in animals considered to be at risk of bleeding because of platelet dysfunction. Those patients with a prolonged BMBT or PFA-100 closure time are considered to be more likely to bleed during surgery than those with times within reference intervals. However, there have been no studies to determine whether a prolonged BMBT or PFA-100 closure time is associated with increased surgical haemorrhage in animals. In a patient with clinical signs referable to platelet dysfunction, suitable precautions should be taken before invasive surgical procedures. These include treatment of the underlying disease in acquired thrombopathias, cessation of drug treatment, attention to strict surgical haemostasis and platelet transfusions. Ideally, platelet-rich plasma or platelet concentrates should be infused, however fresh whole blood is the only form of transfusion therapy readily available to the general practitioner. This should be used judiciously, and ideally all animals should be typed and cross-matched to minimize transfusion reactions. Infusion therapy in inherited thrombopathias is only palliative, and if haemorrhage is severe, euthanasia may be warranted.

References and further reading

Boudreaux MK (2008) Characteristics, diagnosis, and treatment of inherited platelet disorders in mammals. *Journal of the American Veterinary Medical Association* **8**, 1251–1258

Boudreaux MK and Catalfamo JL (2001) Molecular and genetic basis for thrombasthenic thrombopathia in Otterhounds. *American Journal of Veterinary Research* **62**, 1797–1804

Boudreaux MK, Catalfamo JL and Klok M (2007) Calcium-diacylglycerol guanine nucleotide exchange factor 1 gene mutations associated with loss of function in canine platelets. *Translation Research* **150**, 81–92

Boudreaux MK, Kvam K, Dillon AR *et al.* (1996) Type I Glanzmanns thrombasthenia in a Great Pyrenees dog. *Veterinary Pathology* **33**, 503–511

Bowen DJ, Clemmons RM, Meyer DJ and Dorsey-Lee MR (1988) Platelet functional changes secondary to hepatocholestasis and elevation of serum bile acids. *Thrombosis Research* **52**, 649–654

Brassard JA and Meyers KM (1991) Evaluation of the buccal bleeding time and platelet glass bead retention as assays of hemostasis in the dog: the effects of acetylsalicylic acid, warfarin and von Willebrand Factor deficiency. *Thrombosis Haemostasis* **65**, 191–195

Brassard JA and Meyers KM (1994) Von Willebrand factor is not altered in azotemic dogs with prolonged bleeding time. *Journal of Laboratory and Clinical Medicine* **124**, 55–62

Brassard JA, Meyers KM, Person M and Dhein CR (1994) Experimentally induced renal failure in the dog as an animal model for uremic bleeding. *Journal of Laboratory and Clinical Medicine* **124**, 48–54

Brooks MB and Catalfamo JL (2010) Immune-mediated thrombocytopenia, von Willebrand disease and platelet disorders. In: *Textbook of Veterinary Internal Medicine, 7th edn*, ed. SJ Ettinger and EC Feldman, pp.772–783. WB Saunders, Saint Louis

Brooks MB, Catalfamo JL, Brown HA, Ivanova P and Lovaglio J (2002) A hereditary bleeding disorder of dogs caused by a lack of platelet procoagulant activity. *Blood* **99**, 2434–2441

Callan MB, Bennett JS, Phillips DK *et al.* (1995) Inherited platelet δ-storage pool disease in dogs causing severe bleeding: an animal model for a specific ADP deficiency. *Thrombosis and Haemostasis* **74**, 949–953

Callan MB and Giger U (2001) Assessment of point-of-care instrument for identification of primary hemostatic disorders in dogs. *American Journal of Veterinary Research* **62**, 652–658

Colman RW, Clowes AW, George JN, Goldhaber SZ and Marder VJ (2006) Overview of hemostasis. In: *Hemostasis and Thrombosis: Basic principles and clinical practice, 5th edn*, ed. RW Colman, VJ Marder, AW Clowes, JN George and SZ Goldhaber, pp.3–16. JB Lippincott, Philadelphia

Davis B, Tolvio-Kunnican M, Schuller S and Boudreaux MK (2008) Mutation in beta1-tubulin correlates to macrothrombocytopenia in Cavalier King Charles Spaniels. *Journal of Veterinary Internal Medicine* **22**, 540–545

Harrison P (2009) Assessment of platelet function in the laboratory. *Haemostaseologie* **29**, 25–31

Harrison P and Keeling D (2007) Clinical tests of platelet function. In: *Platelets, 2nd edn*, ed. AD Michelson, pp.445–474. Elsevier, Amsterdam

Jennings I, Woods TA, Kitchen S and Walker ID (2008) Platelet function testing: practice among UK National External Quality Assessment Scheme for Blood Coagulation Participants. *Journal of Clinical Pathology* **61**, 950–954

Kristensen AT, Weiss DJ and Klausner JS (1994) Platelet dysfunction associated with immune-mediated thrombocytopenia in dogs. *Journal of Veterinary Internal Medicine* **8**, 323–327

Lewis DC and Meyers KM (1996) Studies of platelet-bound and serum platelet-bindable immunoglobulins in dogs with idiopathic thrombocytopenic purpura. *Experimental Haematology* **24**, 696–701

Lipscomb DL, Bourne C and Boudreaux MK (2000) Two genetic defects in αIIb are associated with Type I Glanzmanns thrombasthenia in a Great Pyrenees dog: a 14 base insertion in exon 13 and a splicing defect on intron 13. *Veterinary Pathology* **37**, 581–588

McMillan R, Tani P, Millard F *et al.* (1987) Platelet-associated and plasma anti-glycoprotein autoantibodies in chronic ITP. *Blood* **70**, 1040–1045

Paniccia R, Antonucci E, Maggini N *et al.* (2009) Assessment of platelet function on whole blood by multiple electrode aggregometry in high-risk patients with coronary artery disease receiving antiplatelet therapy. *American Journal of Clinical Pathology* **131**, 834–842

Parker MT, Collier LL, Kier AB and Johnson GS (1988) Oral mucosa bleeding times of normal cats and cats with Chediak-Higashi syndrome or Hageman trait (factor 12 deficiency). *Veterinary Clinical Pathology* **17**, 9–12

Rao AK (2006) Acquired qualitative platelet defects. In: *Hemostasis and Thrombosis: Basic principles and clinical practice, 5th edn*, ed. RW Colman, VJ Marder, AW Clowes, JN George and SZ Goldhaber, pp.1045–1060. JB Lippincott, Philadelphia

Roth GJ (1992) Platelets and blood vessels: the adhesion event. *Immunology Today* **13**, 100–105

Wei AH, Schoenwelder SM, Andrews RK and Jackson SP (2009) New insights into the haemostatic function of platelets. *British Journal of Haematology* **147**, 415–430

Welles EG, Bourne C, Tyler JW and Boudreaux MK (1994) Detection of activated feline platelets in platelet-rich plasma by use of fluorescein-labeled antibodies and flow cytometry. *Veterinary Pathology* **31**, 553–560

Willis SE, Jackson ML, Meric SM and Rousseaux CG (1989) Whole blood platelet aggregation in dogs with liver disease. *American Journal of Veterinary Research* **50**, 1893–1897

25

Disorders of secondary haemostasis

Reinhard Mischke

Introduction

Inherited disorders of secondary haemostasis (see also Chapter 21) are usually deficiencies of single clotting factors that arise as a result of genetic mutations, although deficiencies in multiple factors may occur (Spurling, 1980; Fogh and Fogh, 1988; Littlewood, 1989; Brooks, 1999). Acquired disorders of coagulation (coagulopathies), are generally deficiencies of multiple factors and may occur in conjunction with platelet disorders (Littlewood, 1992; Couto, 1999).

Clinical approach to coagulopathies

History

The clinical history may be helpful in discriminating between inherited and acquired disorders. Typical features of inherited haemostatic disorders include: first signs of haemorrhage at a young age; and a history of previous bleeding episodes. Older animals presented with haemorrhagic diathesis without previous bleeding episodes are unlikely to have an inherited haemostatic disorder. Adult onset, however, does not exclude a mild hereditary bleeding tendency (Dodds, 2000). Affected relatives further suggest the presence of an inherited haemostatic disorder.

Other important features include exposure to toxins (e.g. anticoagulant rodenticides) or the presence of underlying renal or hepatic disease.

Clinical signs

The nature of abnormal bleeding in animals with coagulation defects is generally similar, irrespective of the specific factor that is deficient, but it is distinct from the clinical signs that result from platelet abnormalities. Typically, patients with coagulation defects are presented with subcutaneous or intramuscular (deep soft tissue) haematomas or haemorrhage at a single site, often without a known history of trauma or after a relatively minor traumatic episode (Littlewood, 1992).

Joint bleeding and subsequent haemarthroses, as well as compression of the spinal cord or peripheral nerves by subdural or organized soft tissue haematomas, respectively, may result in lameness and paralysis (Figure 25.1). Excessive bleeding during teething is often the first sign of an inherited factor deficiency, especially haemophilia (Figure 25.2) Excessive bleeding from the umbilical cord may not be noted by the breeder. Delayed bleeding or rebleeding may occur from venepuncture sites, and excessive haemorrhage may occur during or after surgery (Figure 25.3).

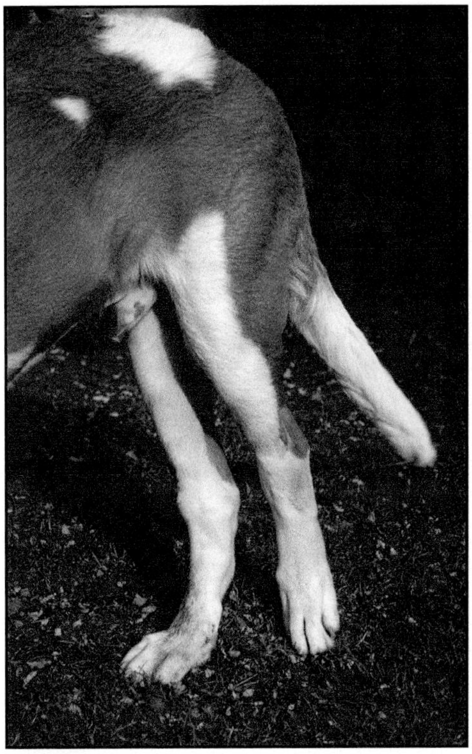

25.1 Lameness caused by bleeding into the stifle joint in a 6-month-old St Bernard with severe haemophilia B.

Bleeding from mucosal surfaces (i.e. epistaxis, oral cavity haemorrhage, haematemesis, haematuria, haematochezia, melaena) and bleeding into body cavities are seen less frequently. Severe haemothorax and haemomediastinum may result in dyspnoea and dullness on chest percussion. Occasionally, severe respiratory compromise may result from submucosal haemorrhage affecting the tracheal and retropharyngeal region (Figures 25.4). Abdominal pain and malaise are the main signs of intraperitoneal or visceral haemorrhage (Littlewood, 2000). Bleeding into body cavities may occasionally lead to sudden death.

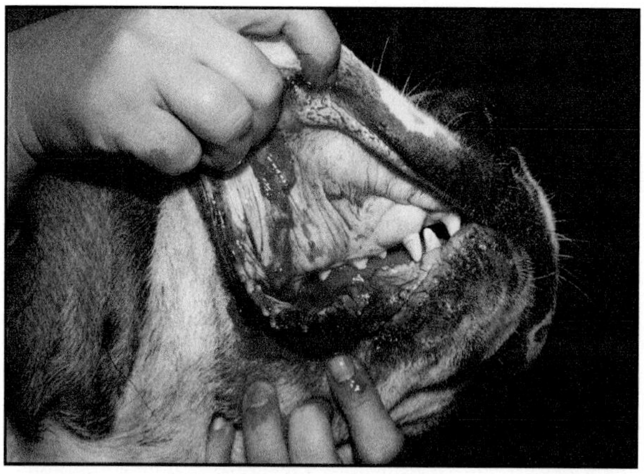

25.2 Massive bleeding during shedding of teeth in a St Bernard with severe haemophilia B (same patient as Figure 25.1).

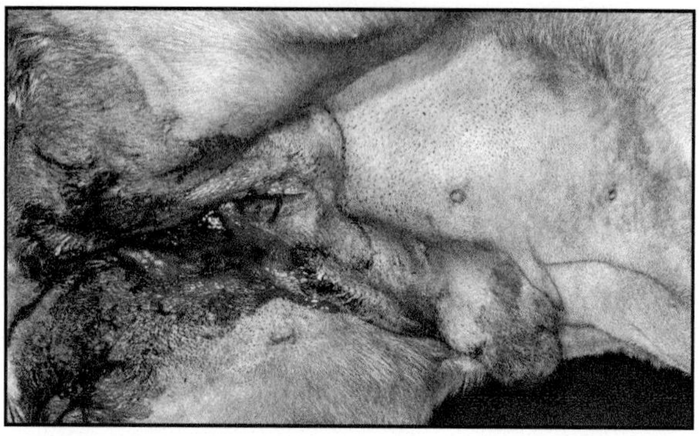

25.3 Haemorrhage following neutering in a male Rhodesian Ridgeback with haemophilia B.

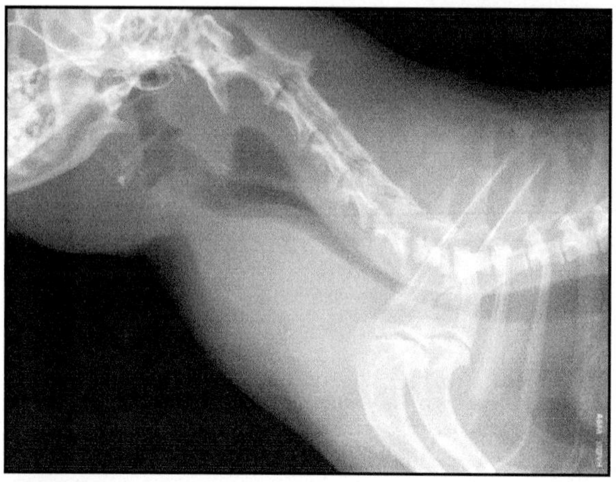

25.4 Radiograph illustrating compression of the trachea by a massive haematoma in the neck of a Dachshund with anticoagulant rodenticide intoxication.

Laboratory investigations

Significant defects of individual clotting factors may be indicated by prolonged clotting or reaction times in global tests of haemostasis (thrombelastography/thrombelastometry, activated clotting time (ACT)) as well as prothrombin time (PT; factor (F)VII, FX, FV, and FII, fibrinogen), activated partial thromboplastin time (aPTT; FXII, FXI, FIX, FVIII:C, FX, FV, and FII, fibrinogen) and thrombin time (fibrinogen) (see Chapter 22). Assays of specific factors, usually coagulometric methods using human deficient plasma, are required to ascertain the exact nature of the coagulation defect (see Chapter 22). Several coagulation defects are defined at the molecular level, and diagnostic testing by polymerase chain reaction (PCR) may accompany coagulation testing. Genetic tests are best for the identification of heterozygous carriers, but they give no information about the residual factor activity, i.e. about the severity of the disease.

Tests of primary haemostasis (platelet count, capillary bleeding time, platelet function tests) are normal in uncomplicated coagulation defects, but the platelet count can decrease as a result of loss during bleeding episodes (e.g. in anticoagulant rodenticide intoxication), or owing to consumption in cases of disseminated intravascular coagulation (DIC).

Therapeutic management

Therapeutic management of bleeding crisis includes:

- Supportive and local, haemostatic measures (including sedation, soft bedding, bandages, compresses, electrocoagulation/vessel ligature)
- Replacement therapy
- Additional medical therapy.

Drugs known to interfere with haemostasis (e.g. platelet aggregation inhibitors such as acetylsalicylic acid) are contraindicated. Gene therapy has been used to bring about long-term correction of haemophilia B in dogs experimentally (Kay et al., 1993; Niemeyer *et al.,* 2009), but it is unlikely that this therapeutic approach will become available for veterinary practice in the near future.

Replacement therapy

In cases of severe internal haemorrhage, haemorrhages with life-threatening consequences (e.g. within the central nervous system, haematomas causing obstruction of the upper airway) or those accompanying essential surgical procedures, replacement therapy is indicated. Ideally, patients with defects of coagulation factors should be treated by replacement of the missing clotting factors. In practice, treatment usually entails giving fresh or fresh frozen plasma (see Chapter 34). Several commercial animal blood-banking facilities provide blood and blood products in North America, the UK and Germany. In addition, several referral institutions maintain donor animals. Theoretically, human factor preparations including recombinant human FVIIa preparations (as non-specific procoagulants or in cases of FVII deficiency), are effective, but they are too expensive and may provoke formation of antibodies (Littlewood and Barrowcliffe, 1987).

With the exception of hypovolaemic patients, whole blood transfusions should not exceed 20 ml/kg body weight to avoid volume overload. This limits the amount of clotting factors that can be administered, and the transfusion of red cells carries the risk of sensitizing the patient (see Chapters 34 and 35). Therefore, if plasma is available, whole blood transfusions should only be given where severe anaemia accompanies the coagulation factor deficiency.

As a guideline, the aim is to increase the activity of the affected clotting factors in the circulation to at least 25–30% of normal to achieve adequate haemostasis. The volume of plasma required to accomplish this depends on the residual factor activity, but in cases of severe factor deficiency at least 15–20 ml/kg of plasma is needed (Figure 25.5).

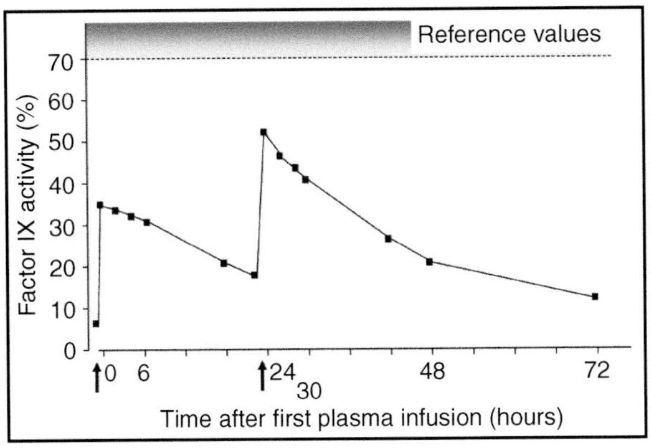

25.5 Factor IX activity in a dog with haemophilia B during repeated treatment with 20 ml/kg fresh frozen plasma (arrows). (Source: Mischke *et al.*, 1996)

The short half-life of individual factors (e.g. FVII, FVIII) may require repeated transfusions (once or twice daily) to maintain individual factor activity at an effective level for long enough to control haemorrhage (Knowler *et al.*, 1994; Mischke *et al.*, 1996). However, limited availability of plasma products may limit the number of transfusions. Sometimes, even a single transfusion may be effective.

Additional medical therapy

Where specific contributory factors or underlying diseases are identified, these must be addressed and treated appropriately. In selected cases of inherited coagulopathies, the additional use of inhibitors of fibrinolysis to support fibrin clot formation at the site of vessel injury has been found to be of benefit. For example, tranexamic acid (not authorized for veterinary use) was effective at a dose of 15–20 mg/kg orally q6–12h (Littlewood, 2000). Broad-spectrum antibiotics are indicated because extravasated blood provides an ideal medium for bacterial growth.

Inherited coagulopathies

An overview of the major features of selected inherited coagulopathies in dogs and cats is given in Figure 25.6.

Factor deficiency	Species and breeds affected	Inheritance	Clinical signs	Abnormal clotting times
Afibrinogenaemia, hypofibrinogenaemia, dysfibrinogenaemia	Bernese Mountain Dog, Lhasa Apso, Hungarian Vizsla, collie	Autosomal incomplete dominant or recessive	Mostly severe bleeding	PT aPTT/ACT TT reduced fibrinogen
II	English Cocker Spaniel, Boxer, Otterhound	Autosomal recessive	Moderate bleeding	PT aPTT/ACT
VII	Beagle, Alaskan Malamute, Miniature Schnauzer and other dog breeds	Autosomal recessive	Usually mild signs	PT
VIII, IX Haemophilia A, B	Dogs and cats, numerous breeds	X-chromosomal recessive	Often severe signs (males), affected females usually asymptomatic carriers	aPTT/ACT
X	American Cocker Spaniel, Jack Russell Terrier, Domestic Shorthair cat	Autosomal dominant (variable penetrance)	Severe clinical signs, high neonatal mortality	PT aPTT/ACT
XI	Kerry Blue Terrier, Springer Spaniel, Pyrenean Mountain Dog, Domestic Shorthair cat	Autosomal recessive	Mild spontaneous bleeding, late, severe post-traumatic bleeding	aPTT/ACT
XII	Domestic Shorthair cat, several dog breeds	Autosomal recessive	No increased bleeding risk, possibly increased thrombotic risk	aPTT/ACT (remarkably prolonged)
Prekallikrein	Labrador Retriever, other dog breeds	Undefined	No increased bleeding tendency	PT aPTT/ACT
Vitamin K-dependent	Devon Rex cat	Autosomal recessive	Moderate bleeding, response to oral vitamin K_1 treatment	PT aPTT/ACT

25.6 Overview of features of selected inherited coagulopathies. ACT, activated coagulation time; aPTT, activated partial thromboplastin time; PT, prothrombin time; TT, thrombin (clotting) time.

Hypofibrinogenaemia

Hereditary fibrinogen deficits can either be associated with a complete lack of fibrinogen (afibrinogenaemia), reduced fibrinogen (hypofibrinogenaemia) or an abnormal fibrinogen (dysfibrinogenaemia). Whereas afibrinogenaemia is incompatible with life, the remaining conditions are usually expressed as a mild bleeding tendency exacerbated by trauma or surgery (Dodds, 2000).

Canine hypofibrinogenaemia was recognized in a family of Bernese Mountain Dogs in which low fibrinogen concentrations were measured with functional and immunological assays. It has also been diagnosed in other breeds such as the Lhasa Apso, Hungarian Vizsla and collies (Dodds, 2000). According to Littlewood (2000), deficiencies of fibrinogen have been identified in several dogs by the coagulation laboratory at the Animal Health Trust, Newmarket. One such case was a 1-year-old male Cocker Spaniel with a fibrinogen concentration of 0.4 g/l (normal range 1–3 g/l), that presented with a history of recurrent episodes of joint stiffness and epistaxis. The clinical examination findings included tachypnoea, pallor and scleral and retinal haemorrhage. Thoracic radiographs revealed alveolar densities caused by pulmonary haemorrhage. The dog subsequently had seizures, and lesions consistent with cerebrovascular infarcts were identified on magnetic resonance imaging (MRI) scans. The acute episode of haemorrhage was managed by plasma transfusions. Prophylactically administered low doses of tranexamic acid (an inhibitor of fibrinolysis, see above) were successful in minimizing the occurrence of bleeding episodes. Both autosomal recessive and incomplete dominant patterns of inheritance of hypofibrinogenaemia have been documented (Fogh and Fogh, 1988). Inherited dysfibrinogenaemia has been reported in an inbred Borzoi colony (Dodds, 2000).

In cases of severe hypofibrinogenaemia (< 0.7 g/l), all group tests (PT, aPTT and thrombin time) are prolonged. Dysfibrinogenaemia is diagnosed if functional assays reveal a decreased fibrinogen concentration whereas immunological or heat precipitation methods reveal a normal concentration.

Factor II deficiency (prothrombin deficiency)

Canine hypoprothrombinaemia is a rare condition, reported in the Boxer, Otterhound and English Cocker Spaniel. The mode of inheritance is autosomal recessive. Mild to moderate bleeding episodes occur, including umbilical bleeding in newborn puppies and epistaxis (Dodds, 2000).

Factor VII deficiency

Canine FVII deficiency is a well recognized bleeding disorder, especially in certain families of laboratory Beagles (Spurling, 1988). The defect is caused by a G96E substitution, and up to one third of the Beagle population carries the defective gene (Wilhelm *et al.*, 2001; Callan *et al.*, 2006). FVII deficiency has also been described in the Alaskan Malamute (Spurling, 1980), a crossbred dog (Macpherson *et al.*, 1999), Alaskan Klee Kai (Kaae *et al.*, 2007) and Miniature Schnauzer (Lillis *et al.*, 2008). The pattern of inheritance is autosomal recessive.

The bleeding tendency is usually mild, which possibly reflects the large contingency reserve of this important clotting factor under physiological conditions. Nevertheless, in rare cases affected animals can show life-threatening haemorrhage and require intensive care (Spurling *et al.*, 1974; Wheeler *et al.*, 1984).

The screening test of the extrinsic pathway, the PT, is prolonged in cases of FVII deficiency, but the aPTT and thrombin time are normal.

FVII deficiency may also be acquired, and isolated FVII deficiency may occur in the early phase of rodenticide poisoning. One case of combined congenital and acquired FVII deficiency has been reported as a result of rodenticide poisoning in an affected Beagle (Daly and Giger, 2007). Hereditary FVII deficiency has not been described in cats thus far.

Factor VIII deficiency (haemophilia A)

Haemophilia A, also known as 'classic' haemophilia, is caused by a deficiency in FVIII and is the commonest of the inherited coagulopathies. This condition is covered in detail in Chapter 28.

Factor IX deficiency (haemophilia B)

Haemophilia B is caused by a deficiency in FIX. This condition is covered in detail in Chapter 28.

Factor X deficiency

Deficiency of FX (Stuart-Power factor) is a rare inherited coagulopathy that has been described in a family of American Cocker Spaniels (Dodds, 1973) and in Jack Russell Terriers (Cook *et al.*, 1993; Dodds, 2000). The mode of inheritance in the American Cocker Spaniel is autosomal dominant with variable penetrance. The severity of bleeding episodes in dogs with FX deficiency is variable. Severely affected dogs with FX activity < 10% are usually stillborn or die as neonates as a result of fatal internal bleeding (Dodds, 2000). Affected American Cocker Spaniels have a high neonatal mortality rate. Less severely affected dogs may survive to adulthood, showing moderate to severe haemorrhagic tendencies. The female Jack Russell Terrier with proven FX deficiency (3–13% of normal) had recurrent episodes of spontaneous and surgical (post tail docking and post ovariohysterectomy) haemorrhage.

The condition has also been identified in a Domestic Shorthair cat that presented with seizures, bleeding associated with jugular venepuncture and after declawing (Gookin *et al.*, 1997). Although not confirmed by imaging techniques, the neurological abnormalities were assumed to have been the result of intracranial haemorrhage, which is reported in some human infants with FX deficiency.

Given that FX is a common pathway defect, individuals with FX levels < 30% usually have a prolonged PT, aPTT and perhaps ACT, but normal thrombin time. The diagnosis is confirmed by a specific FX assay. The FX activity in the affected cat was < 2% (Gookin *et al.*, 1997).

Factor XI deficiency

Deficiency of FXI (plasma thromboplastin antecedent) usually presents with mild clinical signs, but severe and often lethal haemorrhage can occur after surgery or severe trauma. Postsurgical bleeding episodes are often delayed for up to several days (Gentry, 2000). FXI deficiency has been reported in Springer Spaniels and Pyrenean Mountain Dogs (Dodds and Kull, 1971; Dodds, 1977) and in Kerry Blue Terriers (Knowler *et al.*, 1994). The inheritance pattern is autosomal recessive, with FXI activity of < 10% in homozygotes and 25–50% in heterozygotes; the latter are asymptomatic.

A mild congenital FXI deficiency (factor activity 14–18%) was reported in a 6-month-old Domestic Shorthair cat that showed bleeding from its paws following onychectomy, but without prior episodes of haemorrhage (Troxel *et al.*, 2002). In addition, an acquired form of the condition has been reported in a cat, which was attributed to an inhibitor, possibly present owing to systemic lupus erythematosus (Feldman *et al.*, 1983). The fact that FXI deficiency is a defect of the intrinsic pathway is reflected by an isolated prolongation of the aPTT, whereas the PT and thrombin time are normal. The diagnosis is confirmed by a specific FXI assay. A combined fibrinogen and FXI deficiency was detected recently in Maine Coon cats in the UK (Brown, 2008).

Factor XII deficiency

Deficiency of FXII (Hageman factor) is the most common hereditary coagulation factor deficiency in Domestic Shorthair cats (Kier *et al.*, 1980; Peterson *et al.*, 1995). A combined deficiency of FVIII and FXII was encountered in a family of cats (Littlewood and Evans, 1990), in addition to the combined FIX and FXII deficiencies described above (Dillon and Boudreaux, 1988). The pattern of inheritance of FXII deficiency in cats is autosomal recessive, as in humans, with homozygotes having a severe deficiency of FXII activity and heterozygotes having about 50% of normal plasma FXII activity (Kier *et al.*, 1980).

Affected dog breeds include the Standard Poodle and German Shorthaired Pointer (Dodds, 2000). Combined deficiency of FXII and prekallikrein was reported in a 1-year-old Chinese Shar Pei with repeated episodes of intestinal haemorrhage and diarrhoea associated with mild inflammatory bowel disease (Otto *et al.*, 1991). Combined FXII deficiency and von Willebrand's disease (vWD) was described in a family of Miniature Poodles that were affected concurrently with a familial non-spherocytic haemolytic anaemia (Randolph *et al.*, 1986). FXII deficiency was widespread amongst the dogs of the affected family, but only dogs suffering from non-spherocytic haemolytic anaemia had concurrent vWD.

Although a deficiency of FXII results in dramatic prolongation of the aPTT (and ACT), it is not associated with an increased bleeding tendency (Randolph *et al.*, 1986; Littlewood and Evans, 1990). Given that the defect is relatively common in cats, it complicates the performance of diagnostic tests of coagulation in this species. In a family of haemophilic cats, the presence of FXII deficiency complicated the identification of kittens affected with haemophilia A (Littlewood and Evans, 1990). In cases of unexplained prolonged aPTT or ACT, measurement of FXII may be necessary to determine whether a defect of this factor is responsible for the abnormal result.

Prekallikrein deficiency

Prekallikrein deficiency was reported in a 15-year-old dog with chronic haematuria (Chinn *et al.*, 1986). The haematuria was attributed to a renal transitional cell carcinoma, which is consistent with the fact that prekallikrein deficiency rarely causes haemorrhage. As described above, a combined deficiency with FXII has been reported in a dog (Otto *et al.*, 1991).

Vitamin K-dependent coagulopathy

A coagulopathy caused by deficiency of vitamin K-dependent clotting factors (FII, FVII, FIX and FX) was described in three Devon Rex cats in Australia (Maddison *et al.*, 1990). In these cats there was no evidence of exposure to vitamin K-antagonist rodenticides, or of underlying hepatic or gastrointestinal diseases or fat malassimilation. Oral vitamin K_1 treatment resulted in normalization of the clotting factor concentrations. Liver biopsies were taken and it was demonstrated that the coagulation defect was associated with defective hepatic vitamin K metabolism. Gamma-glutamyl carboxylase had a significantly reduced binding affinity for both vitamin K hydroquinone and propeptide (Soute *et al.*, 1992). The condition has also been identified in a Devon Rex cat in the United Kingdom (Littlewood *et al.*, 1995) (Figure 25.7). An autosomal recessive pattern of inheritance is proposed.

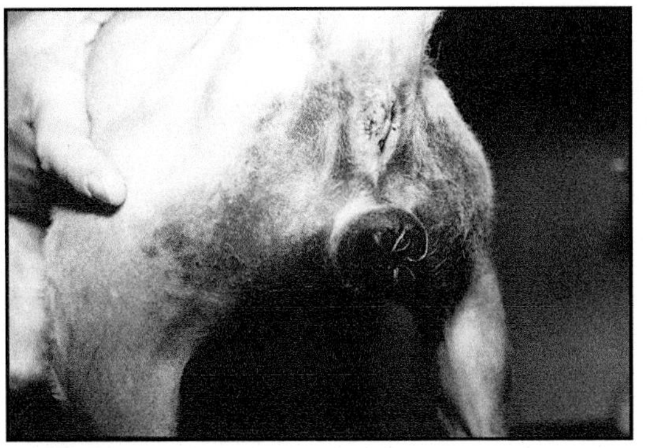

25.7 Vitamin K-dependent coagulopathy of Devon Rex cats: perineal bruising and scrotal haematoma in an affected male cat after surgery. (Courtesy of Steve Shaw)

The clinical signs include prolonged haemorrhage after surgery and trauma, although the risk of bleeding in an individual cat is variable. Cats of both genders are affected. A two- to three-fold prolongation of the PT and aPTT occurs, with reduced activity of all the vitamin K-dependent clotting factors. FII, FIX and FX are reduced to less than 20% of the values in pooled normal plasma in the cat, and FVII to less than 50% of normal.

Treatment with oral vitamin K1, which can be given long term at a dose rate of 5 mg q24h, successfully corrects the abnormalities in clotting factors and controls the bleeding tendency.

The prevalence of the condition in Devon Rex cats is not known, although the PT assay would provide a simple screening test to identify affected animals. These cats could then be removed from breeding programmes, but should be treated prophylactically with vitamin K1 to prevent the risk of haemorrhage (Littlewood, 2000).

Other inherited coagulopathies

Other rare inherited disorders of clotting factors are reported occasionally (Fogh and Fogh, 1988; Peterson *et al.*, 1995; Brooks, 1999).

Acquired coagulopathies

Vitamin K-dependent coagulopathies

Vitamin K antagonism

A common acquired coagulation disorder is caused by depletion of vitamin K-dependent clotting factors resulting from the ingestion of coumarin rodenticides, which are vitamin K antagonists (see Chapter 29).

Vitamin K deficiency

Vitamin K is a fat-soluble vitamin, and deficiencies that result in a coagulopathy may occur secondary to maldigestion and malabsorption in exocrine pancreatic deficiency (Perry *et al.*, 1991), severe infiltrative enteritis (Edwards and Russell, 1987) and bile duct obstruction.

Hepatic disease

Pathogenesis

Liver disease is frequently associated with complex haemostatic disorders as a result of: reduced synthesis of coagulation proteins; consumption of haemostatic components; disturbed vitamin K-dependent carboxylation of coagulation factors; and qualitative platelet changes.

- The liver is the site of synthesis of most of the plasma clotting factors, as well as inhibitors of coagulation, and is the site of conversion of the vitamin K-dependent factors into their active forms. Damage to more than 70–80% of the liver parenchyma may result in deficiencies of protein synthesis, including the production of clotting factors.
- Liver diseases are frequently associated with chronic DIC. This can be promoted or induced by release of tissue factor and/or an impaired clearance function of the mononuclear phagocyte system. The liver is responsible for the removal and inactivation of circulating activated clotting factors.
- Final gamma-carboxylation of FII, FVII, FIX and FX, and proteins C and S, takes place in the liver and depends on vitamin K. Under conditions of vitamin K deficiency or antagonism, only functional inactive coagulation proteins ('proteins induced by vitamin K absence', PIVKA) are present, stored in the liver and finally released into the circulation
- Both qualitative and quantitative alterations in platelets may occur in liver disease. The latter is caused by the inhibitory effects of hyperammonaemia and changes in platelet lipid composition, namely an increased cholesterol to phospholipid ratio, and abnormal phospholipid and fatty acid composition with reduced arachidonic acid content.

Clinical signs

Given that synthesis and consumption induces a balanced decrease of coagulation factors and inhibitors, clinically significant haemorrhagic diatheses are relatively rare. Clinically significant haemostatic abnormalities tend to be associated with acute insults to the liver, although it is considered prudent to check clotting variables before surgery or biopsy in patients with chronic hepatic disease (Badylak, 1988).

Diagnosis

Between 45 and >90% of dogs and cats with liver disease have at least one abnormal blood coagulation test (Badylak *et al.*, 1983; Center *et al.*, 1993; Lisciandro *et al.*, 1998; Prins *et al.*, 2010). Multiple clotting factors are depleted, so prolongation of both PT and aPTT may be seen, but the aPTT is more sensitive (Badylak *et al.*, 1983; Prins *et al.*, 2010). Increased activation makers (e.g. increased D-dimers) are detected as an indicator of chronic DIC (see Chapter 30), probably because activated clotting factors are not cleared from the circulation (Prins *et al.*, 2010).

Defects of the coagulation system that are similar to those occurring in human hepatic cirrhosis have been described in detail in dogs with cirrhosis (Mischke *et al.*, 1998).

Liver disease is indicated by markers of liver cell damage (i.e. increased liver enzyme activities including alanine aminotransferase, gamma glutamyl transferase and, in dogs, alkaline phosphatase) and markers of impaired liver function (e.g. increased bile acids, hyperbilirubinaemia, hypoalbuminaemia). Owing to the multifactorial pathogenesis of coagulation factor defects in liver disease, coagulation factor activities have only limited relevance as indicators of protein synthesis, but may be suited for monitoring of the severity of liver disease and as prognostic parameters.

Treatment

The treatment is primarily supportive, and the prognosis depends on the nature and reversibility of the hepatic disease.

Disseminated intravascular coagulation (DIC)

DIC is a complex syndrome that involves the secondary haemostatic and fibrinolytic system and is characterized by widespread intravascular coagulation within the microcirculation, triggered by underlying diseases that cause activation of the haemostatic system (e.g. neoplasia, septicaemia, shock). This results in the formation of soluble fibrin and microthrombi, with subsequent possible organ failure and/or fibrinolysis with the formation of fibrin(ogen) degradation products (FDPs). The consumption of platelets and clotting factors, together with increased levels of FDPs as potent inhibitors of fibrin formation, and the activation of fibrinolysis, may cause a haemorrhagic diathesis ('consumptive coagulopathy'). Animals with distinct hypofibrinogenaemia/hyperfibrinolysis are particularly likely to show clinical signs (the 'iceberg phenomenon'). The diagnosis is usually based on a panel of abnormal tests, in combination with an underlying disease potentially associated with DIC. The treatment includes management of the underlying disease, fluid therapy and anticoagulant and substitution therapy. The condition, predisposing factors, diagnosis and management are discussed in Chapter 30.

Circulating inhibitors to clotting factors

Lupus anticoagulant

A lupus-type anticoagulant, which in humans is due to the presence of circulating autoantibodies directed against phospholipids, has been reported in one dog with pulmonary thromboembolism and immune-mediated haemolytic anaemia (Stone *et al.*, 1994), as well as in a cat with haemolytic anaemia and hepatic abnormalities (Lusson *et al.*, 1999). This should be considered as a rare cause of unexplained prolonged aPTT or ACT.

Factor inhibitors

The presence of inhibitors (antibodies) of those clotting factors that are deficient in haemophilia is associated with severe forms of haemophilia and can complicate substitution therapy. This has been documented in haemophilic dogs transfused with canine FVIII (Giles *et al.*, 1984; Pijnappels *et al.*, 1986), and antibodies to heterologous FVIII, which cross-react with canine FVIII, have been described in haemophilic dogs that have received human and/or porcine FVIII concentrates (Littlewood and Barrowcliffe, 1987; Littlewood, 1988). Circulating inhibitors of FVIII may also be considered as a rare cause of non-specific haemorrhagic diathesis and/or unexplained prolongation of aPTT.

An acquired coagulopathy associated with the development of inhibitors of FXI has been described in a cat (Feldman *et al.*, 1983).

References and further reading

Badylak SF (1988) Coagulation disorders and liver disease. *Veterinary Clinics of North America: Small Animal Practice* **18**, 87–93

Badylak SF, Dodds WJ and Van Vleet JF (1983) Plasma coagulation factor abnormalities in dogs with naturally occurring hepatic disease. *American Journal of Veterinary Research* **44**, 2336–2340

Brooks M (1999) Hereditary bleeding disorders in dogs and cats. *Veterinary Medicine* **94**, 555–564

Brown R (2008) Haemophilia in Maine Coon cats. *Veterinary Record* **163**, 667

Callan MB, Aljamali MN, Margaritis P *et al.* (2006) A novel missense mutation responsible for factor VII deficiency in research Beagle colonies. *Journal of Thrombosis and Haemostasis* **4**, 2616–2622

Center SA, Crawford MA, Guida L, Erb HN and King J (1993) A retrospective study of 77 cats with severe hepatic lipidosis: 1975–1990. *Journal of Veterinary Internal Medicine* **7**, 349–359

Chinn DR, Dodds WJ and Selcer BA (1986) Prekallikrein deficiency in a dog. *Journal of the American Veterinary Medical Association* **188**, 69–71

Cook AK, Werner LL, O'Neill SL, Brooks M and Feldman BF (1993) Factor X deficiency in a Jack Russell terrier. *Veterinary Clinical Pathology* **22**, 68–71

Couto CG (1999) Clinical approach to the bleeding dog or cat. *Veterinary Medicine* **94**, 450–459

Daly ML and Giger U (2007) A rodenticide exposed and bleeding Beagle dog with hereditary factor VII deficiency. *Journal of Veterinary Emergency and Critical Care* **17**, 170–174

Dillon AR and Boudreaux MK (1988) Combined factors IX and XII deficiencies in a family of cats. *Journal of the American Veterinary Medical Association* **193**, 833–834

Dodds WJ (1973) Canine factor X (Stuart-Power factor) deficiency. *Journal of Laboratory and Clinical Medicine* **82**, 560–566

Dodds WJ (1977) Inherited hemorrhagic defects. In: *Current Veterinary Therapy VI*, ed. RW Kirk, pp.438–445. WB Saunders, Philadelphia

Dodds WJ (2000) Other hereditary coagulopathies. In: *Schalm's Veterinary Hematology, 5th edn*, ed. BF Feldman, JG Zinkl and NC Jain, pp.1030–1036. Lippincott Williams & Wilkins, Baltimore

Dodds WJ and Kull JE (1971) Canine factor XI (plasma thromboplastin antecedent) deficiency. *Journal of Laboratory and Clinical Medicine* **78**, 746–752

Edwards DF and Russell RG (1987) Probable vitamin K-deficient bleeding in two cats with malabsorption syndrome secondary to lymphocytic-plasmacytic enteritis. *Journal of Veterinary Internal Medicine* **1**, 97–101

Feldman BF, Soares CJ, Kitchell BE, Brown CC, O'Neill S (1983) Hemorrhage in a cat caused by inhibition of factor XI (plasma thromboplastin antecedent). *Journal of the American Veterinary Medical Association* **182**, 589–591

Fogh JM and Fogh IT (1988) Inherited coagulation disorders. *Veterinary Clinics of North America: Small Animal Practice* **18**, 231–244

Gentry PA (2000) Factor XI deficiency. In: *Schalm's Veterinary Hematology, 5th edn*, ed. BF Feldman, JG Zinkl and NC Jain, pp.1037–1041. Lippincott Williams & Wilkins, Baltimore

Giles AR, Tinlin S, Hoogendoorn H, Greenwood P and Greenwood R (1984) Development of factor VIII:C antibodies in dogs with hemophilia A (factor VIII:C deficiency). *Blood* **63**, 451–456

Gookin JL, Brooks MB, Catalfamo JL, Bunch SE and Muñana KR (1997) Factor X deficiency in a cat. *Journal of the American Veterinary Medical Association* **211**, 576–579

Kaae JA, Callan MB and Brooks MB (2007) Hereditary factor VII deficiency in the Alaskan Klee Kai dog. *Journal of Veterinary Internal Medicine* **21**, 976–981

Kay MA, Rothenburg S, Landen CN *et al.* (1993) In vivo gene therapy of haematology B sustained partial correction in factor IX-efficient dogs. *Science* **262**, 117–119

Kier AB, Bresnaham JF, White FJ and Wagner JE (1980) The inheritance pattern of factor XII deficiency in domestic cats. *Canadian Journal of Comparative Medicine* **44**, 309–314

Knowler C, Giger U, Dodds WJ and Brooks M (1994) Factor XI deficiency in Kerry blue terriers. *Journal of the American Veterinary Medical Association* **205**, 1557–1561

Lillis SM, Charles JA, Hygate GA, Anderson GA and Parry BW (2008) Inherited factor VII deficiency in Beagles and Miniature Schnauzers in Victoria, Australia and the use of REML analysis to determine heritability of the defect. *Journal of Veterinary Internal Medicine* **22**, 775 (Abstract)

Lisciandro SC, Hohenhaus A and Brooks M (1998) Coagulation abnormalities in 22 cats with naturally occurring liver disease. *Journal of Veterinary Internal Medicine* **12**, 71–75

Littlewood JD (1988) Factor VIII – phospholipid mixtures and factor VIII inhibitors: studies in haemophilic dogs. PhD thesis, University of Cambridge

Littlewood JD (1989) Inherited bleeding disorders of dogs and cats. *Journal of Small Animal Practice* **30**, 140–143

Littlewood JD (1992) Differential diagnosis of haemorrhagic disorders in dogs. *In Practice* **14**, 172–180

Littlewood JD (2000) Disorders of secondary haemostasis. In: BSAVA

Manual of Canine and Feline Haematology and Transfusion Medicine, ed. M Day *et al.*, pp.209–215. BSAVA Publication, Gloucester

Littlewood JD and Barrowcliffe TW (1987) The development and characterisation of antibodies to human factor VIII in haemophilic dogs. *Thrombosis and Haemostasis* **57**, 314–321

Littlewood JD and Evans RJ (1990) A combined deficiency of factor VIII and contact activation defect in a family of cats. *British Veterinary Journal* **146**, 30–35

Littlewood JD, Shaw SC and Coombes LM (1995) Vitamin K-dependent coagulopathy in a British Devon Rex cat. *Journal of Small Animal Practice* **36**, 115–118

Lusson D, Billiemaz B and Chabanne JL (1999) Circulating lupus anticoagulant and probable systemic lupus erythematosus in a cat. *Journal of Feline Medicine and Surgery* **1**, 193–196

Macpherson R, Scherer J, Ross ML and Gentry PA (1999) Factor VII deficiency in a mixed breed dog. *Canadian Veterinary Journal* **40**, 503–505

Maddison JE, Watson ADJ, Eade IG and Exner T (1990) Vitamin K-dependent multifactor coagulopathy in Devon Rex cats. *Journal of the American Veterinary Medical Association* **197**, 1495–1497

Mischke R, Hänies R, Deniz A and Hart S (1996) Hemophilia B in a mixed breed male dog: treatment of a hemorrhagic crisis with fresh frozen plasma. *Deutsche Tierärztliche Wochenschrift* **103**, 3–6 (in German)

Mischke R, Pohle D, Schoon HA, Fehr M and Nolte I (1998) Changes in blood coagulation in dogs with hepatic cirrhosis. *Deutsche Tierarztliche Wochenschrift* **105**, 43–47 (in German)

Niemeyer GP, Herzog RW, Mount J *et al.* (2009) Long-term correction of inhibitor-prone hemophilia B dogs treated with liver-directed AAV2-mediated factor IX gene therapy. *Blood* **113**, 797–806

Otto CM, Dodds WJ and Greene CE (1991) Factor XII and partial prekallikrein deficiencies in a dog with recurrent gastrointestinal hemorrhage. *Journal of the American Veterinary Medical Association* **198**, 129–131

Perry LA, Williams DA, Pidgeon GL and Boosinger TR (1991) Exocrine pancreatic insufficiency with associated coagulopathy in a cat. *Journal of the American Animal Hospital Association* **27**, 109–114

Peterson JL, Couto CG and Wellman ML (1995) Hemostatic disorders in cats: a retrospective study and review of the literature. *Journal of Veterinary Internal Medicine* **9**, 298–303

Pijnappels MIM, Briet E, van der Zweet GT *et al.* (1986) Evaluation of the cuticle bleeding time in canine haemophilia A. *Thrombosis and Haemostasis* **55**, 70–73

Prins M, Schellens CJ, van Leeuwen MW, Rothuizen J and Teske E (2010) Coagulation disorders in dogs with hepatic disease. *The Veterinary Journal* **185**, 163–168

Randolph JF, Center SA and Dodds WJ (1986) Factor XII deficiency and von Willebrand's disease in a family of miniature poodle dogs. *Cornell Veterinarian* **76**, 3–10

Soute BA, Ulrich MM, Watson AD *et al.* (1992) Congenital deficiency of all Vitamin-K-dependent blood coagulation factors due to a defective vitamin-K-dependent carboxylase in Devon Rex cats. *Thrombosis and Haemostasis* **68**, 521–525

Spurling NW (1980) Hereditary disorders of haemostasis in dogs: a critical review of the literature. *Veterinary Bulletin* **50**, 151–173

Spurling NW (1988) Hereditary blood coagulation factor-VII deficiency: A comparison of the defect in beagles from several sources. *Comparative Biochemistry and Physiology Part A: Physiology* **89**, 461–464

Spurling NW, Peacock R and Pilling T (1974) The clinical aspects of canine factor-VII deficiency including some case histories. *Journal of Small Animal Practice* **15**, 229–239

Stone MS, Johnstone IB, Brooks M, Bollinger TK and Cotter SM (1994) Lupus-type "anticoagulant" in a dog with hemolysis and thrombosis. *Journal of Veterinary Internal Medicine* **8**, 57–61

Troxel MT, Brooks MB and Esterline ML (2002) Congenital factor XI deficiency in a domestic shorthair cat. *Journal of the American Animal Hospital Association* **38**, 549–553

Wheeler SL, Weingand KW, Thrall MA *et al.* (1984) Persistent uterine and vaginal hemorrhage in a beagle with factor VII deficiency. *Journal of the American Veterinary Medical Association* **185**, 447–448

Wilhelm C, Czwalinna A, Wermes C *et al.* (2001) Isolation and characterisation of the canine factor VII gene of the Beagle dog with factor VII deficiency. XVIII. Annual Congress ISTH, Paris, France, *Thrombosis and Haemostasis, Suppl. July 2001*, Abstr. P577

26

Immune-mediated thrombocytopenia

Carrie White and Ann Hohenhaus

Introduction

The most common cause of severe thrombocytopenia is immune-mediated thrombocytopenia (IMTP). Retrospective studies of large populations of thrombocytopenic patients have revealed that 5% of dogs and 2% of cats had primary IMTP (Grindem *et al.*, 1991; Jordan *et al.*, 1993; Botsch *et al.*, 2009). IMTP is defined by a low platelet count, normal bone marrow function, the absence of other causes of thrombocytopenia and response to immunosuppressive therapy. IMTP can be primary, also termed idiopathic, or can occur secondary to an antigenic stimulus.

Pathogenesis of primary and secondary IMTP

IMTP is a disease in which antibodies cause the premature destruction of platelets, resulting in a significantly shortened platelet lifespan and thrombocytopenia. Antibodies may be directed at autoantigens on the platelet surface (autoantibodies), at foreign adsorbed antigens, at platelet antigen that has been altered as a result of underlying disease, or they can exist as adherent immune complexes. With primary IMTP, the reason for autoantibody production is unknown, and the immune system recognizes platelets as foreign antigens.

With secondary IMTP, there is an identifiable cause for the antibody production. Most commonly infectious agents or drugs bind to the platelet membrane, act as haptens, and antibodies are produced against the platelet–hapten combination. Autoantibodies are usually IgG and are directed toward epitopes on the glycoprotein IIb/IIIa complex (integrin $\alpha_{IIb}\beta_3$), the most abundant and immunogenic platelet surface glycoprotein, but they can also be directed toward epitopes on glycoproteins Ib/V/IX, Ia/IIa and IV (Lewis and Meyers, 1996a). It is also possible for antibodies to react with more than one glycoprotein. Antibody binding to the platelet surface results in the increased clearance of the antibody-coated platelets by macrophages in the reticuloendothelial system. Platelet destruction by splenic macrophages may be enhanced by the presence of P-selectin on the platelet membrane, because P-selectin mediates the adherence of IgG to monocytes and macrophages (Turner and Hadley, 2003). Some human patients with IMTP have been shown to have increased platelet-associated complement component C3, which suggests that complement may play a role in the pathogenesis of IMTP via opsonization or cytolysis of platelets.

IMTP can occur concurrently with other immune-mediated conditions, such as immune-mediated haemolytic anaemia (IMHA; the combined disease is known as Evans' syndrome), immune-mediated neutropenia (IMNP), or systemic lupus erythematosus (SLE).

The most common reason for the haemorrhage that can be observed in patients with IMTP is thrombocytopenia, but it has been proposed that thrombopathia may also play a role. One study revealed that the antibodies that cause thrombocytopenia in dogs with IMTP may cause platelet dysfunction in addition to platelet destruction (Kristensen *et al.*, 1994). However, others believe that the platelets that remain in these dogs are larger and more haemostatically competent (Lewis and Meyers, 1996b). This latter theory is supported by the fact that dogs with IMTP often have an elevated mean platelet volume (MPV), and life-threatening haemorrhage is actually relatively uncommon despite very low platelet counts (Lewis and Meyers, 1996b).

Acquired amegakaryocytic thrombocytopenia

Acquired amegakaryocytic thrombocytopenia (AATP) is a rare disease that involves immune-mediated destruction of megakaryocytes. Similar to IMTP, this disease can be primary (idiopathic) or can occur secondary to stimuli such as drugs, neoplasia, megakaryocytic stem cell dysfunction or infectious diseases (including those caused by *Borrelia burgdorferi* and *Ehrlichia canis*) (Lachowitz *et al.*, 2004). AATP is thought to result either from an intrinsic defect at the level of the colony forming unit–megakaryocyte (CFU-M), or a circulating cytotoxic autoantibody directed against the CFU-M.

Causes of secondary IMTP

IMTP has been reported to occur secondary to

neoplasia (e.g. lymphoma, haemangiosarcoma, leukaemia, hepatic tumours, mammary gland tumours), vaccination, specific infection (monocytic ehrlichiosis, angiostrongylosis, anaplasmosis, leptospirosis, borreliosis, babesiosis, leishmaniosis), inflammatory disease (e.g. prostatitis, endometritis, abscesses, pyometra), systemic immune-mediated disease (SLE), drugs, or following a blood transfusion (Breitschwerdt, 1988; Putsche and Kohn, 2008) (Figure 26.1).

Drugs
• Antibiotics: cefalothin, novobiocin, oxytetracycline, ristocetin, erythromycin, streptomycin, penicillin, rifamycin • Antimicrobial agents: sulphonamides, dinitrophenol, quinine, organic arsenicals, dapsone • Anti-inflammatories: paracetamol, aspirin, phenylbutazone, gold salts • Cardiovascular drugs: digitoxin, digoxin, nitroglycerin, methyldopa, dopamine, hydralazine, quinidine • Diuretics: thiazide derivatives • Hormones: oestrogens • Miscellaneous: vaccines, protamine sulphate, heparin, phenobarbital, diazepam, para-aminosalicylic acid, desipramine, chlorphenamine, lidocaine, oxaliplatin
Infections
• Rickettsial: *Ehrlichia canis, Rickettsia rickettsii, Anaplasma phagocytophilum, Borrelia burgdorferi* • Viral: distemper; feline infectious peritonitis; feline leukaemia virus, feline immunodeficiency virus • Parasitic: *Angiostrongylus vasorum* • Bacterial: *Leptospira* spp., prostatitis, endometritis, abscesses, pyelonephritis • Protozoal: *Leishmania* spp., *Babesia* spp.
Systemic autoimmune disease
• Systemic lupus erythematosus
Neoplasia
• Lymphoma • Haemangiosarcoma • Leukaemia • Hepatic tumours • Mammary gland tumours
Miscellaneous
• Following blood transfusion • Heatstroke

26.1 Potential causes of secondary IMTP. (Data from Thomason and Feldman, 1985; Kohn *et al.*, 2006; Thomas, 2010)

Drug-induced IMTP

Any drug can potentially provoke IMTP (Lewis and Meyers, 1996b). Antibodies will bind to complexes of a drug or drug metabolite that are bound to platelet glycoproteins (most often glycoprotein IIb/IIIa, glycoprotein Ib/IX, or both). If a drug is given for the first time, the onset of thrombocytopenia typically occurs at least 1 week after the drug is started. If a patient is already sensitized to a drug, the onset of thrombocytopenia can be very rapid following re-exposure. Platelet counts should increase 3–4 days after withdrawal of the drug (Aster and Bougie, 2007). Drug-induced secondary IMTP can be difficult to diagnose definitively because specific testing is not available; however, it should be suspected in patients with a sudden and significant drop in platelet count following drug exposure. The thrombocytopenia associated with drug-induced secondary IMTP is often severe, with 85–90% of human patients having a nadir of less than 20×10^9 platelets/l.

Infection-induced IMTP

Infectious agents can induce IMTP by several mechanisms, including altering immune regulation, exposing antigenic sites on the platelet surface, or via immune complex injury to the platelet membrane (Breitschwerdt, 1988). Thrombocytopenia is a common laboratory finding in dogs with rickettsial diseases; however, the cause of the thrombocytopenia is multifactorial, and may vary according to the infecting species. There are many other infectious agents that have been found to trigger secondary IMTP (Figure 26.1).

Neoplasia-induced IMTP

Thrombocytopenia is relatively common observation in dogs and cats with neoplasia (Jordan *et al.*, 1993; Grindem *et al.*, 1994). While the aetiology of the thrombocytopenia is multifactorial, immune-mediated platelet destruction may play a role. Immune-mediated platelet destruction has been documented in human patients with several types of solid tumour, including ovarian papillary cystadenoma, vaginal squamous cell carcinoma, pulmonary squamous cell carcinoma, basal cell carcinoma, prostatic adenocarcinoma, ductal cell carcinoma of the breast, ovarian adenocarcinoma and pulmonary adenocarcinoma. While the exact pathogenesis of neoplasia-induced secondary IMTP is unknown, it is believed that antibodies or antigen–antibody complexes formed against tumour antigens may either bind to the platelet surface non-specifically or cross-react with platelet antigen.

Miscellaneous causes of secondary IMTP

Thrombocytopenia can be observed in human patients with severe liver disease. Human patients with hepatic cirrhosis have been demonstrated to have a similar profile of the anti-GPIIb/IIIa autoantibody response to patients with IMTP. This suggests that autoantibody-mediated platelet destruction may contribute, at least in part, to cirrhotic thrombocytopenia (Kajihara *et al.*, 2003).

Clinical approach to primary IMTP

IMTP has been reported in dogs ranging in age from 4 months to 14 years, although the majority of dogs present as adults, with a median age at the time of diagnosis of 4–5 years of age (Grindem *et al.*, 1991; Putsche and Kohn, 2008). Cats with IMTP can also be of any age, ranging from 2–12 years, although they are most often young adult to middle-aged at the time of diagnosis (Bianco *et al.*, 2008; Wondratschek *et al.*, 2010). Bitches are affected more often than male dogs (Williams and Maggio-Price, 1984; Jackson and Kruth, 1985; Grindem *et al.*, 1991; Putsche and Kohn, 2008; Botsch *et al.*, 2009), and several breeds, including Cocker Spaniels, Old English Sheepdogs, Golden Retrievers and Poodles, among others, have been overrepresented in studies of canine IMTP (Wilkins *et al.*, 1973; Williams and Maggio-Price, 1984; Jackson and Kruth, 1985; Jans *et al.*, 1990; Grindem *et al.*, 1991). No definitive sex or breed predispositions have been observed in cats.

Presenting signs

Patients with IMTP can present with a wide variety of clinical signs, or they may be completely asymptomatic. In one study, 70% of patients with IMTP had clinical evidence of bleeding on initial examination (Putsche and Kohn, 2008). Increased bleeding tendency is most likely when platelet counts are less than 30–50 × 10^9/l (Williams and Maggio-Price, 1984). The most common type of bleeding to occur in thrombocytopenic patients is surface or capillary bleeding, which can manifest as petechiae (Figures 26.2 and 26.3), ecchymoses (Figure 26.4), melaena, haematuria, epistaxis (Figure 26.5), retinal haemorrhages, haematemesis, haemoptysis, haematochezia or prolonged bleeding following surgery or whelping (Wilkins *et al.*, 1973; Williams and Maggio-Price, 1984).

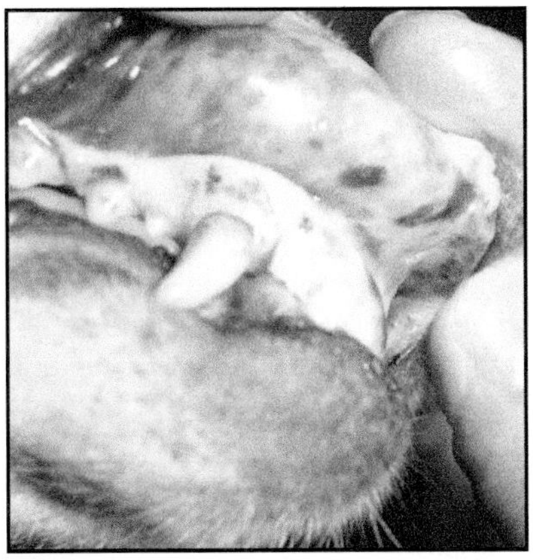

26.2 Petechiation of the buccal mucosa in a dog with primary IMTP.

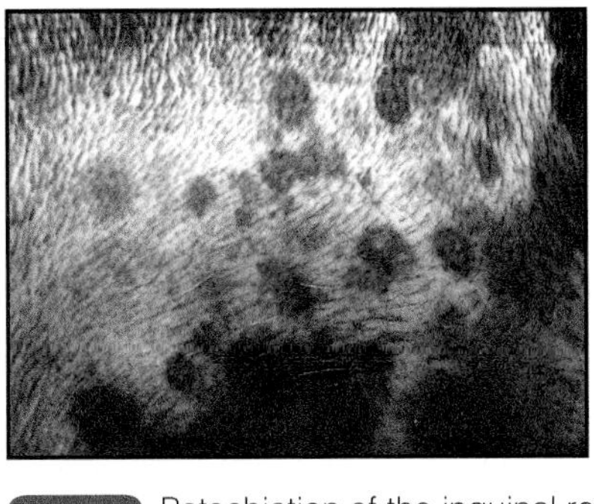

26.3 Petechiation of the inguinal region in a dog with primary IMTP.

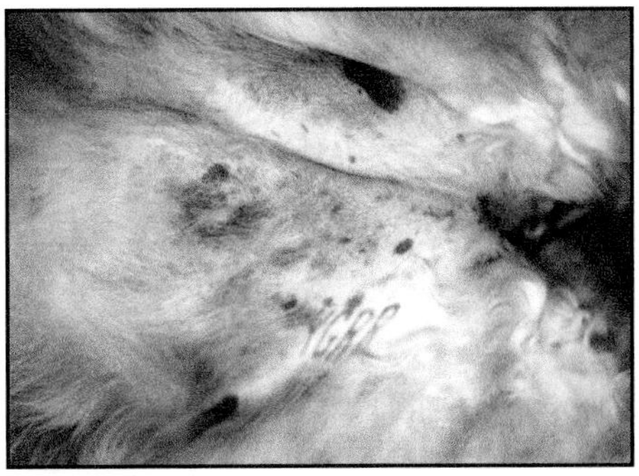

26.4 Ecchymoses on the ventral abdomen of a dog with primary IMTP.

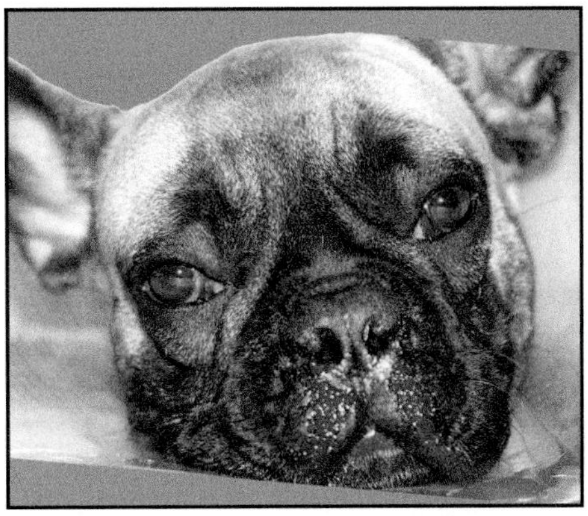

26.5 Epistaxis, as observed in this dog with primary IMTP, is a relatively common manifestation of severe thrombocytopenia.

Less commonly, bleeding can occur into body cavities, resulting in haemarthrosis, central nervous system signs (Figure 26.6) and dyspnoea. Rarely, fever, splenomegaly and lymphadenomegaly can be observed (Wilkins *et al.*, 1973; Williams and Maggio-Price, 1984; Putsche and Kohn, 2008). The presence of haemoptysis has been associated with a poor outcome in dogs and cats (Bianco *et al.*, 2008).

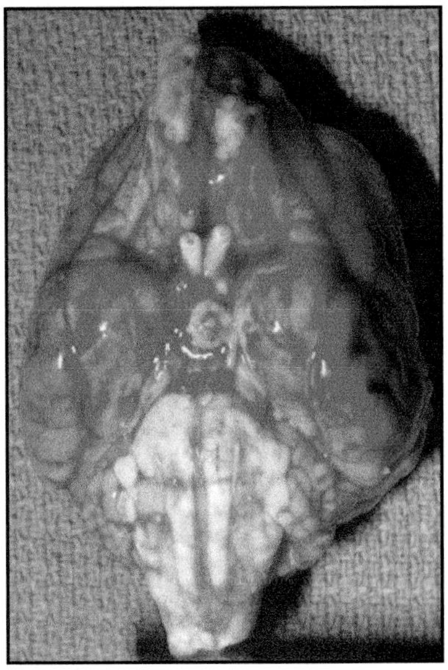

26.6 The brain of a dog with primary IMTP that died of intracranial haemorrhage.

Cats with IMTP have clinical bleeding less commonly. This may be because cats have a very efficient haemostatic system, and seem to tolerate lower numbers of platelets better than dogs (Wondratschek *et al.*, 2008). Cats with clinical bleeding present most often with spontaneous surface bleeding or haematomas (Figure 26.7).

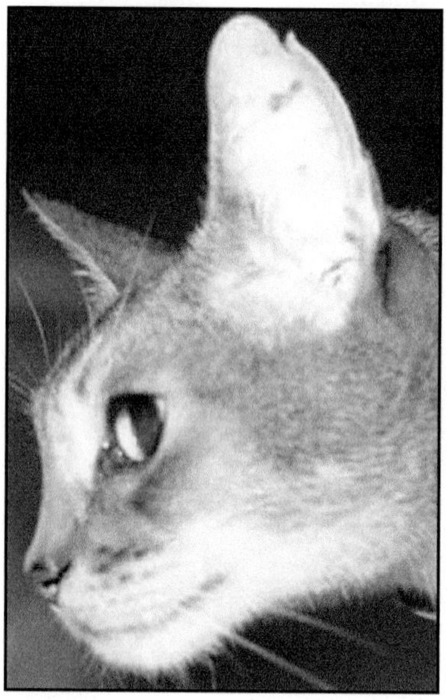

26.7 Clinical bleeding is less commonly observed in thrombocytopenic cats compared with dogs. Petechiation of the pinna of a cat with primary IMTP.

Laboratory results in IMTP

Historically, the diagnosis of IMTP has been based on the following criteria (Lewis and Meyers, 1996b):

- Severity of thrombocytopenia
- Microthrombocytosis or platelet fragmentation
- Normal to increased megakaryocytes in the bone marrow
- Detection of platelet-bound antibodies
- Increased platelet counts following immunosuppressive glucocorticoid therapy
- Exclusion of other aetiologies for thrombocytopenia.

Platelet enumeration

Thrombocytopenia detected on a complete blood count (CBC) must be confirmed by a manual platelet count in order to rule out pseudothrombocytopenia. Common causes for pseudothrombocytopenia include the use of automated haematology analysers, traumatic venepuncture, platelet activation or platelet clumping. Blood smear examination allows the evaluation of an estimated platelet count, platelet size and structure (Figure 26.8). Platelet clumps often form at the feathered edge, and can lower the total platelet count significantly. The platelet count can be estimated by multiplying the mean number of platelets per high power (×100 oil immersion) field in 10 fields by 15×10^9/l. The presence of 10–12 platelets per high power field generally indicates an adequate platelet count. Most dogs with IMTP will

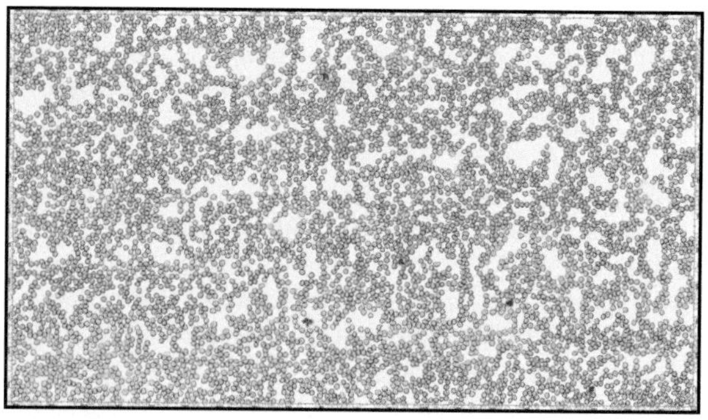

26.8 A blood smear from a severely thrombocytopenic patient with a manual platelet count of 2×10^9/l. Note the complete lack of platelets on this blood smear (x100 objective).

have severe thrombocytopenia, with platelet counts often below 30×10^9/l, and dogs with primary IMTP tend to have lower platelet counts than dogs with secondary IMTP or thrombocytopenia due to non-immune causes (Grindem *et al.,* 1991). The same is not true in cats with IMTP, with no significant difference in platelet count between cats with primary IMTP and cats with thrombocytopenia associated with other aetiologies (Jordan *et al.*, 1993).

Platelet indices

Variable platelet volume (MPV) and platelet distribution width (PDW) can be observed in patients with IMTP. These platelet indices have an inverse relationship with platelet count, and thus thrombocytopenic patients may have increased MPV and PDW values, associated with a regenerative response in the bone marrow. However, this is not a specific finding for IMTP, and these platelet indices are unlikely to aid in determining the underlying cause of thrombocytopenia. In addition, some studies have suggested that primary IMTP is more commonly associated with normal to decreased MPV values, particularly early in the course of disease, as a result of immune-mediated platelet injury. The presence of reticulated platelets (immature platelets with increased RNA content that stains with thiazole orange) indicates ongoing platelet production, and thus IMTP patients may have increased reticulated platelet counts. However, the absence of reticulated platelets does not necessarily indicate megakaryocytic hypoplasia.

Other CBC abnormalities

The remainder of the CBC may be normal, or may reveal additional abnormalities. Dogs with IMTP are not uncommonly anaemic (57% of dogs in one study; Putsche and Kohn, 2008), and may have a leucocytosis (40% of dogs in one study; Putsche and Kohn, 2008). Anaemia can occur as a result of bleeding or concurrent IMHA. The coagulation profile should be normal, unless the patient has disseminated intravascular coagulation (DIC). In cats with IMTP, a neutrophil–platelet association has been observed on peripheral blood smears. In these patients, neutrophils appear to contain or have platelets adhering to their membranes. In addition, bone marrow cytology in some cats has revealed neutrophil–megakaryocyte associations and emperipolesis, or the non-phagocytic engulfment of neutrophils by megakaryocytes (Bianco *et al.,* 2008).

Bone marrow evaluation

Bone marrow aspiration cytology has been considered to be equivocal in the diagnosis of canine IMTP. Recent evidence suggests that bone marrow cytology may be of limited diagnostic value in the majority of cases of primary IMTP (Miller and Lunn, 2007).

In human medicine, it is believed that the evaluation of bone marrow cytology in patients with IMTP is often of little diagnostic value. The American Society of Hematology currently does not recommend the evaluation of bone marrow cytology in adults under 60 years old who have a presentation typical for IMTP. Bone marrow evaluation tends to be reserved for older patients, those with atypical features or additional cytopenias, or those who do not respond appropriately to therapy.

In animals, it has been shown that bone marrow cytology is of limited utility because non-megakaryocytic bone marrow disease leading to severe thrombocytopenia is unlikely in the absence of other peripheral cytopenias (Miller and Lunn, 2007). Given that the majority of patients with IMTP have thrombocytopenia that is considered to be severe, it can be postulated that bone marrow cytology is likely to be of little diagnostic value in the majority of patients with primary IMTP. However, in animals that do exhibit other cytopenias, or that are refractory to therapy, bone marrow evaluation may be warranted. The presence of two or three megakaryocytes in a large bone marrow spicule is usually considered adequate. A healthy bone marrow will respond to immune-mediated platelet destruction by increasing megakaryocyte number; thus, most patients with primary IMTP will have normal to increased numbers of megakaryocytes on bone marrow cytology (Figure 26.9). Thrombocytopenia is not considered a contraindication to performing bone marrow aspiration or even core biopsy, because significant bleeding is rare, and can generally be controlled with local pressure. Patients with AATP have significantly decreased numbers of megakaryocytes in the bone marrow (Figure 26.10), and may have anti-platelet antibodies detected by flow cytometry (Lachowitz *et al.*, 2004).

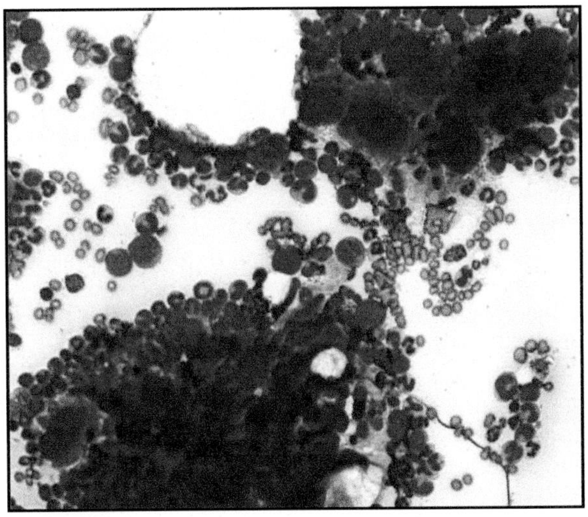

26.9 Bone marrow cytology from a patient with primary IMTP revealing megakaryocytic hyperplasia, which is an appropriate marrow response to peripheral thrombocytopenia (x100 objective).

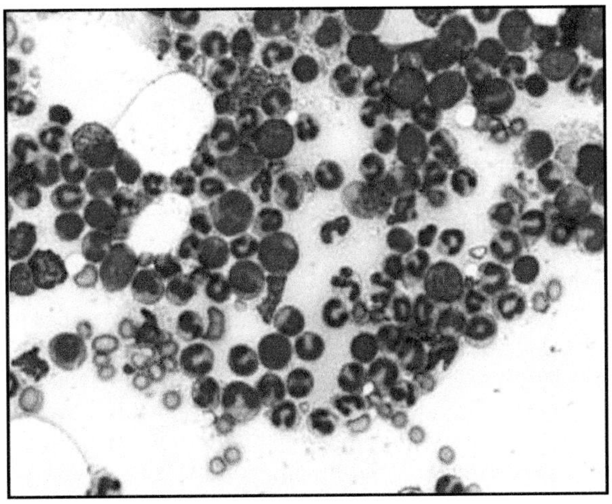

26.10 Bone marrow cytology from a patient with acquired amegakaryocytic thrombocytopenia. Note the lack of megakaryocytes in this patient's bone marrow (x100 objective).

Platelet antibody testing

Confirming a suspected case of primary IMTP can be difficult, because at this time reliable direct platelet-bound antibody testing is only performed in specialist laboratories. As a result, the diagnosis is often made after ruling out causes of secondary IMTP, and a positive response to immunosuppressive therapy.

The platelet factor 3 (PF3) test establishes the presence of antibodies directed against the platelet membrane. This is an indirect functional assay, because immune-mediated platelet injury (via anti-platelet antibodies) results in the release of PF3. This test has a low sensitivity of 28%, and is no longer conducted by most laboratories.

Multiple tests utilizing enzyme-linked immunosorbent assay (ELISA) or flow cytometry exist for measuring platelet-bound antibodies, however these tests show marked variability in sensitivity and specificity. Platelet surface-associated antibodies can be measured directly, or indirectly by measuring circulating platelet bindable antibodies in serum. The direct assay has greater sensitivity (94%) than the indirect assay (34%) (Lewis *et al.*, 1995). The likely reason for this discrepancy is that most anti-platelet antibodies exist bound to platelets and not free in circulation. Neither test is highly specific, because the platelet bound or platelet bindable antibody may consist of autoantibodies (as is the case in primary IMTP) or could be immune complexes or antibodies associated with foreign antigens that are adsorbed to the platelet surface. As a result of this, positive results can be observed with both primary IMTP and conditions that induce thrombocytopenia by secondary IMTP (see Figure 26.1) (Grindem *et al.*, 1991; Kristensen *et al.*, 1994; Lewis *et al.*, 1995). The direct assay offers the advantage of significantly improved sensitivity, and is preferred over the indirect assay. Both of these assays may become negative following the institution of therapy. Platelet-bound antibody tests have also been used to diagnose primary and secondary IMTP in cats (Kohn *et al.*, 2006; Wondratschek *et al.*, 2010).

Antibodies against megakaryocytes can be measured using immunofluorescence applied to bone marrow cytology (megakaryocyte immunofluorescence assay). Direct immunofluorescence of megakaryocytes has been used in the diagnosis of primary IMTP in a cat.

False positive results for all of these diagnostic tests can be seen as a result of technical error or cross-reactivity of other serum antibodies with platelets, and false negative results can be observed with technical error, excessive *in vivo* serum antibody binding to platelets, insufficient platelet number (for direct assays), or lack of serum antibody binding to heterologous platelets (for indirect assays). In addition, all of these assays are unable to differentiate primary from secondary IMTP, and are only offered by selected laboratories.

Thromboelastography

Thromboelastography (TEG), a diagnostic modality that assesses global haemostasis, is being used with greater frequency for the evaluation of patients with suspected hypercoagulability or coagulopathy. Severe thrombocytopenia will affect the TEG tracing by decreasing clot strength and rigidity. As a result, patients with very low platelet counts may have decreased maximum amplitude (MA) and G values (Figure 26.11).

Management of IMTP

General care

Severely thrombocytopenic patients must be handled carefully so as not to induce any bleeding. Jugular venepuncture, either for a blood sample or catheterization, should be avoided, and direct pressure should be applied to any venepuncture or injection sites to ensure adequate haemostasis. Medications should be given intravenously or orally, eliminating the potential for bleeding from subcutaneous or intramuscular injections. These patients should be strictly cage rested, so as to minimize the risk of injury and haemorrhage. Visible evidence of bleeding (petechiae, ecchymoses) should be monitored frequently to assess for progression or the development of new lesions.

Medication

While new therapies are being used more frequently in the treatment of IMTP, the mainstay of treatment in these patients is the administration of glucocorticoids.

Glucocorticoids

Studies with indium-labelled platelets suggest that the mechanisms of action of prednisolone may include increased effective platelet production, impaired megakaryocyte–antibody binding, and interference with the immediate reticuloendothelial macrophage removal of platelets from the bone marrow. Additional benefits of glucocorticoids may include splenic contraction, which releases platelets into circulation, and the stabilization of vascular membranes, thereby decreasing excessive platelet consumption. Glucocorticoids are desirable because they have a rapid onset of action. Glucocorticoid therapy is generally started with prednisolone at 2 or 4 mg/kg orally q24h for dogs and cats, respectively, or dexamethasone at 0.2 mg/kg i.v. q24h for dogs

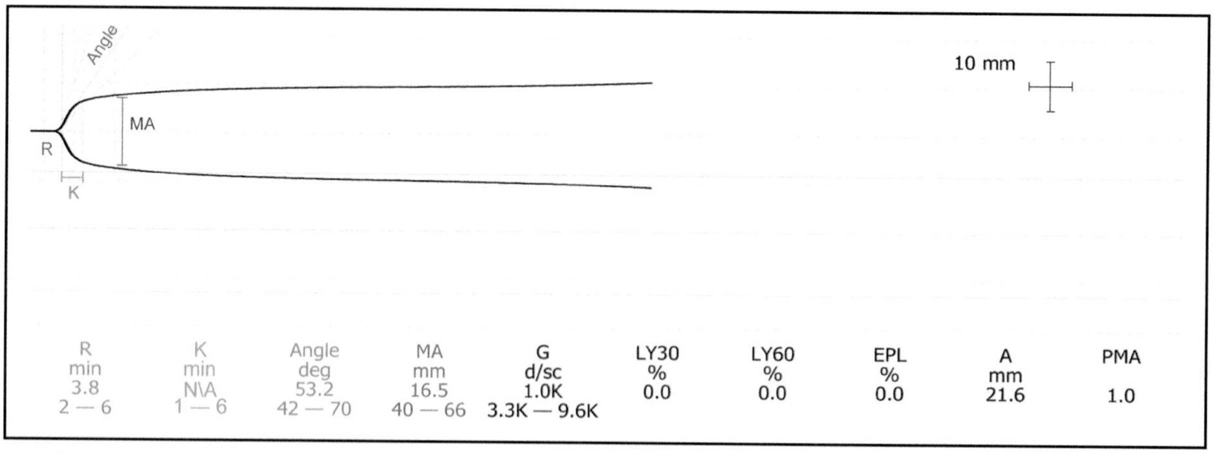

26.11 Thromboelastography (TEG) tracing from a severely thrombocytopenic patient with primary immune-mediated thrombocytopenia. R is the reaction time (evaluates the intrinsic pathway); K is the clot formation time (measures the rapidity of clot development); Angle indicates the rate of clot formation; MA is the maximum amplitude (reflects final clot strength); G is a calculation that takes into account the MA, and reflects the overall coagulant state as normo-, hyper- or hypocoagulant. ($G = 5000 \times MA / (100 - MA)$). Normal reference intervals are listed below each value. In this patient, the MA is significantly decreased as a result of thrombocytopenia, which would yield decreased clot strength. The 10 mm scale bar shows the exact measurements of the tracing (in case the image is magnified or made smaller on reproduction).

and 0.2–1 mg/kg for cats. Patients are generally maintained on an oral dose of prednisolone that is slowly tapered to the minimum effective dose based on platelet count and clinical signs. Pulsed high dose dexamethasone therapy has been evaluated in humans with chronic IMTP. The results, however, have been inconsistent, with some patients achieving full remission while others have shown a poor response. Some cats with primary IMTP that have been refractory to oral prednisolone therapy have responded to oral or intravenous dexamethasone therapy (Bianco *et al.*, 2008).

Additional therapies

The lack of prospective randomized controlled clinical trials evaluating therapies in the treatment of IMTP, combined with the fairly reliable response to glucocorticoids, make the use of additional agents a matter of clinician preference.

Many clinicians use additional therapies such as long-term steroid-sparing agents, or rescue therapies in cases of acute, severe IMTP. Adjunctive immunosuppressive therapies that have been used in canine patients with primary IMTP include cyclophosphamide (50 mg/m^2 orally q24h for 4 days/week), ciclosporin (5–15 mg/kg orally q12–24h), azathioprine (2 mg/kg orally q24–48h) and leflunomide (2–4 mg/kg orally q 24h). Ciclosporin (5–7.5 mg/kg orally q12h) and chlorambucil (2 mg/m^2 orally q24–48h) may be effective in the treatment of IMTP in cats.

Human intravenous immunoglobulin (IVIG) has been evaluated in the treatment of acute IMTP in dogs. The mechanism of action of IVIG involves the blockade of Fc receptors on mononuclear phagocytic cells, thereby decreasing platelet clearance. A prospective controlled study revealed a significant reduction in platelet count recovery time and duration of hospitalization in dogs with acute IMTP that received IVIG in addition to prednisolone when compared with those that received prednisolone alone (Bianco *et al.*, 2009). IVIG is likely only to be helpful in the acute management of IMTP, because its half-life in healthy dogs is only 7–9 days. Adverse reactions to the administration of a single dose of IVIG are rare. They are reported to occur in fewer than 5% of human patients who receive transfusions, and in the veterinary literature only one dog has been reported to vomit during an IVIG transfusion. However, because IVIG is derived from human plasma, there is a risk of inciting an allergic reaction or immune complex formation with subsequent IVIG transfusions. The recommended dose is 0.5–1.5 g/kg. While the main drawback to IVIG therapy is cost, it has been proposed that the cost of this product may be offset by a shorter hospitalization period and fewer blood product transfusions.

Vincristine can also be used in the treatment of acute IMTP. The exact mechanism by which vincristine increases platelet count is unknown, however proposed mechanisms include accelerated platelet production via megakaryocyte fragmentation and impaired platelet destruction. A prospective study revealed a more rapid increase in platelet count and shorter hospitalization period in dogs with IMTP that received vincristine and prednisone when compared with dogs that received prednisolone alone (Rozanski *et al.*, 2002). It has been suggested that vincristine may affect platelet function adversely; however, clinical studies of dogs with IMTP that received vincristine have not supported this (Rozanski *et al.*, 2002). The recommended dose for dogs with IMTP is 0.02 mg/kg i.v., and this dose seems to be well tolerated. To the authors' knowledge, the use of vincristine has not been evaluated in cats with IMTP. Danazol (5 mg/kg orally q12h), a synthetic analogue of androgenic steroids and progesterone, has been used successfully in the treatment of canine IMTP, but is not widely applied for this purpose. Danazol has been helpful in isolated cases of IMTP, and its use may be considered if other therapies have failed.

Response to therapy

Platelet counts reach normal levels within 3–7 days of starting treatment in most dogs that respond to therapy. If no response to therapy is noted in this time span, the addition of another agent should be considered. The complications of long-term immunosuppressive therapy can be significant, and secondary infections, which can be fatal, have been reported in immunosuppressed IMTP patients. Additional potential complications include gastrointestinal ulceration, polyuria/polydipsia and panting in dogs, and diabetes mellitus in cats.

Splenectomy

Splenectomy is performed in humans with chronic IMTP. Most studies reveal a complete response in more than 50% of patients with chronic IMTP. Mortality from splenectomy tends to be low in humans with IMTP who are young and otherwise healthy, with most patients, surprisingly, not requiring transfusion pre- or postoperatively. While the veterinary literature regarding splenectomy for the treatment of IMTP is sparse, it may potentially be a valuable treatment option for these patients (Jans *et al.*, 1990). Although it can be difficult to determine which canine patients with IMTP may respond favourably to splenectomy, human studies have shown that a positive response to IVIG is a sensitive and specific predictor of response to splenectomy.

Treatment of infection-induced secondary IMTP

The predominant treatment for infection-induced secondary IMTP includes proper antimicrobial therapy, and in most cases doxycycline should be instituted empirically while infectious disease tests are pending. Immunosuppression may be necessary in some cases to halt antibody-mediated platelet destruction, and should be considered in patients with moderate to severe bleeding (Breitschwerdt, 1988). Immunosuppressive therapy can play a valuable role in the initial stabilization of a critically thrombocytopenic patient, and can allow time for pathogen-specific drug therapy to take effect, and for the results of infectious disease testing to be received. Immunosuppressive therapy, however, should only be used for as long as it is deemed necessary, while antimicrobials are continued for the longer term (Breitschwerdt, 1988).

Treatment of drug-induced secondary IMTP

The treatment for drug-induced secondary IMTP includes immediate withdrawal of the drug and transfusions of platelet products if a patient is symptomatic as a result of thrombocytopenia. Human patients with drug-induced secondary IMTP are often treated with glucocorticoids; however, there is no definitive evidence that this is beneficial. Once a patient is sensitized to a drug, it is likely that the sensitization is permanent, so patients should avoid such medications indefinitely. Pharmacological equivalents that have different chemical structures can be substituted.

Treatment for AATP consists of immunosuppressive therapies if the disease is idiopathic, and antimicrobials if secondary to an infectious process.

Supportive therapies

Transfusion of platelet-containing products (e.g. fresh whole blood, platelet-rich plasma, platelet concentrate) is rarely indicated in patients with IMTP, because the transfused platelets are destroyed within minutes to hours of being infused. However, they can be useful in helping to control or prevent life-threatening bleeding, such as intracranial bleeding, in the acute period until other therapies have taken effect. It is not uncommon for severely affected patients to become anaemic as a result of bleeding. Fresh whole blood (blood that has been collected and transfused within 8 hours) has the benefit of providing both red blood cells and platelets. Alternatively, Oxyglobin can increase oxygen-carrying capacity effectively in patients that are anaemic secondary to IMTP-induced bleeding (see Chapter 36).

Many patients with IMTP will suffer from gastrointestinal bleeding, most commonly as a result of their thrombocytopenia, however glucocorticoid-induced ulceration can also occur. H2 receptor antagonists or proton pump inhibitors with sucralfate should be used in these patients.

Prognosis

The prognosis for canine patients with primary IMTP is considered guarded to good, with mortality rates ranging from 3 to 30% (Jans *et al.*, 1990; Putsche and Kohn, 2008). While there are fewer studies on cats with primary IMTP, the published mortality rates are 20–25% (Bianco *et al.*, 2008; Wondratschek *et al.*, 2010). Death during the initial episode or relapses usually results from uncontrollable haemorrhage. Relapse rates in dogs range from 26 to 47% (Williams and Maggio-Price, 1984; Jans *et al.*, 1990; Putsche and Kohn, 2008). No specific factors observed during the initial management of IMTP have been correlated with the likelihood of relapse (Jans *et al.*, 1990). The prognosis for primary AATP is poor; however, it can be good for AATP secondary to infection in patients who respond to antibiotics (Williams and Maggio-Price, 1984; Lachowitz *et al.*, 2004).

References and further reading

Aster RH and Bougie DW (2007) Drug-induced immune thrombocytopenia. *New England Journal of Medicine* **357**, 580–587

Bianco D, Armstrong PJ and Washabau RJ (2008) Presumed primary immune-mediated thrombocytopenia in four cats. *Journal of Feline Medicine and Surgery* **10**, 495–500

Bianco D, Armstrong PJ and Washabau RJ (2009) A prospective, randomized, double-blinded, placebo-controlled study of human intravenous immunoglobulin for the acute management of presumptive primary immune-mediated thrombocytopenia in dogs. *Journal of Veterinary Internal Medicine* **23**, 1071–1078

Botsch V, Kuchenhoff H, Hartmann K *et al.* (2009) Retrospective study of 871 dogs with thrombocytopenia. *Veterinary Record* **164**, 647–651

Breitschwerdt EB (1988) Infectious thrombocytopenia in dogs. *Compendium on Continuing Education for the Practicing Veterinarian* **10**, 1177–1186

Grindem CB, Breitschwerdt EB, Corbett WT *et al.* (1991) Epidemiologic survey of thrombocytopenia in dogs: a report on 987 cases. *Veterinary Clinical Pathology* **20**, 38–43

Grindem CB, Breitschwerdt EB, Corbett WT *et al.* (1994) Thrombocytopenia associated with neoplasia in dogs. *Journal of Veterinary Internal Medicine* **8**, 400–405

Jackson ML and Kruth SA (1985) Immune-mediated hemolytic anemia and thrombocytopenia in the dog: a retrospective study of 55 cases diagnosed in 1969 through 1983 at the Western College of Veterinary Medicine. *Canadian Veterinary Journal* **26**, 245–250

Jans HE, Armstrong PJ and Price GS (1990) Therapy of immune mediated thrombocytopenia: a retrospective study of 15 dogs. *Journal of Veterinary Internal Medicine* **4**, 4–7

Jordan HL, Grindem CB and Breitschwerdt EB (1993) Thrombocytopenia in cats: a retrospective study of 41 cases. *Journal of Veterinary Internal Medicine* **7**, 261–265

Kajihara M, Kato S, Okazaki Y *et al.* (2003) The role of autoantibody-mediated platelet destruction in thrombocytopenia in patients with cirrhosis. *Hepatology* **37**, 1267–1276

Kohn B, Linden T and Leibold W (2006) Platelet-bound antibodies detected by a flow cytometric assay in cats with thrombocytopenia. *Journal of Feline Medicine and Surgery* **8**, 254–260

Kristensen AT, Weiss DJ, Klausner JS *et al.* (1994) Detection of antiplatelet antibody with a platelet immunofluorescence assay. *Journal of Veterinary Internal Medicine* **8**, 36–39

Lachowitz JL, Post GS, Moroff SF *et al.* (2004) Acquired amegakaryocytic thrombocytopenia – four cases and a literature review. *Journal of Small Animal Practice* **45**, 507–514

Lewis DC and Meyers KM (1996a) Studies of platelet bound and serum bindable immunoglobulins in dogs with idiopathic thrombocytopenic purpura. *Experimental Hematology* **24**, 696–701

Lewis DC and Meyers KM (1996b) Canine idiopathic thrombocytopenic purpura. *Journal of Veterinary Internal Medicine* **10**, 207–218

Lewis DC, Meyers KM, Callan B *et al.* (1995) Detection of platelet-bound and serum platelet-bindable antibodies for diagnosis of idiopathic thrombocytopenic purpura in dogs. *Journal of the American Veterinary Medical Association* **206**, 47–51

Miller MD and Lunn KF (2007) Diagnostic use of cytologic examination of bone marrow from dogs with thrombocytopenia: 58 cases (1994–2004). *Journal of the American Veterinary Medical Association* **231**, 1540–1544

Putsche JC and Kohn B (2008) Primary immune-mediated thrombocytopenia in 30 dogs (1997–2003). *Journal of the American Animal Hospital Association* **44**, 250–257

Rozanski EA, Callan MB, Hughes D *et al.* (2002) Comparison of platelet count recovery with use of vincristine and prednisone or prednisone alone for treatment for severe immune-mediated thrombocytopenia in dogs. *Journal of the American Veterinary Medical Association* **220**, 447–481

Thomas KJ and Feldman BF (1985) Immune-mediated thrombocytopenia: diagnosis and treatment. *Compendium on Continuing Education for the Practicing Veterinarian* **7**, 569–576

Thomas JS (2010) Non-immune-mediated thrombocytopenia. In: *Schalm's Veterinary Hematology, 6th edn,* ed. DJ Weiss and J Wardrop, pp.597–603. Wiley Blackwell Publishing, Iowa

Turner CP and Hadley AG (2003) The role of p-selectin in the immune

destruction of platelets. *British Journal of Haematology* **121**, 623–631
Wilkins RJ, Hurvitz AI and Dodds-Laffin WJ (1973) Immunologically mediated thrombocytopenia in the dog. *Journal of the American Veterinary Medical Association* **163**, 277–282
Williams DA and Maggio-Price L (1984) Canine idiopathic thrombocytopenia: clinical observations and long-term follow-up in 54 cases. *Journal of the American Veterinary Medical Association* **185**, 660–662
Wondratschek C, Weingart C and Kohn B (2010) Primary immune-mediated thrombocytopenia in cats. *Journal of the American Animal Hospital Association* **46**, 12–19

27

von Willebrand's disease

Tracy Stokol

Introduction

von Willebrand's disease (vWD) is caused by a deficiency of, or abnormality in, a large plasma glycoprotein called von Willebrand factor (vWf). It is the most common inherited disorder of haemostasis in dogs, but has been diagnosed only rarely in cats. vWD has been detected in over 50 breeds of dog, with a high prevalence in Dobermanns, Pembroke Welsh Corgis, Manchester Terriers, Shetland Sheepdogs and Scottish Terriers. Some of these animals display excessive haemorrhage attributable to vWD. Knowledge of the pathogenesis, diagnosis and treatment of vWD is therefore essential for practitioners.

Structure and function of von Willebrand factor

In humans, vWf is produced by endothelial cells and megakaryocytes. These cells store vWf in specific organelles called Weibel–Palade bodies (endothelial cells) or α-granules (megakaryocytes). These organelles release vWf in response to endothelial damage and various agonists, including thrombin and histamine. Plasma levels of vWf are maintained by constitutive secretion of vWf from endothelial cells. These cells also secrete vWf directly into the subendothelial matrix, where it binds to matrix components such as type VI collagen and elastin-associated microfibrils. In plasma, vWf circulates in a non-covalently bound complex with coagulation factor VIII (FVIII). Because these two proteins are found as a complex, vWf was formerly called FVIII-related antigen, but this term is misleading and now obsolete. In dogs, vWf is produced by endothelial cells, with a negligible amount detectable in platelets (in contrast to human platelets).

vWf is composed of a series of protein polymers called multimers, which consist of repeating subunits linked by disulphide bonds. Each subunit contains separate binding sites for platelet glycoprotein receptors, CD42 (GPIb) and CD41/CD61 (GPIIb-IIIa or $\alpha_{IIb}\beta_3$), and subendothelial matrix components (e.g. collagen). The number of subunits in each multimer varies, imparting a range of molecular weights (from 0.5–20 million Daltons) to the multimers. The multimeric structure is important because higher molecular weight multimers, owing to their large size and multiple binding sites, are the most effective in haemostasis.

vWf is essential in primary haemostasis where it functions primarily as a glue, permitting adhesion of circulating platelets (via CD42 or GPIb) to exposed collagen in the subendothelial matrix under high shear forces (Figure 27.1; also see Chapter 21). vWf also has minor roles in platelet aggregation (bridging adjacent platelets via the integrin CD41/CD61) and fibrin incorporation into the platelet plug (via CD42).

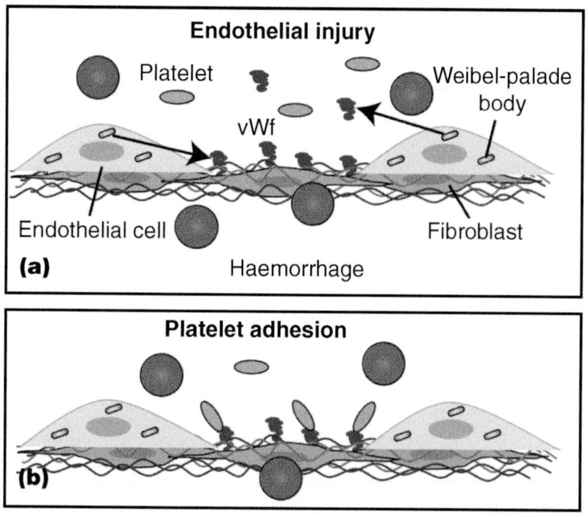

27.1 The role of von Willebrand factor (vWf) in primary haemostasis. Platelet adhesion is the initiating event in primary haemostasis and is mediated by vWf in blood vessels with high shear rates. **(a)** Vessel injury exposes vWf that is prebound to subendothelial matrix proteins (collagen, fibronectin and vitronectin) and induces secretion of vWf from stores within Weibel–Palade bodies of endothelial cells. Stored vWf consists mostly of the more active high molecular weight multimers and is secreted preferentially into the subendothelial matrix. Plasma vWf also binds to subendothelial matrix proteins upon vessel injury. **(b)** Platelets adhere to the vessel wall through vWf, which acts as a bridge between the platelet glycoprotein receptor complex, GP1b-V-IX (not shown), and exposed subendothelial matrix protein components. GPIb-V-IX does not require prior activation before engaging vWf. Once bound, platelets become activated, change shape and release platelet agonists (e.g. adenosine diphosphate (ADP), thromboxane A_2), which serve to recruit and activate new platelets to the injured site. Recruited platelets form aggregates via binding of fibrinogen to the $\alpha_{IIb}\beta_3$ integrin receptor (CD41/61) on adjacent platelets, which then forms a primary platelet plug (not shown) (see Chapter 21).

Any quantitative or qualitative abnormality in vWf thus causes inadequate platelet plug formation, resulting in excessive haemorrhage from injured vessels.

Disease mechanism and classification

vWD is an inherited disorder that is classified into three different types based on vWf concentration and multimeric structure (Figures 27.2 and 27.3). The disease is inherited as an autosomal trait and is probably recessive in dogs with types I and III vWD. However, the inheritance pattern is still under dispute (i.e. inheritance may be dominant with incomplete penetrance in some dog breeds with type I vWD) or unknown (type II vWD). Several breed-specific point mutations or deletions in the vWD gene have been identified in dogs. A point mutation at a splice site in intron 16 generates a premature stop codon, with no protein production, in Dutch Kooiker dogs with type III vWD (Rieger *et al.*, 1998). A single nucleotide mutation in exon 28 was identified (but not proven to be causative) in German Shorthaired Pointers with type II vWD (Kramer *et al.* 2004). A single base deletion in exon 4 causes a frameshift mutation and a *de novo* stop codon, resulting in a severely truncated protein (and no protein production) in Scottish Terriers with type III vWD (Venta *et al.*, 2000). Acquired forms of vWD are rarely recognized in dogs. There is no definitive proof of a causal association between hypothyroidism and acquired vWD in dogs (Panciera and Johnson, 1994, 1996; Heseltine *et al.*, 2005). Abnormal vWf with decreased amounts of high molecular weight multimers (similar to inherited type II vWD) has been identified in dogs with mitral valve insufficiency (Tarnow *et al.*, 2005). The cause of the altered multimeric composition of vWf in these dogs is unknown. It may be due to increased proteolysis from high shear forces generated by valvular dysfunction, which activates the enzyme (ADAMTS-13) that normally degrades the higher molecular weight multimers of vWf. Affected dogs do have abnormal platelet function but do not appear to bleed excessively, thus the clinical consequence of this vWf abnormality is unknown.

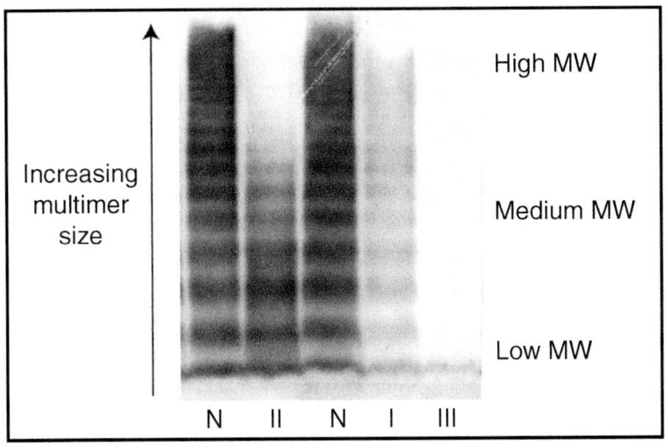

27.2 Multimeric structure of von Willebrand factor (vWf). The classification of von Willebrand's disease (vWD) into three types is based on the multimeric composition of the protein as determined by sodium dodecyl-sulphate agarose gel electrophoresis. This technique separates out the multimers on the basis of size (molecular weight MW). Dogs with type I vWD have a quantitative defect in vWf but multimeric composition is normal. Dogs with type II vWD have a quantitative defect in vWf and are lacking the high molecular weight multimers. Dogs with type III vWD have an absolute deficiency of vWf. N indicates that the sample comes from a normal dog.

Clinical signs

vWD manifests with clinical signs typical of a primary haemostatic disorder (see Chapter 21), i.e. excessive bleeding from mucosal surfaces that are rich in fibrinolysins, including gingival haemorrhage, epistaxis, melaena, haematuria and uterine haemorrhage. Excessive haemorrhage after surgery or

	Breeds [a]	vWf:Ag	Multimeric structure	Genetic defect	Clinical signs
Type I	Dobermann (85%), Pembroke Welsh Corgi (43%), Manchester Terrier (41%), Bernese Mountain Dog (17%), Poodle (10%), and others	<50%	Normal	Intron splice site (www.vetgen.com)	Variable, depends on vWf:Ag and other unknown factors Dogs with vWf:Ag < 25–40% are 'at risk' of bleeding
Type II	German Shorthaired and Wirehaired Pointers, Deutsch Drahthaar	<50% Usually <15%	Abnormal: Decreased large MW multimers	Point mutation in exon 28? (German Shorthaired Pointer)	Severe
Type III	Scottish Terrier (10%), Shetland Sheepdog (10%), Dutch Kooiker dog and others	<1% in affected <50% in carriers	NA: Little to no protein present in plasma or endothelial cells of affected dogs	Deletion in exon 4 (Scottish Terrier) Intron 16 splice site (Dutch Kooiker)	Severe only in homozygotes. Heterozygotes are asymptomatic or mildly symptomatic (Shetland Sheepdog) carriers

27.3 Types of inherited von Willebrand's disease in dogs, classified on the basis of the concentration and multimeric structure of von Willebrand factor antigen (vWf:Ag). MW, Molecular weight; NA, Not applicable. [a] Percentages in parentheses indicate reported prevalence rates (heterozygous carriers and homozygotes, as per www.vetgen.com, 2010)

trauma (including clipping of claws) is often the first presenting sign in dogs (Figure 27.4). Petechiae, however, are observed infrequently in dogs with vWD (in contrast to those with thrombocytopenia), which may be a useful diagnostic clue when trying to differentiate clinically between primary haemostatic disorders. Other signs that have been attributed to vWD include lameness, intracranial haemorrhage and poor wound healing. The disease can be diagnosed at any age, but is typically detected in young dogs, especially in countries where early neutering is practised and in breeds subjected to cosmetic surgery at a young age. Given that vWD is inherited as an autosomal trait, males and females are affected equally.

The clinical expression of vWD is variable, with many affected dogs not showing any evidence of excessive bleeding. Excessive bleeding is difficult to document and quite subjective. Clinical assessment of haemorrhage may be improved through application of a scoring system (Burgess *et al.*, 2009a). A study was performed in a large group of dogs with and without vWD and it was demonstrated that the bleeding score (based on a defined questionnaire) was not predictive of vWD status. Despite this, there is a documented association between the clinical expression and the concentration of vWf or type of vWD (Figure 27.5), with the likelihood of haemorrhage being higher with lower vWf concentrations. In contrast, the genetic defect or status (heterozygous or homozygous) has not been linked conclusively to disease expression. The critical threshold of vWf:Ag (i.e. the concentration below which a dog is considered 'at risk' of haemorrhage) varies from 25–40% in dogs with type I vWD, although not all dogs with concentrations below this threshold will bleed excessively. This indicates that other variables affect the clinical manifestation of vWD, however these factors remain largely unknown. Furthermore, some dogs may haemorrhage despite vWf concentrations above this threshold. It is arguable whether this haemorrhage can be truly attributed to vWD and, in many cases, affected animals have concurrent thrombocytopenia or underlying disease, or drug therapy that may affect platelet function (see Chapter 24). An absolute deficiency (type III vWD) or abnormal multimeric structure (type II vWD, which is combined with low vWf:Ag concentrations) of vWf

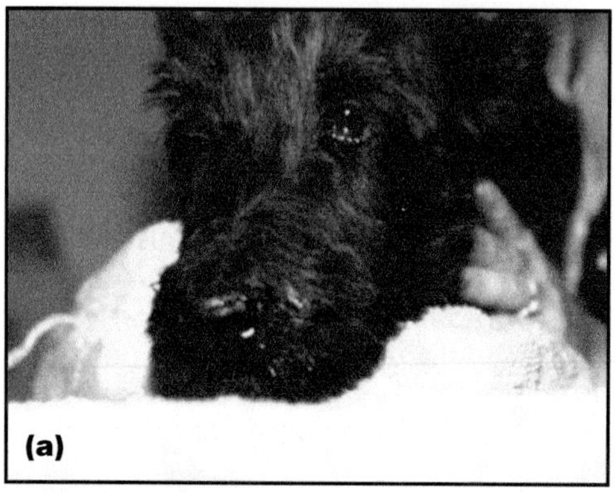

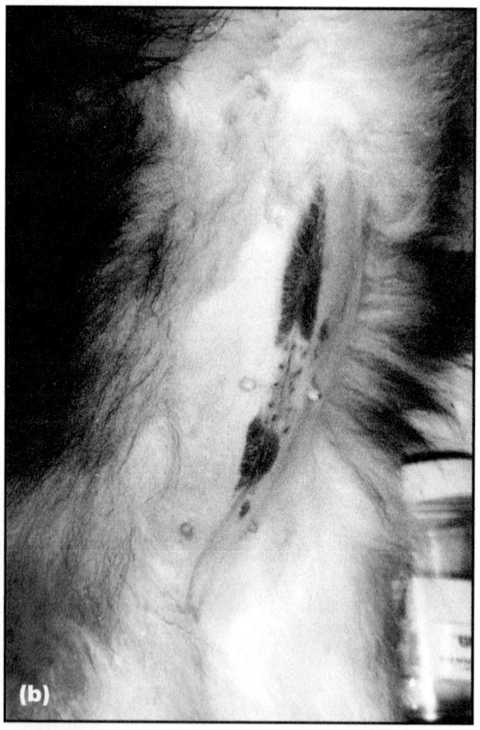

27.4 Clinical signs associated with von Willebrand's disease (vWD). **(a)** Spontaneous epistaxis in a Scottish Terrier with severe type III vWD (< 1% vWf:Ag). **(b)** Post-surgical bruising around the suture line in a Shetland Sheepdog with type III vWD. (Courtesy of Dr Marjory Brooks, Comparative Coagulation Laboratory, Cornell University)

Assay	Anticipated results in von Willebrand's disease	Notes
Screening tests for primary haemostasis		
In vivo: Buccal mucosal bleeding time	> 4 minutes	Use with caution in dogs with suspected type II or III vWD. Affected dogs may have infinite bleeding times, suffer from rebleeding, and induced bleeding may be difficult to control. Direct measurement of vWf:Ag preferred
In vitro: PFA-100: ADP closure time	> 2 minutes	
Diagnostic tests for vWD		
ELISA for vWf:Ag concentration	< 50%	Available from Animal Health Trust or Animal Health Diagnostic Center, Cornell University
Genetic mutation	Present	Available at VetGen LLC, Animal Health Trust or Laboklin
Collagen binding assay	< 60%	Available at Animal Health Diagnostic Center, Cornell University

27.5 Available tests for von Willebrand's disease (vWD). The screening tests are neither sensitive nor specific for vWD; thus, abnormal results do not always indicate underlying vWD (see Chapter 21).

causes severe haemorrhage in affected dogs. Given that acquired diseases or drugs may precipitate or worsen haemorrhage in any dog with vWD, bleeding does not always manifest at a young age.

Diagnostic tests

Various tests are available to facilitate diagnosis of vWD. These include general tests of primary haemostasis, which are useful as screening tests for vWD, and specific tests for vWD diagnosis (i.e. vWf:Ag concentrations or genetic analysis; Figure 27.5). Only some of these tests will be described in more detail below. Multimeric analysis of vWf is typically performed as a research tool, having been replaced by the more widely available collagen-binding assay (CBA) for diagnosis of type II vWD. Routine coagulation assays, either performed patient-side (e.g. activated coagulation time) or in a diagnostic laboratory (activated partial thromboplastin time and prothrombin time) are usually within reference intervals and cannot be used to screen for vWD.

The choice of a screening or diagnostic test depends largely on clinician preference and the clinical situation. For dogs (particularly of a predisposed breed) that present with clinical signs of excessive haemorrhage attributable to a primary haemostatic disorder AND that have platelet counts and routine coagulation assay results within reference intervals, a screening test for vWD or direct measurement of vWf:Ag concentration is indicated. Screening tests that could be performed in this scenario include the *in vivo* buccal mucosal bleeding time (BMBT) and platelet function testing with platelet function analysers (e.g. PFA-100) (Callan and Giger, 2002; Burgess *et al.*, 2009a,b), depending on availability. However, if the results of these general tests of primary haemostasis are abnormal, specific testing for vWD is still required to determine whether vWD is responsible for the observed clinical signs. Given that vWf:Ag concentrations do correlate with clinical expression, a vWf:Ag measurement could be performed without the need for these screening tests.

For assisting dog breeders with optimal breeding strategies, detection of carriers is best performed using genetic analysis for the specific mutation, if it has been identified in the breed in question. If the genetic mutation has not been identified or no other genetic tools (haplotype mapping) are available, carrier detection will rely on vWf:Ag concentrations. This is not optimal because there is an overlap in vWf:Ag concentrations between carriers and affected dogs. Note that genetic analysis should not be used as the sole diagnostic test for vWD in a bleeding animal, because genetic status cannot be used to predict vWf:Ag concentrations and there is no evidence linking genetic status to excessive haemorrhage.

Buccal mucosal bleeding time

The BMBT is an *in vivo* test of primary haemostasis in any dog. It can be used as a screening test for vWD, but is not sensitive or specific for this disorder. The BMBT requires a specific device (e.g. Surgicutt, Simplate) and should be done by a single skilled operator, because it is subject to marked operator variability (Sato *et al.*, 2000). Given that type I vWD is highly prevalent in Dobermanns, with up to one third of affected dogs being at risk of haemorrhage (Stokol *et al.*, 1995), the BMBT may be used as a presurgical assessment for vWD in Dobermanns of unknown vWD status, or those with vWf:Ag concentrations below a critical threshold, particularly dogs with a history of bleeding episodes (Figure 27.6). A prolonged BMBT (> 4 minutes) warrants prophylactic treatment. However, normal surgical haemostasis should not be assumed for a dog with a normal BMBT because the BMBT is not predictive of haemorrhage, and surgical drugs (e.g. phenothiazines and anaesthetic agents) may impair platelet function, precipitating surgical bleeding in dogs with mildly decreased vWf:Ag concentrations. The BMBT should be used with care as a screening test (presurgical or otherwise) in dogs with suspected type II or III vWD. Affected dogs can have infinite BMBTs, may suffer from rebleeding and it may be difficult to stop the induced haemorrhage without replacement therapy or local treatment (such as fibrin glue).

von Willebrand factor antigen concentrations

The vWf concentration is measured with antibody-based immunological assays, typically enzyme-linked immunosorbent assays (ELISAs), which detect antigenic epitopes on the protein (hence the term vWf:Ag). Animals with vWf:Ag concentrations < 50% are considered to have vWD; those with vWf:Ag concentrations > 70% are considered 'free' of the disease. Animals with results between these

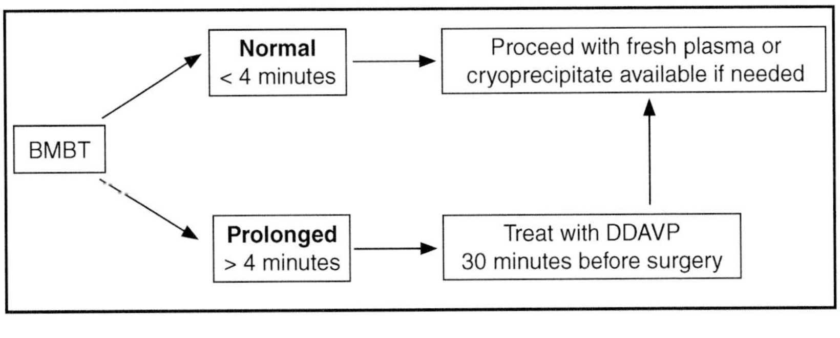

27.6 Flowchart outlining the use of the buccal mucosal bleeding time (BMBT) as a screening test and desmopressin (DDAVP) as prophylactic therapy before elective surgery in dogs of unknown von Willebrand's disease status or those with vWf:Ag concentrations below a critical threshold (< 25–40%, i.e. 'at risk' of haemorrhage). This chart is not recommended for use in dogs with suspect or known type II or III vWD.

values are 'equivocal' or 'indeterminate'. As mentioned above, vWf:Ag testing is preferred for the diagnosis of vWD in a bleeding animal, whereas genetic testing (if available) is superior for detection of carriers. It must be noted that strict attention should be paid to sample collection and handling for measurement of vWf:Ag, and the test should be optimized for detection of vWf:Ag in animal plasma (not all vWf:Ag assays are created equal; Figure 27.7). Sample mishandling can result in falsely increased or decreased vWf:Ag concentrations due to *in vitro* proteolysis which exposes or degrades antigenic epitopes (in an unpredictable manner), respectively. In type I vWD, critical thresholds of vWf:Ag concentrations can be used as an approximate guide for haemorrhagic risk or response to transfusion therapy, however the results do not always correlate with clinical signs (Stokol *et al.*, 1995; Burgess *et al.*, 2009a). The vWf:Ag concentration can also increase in certain situations, and vWf:Ag concentrations above reference intervals have been used as an indirect marker of endothelial injury in cats with cardiomyopathy and dogs with sepsis (Stokol *et al.*, 2008; Rogers and Rozanski, 2010). High concentrations may also be seen as part of the acute phase response.

Sample collection
• Minimize stress and venous stasis • Correct ratio of blood to citrate [a] (9:1): no under- or over-filling • Clean venepuncture
Sample submission
• Centrifuge immediately and separate plasma from cells • Submit to laboratory immediately (keep cool, at 4°C, during transport)
Sample storage
• < 24 hours: 4°C • > 24 hours: at or below –20°C (no frost-free freezers), submit frozen on ice packs (or dry ice if in transit for > 24 hours)
Other
• If needed, thaw at 37°C and assay immediately

27.7 Sample collection and submission guidelines for measurement of vWf:Ag concentration. [a]Citrate concentration (3.2 or 3.8%) does not alter vWf:Ag concentration, but can affect PFA-100 closure times.

Collagen-binding assay (CBA)

This functional assay is based on the ability of plasma vWf to bind to immobilized collagen in a modified ELISA. The CBA results correlate with vWf:Ag concentrations in an approximate 1:1 vWf:Ag to CBA ratio in healthy dogs and dogs with type I vWD. The assay can be used as a screening test for type II vWD, because the CBA is disproportionally lower than the vWf:Ag concentration (resulting in a vWf:Ag to CBA ratio > 1:1) because the protein is structurally abnormal (Sabino *et al.*, 2006; Burgess *et al.*, 2009a,b).

Treatment

Treatment for vWD is palliative, with the goal being short-term prevention or control of haemorrhage. This is best accomplished by infusion of plasma products that contain high concentrations of vWf, although desmopressin, a drug that increases plasma vWf:Ag concentrations, can also be used. Local haemostatic measures, e.g. application of fibrin glue, can be useful for surgical haemostasis or localized haemorrhage (e.g. induced by a BMBT), but vWf replacement is usually required for treatment of bleeding episodes associated with vWD. Note that it is far easier to prevent haemorrhage than to treat haemorrhage once it has begun (prophylaxis is paramount for elective surgical procedures). Drugs that are known to inhibit platelet function, such as non-steroidal anti-inflammatory agents or aspirin, should be avoided in animals with vWD.

Thyroid supplementation should not be used for treatment or prophylaxis in vWD, unless dogs are proven to be hypothyroid by thyroid function testing.

Cryoprecipitate

The product of choice for prevention or cessation of haemorrhage in vWD is cryoprecipitate, a concentrated form of vWf and FVIII. Cryoprecipitate provides the greatest amount of vWf in a small plasma volume and is associated with few side effects. It is also more effective at increasing plasma vWf:Ag concentrations and shortening the BMBT than other blood products (see Chapter 34 for preparation of these blood products). Fresh or fresh frozen plasma is a good alternative to cryoprecipitate, but is associated with more non-haemolytic transfusion reactions, particularly with fast infusion rates. Unnecessary transfusions of whole blood (in non-anaemic patients) should be avoided to prevent sensitization of the recipient to foreign antigens and to minimize the risk of future transfusion reactions (particularly because many of these dogs may suffer recurrent bouts of haemorrhage and require multiple transfusions). Figure 27.8 provides guidelines for transfusion therapy in vWD.

Desmopressin

Desmopressin (1-deamino-8-arginine vasopressin; DDAVP) is a synthetic analogue of arginine vasopressin (antidiuretic hormone). Desmopressin increases plasma vWf:Ag concentrations by inducing vWf release from Weibel–Palade bodies in endothelial cells. This drug will only work in dogs with stores of vWf (i.e. type I vWD) and is thus ineffective in dogs with type III vWD. Repeated injections produce a diminishing response owing to store depletion, therefore the drug has limited use in the treatment of haemorrhagic episodes in vWD. Desmopressin is recommended for use as presurgical prophylaxis in dogs of unknown vWD status or those with vWf:Ag concentrations below a critical threshold (see Figure 27.6). Synthetic vasopressin is available in tablet form or as an aqueous solution for injection. Intranasal preparations are also available as solutions or sprays, which are more cost-effective than

Product	Volume	Frequency	Comments
Cryoprecipitate	1 unit [a] per 10 kg	q4–12h (as needed)	Unit definition varies between suppliers. **Prophylaxis**: Give just before surgery and repeat if surgery > 2 hours, then as needed
Fresh or fresh frozen plasma	6–12 ml/kg 15–20 ml/kg if severe haemorrhage	q8–12h	Use a slow infusion rate to avoid reactions. **Prophylaxis**: As for cryoprecipitate
Fresh whole blood	12–20 ml/kg	q24h	Avoid unless animal is anaemic and hypoxic (components still preferred)

27.8 Guidelines for the prevention or treatment of haemorrhagic episodes associated with von Willebrand's disease. [a] 1 unit is that derived from 200 ml of fresh or fresh frozen plasma.

the aqueous solution for injection. The intranasal preparations are injected subcutaneously 30 minutes before surgery, at a dose of 1 µg/kg diluted to 1 ml volume with sterile saline. This dose may shorten the BMBT in Dobermanns with vWD for up to 4 hours. However, the response to the drug is unpredictable (although the response in individual dogs is repeatable) and some dogs may not respond at all. Thus, DDAVP should not be relied upon to achieve surgical haemostasis; plasma or cryoprecipitate should be available in the event of excessive surgical haemorrhage.

Disease control

Control of the disease is dependent on genetic testing, with removal of carriers from breeding programmes. This can only be done in breeds in which a causative mutation has been identified. Genetic testing for vWD can potentially eliminate the disease in specific breeds (van Oost *et al.*, 2004), although the possibility of *de novo* mutations always exists. However, given that some dogs with vWD are considered too valuable to remove from the breeding pool, it is unlikely the disease will be eliminated from many breeds.

References and further reading

Brooks MB and Catalfamo JL (2010) von Willebrand Disease. In: *Schalm's Veterinary Hematology, 6th edn*, ed. DJ Weiss and KJ Wardrop, pp.612–618. Wiley-Blackwell, Ames, Iowa

Burgess HJ, Woods JP, Abrams-Ogg ACG and Wood RD (2009a) Use of a questionnaire to predict von Willebrand disease status and characterize hemorrhagic signs in a population of dogs and evaluation of a diagnostic profile to predict risk of bleeding. *Canadian Journal of Veterinary Research* **73**, 241–251

Burgess HJ, Woods JP, Abrams-Ogg ACG and Wood RD (2009b) Evaluation of laboratory methods to improve characterization of dogs with von Willebrand disease. *Canadian Journal of Veterinary Research* **73**, 252–259

Callan MB and Giger U (2002) Effect of desmopressin acetate administration on primary hemostasis in Doberman Pinschers with type-1 von Willebrand disease as assessed by a point-of-care instrument. *American Journal of Veterinary Research* **63**, 1700–1706

Heseltine JC, Panciera DL, Troy GC *et al.* (2005) Effect of levothyroxine administration on hemostatic analytes in Doberman Pinschers with von Willebrand disease. *Journal of Veterinary Internal Medicine* **19**, 523–527

Kramer JW, Venta PJ, Klein SR *et al.* (2004) A von Willebrand's factor genomic nucleotide variant and polymerase chain reaction diagnostic test associated with inheritable type-2 von Willebrand's disease in a line of German shorthaired pointer dogs. *Veterinary Pathology* **41**, 221–228

Panciera DL and Johnson GS (1994) Plasma von Willebrand factor antigen concentration in dogs with hypothyroidism. *Journal of the American Veterinary Medical Association* **205**, 1550–1553

Panciera DL and Johnson GS (1996) Plasma von Willebrand factor antigen concentrations and buccal mucosal bleeding time in dogs with experimental hypothyroidism. *Journal of Veterinary Internal Medicine* **10**, 60–64

Rieger M, Schwarz HP, Turecek PL *et al.* (1998) Identification of mutations in the canine von Willebrand factor gene associated with type III von Willebrand disease. *Thrombosis and Haemostasis* **80**, 332–337

Rogers CL and Rozanski EA (2010) Von Willebrand factor antigen concentration in dogs with sepsis. *Journal of Veterinary Internal Medicine* **24**, 229–230

Sabino EP, Erb HN and Catalfamo JL (2006) Development of a collagen-binding activity assay as a screening test for type II von Willebrand Disease in dogs. *American Journal of Veterinary Research* **67**, 242–249

Sato I, Andersen GA and Parry BW (2000) An interobserver and intraobserver study of buccal mucosal bleeding times in Greyhounds. *Research in Veterinary Science* **68**, 41–45

Stokol T, Brooks MB, Rush JE *et al.* (2008) Hypercoagulability in cats with cardiac disease. *Journal of Veterinary Internal Medicine* **22**, 546–552

Stokol T, Parry BW and Mansell PD (1995) von Willebrand's disease in Dobermann dogs in Australia. *Australian Veterinary Journal* **72**, 257–262

Tarnow I, Kristensen AT, Olsen LH *et al.* (2005) Dogs with heart diseases causing turbulent high-velocity blood flow have changes in platelet function and von Willebrand factor multimer distribution. *Journal of Veterinary Internal Medicine* **19**, 515–522

Torres R and Fedoriw Y (2009) Laboratory testing for von Willebrand disease: toward a mechanism-based classification. *Clinical and Laboratory Medicine* **29**, 193–228

van Oost BA, Versteeg SA and Slappendel RJ (2004) DNA testing for type III von Willebrand disease in Dutch Kooiker dogs. *Journal of Veterinary Internal Medicine* **18**, 282–288

Venta PJ, Yuzbasiyan-Gurkan V, Brewer GJ and Schall WD (2000) Mutation causing von Willebrand's disease in Scottish Terriers. *Journal of Veterinary Internal Medicine* **14**, 10–19

28

Haemophilia A and B

Marjory B. Brooks

Introduction

Haemophilia A and B are hereditary, X-linked bleeding disorders caused, respectively, by deficiencies of coagulation factors FVIII and FIX. The key clinical feature of haemophilia (i.e. a severe familial bleeding tendency that afflicts males) has been recognized since biblical times. The most famous carrier of haemophilia, Queen Victoria, transmitted the 'royal disease' through her children to the monarchies of Spain, Germany and Russia. Haemophilia A and B were differentiated as distinct single factor deficiencies in the 1950s. Molecular genetic analyses, begun in the 1980s and continuing to date, have revealed hundreds of unique FVIII and FIX mutations in unrelated affected families.

Haemophilia is among the most common hereditary human disorders, with a worldwide incidence of approximately 1 per 5000 male births for haemophilia A, and approximately 1 per 30,000 male births for haemophilia B. Both haemophilia A and B have been identified in domestic animals and, as in humans, haemophilia A is by far the more common form. The clinical features of haemophilia in dogs and cats are similar to their human disease counterparts. With recent advances in veterinary transfusion medicine, successful management of canine and feline cases has become a possibility.

Function of factors VIII and IX

FVIII and FIX play a critical role in coagulation by acting as a signal amplifier to generate the burst of thrombin that transforms plasma fibrinogen into an insoluble fibrin clot (see Chapter 21). FIX, a serine protease factor, and FVIII, its cofactor, assemble with calcium on a phospholipid surface to form an active enzyme complex referred to as the 'intrinsic tenase' complex. This complex is highly efficient in generating active FX (FXa), which in turn catalyses the rapid production of a large amount of thrombin. Assembly of the intrinsic tenase complex depends on the initial cleavage of FIX to its active form (FIXa) and the disassociation of FVIII from its carrier protein, von Willebrand factor (vWF), with subsequent activation to form FVIIIa. *In vivo*, these reactions occur on membrane surfaces. FIXa and FVIIIa bind to the surface of activated platelets whereupon they cleave their substrate, FX (Figure 28.1). A fully functional intrinsic tenase complex requires that the FVIII and FIX molecules are capable of interacting not only with each other, but with other haemostatic proteins (e.g. FX, FXI, thrombin), membrane phospholipids and calcium. Mutations within the genes encoding FVIII (*F8*) or FIX (*F9*) that interfere with any of these interactions result in delayed or inadequate thrombin generation, and ultimately in ineffective fibrin clot formation and clinical signs of a bleeding diathesis.

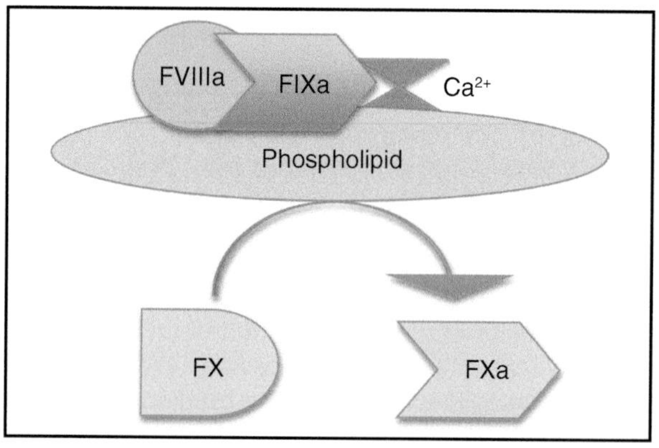

28.1 The intrinsic tenase coagulation complex. The serine protease FIXa assembles on a phospholipid membrane surface with calcium and its cofactor, FVIIIa, to form an active enzyme complex. The tenase complex interacts with its substrate, the zymogen FX, to induce rapid generation of the enzyme, FXa.

Prevalence and inheritance of haemophilia

Haemophilia A and B are the most common hereditary bleeding diatheses caused by coagulation factor deficiencies in dogs and cats, with observed case ratios of approximately 4 to 1 favouring haemophilia A. Hereditary FXII deficiency (Hageman trait) is more common in cats in the United States than haemophilia; however, FXII deficiency does not cause abnormal haemorrhage and the prevalence of the trait outside the United States is unknown. Case series and case reports of haemophilia reveal that the defect is not restricted to a single breed or inbred line, rather haemophilia appears in many different purebred and mixed-breed dogs and cats. Haemophilia A was diagnosed in 31 distinct breeds and mixed-breed dogs in a consecutive series of

102 cases of canine haemophilia A diagnosed through the author's laboratory (Figure 28.2). Similar breed heterogeneity is found in haemophilia B. Frequent *de novo* mutations in *F8* and *F9* are known to cause haemophilia in humans, and the same processes probably underlie the occurrence of haemophilia in dogs and cats. Importantly, the clinical suspicion of haemophilia should not be restricted to breeds with previously diagnosed cases, because new cases may arise in any purebred or mixed-breed family.

Haemophilia A and B are X-linked recessive traits. Males with an *F8* or *F9* mutation that impairs factor activity will invariably express a bleeding tendency, whereas female carriers, with one mutant and one functional gene, are clinically normal. Haemophilia is most often propagated when asymptomatic carrier females are bred. In these litters, on average, half the male pups will be affected with haemophilia and half the females will be carriers (Figure 28.3a). Although males with severe forms of haemophilia often succumb before 1 year of age and

Group	Affected breeds
Gundogs (Sporting dogs)	American Cocker Spaniel, Golden Retriever, Labrador Retriever
Hounds	Basset Hound, Beagle, Dachshund, Redbone Coonhound
Working dogs	Boxer, Great Dane, Husky, Rottweiler
Terriers	Airedale Terrier, Jack Russell Terrier, Soft-coated Wheaten Terrier, West Highland White Terriert
Toy dogs	Chihuahua, Japanese Chin, Maltese, Pekinese, Pug, Yorkshire Terrier
Utility dogs	Akita, Boston Terrier, Keeshond, Lhasa Apso, Poodle, Shih Tzu
Pastoral dogs (Herding)	Australian Shepherd Dog, German Shepherd Dog, Shetland Sheepdog
Miscellaneous	Coton de Tulear

28.2 Breeds that presented with canine haemophilia A over a 2-year period. The cases were compiled from submissions to the Comparative Coagulation Laboratory at Cornell University from February 2006 to February 2008. Diagnoses of haemophilia A (three to five cases per month) represent approximately 1% of the monthly submissions for canine coagulation testing.

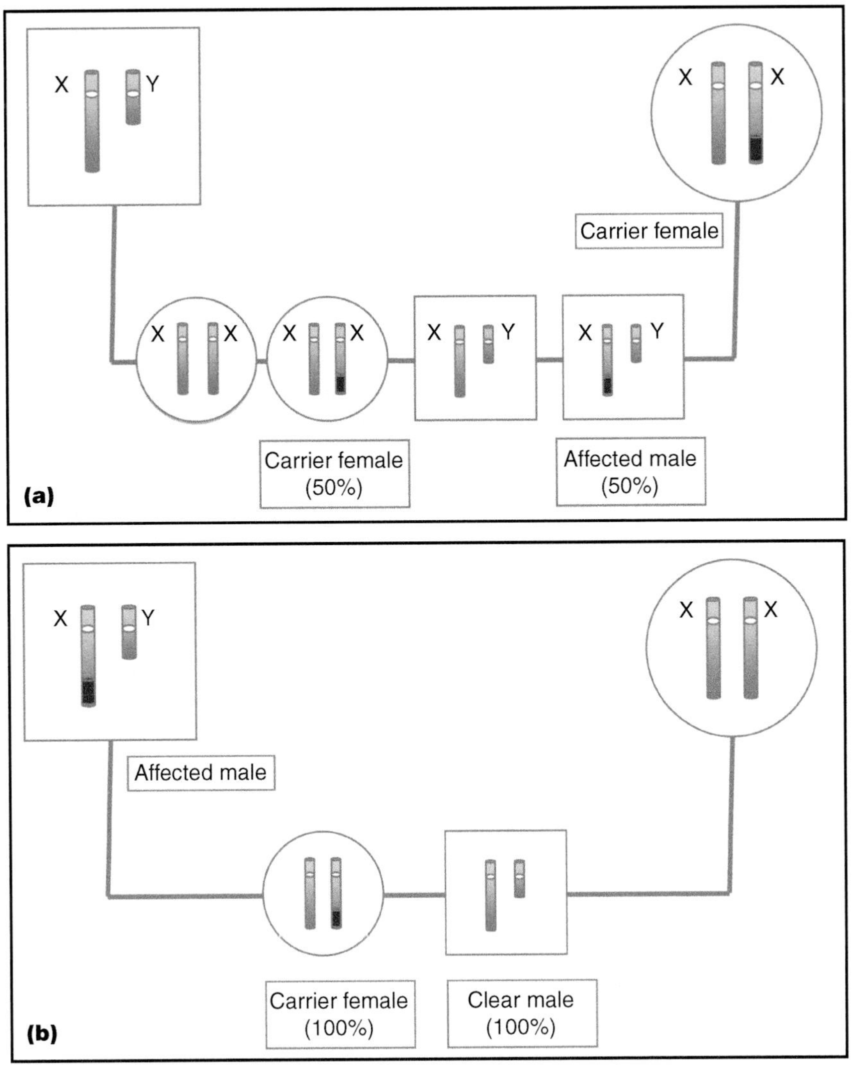

28.3 X-linked inheritance of haemophilia A and B. **(a)** Propagation of haemophilia by a carrier female. Carrier females transmit a mutant gene (depicted as a dark bar on the X chromosome) on average to half their sons and half their daughters. The sons that inherit this mutation are affected with haemophilia and the daughters are haemophilia carriers. **(b)** Propagation of haemophilia by an affected male. Males with mild to moderate haemophilia may survive to reproductive age. If bred to an unaffected female, all the daughters of an affected male are carriers of haemophilia and all the sons are clear.

are rarely used for breeding, males with clinically milder forms of haemophilia may survive to adulthood. The use of haemophilic males as stud dogs can lead to widespread transmission of haemophilia through their carrier daughters (Figure 28.3b). Haemophilia A was propagated in German Shepherd Dogs by a popular founder sire, with cases related to this male diagnosed in Europe, the United Kingdom, Australia and North America. More recently, mild haemophilia B in North American German Wirehaired Pointers was traced to founder sires in Germany, and a mild form of haemophilia A has been propagated in Golden Retrievers by carrier females and affected males. The X-linked recessive transmission pattern of haemophilia may lead to delays in diagnosis, because carrier females do not express a bleeding tendency and litters with few males may not include any affected pups. Litters sired by affected males produce no affected offspring, so the trait may appear to 'skip' generations, with new cases appearing only after the carrier daughters produce affected sons.

Clinical signs

Haemophilia should be high on the differential diagnosis list for any male with severe or unexplained haemorrhage. Presenting signs of haemophilia typically include lameness due to haemarthrosis (Figure 28.4a), intramuscular and subcutaneous haematoma formation (Figure 28.4b), and prolonged bleeding from minor wounds and from the gingivae at tooth eruption sites. Milder forms of haemophilia may become apparent only after surgery or trauma, whereas more severe forms are characterized by recurrent and apparently spontaneous haemorrhagic events. Severe haemophilia usually manifests within the first few months of life and these animals are dependent on transfusion for survival. Death may result from haemorrhage into critical anatomical sites (e.g. central nervous system, respiratory tract) or from hypovolaemic shock and blood loss anaemia. The key to timely diagnosis of haemophilia requires an initial suspicion that joint swellings or fluid effusions in any body cavity or potential space may represent haemorrhage, which in turn prompts collection of samples for coagulation testing.

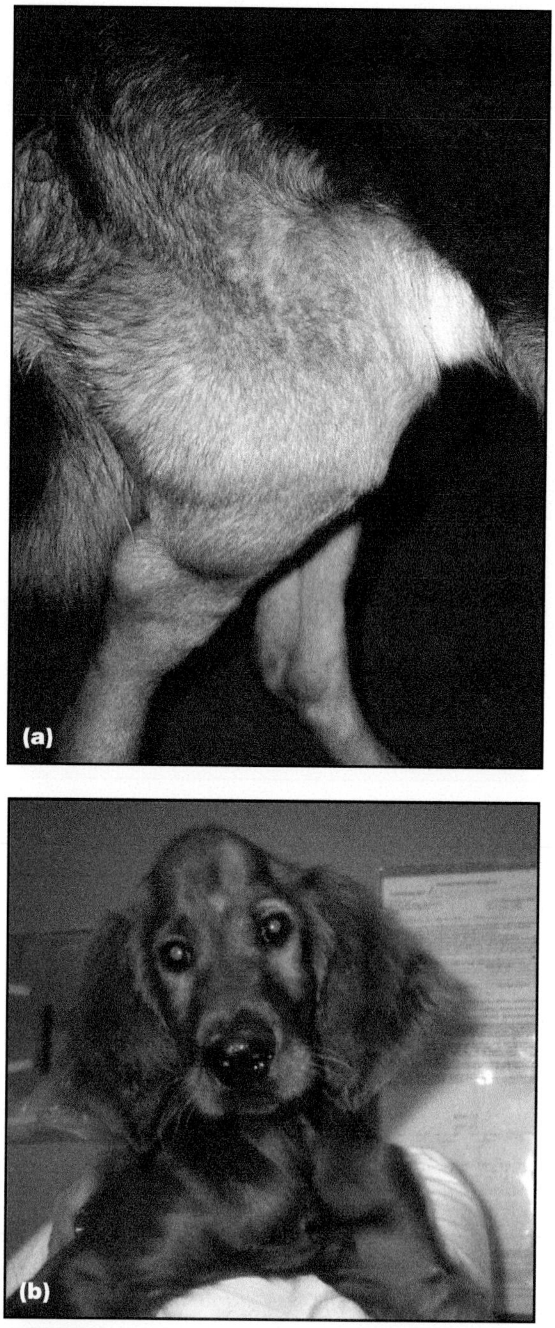

28.4 Clinical signs of haemophilia. **(a)** Haemarthrosis of the stifle joint and thigh muscle haematoma in a mixed-breed dog affected with severe haemophilia B (factor IX activity < 1%). **(b)** Dorsal temporal muscle haematoma in an Irish Setter puppy affected with severe haemophilia A (factor VIII activity < 1%).

Diagnosis

Coagulation assays that measure the rate of fibrin clot formation *in vitro* are the primary means for screening and definitive diagnosis of haemophilia. An initial patient assessment that includes a platelet count and point-of-care coagulation screening tests will help to identify rapidly those patients with factor deficiencies and direct more detailed evaluation of the coagulation cascade (see Chapter 22). FVIII and FIX promote thrombin generation and subsequent fibrin clot formation by catalysing a key step in the intrinsic coagulation pathway (Figure 28.5). A lack of either factor slows the clotting endpoint in screening tests of the intrinsic pathway (e.g. activated clotting time (ACT) and activated partial thromboplastin time (aPTT)). A long clotting time in the aPTT with normal values for prothrombin time, thrombin time and fibrinogen are the hallmarks of haemophilia. Deficiencies of FVIII and FIX will alter the kinetics of fibrin formation as detected by thromboelastometry; however, the use of tissue factor activators reduces the sensitivity of this methodology for the detection of intrinsic pathway defects (Figure 28.6).

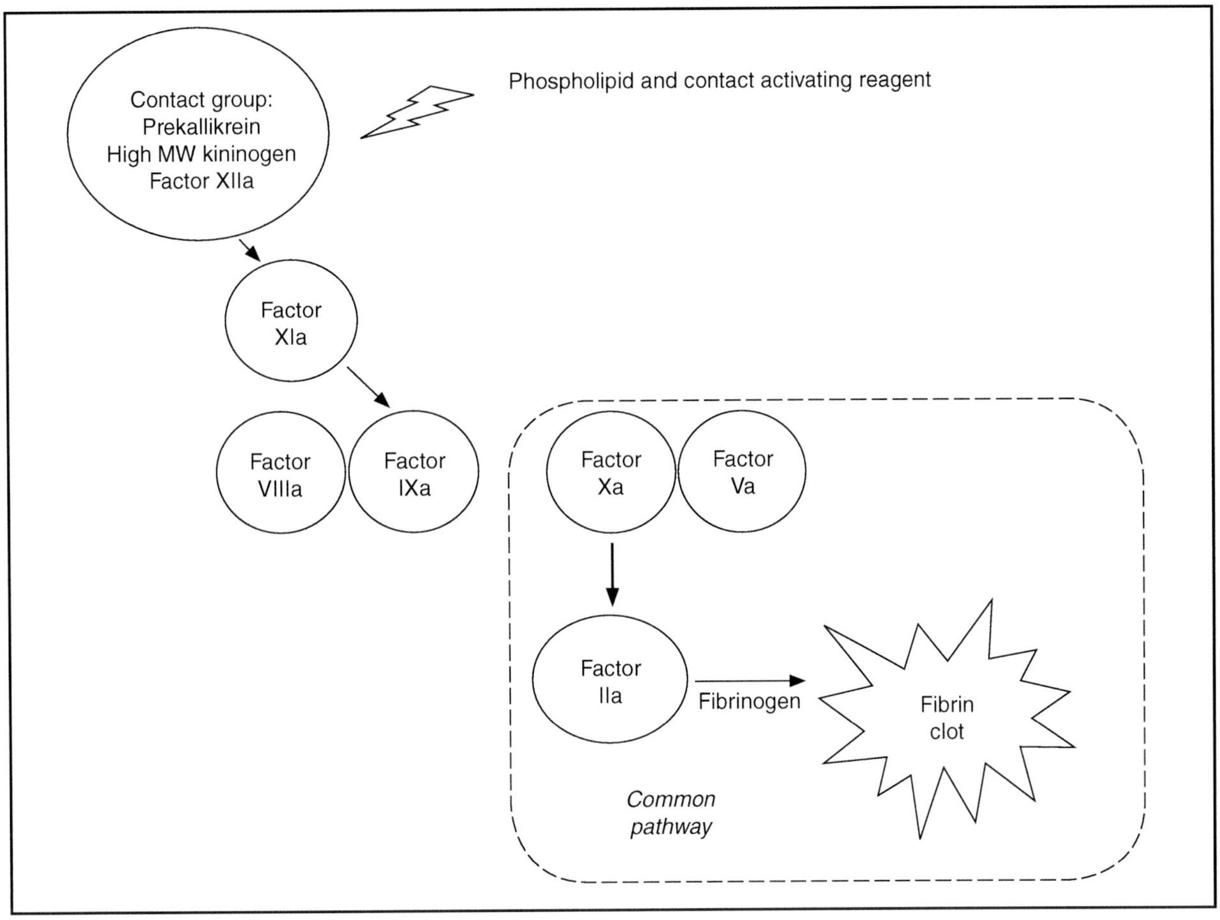

28.5 Intrinsic coagulation pathway. The intrinsic pathway leading to *in vitro* fibrin formation is initiated by pre-incubation of plasma with a reagent containing phospholipid and a particulate surface. Upon the addition of calcium, activation of the contact pathway proceeds through a series of steps culminating in the common pathway (outlined by a dashed line), which produces a burst of thrombin (factor IIa) that cleaves fibrinogen to form an insoluble fibrin clot. MW, molecular weight.

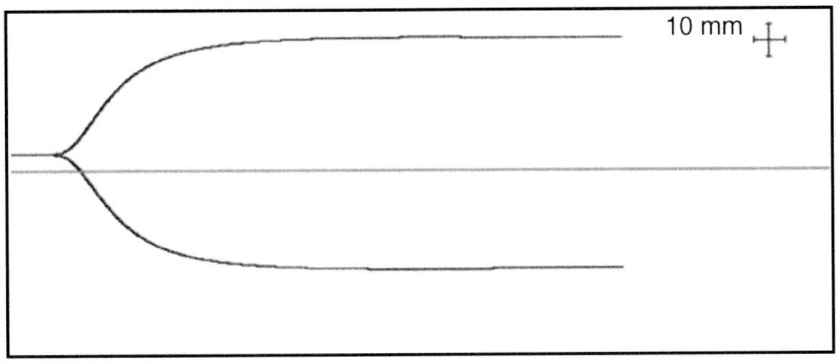

28.6 Thromboelastography (TEG) tracings from a dog with severe haemophilia A. Superimposed tracings depict assays performed on whole blood samples activated by the addition of a tissue factor reagent (black tracing) or with no activating agent (green tracing). The activated sample shows only a slight delay in the time for initial fibrin formation (denoted by the first separation of the solid black line into two mirror images), and has no abnormalities in TEG parameters denoting fibrin clot strength. In contrast, in the absence of tissue factor to bypass the intrinsic pathway, a stable fibrin clot fails to form in the reaction cup (denoted by the single flat green line).

Further differentiation between haemophilia A and B is based on specific measurement of FVIII and FIX coagulant activities (FVIII:C, FIX:C). Clinical expression of the bleeding diathesis relates to residual factor activity. In general, the most severe forms of haemophilia are characterized by FVIII:C or FIX:C values < 2% of normal, whereas values ranging from 2–20% are associated with clinically moderate to mild haemophilia. The sensitivity of aPTT screening tests to detect mild factor deficiencies varies among testing laboratories. In addition, the assay systems optimized to measure human factors require modification to provide accurate measures of FVIII:C and FIX:C in dogs and cats. Factor assays should be configured with same-species standards to account for relative species differences in procoagulant enzyme and coenzyme activities. Determination of FVIII or FIX protein concentration (rather than activity) is used infrequently for clinical diagnosis. Commercial tests configured with cross-reactive antibodies are not widely available and the methods for quantitative determination do not facilitate rapid test turnaround times. Moreover, quantitative protein assays will not detect haemophiliacs that have dysfunctional factor variants.

Management of haemophilia

Transfusion therapy

Transfusion to supply FVIII or FIX is the primary mode of therapy to control or prevent haemorrhage in affected dogs and cats (see Chapters 34 and 35). Rapid replacement of the deficient factor supports fibrin formation sufficient to form a haemostatic plug. The use of blood components allows for more selective factor replacement with lower volumes than whole blood transfusion. Fresh frozen plasma (FFP) supplies both FVIII and FIX, whereas cryoprecipitate is a plasma concentrate that contains FVIII, and the residual plasma cryosupernatant is a source of FIX. Fresh whole blood transfusions may be given to replace active factors and red cell mass in patients with blood loss anaemia and hypovolaemic shock. However, in cases that require repeated transfusion to sustain haemostatic factor levels, the use of whole blood carries a high risk of inducing volume overload or alloimmunization to donor red cell antigens.

The appropriate transfusion volume and interval for each patient depends on a number of different criteria, including the patient's residual baseline factor activity, the extent and anatomical site of active haemorrhage or planned surgical intervention, and any underlying conditions that may further impair haemostasis (e.g. thrombocytopenia, exposure to anti-platelet drugs). In most cases, transfusion of 10–12 ml/kg of FFP with a transfusion interval of 6–8 hours will supply adequate factor replacement to sustain haemostasis without causing volume overload. Higher initial volumes (e.g. 15–20 ml/kg) and shorter intervals may be needed for animals in acute haemorrhagic crisis or as preoperative prophylaxis for major surgery.

Clinical status is the most important indicator of appropriate transfusion response. While point-of-care coagulation assays (e.g. ACT or aPTT) can aid in patient monitoring, resolution of signs of haemorrhage and confirmation of stable or rising haematocrit and plasma protein levels are more useful parameters to guide transfusion. FVIII and FIX have relatively short half-lives of < 24 hours, therefore patients with severe factor deficiencies almost invariably require more than a single transfusion when undergoing invasive procedures or to resolve blood loss anaemia. Repeated transfusions over a period of 2–3 days may be needed to control a haemorrhagic episode. The development of anticoagulant inhibitory antibodies is a rare, but severe, complication of factor replacement therapy that is well characterized in humans and has been reported in dogs with haemophilia A and B. Inhibitory antibodies cause transfusion resistance, which in some cases can be overcome with high volume plasma or plasma concentrate transfusion. Maintenance of good quality of life for patients with severe haemophilia (factor activities < 2%) may be difficult because of recurrent haemorrhage. Many of these patients are euthanased, or develop fatal haemorrhage, before 1 year of age.

Non-transfusion therapy

Given that haemophilia is a life-long bleeding disorder, husbandry and management practices should be aimed at minimizing the chances of injury and joint stress. It is best to avoid any invasive procedures, including intramuscular injections, and drugs that impair platelet function or anticoagulants (e.g. non-steroidal anti-inflammatory agents, dextran, hetastarch, heparin). The synthetic vasopressin analogue, desmopressin (DDAVP, desamino 8-D-arginine vasopressin), induces the release of VWF from intracellular stores and is used as an adjunct to transfusion therapy for human patients with mild haemophilia A. In the author's experience, haemophilic dogs treated with desmopressin have shown no clinical response and no increase in FVIII:C. The management of haemophilia in human patients may also include administration of lysine analogue antifibrinolytic agents. Aminocaproic acid and tranexamic acid act to inhibit plasmin-mediated fibrinolysis and are most often used, with factor concentrates, after surgical and dental procedures. The use of antifibrinolytic agents to reduce the transfusion requirements of haemostatic defects in animals, however, has not been investigated thoroughly. Aminocaproic acid is generally given to humans at an initial loading dose of 100 mg/kg i.v., followed by an hourly dose of 30 mg/kg for up to 8 hours. Tranexamic acid is typically given at an initial dose of 10 mg/kg i.v., and then maintained for up to 7 days postoperatively at a dose of 25 mg/kg orally q8h.

Human-derived and recombinant FVIII and FIX concentrates, and recombinant human FVIIa (rhFVIIa), have been shown to support fibrin generation and correct the bleeding tendency transiently in research dogs used as animal models of haemophilia. The high cost and immunogenicity of these concentrates, however, limit their clinical utility in veterinary practice.

Genetic counselling

New cases of haemophilia A and B apparently arise in previously unaffected pedigrees through frequent spontaneous mutation events in *F8* and *F9*. Complex inversion mutations that involve repetitive regions within intron 22 of the human *F8* gene account for close to half of all severe haemophilia A in families with newly diagnosed cases. A similar mutation mechanism has been reported in dogs, and it is possible that the relatively high incidence of haemophilia A in dogs and cats results from recurrent *de novo* gene rearrangements. Distinct point mutations in *F9* have been reported in haemophilic dogs and cats, and large insertions and deletions have also been identified in different breed-variants of canine haemophilia B. This molecular genetic heterogeneity complicates the development of genetic tests for haemophilia, because each affected breed or line may have its own unique mutation.

Nevertheless, pedigree review and selective breeding are useful in limiting the propagation of haemophilia within any breed. Affected males and clear males can be differentiated accurately on the basis of their levels of FVIII:C or FIX:C. Obligate carrier females are then identified as the dams (and daughters) of affected males (see Figure 28.3). The female siblings of an affected male have a 50% chance of inheriting a haemophilia-causing mutation from the carrier dam. Obligate and suspect carrier females can be neutered safely and they have no restrictions in use other than breeding, because they do not express a bleeding tendency. Indirect detection of carriers, based on the use of DNA microsatellite markers linked to the *F8* or *F9* genes, has been reported to aid in the detection of carriers of haemophilia. Progeny testing also provides probabilistic estimates of carrier status for suspect females. Providing that all male puppies are screened (by aPTT and/or factor assays), females that produce four or more unaffected male puppies are predicted to have a less than 10% chance of being a carrier, whereas six or more unaffected male puppies reduces the probability of carrier status to less than 2%.

References and further reading

Brooks MB, Barnas JL, Fremont J *et al.* (2005) Cosegregation of a factor VIII microsatellite marker with mild hemophilia A in Golden retriever dogs. *Journal of Veterinary Internal Medicine* **19**, 205–210

Brooks MB, Gu W, Barnas JL *et al.* (2003) A Line 1 insertion in the factor IX gene segregates with mild hemophilia B in dogs. *Mammalian Genome* **14**, 788–795

Brooks MB, MacNguyen R, Hall R *et al.* (2008) Indirect carrier detection of canine hemophilia A using FVIII microsatellite markers. *Animal Genetics* **39**, 278–283

Fogh JM (1988) A study of hemophilia A in German Shepherd dogs in Denmark. *Veterinary Clinics of North America: Small Animal Practice* **18**, 245–254

Goree M, Catalfamo JL, Aber S *et al.* (2006) Characterization of the mutations causing hemophilia B in 2 domestic cats. *Journal of Veterinary Internal Medicine* **19**, 200–204

Lee AP, Boyle CE, Savidge GF *et al.* (2005) Effectiveness in controlling haemorrhage after dental scaling in people with haemophilia by using tranexamic acid mouthwash *British Dental Journal* **198**, 33–38

Levy JH (2008) Pharmacologic methods to reduce peri-operative bleeding. *Transfusion* **48**, 31S–38S

O'Kelley, Whelan MF and Brooks MB (2009) Factor VIII inhibitors complicating treatment of postoperative bleeding in a dog with hemophilia A. *Journal of Veterinary Emergency and Critical Care* **19**, 381–385

Stokol T and Parry B (1998) Efficacy of fresh frozen plasma and cryoprecipitate in dogs with von Willebrand's disease or hemophilia A. *Journal of Veterinary Internal Medicine* **12**, 84–92

Useful websites

Canadian Hemophilia Society. Comprehensive Care Standards. http://www.hemophilia.ca/en/care-and-treatment/comprehensive-care-standards/

Comparative Coagulation Laboratory. Animal coagulation factor assays and information on haemophilia in animals. http://ahdc.vet.cornell.edu/Sects/coag/

GeneTests at NCBI. Medical genetics information resource. http://www.ncbi.nlm.nih.gov/sites/GeneTests/?db=GeneTests

HAMSTeRS. The Haemophilia A mutation, structure, test and resource site. Compilation database of human factor VIII mutations. http://hadb.org.uk

National Institutes of Health. On-line Mendelian Inheritance in Man (OMIM) and On-line Mendelian Inheritance in Animals (OMIA). Information on the inheritance, expression, and genetic basis of haemophilia A and B in human beings and animals. http://www.ncbi.nlm.nih.gov/sites/gquery

29

Anticoagulant rodenticide intoxication

Alexandre Proulx and Cynthia M. Otto

Introduction

Rodenticides are one of the most common pesticides ingested by companion animals, with dogs being poisoned more commonly than cats (Peterson and Talcott, 2006). The four major types of rodenticide currently in use are: vitamin K antagonists (which represent approximately 90% of all rodenticide intoxications in the United States); calciferols; metal phosphides; and bromethalin. Intoxication with these products leads to coagulopathy, hypercalcaemia, cardiovascular collapse and neurological disorders, respectively. This chapter focuses on vitamin K antagonist exposure and intoxication.

Role of vitamin K in haemostasis

Vitamin K plays an important role in haemostasis, mainly by activating the coagulation factors of secondary haemostasis via carboxylation. These include procoagulant factors (prothrombin (factor II), factors (F)VII, IX, X) and anticoagulant proteins (protein C, protein S). They are all synthesized in their inactivated form by the liver. In order to become activated, these proteins require the modification of a glutamic amino acid to a carboxylated form, which in turn requires the presence of vitamin K. In humans, the half-lives of specific coagulation factors are variable, with FVII having the shortest half-life (6.2 hours) (Hellemans *et al.*, 1963). In dogs FVII is also recognized as having the shortest half-life (Gaston and Spivack, 1968). In cats there are no published studies documenting the effects of anticoagulant rodenticides on specific coagulation factors, but in both dogs and cats the prothrombin time is the first test to be prolonged. Vitamin K itself is activated via hepatic reduction and epoxidation. Figure 29.1 illustrates the relationship between these different enzymatic reactions.

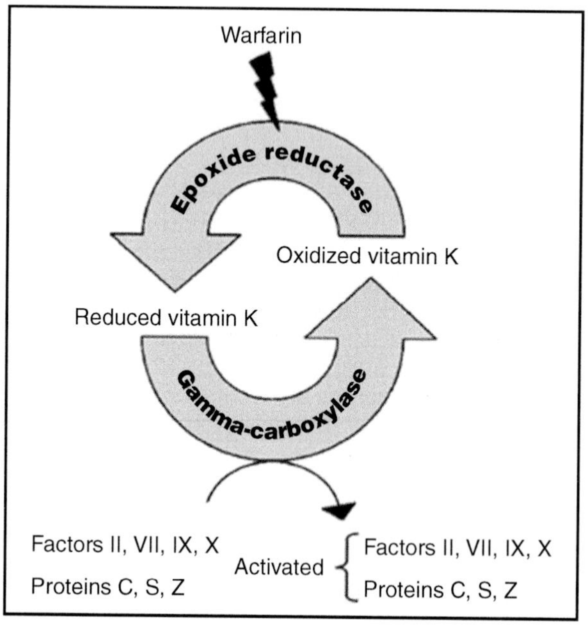

29.1 Inter-relationship of the vitamin K recycling enzymatic pathway and anticoagulant rodenticides.

Anticoagulant rodenticides

The intoxication of cattle by mouldy sweet clover led to the discovery of coumarin. Subsequently, warfarin was synthesized and then marketed widely as a rodenticide. With its increasing use, rodent species developed resistance to warfarin. Compounds effective against warfarin-resistant rodents were then developed. These second-generation anticoagulant rodenticides include brodifacoum, bromadiolone, chlorophacinone, coumachlor, coumatretralyl, coumafuryl, difenacoum, difethialone, diphenadione (synonym: diphacinone), flocoumafen, pindone and valone. Because second-generation anticoagulant rodenticides are more potent and/or longer acting than warfarin, ingestion is associated with a greater potential toxicity. Rodenticide formulations include grain-based pellets, mini-pellets, paraffin-wax blocks, meal baits, dry concentrates, water bait, tracking powder, ground spray, whole and broken grains, nylon pouches, coated talc and dust. Most rodenticides that are available commercially for household use are dyed blue or green, but some, especially those used in agriculture and industry, are colourless. The active ingredient is usually present in concentrations ranging from 0.05–0.25%.

Exposure and clinical signs

Animals with anticoagulant rodenticide ingestion may be brought for veterinary care if the owner observed the ingestion (exposure) or if the pet is showing clinical signs secondary to haemorrhage (intoxication). The approach to the case will depend on whether there is exposure or intoxication.

Exposure

Based on the limited reports (Kohn *et al.*, 2003; Berny *et al.*, 2010) cats seem to be much less likely to ingest rodenticide; however dogs or cats with recent ingestion of an anticoagulant rodenticide will not demonstrate any associated clinical signs. In one experimental study of warfarin intoxication in dogs, the onset of bleeding was not observed until approximately 3.5 days after ingestion, the time required (two half-lives) to deplete prothrombin (Woody *et al.*, 1992). The owner's observation or suspicion of ingestion dictates treatment.

Intoxication

Overall, rodenticide intoxication occurs 5–20 times more often in dogs than in cats. Affected cats are more likely to be those with outdoor access (Kohn *et al.*, 2003). Dogs and cats with known or suspected rodenticide intoxication can display a wide variety of clinical signs associated with haemorrhage. These signs typically occur approximately 3.5 days after ingestion. Some astute owners may observe the presence of the green or blue dye in the faeces prior to the onset of signs. Occult haemorrhage can make the diagnosis of anticoagulant rodenticide intoxication challenging. Depletion of activated prothrombin is thought to be the main reason for development of haemorrhage with rodenticide intoxication (Woody *et al.*, 1992). The most common clinical signs are caused by the failure of secondary haemostasis (see Chapter 25).

Cavitary haemorrhage typically occurs into the pleural, mediastinal, pericardial, peritoneal and retroperitoneal spaces. In addition animals can bleed into their joints, urinary tract, gastrointestinal tract or respiratory tract (Figures 29.2 to 29.4).

Extensive haemorrhage into any cavity can result in signs of haemorrhagic shock, tachycardia, tachypnoea, pale mucous membranes, lethargy and cold

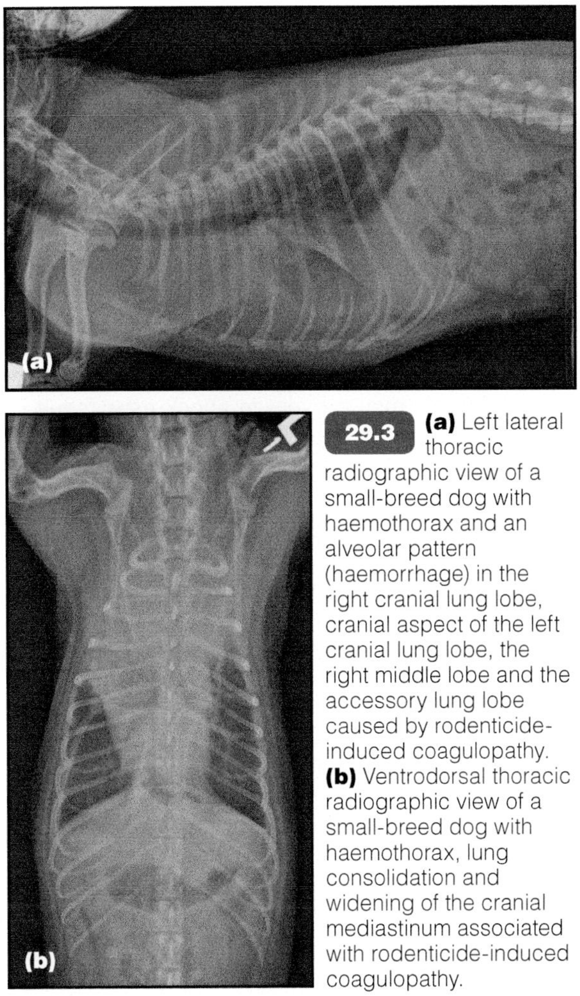

29.3 **(a)** Left lateral thoracic radiographic view of a small-breed dog with haemothorax and an alveolar pattern (haemorrhage) in the right cranial lung lobe, cranial aspect of the left cranial lung lobe, the right middle lobe and the accessory lung lobe caused by rodenticide-induced coagulopathy. **(b)** Ventrodorsal thoracic radiographic view of a small-breed dog with haemothorax, lung consolidation and widening of the cranial mediastinum associated with rodenticide-induced coagulopathy.

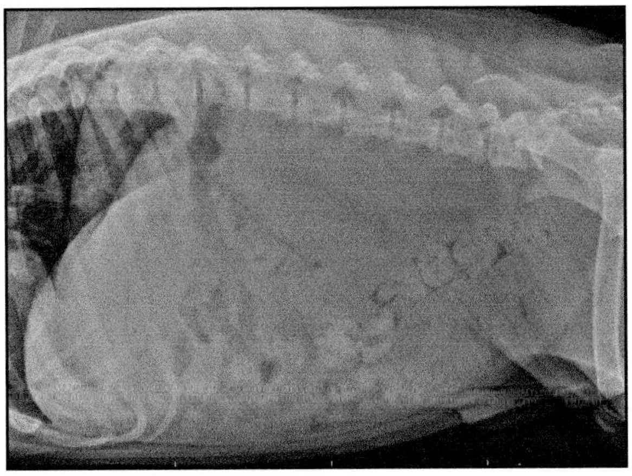

29.2 Right lateral abdominal radiographic view of a medium-breed dog with haemoretroperitoneum.

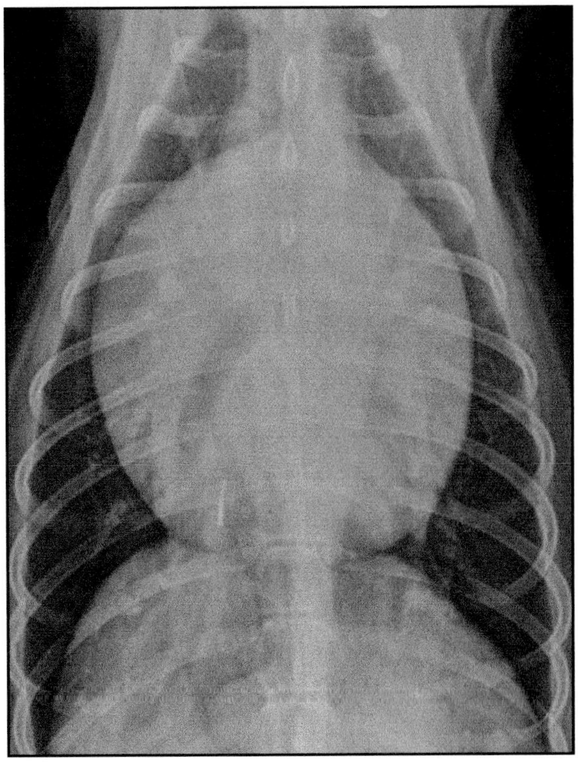

29.4 Ventrodorsal thoracic radiographic view of a medium-breed dog with haemopericardium.

extremities. Haemorrhage into the pleural space leads to a short and shallow respiratory pattern and is associated with dull ventral breath sounds on auscultation. Peritoneal haemorrhage manifests as abdominal distension, potentially leading to an increased respiratory rate from increased pressure on the diaphragm. In addition, a fluid wave can sometimes be appreciated on abdominal palpation when a large amount of haemorrhage is present. Pericardial haemorrhage causes tachycardia and pulsus paradoxus, and an electrical alternans may be appreciated on the electrocardiogram (ECG). Depending on the volume or rapidity of haemorrhage, animals may present in shock as a result of cardiac tamponade and diastolic (filling) failure. In patients with mediastinal or retroperitoneal haemorrhage, the clinical signs may be non-specific or related to haemorrhagic shock if the bleeding is sufficiently severe.

Pulmonary parenchymal haemorrhage usually causes tachypnoea, tachycardia and dyspnoea. On auscultation, the breath sounds may be normal, or increased breath sounds and crackles may be evident. Lameness, joint swelling and gait abnormality can be associated with haemarthrosis. Haematuria and haemorrhagic vaginal discharge can be associated with bleeding from the urogenital tract. Fascial plane haemorrhage and haematomas can be associated with swelling and discomfort of the affected area.

Signs that are typically associated with abnormal primary haemostasis and have also been reported with anticoagulant rodenticide intoxication include melaena, haematochezia, haematemesis, epistaxis, and petechiae or ecchymoses of mucous membranes and skin.

Diagnosis

Exposure

Exposed patients are defined as those with documented ingestion reported by the owners or by observation of rodenticide (green or blue dye) in the vomitus or faeces (Figure 29.5). Because other types of rodenticide exist, documenting the name of the active ingredient is essential.

29.5 Green vomitus after ingestion of rodenticide and induction of emesis.

Intoxication

In patients with suspected intoxication, the first diagnostic step is to confirm a bleeding disorder (see Figure 29.6). More general diagnostic procedures are included in Figure 29.7.

Test	Role
Prothrombin time (PT)	Measures the extrinsic and common pathway coagulation factors (FII, V, VII, X and fibrinogen). Because FVII has the shortest half-life of all vitamin K-dependent clotting factors, PT is the first measure to be prolonged (Hellemans *et al.*, 1963)
Activated partial thromboplastin time (aPTT)	Measures the intrinsic and common pathway coagulation factors. Although this test may be normal in the early stage of intoxication, it will become prolonged later during the clinical phase
Activated clotting time (ACT)	Measures the intrinsic and common pathway coagulation factors. Changes in ACT are usually similar to changes in aPTT
Thrombin time (TT)	Useful to rule out hypofibrinogenaemia and dysfibrinogenaemia. A normal TT in the light of severely prolonged PT and aPTT is highly suggestive of rodenticide intoxication
Proteins induced by vitamin K antagonism or absence test (PIVKA)	Measures modification of the PT by diluting the patient's plasma. Although it may be more sensitive than the PT, its clinical utility is limited because it is only offered by some laboratories and therefore has a longer turnaround time
Thromboelastography (TEG)	Provides an assessment of the rate of formation and strength of the clot. TEG is a useful point-of-care tool to identify hypo- and hypercoagulable states. The sample must be analysed shortly after collection, which requires specialized in-house testing capability and limits its broad applicability

29.6 Confirmatory tests for bleeding disorders.

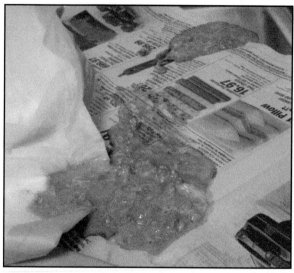

Test	Role
Complete blood count (CBC)	Likely to show non-specific changes such as mild to severe anaemia (due to blood loss) and mild to moderate thrombocytopenia (due to consumption). The anaemia is typically normocytic, normochromic and non-regenerative initially. Regeneration (i.e. reticulocyte count > 40 x 10^9/l, polychromasia) occurs approximately 3–5 days after haemorrhage, and the degree of regeneration depends on the severity and chronicity of the blood loss
Serum chemistry	Likely to show non-specific abnormalities such as panhypoproteinaemia and an increase in blood urea nitrogen (BUN) in patients with gastrointestinal haemorrhage
Imaging	Radiographic and/or ultrasonographic changes may be appreciated in clinical patients, depending on the location of the haemorrhage. Figures 29.2–29.4 represent some examples of images obtained from cases of rodenticide intoxication
Analytical methods	Used to identify specific anticoagulant rodenticides in serum, plasma, liver, other tissues and bait. High-performance liquid chromatography (HPLC) and gas chromatography–mass spectrometry (GC–MS) methods are the most commonly used. These tests are available in certain veterinary laboratories. The range of compounds tested depends on the institution. Most laboratories detect concentrations as low as parts per billion (ppb) and therefore can detect positive plasma concentrations very early in the course of intoxication. Direct measurement of the toxic compound or its metabolites is the only confirmatory test available

29.7 General tests for the diagnosis of rodenticide toxicity.

Management

Exposure

The mainstay of treatment for dogs and cats with recent (< 6 hours) exposure to anticoagulant rodenticide is decontamination. Although induction of emesis is a controversial practice in human medicine (Green *et al.*, 2008), it has been shown to be of relatively low risk and is considered beneficial in veterinary cases of anticoagulant rodenticide toxicity (Pachtinger *et al.*, 2008). In animals with known rodenticide exposure in which induction of emesis cannot be performed, gastric lavage may be considered. However, gastric lavage is associated with an increased risk of aspiration pneumonia because of the need for sedation, leading to decreases in consciousness and the deglutition reflex. Similar to recommendations in human medicine, activated charcoal should be given to animals with rodenticide intoxication (Peterson and Talcott, 2006).

Induction of emesis

Decreased mentation leading to loss of the gag reflex, increased intracranial pressure, recent abdominal surgery, megaoesophagus, significant cardiac disease or epilepsy are all absolute contraindications to the induction of emesis (Schildt and Jutkowitz, 2008). In addition, if other agents such as hydrocarbons, acids, alkalis, caustic agents or sharp objects were ingested with the rodenticide, emesis should not be induced. If the rodenticide ingestion occurred more than 6 hours prior to presentation, induction of emesis is unlikely to be of any benefit because normal gastric emptying is likely to have occurred and the peak level of absorption of most anticoagulant rodenticides is < 6 hours (Peterson and Talcott, 2006).

In dogs, apomorphine, a centrally active emetic agent, is used most commonly. At 0.015–0.03 mg/kg i.v., apomorphine produces consistent emesis within 15 minutes of administration (Schildt and Jutkowitz, 2008). Alternatively, apomorphine can be administered subcutaneously or intramuscularly at a dose of 0.04–0.1 mg/kg (Plumb, 2005; El Bahri, 2006) although absorption may be slow or unpredictable (Peterson and Talcott, 2006). The subconjunctival tablet form of apomorphine is also available through compounding pharmacies and is similarly effective. Approximately 0.25 mg/kg should be placed in the subconjunctival sac and then flushed out with saline eye wash after emesis has occurred to avoid excessive corneal irritation (Plumb, 2005). The injectable formulation or the tablet dissolved in saline can also be administered into the subconjunctival sac. Most textbooks caution against the use of apomorphine in cats (Plumb, 2005). High doses (2 mg/kg) are associated with hallucinations and fear; however, low dose apomorphine (0.02 mg/kg i.v.) has been suggested as an effective emetic (Peterson and Talcott, 2006).

Alpha$_2$-agonists typically induce vomiting by stimulating the chemoreceptor trigger zone in the early sedative stage. Xylazine induces emesis in as many as 50% of dogs and 90% of cats (Sinclair, 2003). The drug may cause deleterious side effects including bradycardia, dysrhythmias and muscle tremors but these can be minimized by reversing the drug with yohimbine hydrochloride at a dosage of 0.25–0.5 mg/kg once emesis has occurred. The recommended dose of xylazine is 0.44–1.1 mg/kg i.m. or s.c. (Schildt and Jutkowitz, 2008). With medetomidine sedation, vomiting was observed in 8–20% of dogs and up to 90% of cats (Sinclair, 2003). The recommended dosage is provided by the manufacturer in the form of a bodyweight chart. Both agents can be reversed using atipamezole at a dosage of 3750 $\mu g/m^2$ i.v. or 5000 $\mu g/m^2$ i.m.; conversion charts from m^2 to bodyweight are typically available from the manufacturer. For ease of dosing when using atipamezole (typical concentration of 5 mg/ml) to reverse medetomidine (typical concentration of 1 mg/ml), an equal volume (ml for ml) can be administered because it requires 5 mg of atipamezole to reverse 1 mg of medetomidine

Hydrogen peroxide (3%) administered orally at a dose of 1–2 ml/kg is an alternative, albeit less reliable, emetic (Schildt and Jutkowitz, 2008). Because of its low cost and wide availability it can easily be used at home by owners. Its emetic property is mediated by gastric irritation. Therefore, repeated administration can lead to mucosal irritation, ulceration and ptyalism. Any recommendation for home induction of emesis should be accompanied by a clear explanation of the contraindications and risks of inducing emesis and should not delay veterinary care.

Syrup of ipecacuanha ('ipecac') is derived from the roots of certain plants and is composed mainly of two alkaloids: emetine and cephaeline. Emesis is mediated by gastric irritation and stimulation of the chemoreceptor triggering zone. It has unreliable effects in dogs and may cause prolonged vomiting, delaying the administration of activated charcoal (Schildt and Jutkowitz, 2008). Additional side effects include diarrhoea, drowsiness and cardiotoxicity. Given the potential hazards and the availability of more effective agents, syrup of ipecacuanha is not recommended.

Activated charcoal

Activated charcoal is an absorptive compound with a large surface area that absorbs multiple toxins and allows their elimination via defecation. It is often combined with a cathartic to hasten elimination. If activated charcoal remains in the bowel for an extended period of time, release of the toxin and subsequent systemic absorption is possible. Some animals swallow activated charcoal preparations willingly, but food can be added to it to increase palatability (Figure 29.8). Activated charcoal can also be administered orally via a syringe in compliant animals, but extra care must be taken to avoid aspiration because it can lead to severe osmotic and chemical pneumonitis (Schildt and Jutkowitz, 2008). The recommended dose of activated charcoal is 2–8 g/kg. Repeated dosing every 4–8 hours may be beneficial because anticoagulant rodenticides undergo enterohepatic recirculation. Excessive administration of activated charcoal may cause diarrhoea, leading to metabolic abnormalities such as acidosis from bicarbonate loss. Formulations that include a cathartic may predispose to hypernatraemia as a result of unreplaced free water loss (Allerton and Strom, 1991).

29.8 Administration of activated charcoal in food.

Long-term management

There are two potential approaches to long-term therapy following anticoagulant rodenticide exposure, either empirical vitamin K_1 therapy or assessment of coagulation defects at 48 hours and administration of vitamin K_1 in cases with confirmed coagulation defects. The most common strategy is to provide empirical vitamin K_1 therapy. It should be administered at a dose of 2.5 mg/kg orally q12h for 4–6 weeks, depending on the type of rodenticide (Plumb, 2005). Given that vitamin K_1 is lipophilic, it should be administered with a small meal to maximize its absorption. This approach requires compliance by the owner and can be expensive, depending on the size of the dog. A prothrombin time (PT) test 48 hours after completion of the course of vitamin K_1 is recommended to determine whether continued treatment with vitamin K_1 is required.

In the second approach to anticoagulant rodenticide exposure, vitamin K therapy is delayed until confirmation of intoxication. Decontamination using an emetic agent and/or activated charcoal is still recommended if the ingestion occurred less than 6 hours before presentation. The animal is then discharged without administration of vitamin K_1. A PT test is performed approximately 48 hours after decontamination to assess for coagulopathy. If the PT is prolonged by > 25%, vitamin K therapy should be instituted. If the PT is mildly prolonged (i.e. < 25%), it should be repeated 24 hours later. In a retrospective study evaluating this approach, only 7.3% of 151 dogs required vitamin K_1 treatment (Pachtinger *et al.*, 2008). The safety of this approach relies on the fact that FVII is depleted at 48 hours, causing a prolonged PT time, but other factors are not yet affected, so clinical bleeding typically does not occur until 3.5 to 5 days after ingestion. The depletion of FII (prothrombin) takes approximately 3.5 days and this is the factor thought to be associated with the onset of clinical signs (Woody *et al.*, 1992). Of all the dogs with a prolonged PT time at the 48 hour re-examination, no dog had clinical signs of bleeding at the time of the testing. This strategy allows vitamin K_1 therapy to be used only in patients that require treatment and before the onset of clinical signs.

Intoxication

Critical care

In patients with haemorrhage, stabilizing treatments are most important. Vital signs (i.e. heart rate, respiratory rate, mucous membrane colour, capillary refill time and temperature), blood pressure, venous lactate and pulse oximetry can help determine the need for crystalloids and colloids. Oxygen therapy

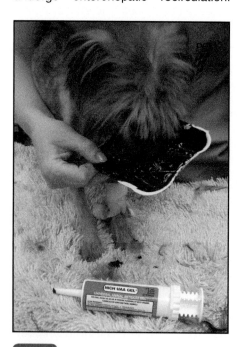

can be provided with flow-by mask or oxygen cage; however, the most important factor in determining oxygen delivery will be the level of haemoglobin. Packed red blood cells may be necessary for patients with evidence of clinical hypoxaemia from anaemia or for a patient in haemorrhagic shock (anaemia, hypoxaemia, hypotension, tachycardia, tachypnoea and lactic acidosis).

Aggressive treatment of the coagulopathy is warranted in these patients. Vitamin K_1 should be administered subcutaneously at a dose of 2.5 mg/kg q12h for the first 24–48 hours. The intramuscular route should be avoided because of the risk of haemorrhage, and the intravenous route should be avoided because of the risk of anaphylactic reactions (recommendations developed in the USA). Transfusion of fresh frozen plasma (FFP) is indicated because production of new coagulation factors will not occur until approximately 6 hours after the initiation of vitamin K_1 therapy and because persistent haemorrhage causes consumption of coagulation factors. The recommended dose of FFP is 10 ml/kg over a 4–6-hour period. The frequency of blood product transfusion should be based on the patient's packed cell volume and coagulation times. It is often necessary to transfuse with FFP every 6–8 hours (Brown and Waddell, 2008). In dogs that have received prior transfusions of red blood cell products, a cross-match should be performed to confirm compatibility between the donor and the recipient. In naïve patients, blood typing (for at least DEA 1.1) is ideal before any transfusion. If blood typing is not available, transfusion of DEA 1.1-negative blood is recommended in dogs. Because of the severe lethal anaphylactic reaction with incompatible transfusion in cats, blood typing is imperative (see Chapters 34 and 35).

In patients with cavitary bleeding, centesis should only be done in life-threatening conditions (i.e. pleural haemorrhage with impaired ventilation or pericardial haemorrhage with severe cardiovascular impairment), because of the risk of worsening haemorrhage following the procedure. Typically, peritoneal haemorrhage does not require abdominocentesis. Moreover, allowing protein reabsorption via lymphatic drainage is beneficial for subsequent management.

Care should be taken when handling patients with coagulopathies. Trauma and restraint should be minimized, as should subcutaneous injections and venepuncture of large vessels such as the jugular vein.

Prognosis

Exposure

Patients with witnessed ingestion treated by decontamination followed by activated charcoal have an excellent prognosis and very few animals require vitamin K therapy (Pachtinger *et al.*, 2008).

Intoxication

The prognosis for asymptomatic patients treated adequately with a proper course of vitamin K is typically excellent. The prognosis for symptomatic patients is usually good to excellent with appropriate treatment. However, patients with pulmonary, cerebral, intracranial or spinal haemorrhage have a worse prognosis. The cost for adequate treatment is variable and depends on the need for blood product transfusions.

References and further reading

Allerton JP and Strom JA (1991) Hypernatremia due to repeated doses of charcoal-sorbitol. *American Journal of Kidney Diseases* **17**, 581–584

Berny P, Caloni F, Croubels S *et al.* (2010) Animal poisoning in Europe. Part 2: Companion animals. *The Veterinary Journal* **183**, 255–259

Brown AJ and Waddell LS (2008) Rodenticides. In: *Small Animal Critical Care Medicine*, ed. D Silverstein and K Hopper, pp. 346–350. Saunders, St Louis

El Bahri L (2006) Pharm profile: Apomorphine. *Compendium on Continuing Education for the Practicing Veterinarian* **28**, 653–657

Gaston LW and Spivack AR (1968) Preparation of canine factor VII deficient substrate plasma. *The Journal of Laboratory and Clinical Medicine* **72**, 548–555

Green S, Harris C and Singer J (2008) Gastrointestinal decontamination of the poisoned patient. *Pediatric Emergency Care* **24**, 176–189

Hellemans J, Vorlat M and Verstraete M (1963) Survival time of prothrombin and factors VII, IX and X after completely synthesis blocking dose of coumarin derivatives. *British Journal of Haematology* **9**, 506–512

Kohn B, Weingart C and Giger U (2003) Haemorrhage in seven cats with suspected anticoagulant rodenticide intoxication. *Journal of Feline Medicine and Surgery* **5**, 295–304

Pachtinger GE, Otto CM and Syring RS (2008) Incidence of prolonged prothrombin time in dogs following gastrointestinal decontamination for acute anticoagulant rodenticide ingestion. *Journal of Veterinary Emergency and Critical Care* **22**, 285–291

Peterson ME and Talcott PA (2006) *Small Animal* Toxicology, pp.131 and 563–577. Saunders, Philadelphia

Plumb DC (2005) *Plumb's Veterinary Drug Handbook.* Blackwell, Ames

Schildt JC and Jutkowitz LA (2008) Approach to poisoning and drug overdose. In: *Small Animal Critical Care Medicine*, ed. D Silverstein and K Hopper, pp. 326–329. Saunders, St Louis

Sinclair MD (2003) A review of the physiological effects of α_2-agonists related to the clinical use of medetomidine in small animal practice. *Canadian Veterinary Journal* **44**, 885–897

Woody BJ, Murphy MJ and Ray AC (1992) Coagulopathic effects and therapy of brodifacoum toxicosis in dogs. *Journal of Veterinary Internal Medicine* **6**, 23–28

30

Disseminated intravascular coagulation

Bo Wiinberg and Annemarie T. Kristensen

Introduction

Disseminated intravascular coagulation (DIC) is a complicated and dynamic haemostatic syndrome characterized by simultaneous variable imbalances of several components of the haemostatic system. Consequently, the clinical signs vary from none to overt signs of bleeding, and DIC may be chronic and compensated (non-overt) or acute and uncompensated (overt), with compromised haemostasis, characterized by severe hypotension and multiple organ failure. Until now, the diagnosis in veterinary medicine has not been standardized and no laboratory tests have been available to predict the response to treatment in patients with DIC, and therefore the diagnosis is often uncertain and treatment has largely remained empirical.

Aetiology of DIC

DIC always occurs secondary to an underlying disease, which causes an uncontrolled systemic inflammatory response. The initiating event may be procoagulant (e.g. circulating thrombin or tissue factor), profibrinolytic (e.g. circulating plasmin), or a direct enzymatic activation (e.g. toxicity). DIC is associated with a wide variety of disorders and aetiologies such as obstetrical complications, intravascular haemolysis, sepsis, viraemia, burns, trauma, vascular disease and malignancies, in particular secondary to distant metastasis. The majority of these diseases activate coagulation either by producing endogenous tissue factor (TF) directly, which interacts with factor (F)VII, or alternatively by causing endothelial damage with secondary release or exposure of TF to the circulating blood.

Pathophysiology

Examination of the evolutionary tree gives a hint that the haemostatic and inflammatory systems are perhaps related more intricately than might be perceived at first glance. In some invertebrates, clotting and inflammation are mediated by a single cell system, the haemocyte, and the haemopoietic stem cells are located in the lymph nodes. Moving up the evolutionary ladder to the horseshoe crab (*Limulus polyphemus*), clotting is initiated by endotoxin, which causes the blood corpuscles to aggregate. In the last decade it has become increasingly clear that inflammation and haemostasis are also intricately linked in vertebrates, and that both systems play vital roles in host defence. Thus cells and inflammatory mediators of the immune system are capable of triggering coagulation pathways, and coagulation proteases, on the other hand, have significant immunomodulatory effects, and this cross-talk between haemostasis and inflammation is essential in the progression of DIC.

The pathophysiology of DIC is summarized in Figure 30.1. The *in vivo* activation of coagulation is triggered by the binding of FVIIa to exposed TF, which is expressed constitutively on the adventitial cells and pericytes surrounding the blood vessels. Tissue injury that disrupts the endothelial lining of the vessels is normally needed to activate coagulation. However, in inflammatory or pathological states, monocytes, endothelium and perhaps even platelets can be stimulated to express TF. The binding of TF to FVIIa and FXa in turn initiates intracellular signal transduction pathways, which induce the production of transcription factors necessary for the synthesis of adhesion proteins, proinflammatory cytokines and growth factors.

The activation of coagulation through endothelial damage, tissue damage or platelet/erythrocyte damage ultimately leads to increased thrombin formation. Thrombin cleaves fibrinopeptides A and B from fibrinogen, which is thus transformed to active fibrin monomers. Initially the effect of thrombin is limited by endogenous anticoagulants, such as antithrombin (AT) or protein C (PC). However with massive activation of thrombin, the endogenous anticoagulants are quickly consumed, and the ensuing systemic activation of thrombin leads to widespread fibrin polymerization with subsequent micro- and macrovascular thrombosis, which impedes blood flow and ultimately leads to ischaemia with further tissue and/or organ damage. As the fibrin is deposited in the microvasculature, it also traps platelets in the developing clot, leading to consumption of circulating platelets and eventually thrombocytopenia. Through the activation of FXIIa, prekallikrein is activated to kallikrein, which cleaves plasminogen, resulting in free plasmin. Plasmin effectively breaks down several clotting factors and leads to an increase in circulating fibrin degradation products (FDPs) and D-dimer fragments from the

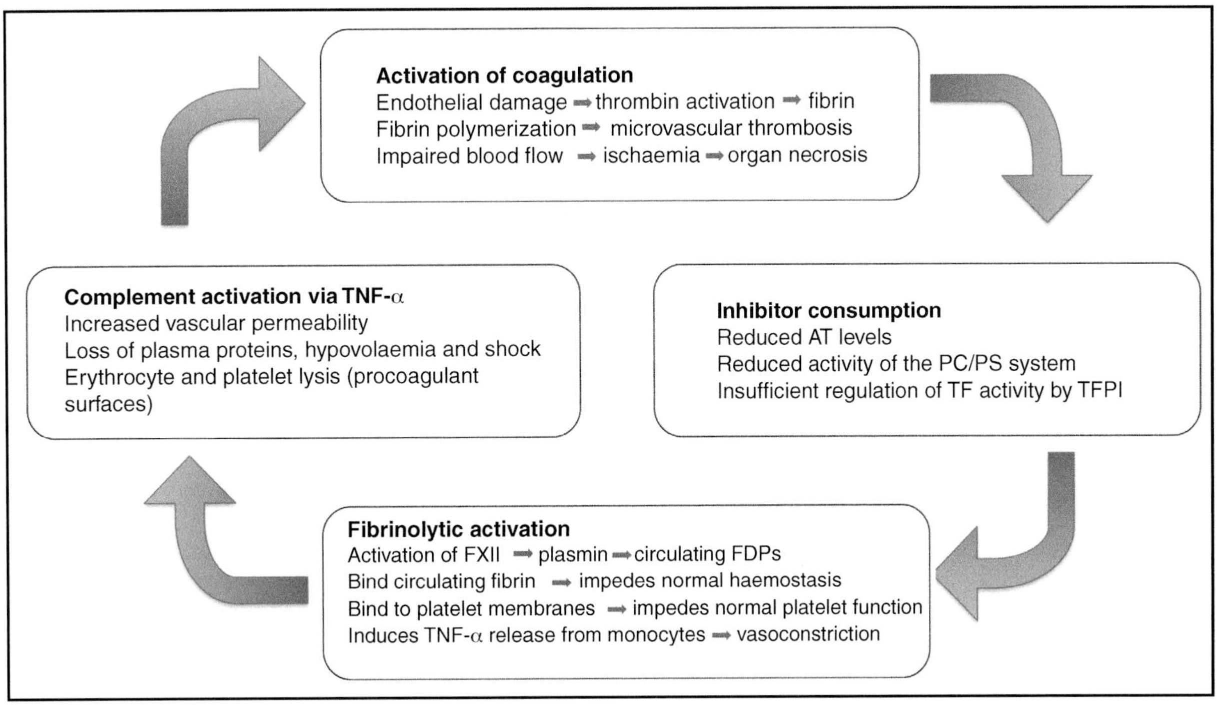

Activation of coagulation
Endothelial damage → thrombin activation → fibrin
Fibrin polymerization → microvascular thrombosis
Impaired blood flow → ischaemia → organ necrosis
Complement activation via TNF-α
Increased vascular permeability
Loss of plasma proteins, hypovolaemia and shock
Erythrocyte and platelet lysis (procoagulant surfaces)
Inhibitor consumption
Reduced AT levels
Reduced activity of the PC/PS system
Insufficient regulation of TF activity by TFPI
Fibrinolytic activation
Activation of FXII → plasmin → circulating FDPs
Bind circulating fibrin → impedes normal haemostasis
Bind to platelet membranes → impedes normal platelet function
Induces TNF-α release from monocytes → vasoconstriction

30.1 Pathophysiology of disseminated intravascular coagulation (DIC) as proposed by Bick (2003). AT, antithrombin; FDPs, fibrin degradation products; PC, protein C; PS, protein S; TF, tissue factor; TFPI, tissue factor pathway inhibitor; TNF-α, tumour necrosis factor-α.

cleavage of fibrinogen and fibrin. The resulting FDPs can bind circulating fibrin directly before it is able to polymerize, and thus they potentially disrupt normal haemostasis, which can lead to an overt coagulopathy. Furthermore, the D and E fragments from cross-linked fibrin degradation have high affinity for platelet membranes, to which they bind and cause platelet functional defects, which may attenuate the abnormal coagulation function further and exacerbate clinical haemorrhage.

To complicate matters further, FDPs and thrombin induce release of the pro-inflammatory cytokines interleukin (IL)-1, IL-6 and tumour necrosis factor (TNF)-α from monocytes. These cytokines in turn activate, among others, thrombomodulin, selectin, and importantly endothelin, which causes vasospasm, vasoconstriction, and ultimately contributes to vascular occlusion, ischaemia and organ damage. The IL-1 and TNF-α also induce up-regulation of TF on monocytes and neutrophils, which leads to further activation of coagulation. Monocyte and neutrophil recruitment and expression of TF in inflammation is further up-regulated via interaction with P-selectin expressed on the surface of activated platelets. The increase in circulating TNF-α also leads to complement activation, which results in erythrocyte and platelet lysis with subsequent release of cell membrane phospholipids and procoagulant surfaces for further propagation of coagulation. The activation of the complement system increases vascular permeability, leading to further loss of plasma proteins, and to hypotension and shock. The increased vascular permeability is attenuated by the kinin system, which is activated by kallikrein simultaneously with cleavage of plasminogen, which all leads to increased endothelial and tissue damage, exposure of collagen and TF, with further activation of FXII, and thus a 'vicious circle' develops.

It is evident that DIC is driven by a massive activation of thrombin, stimulated by inflammation, which causes fibrin deposition and microvascular thrombosis with concurrent consumption of coagulation factors and entrapment of platelets. As a normal defence mechanism, plasmin is activated, which in this situation leads to a detrimental rise in circulating FDPs. The result is inhibition of fibrin polymerization and defective platelet function, which both increase the risk of haemorrhage. With this complex and unpredictable series of events in mind, it is easy to understand why many patients experience both thrombosis and haemorrhage and to appreciate the clinical challenges in diagnosing and treating DIC.

Biomarkers

The highly intricate and variable pathophysiology of DIC, partly caused by the large variability in the initiating disorders, together with the unpredictability of the host response, often results in a lack of consistency in clinical manifestations of DIC. Consequently there has been a lack of consensus on the specific approach to the diagnosis of DIC, and a lack of specific evidence-based therapeutic modalities.

In an attempt to standardize the diagnosis, Roger L. Bick has defined the minimal criteria for the diagnosis of DIC in humans (Bick, 2003). Bick defines DIC as a systemic thrombohaemorrhagic disorder, seen in association with well defined clinical situations in patients suffering from an underlying disease known to predispose to DIC. Furthermore the following four criteria must be satisfied:

- Laboratory evidence of procoagulant activation
- Laboratory evidence of fibrinolytic activation
- Laboratory evidence of inhibitor consumption
- Biochemical evidence of organ damage or failure.

The laboratory assays that provide evidence of these criteria are listed in Figure 30.2 and discussed briefly below.

Procoagulant activation
• PT • aPTT • Platelet count • TAT • D-dimer • Prothrombin fragment 1+2
Fibrinolytic activation
• D-dimer • FDP • Plasmin • Plasminogen
Inhibitor consumption
• AT • PC • PS • α_2-antiplasmin • TAT

30.2 Examples of assays available in veterinary medicine for the diagnosis of disseminated intravascular coagulation (DIC). aPTT, activated partial thromboplastin time; AT, antithrombin; FDPs, fibrin degradation products; PC, protein C; PS, protein S; PT, prothrombin time; TAT, thrombin antithrombin; TFPI, tissue factor pathway inhibitor.

Evidence of procoagulant activation

The prothrombin time (PT) is prolonged in only 50–75% of dogs with DIC. Thus the PT is normal in up to 50% of affected dogs, and therefore it is an unreliable solitary marker for DIC. The reason for the normal PT in many patients with DIC is probably related to the circulation of elevated amounts of activated thrombin or FXa.

As mentioned previously, plasmin degrades coagulation factors (FV, FVIII, FIX and FXI), which can cause the activated partial thromboplastin time (aPTT) to be prolonged. Furthermore the aPTT is prolonged when fibrinogen is below 1 g/l and may be inhibited by FDP inhibition of fibrin polymerization. In spite of all these factors affecting aPTT, in addition to ongoing consumption of coagulation factors, the aPTT is prolonged in only about 50–60% of canine patients with DIC. Furthermore, the aPTT can be prolonged in patients without any identifiable reason other than systemic inflammation, which means that it can be tricky to identify the precise cause. A plausible explanation for the low efficacy of aPTT as a test of global haemostatic capability may be that the assay was designed originally for a completely different purpose, namely as a screening tool for the identification of patients with haemophilia.

The platelet count is usually decreased to a variable extent in dogs with DIC, and studies in humans have shown that platelet function tests are often abnormal, probably due to FDP coating platelet membranes. Increased platelet turnover, with decreased survival, is normal in patients with DIC. A falling trend in combination with an absolute platelet count is much more useful than a fixed cut-off value alone, because a platelet count that is decreasing over time in a patient with normal bone marrow activity is indicative of increased consumption of platelets, even though the absolute count may still be within the normal range.

Immunoassays for prothrombin fragment 1+2 provide a specific measure of thrombin generation and offer potential value in detecting activation of the coagulation system and in monitoring anticoagulant therapy.

Platelet factor 4 (PF4) is a small protein released from the alpha-granules of blood platelets, which binds strongly to and neutralizes the anticoagulant properties of heparin. PF4 is an interesting marker, because it is indicative of increased platelet activity; however, it is not specific for DIC and may be elevated in human patients with pulmonary thromboembolism (PTE), deep vein thrombosis (DVT) or myocardial infarction. The use of PF4 as a marker for the effect of treatment may be feasible, because PF4 activity will decrease if antithrombotic treatment is effective in stopping the intravascular clotting process.

Evidence of increased fibrinolytic activity

FDPs/D-dimers have mainly negative predictive value in thromboembolic disease. They are indicative of increased plasmin activity, but are non-specific for thromboembolic disease. They are elevated in 80–100% of dogs with DIC, but may also be elevated for many reasons other than thromboembolic disease.

Specific molecular markers of fibrinolysis are present in patients with thrombosis or DIC. Tests for these markers are available commercially but, except for D-dimer and FDP, they are not commonly used clinically. Such tests include quantification of plasminogen, α_2-anti-plasmin, plasmin–antiplasmin complexes (PAP) and plasmin activator inhibitor-1. When fibrinolysis is activated, plasminogen levels may decrease as plasminogen is converted into plasmin. As plasmin degrades fibrin, FDP and D-dimers are formed. As plasmin is formed, antiplasmin binds to plasmin, forming a plasmin–anti-plasmin (PAP) complex, which thereby inhibits plasmin in order to prevent excessive fibrinolysis.

Evidence of inhibitor consumption

Antithrombin (AT), protein C (PC), protein S (PS) and tissue factor pathway inhibitor (TFPI) are the most commonly used markers of endogenous inhibitor consumption. As thrombin is formed, AT binds to thrombin to form a thrombin–antithrombin complex (TAT), which thereby inhibits thrombin in order to prevent excessive clotting. In many studies, AT is perceived to be a very important marker for DIC because, in DIC, circulating AT is bound by thrombin and activated clotting factors, which results in the measurable AT activity being significantly decreased. In general, there is a close correlation between AT and TAT; however, situations have been described in which increased levels of TAT complexes were not associated with decreased AT activity in DIC, and TAT is perhaps a more direct measure of AT anticoagulant activity than AT levels measured directly.

Diagnosis

In the last decade the International Society of Thrombosis and Haemostasis (ISTH), through the Scientific and Standardization Committee on DIC, has used Bick's theory to develop a practical diagnostic approach for the diagnosis of DIC in human patients. The work of the ISTH committee was based on the assumption that DIC is characterized by the generation of fibrin-related products and that it is associated with an acquired disorder of the microvasculature. Based on this, simple diagnostic models for the diagnosis of overt and non-overt DIC in human patients have been developed. With the lack of a gold standard, these diagnostic algorithms have been based on consensus statements (Taylor *et al.*, 2001). Prospective evaluations of the scoring systems are ongoing, and because post-mortem fibrinolysis makes necropsy an insensitive diagnostic criterion, these studies use a broad panel of analyses of haemostasis proposed by Bick as the gold standard. Initial pilot studies evaluating the sensitivity and specificity of these scoring systems have shown promising results.

There is general agreement in veterinary medicine that DIC should be diagnosed only if a patient is suffering from a disease known to predispose to DIC, such as systemic infection (bacterial sepsis, viraemia, parasitic infection), cancer, immune-mediated haemolytic anaemia, pancreatitis, shock or massive traumatic injuries. However, the laboratory diagnosis of DIC in dogs and cats is non-standardized, and the haemostatic function tests used in veterinary medicine are not consistent. The diagnosis of DIC in animals is therefore currently based on clinical findings, including petechiae, haematomas, wound bleeding, acral cyanosis, gangrene, fever, hypotension, hypoxia, acidosis and proteinuria. It is important to note that many of these clinical signs do not present until the late stages of DIC. Establishment of a definitive diagnosis is based further on the compilation of a variable number of abnormal haemostatic laboratory test results. Most veterinary studies have used the diagnostic criterion 'any three or more abnormal coagulation parameters equals DIC'. The core problem with such a diagnostic approach is that, although it may be sensitive, it is entirely non-specific for the diagnosis of a complex syndrome such as DIC. Non-specific diagnosis makes it impossible to standardize diagnosis, monitoring or treatment, or to conduct clinical studies to improve the outcome of animals with DIC.

Tests

Although there is a trend in the panel of tests used to diagnose DIC in these studies, there is currently no consensus on the minimal diagnostic criteria in veterinary medicine. The lack of consensus is especially evident when it comes to the early diagnosis of non-overt DIC, and few prospective veterinary studies have sought to establish criteria similar to those defined by the ISTH for human DIC. Several veterinary studies have evaluated the prognostic value of single tests, such as aPTT, PT, fibrinogen, D-dimers/FDPs, erythrocyte morphology and platelet count. The aPTT and PT have been used in most studies, but there has been some inconsistency in whether prolongation should be measured as a ratio or an absolute number. Several studies have confirmed that PT is the more sensitive of the two tests in diagnosing DIC. Some studies have measured prolongation in absolute terms, but given that the test result depends on the assay and type of activator used, the assessment of test results is probably more accurate if they are evaluated as a relative increase compared with the reference population, as with the human international normalization ratio (INR) standard.

Plasma levels of fibrinogen are increased in the early stages of the inflammatory response. During long periods of inflammation, fibrinogen stores are depleted and the concentration of circulating plasma fibrinogen may become lower than normal. Consequently, dogs with DIC may have either high or low plasma fibrinogen levels, depending on the time point of measurement. Given that they are degradation products from the breakdown of fibrin, FDPs theoretically should be increased in patients with DIC. However, because fibrinogen is an acute phase reactant, FDPs may be increased as a consequence of any inflammatory state, and several studies have shown that an increase in FDPs alone is a poor marker for DIC. D-dimers are probably the single most accurate marker of DIC. The test is very sensitive when used to detect thromboembolic disease and breakdown of microthrombi, but unfortunately is not very specific. Fragmentation of erythrocytes (schistocytes) may be indicative of fibrin deposition in the microvasculature, but altered erythrocyte morphology in the presence of a low platelet count has been found to be non-specific for DIC in dogs, although many studies have used low platelet counts as a criterion for the diagnosis of DIC, because platelets are consumed in the hypercoagulable state of the disease. Measurement of AT has had limited use in veterinary medicine until now, but it has been shown to be very useful for determination of fibrinolytic activity. Measurement of protein

C was used in one study, but PS and TAT have not been used thus far in the diagnosis of DIC in veterinary medicine.

Standardization

Consensus on the diagnostic criteria for DIC would provide an important basis for optimization of treatment in dogs, and would make it possible to conduct multi-centre therapeutic studies with the minimum risk of systematic misclassification of patients. Furthermore, early diagnosis of DIC would facilitate prompt and precise treatment and increase the chance of survival.

Recent veterinary studies have attempted to standardize the diagnosis of DIC in dogs, using comparable methods to those used in human medicine. The first study attempted to establish whether the diagnosis of DIC in dogs could be approached on the basis of the ISTH criteria for diagnosis in human patients, and also aimed to establish which coagulation assay should or could be used for such a diagnostic approach (Wiinberg *et al.*, 2010). The objectives of the study were: to develop a simple, sensitive and specific diagnostic model for canine DIC based on the ISTH diagnostic criteria; and to validate the model prospectively in an independent population of dogs in order to assess its diagnostic accuracy. To develop the scoring system, 100 dogs admitted consecutively to an intensive care unit (ICU) with diseases predisposing to DIC were enrolled prospectively (Group A). The validation involved 50 dogs diagnosed consecutively with diseases predisposing to DIC that were admitted to a different ICU (Group B). The final diagnostic model was based on aPTT, PT, D-dimers and fibrinogen, but, surprisingly, not platelet count. The model had a diagnostic sensitivity and specificity of 90.9% and 90.0%, respectively. The diagnostic accuracy of the model was sustained in the prospective evaluation in Group B (sensitivity 83.3%, specificity 77.3%).

This study demonstrates that it is possible to design an objective diagnostic model for canine DIC based on generally available assays. The results suggest further that it is possible to develop a scoring algorithm for the diagnosis of DIC in dogs which is standardized and superior to the current non-specific approach to diagnosis in veterinary medicine. With further validation, this model could make it possible to conduct multi-centre therapeutic studies with less misclassification of canine patients, and to optimize the treatment of canine DIC.

Tissue factor-activated thromboelastography

Owing to the considerable variation in the coagulation profile in DIC, it is difficult to assess the overall haemostatic capability of a dog or cat and to choose appropriate therapy. A recent veterinary study attempted to resolve this issue by characterizing the overall haemostatic state in dogs with DIC (Wiinberg *et al.*, 2008). Tissue factor-activated thromboelastography (TF-TEG) was used to separate 50 dogs diagnosed with DIC into three subgroups: hypocoaguability, normal coagulability, and hypercoagulability. The diagnosis of DIC was based on the evaluation of an extended coagulation panel by three human medical and veterinary experts. Haemostatic dysfunction was observed on the TF-TEG profile in 33/50 of the dogs. Of the 50 dogs, 22 showed hypercoagulability, whereas only 11/50 showed hypocoagulability based on the TF-TEG G value alone. The TEG G value is a measure of total clot strength and it is calculated with the formula: $G = (5000 \times MA)/(100 - MA)$. There were significant differences in k, α and MA values (see Chapter 22) between dogs with normal coagulability and those with hypo- and hypercoagulability, and there was a significant difference in mortality rate between dogs with hypo- (64%) and hypercoagulability (32%) (relative risk = 2.2). Dogs that died also had significantly lower AT and higher D-dimer values than the dogs that survived, indicating that these dogs may have been prothrombotic. The conclusion of the study was that TF-TEG documented, for the first time, that the most common overall haemostatic abnormality in dogs diagnosed with DIC is hypercoagulability and that there is a significant difference in survival between dogs with hyper- and hypocoagulability. The results of the study suggest that TF-TEG is valuable in the assessment of overall haemostatic function in dogs diagnosed with DIC.

Treatment

Routine therapies

The optimum treatment of DIC is poorly defined and occasionally even controversial. There is also a common misconception that treatment is futile and that the patient will die irrespective of treatment. However, this is incorrect and is probably due to the lack of published studies on the therapy, morbidity and mortality of animals with DIC. Difficulties in selecting an appropriate therapy often arise as a result of the diverse aetiologies and clinical manifestations of DIC. This means that a certain therapeutic approach may be suitable for one type of aetiology, but not for another, and a certain therapy may be suitable for haemorrhage but not thrombosis. Often, the treatment is based on expert opinion, and the use of heparin is an excellent example of this. Some clinicians will give heparin in every case, even though there is no objective scientific evidence to support its beneficial effect, while other clinicians strongly discourage the use of heparin although there is also no documentation of adverse effects.

A logical approach to the treatment of DIC (Figure 30.3) involves five components:

- Individualize treatment
- Treat/remove the underlying cause
- Stop any intravascular clotting process
- Use blood component therapy as indicated
- Inhibit/reverse residual fibrinolysis.

Individualized treatment

It is clear from an understanding of the complex

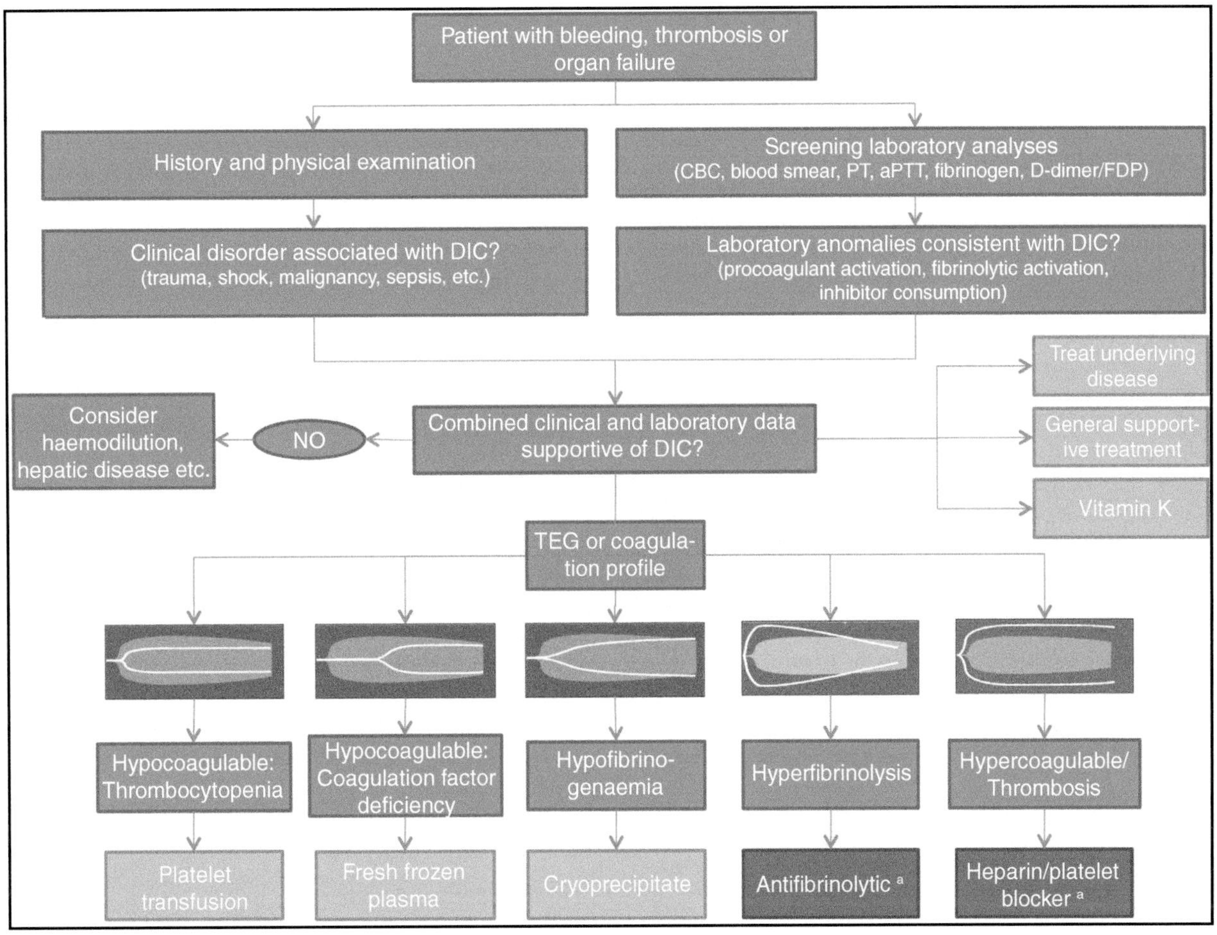

30.3 Diagnostic and therapeutic decision tree for patients with disseminated intravascular coagulation (DIC). aPTT, activated partial thromboplastin time; AT, antithrombin; CBC, complete blood count; FDP, fibrin degradation products; PT, prothrombin time; TEG, thromboelastography. [a] Controversial treatment.

aetiology, pathophysiology and diverse clinical picture that therapy must be individualized, logical and aggressive if it is to be successful.

Treating the underlying cause

Early intervention is needed for the effective treatment of patients with DIC and it is essential that the underlying cause is treated aggressively, because DIC is likely to persist until the initiating cause is eliminated. This treatment often involves shock therapy, fluid resuscitation, maintenance of blood pressure, surgery, antibiotics, chemotherapy, etc.

Clot prevention

Treatment to stop clotting includes administration of unfractionated heparin, low molecular weight heparin, anti-platelet drugs (e.g. aspirin) or antithrombin. Heparin is the drug used most commonly for the prevention and treatment of acute thromboembolic diseases. Heparin can prevent venous thromboembolism in patients with trauma, and consequently it might be hypothesized that it would also be suitable as a prophylactic agent against DIC. Heparin has been shown partly to inhibit activation of coagulation in DIC through increased release of TFPI from endothelial cells, and to increase TFPI gene expression. In human trials with both fractionated and unfractionated heparin, both were shown to: decrease activation of coagulation significantly; reduce prothrombin fragment 1+2 and polymerized fibrin; decrease the number of monocytes expressing TF; and increase plasma TFPI values after infusion of lipopolysaccharide (LPS), compared with a placebo group. There is, however, no documented evidence for the effectiveness of heparin with regard to survival, and it is doubtful whether heparin has a positive effect on clinically diagnosed DIC. In some cases, especially in patients with sepsis, heparin may even aggravate DIC and multiple organ dysfunction syndrome (MODS). This was illustrated in a model of sepsis using caecal ligation and puncture in rats, where heparin infusion caused an increase in mortality from 13% in the placebo group to 75% in the heparin group. An additional problem is that heparin increases the risk of severe bleeding in cases of DIC. In human patients it has been demonstrated that the administration of small doses of heparin to patients with DIC worsens thrombocytopenia, increases AT consumption and increases the bleeding tendency. Heparin should be avoided during AT replacement, in order to permit AT to modulate sepsis-induced inflammatory responses. As mentioned, heparin should be used with extreme caution in patients with DIC. The treatment is not evidence based, and both dosage ranges and methods vary widely depending on the clinician/author. The suggested dosage of unfractionated heparin (UFH) is 50–100 IU/kg s.c. q6–8h. The dose should start low and should be increased until aPTT measured 3 hours after injection is prolonged to 1.5–2 times the normal range. Treatment with UFH must be tapered over 48 hours to avoid rebound hypercoagulability. The suggested dosage of the low molecular weight heparin (LMWH) dalteparin is 150 IU/kg s.c. q8h. Treatment with LMWH cannot be monitored with aPTT, but the risk of adverse bleeding is lower than for UFH and the treatment does not need to be tapered.

Blood component therapy

While treating the underlying disease, supportive therapy is instituted to accommodate the acute need to maintain normal haemostatic capability in the patient. Traditionally this is achieved through transfusion with fresh frozen plasma (FFP), with the intent of administering protease inhibitors and other endogenous substances contained in plasma that have inhibitory effects on the haemostatic and inflammatory processes. However, substances that have an enhancing effect on these processes are also included in FFP and consequently there is a risk of an exacerbation rather than an improvement in the condition of the patient. Erythrocyte transfusions are given in cases of anaemia, and the use of platelet concentrates is warranted if there is evidence of marked thrombocytopenia and increased bleeding tendency. It is believed by some that the lack of platelets and coagulation factors in patients with DIC contributes to the slowing down of the thrombotic process, and as such, may be considered a favourable reaction to hyperactivation of the haemostatic system. Administration of these haemostatic components should therefore be reserved for cases in which there are reasonable reasons to assume that serious bleeding complications can arise.

Reverse residual fibrinolysis

Anti-fibrinolytics should generally be avoided in cases of DIC, because they impede the breakdown of microthrombi, thus increasing the risk of MODS. The use of anti-fibrinolytic drugs to treat DIC is therefore only justified in cases of acute DIC with a marked bleeding tendency caused by documented high fibrinolytic activity, such as may be seen on TEG analysis.

Novel therapies

With the knowledge that thrombin and the endothelium play key roles in the evolution of DIC, drugs that modulate these components have received growing attention in recent years.

Antithrombin

AT is a natural anticoagulant that is present in plasma and on the surface of the endothelium. It has anti-inflammatory effects, and studies have shown that low levels of AT have a negative effect on the prognosis of patients with sepsis and DIC. Animal experiments and a number of small clinical trials have demonstrated a beneficial effect of AT in DIC, in humans, rats and baboons. The aims of the clinical trials have primarily been to clarify whether AT can counteract hypercoagulability and intravascular fibrin formation. AT modulates the interaction between endothelial cells and leucocytes by reducing leucocyte activation and adhesion. It stimulates the release of prostacyclin from endothelial cells, reduces platelet aggregation and decreases proinflammatory cytokine production. AT also directly inhibits the release of IL-6 and the expression of TF by endothelial cells. Interestingly, AT must bind to glycosaminoglycan (GAG) on leucocytes or endothelium in order to exert its anticoagulant and anti-inflammatory effects. In patients with sepsis and DIC, AT substitution prevents MODS. Meta-analysis of these studies suggests that AT treatment may reduce mortality if concomitant treatment with heparin is avoided. This creates a dilemma for the clinician who is treating a patient with heparin in order to maximize the anticoagulant effects of AT, because in doing so, the potentially important anti-inflammatory effects of AT may be lost. Animal studies have shown that high plasma AT concentrations are needed to obtain an optimal effect, and consequently a number of clinical studies have aimed to achieve plasma concentrations of 120–200% of normal.

Tissue factor inhibitors

Inhibitors of TF have been examined in trials involving patients with sepsis, which have shown that infusion of TFPI inhibits the activation of coagulation successfully and completely, but fails to influence leucocyte activation, chemokine release, endothelial activation or the acute phase response. The results indicate that inhibition of coagulation by TFPI does not affect the activation of inflammation in patients with endotoxaemia, and although preliminary trials have been promising, treatment with TFPI has yet to be proven to have a positive effect on outcome. Given that TFPI only inhibits the binding of FXa to the TF/FVIIa complex, the results indicate that the TF/FVIIa complex alone might be sufficient for activation of intracellular signalling pathways that activate inflammation. Therefore an alternative is to block the surface receptor of TF completely with innate FVIIa or an antibody against TF. Such an approach has been tried in rabbits and baboons, where a low concentration of inactivated FVIIa inhibited the endotoxin-induced decrease in platelet count and fibrinogen levels, and inhibited fibrin deposition in the kidneys.

Activated protein C

The activated PC (APC) pathway has significant anti-inflammatory actions; it acts indirectly via inactivation of thrombin by thrombomodulin (TM). The APC inactivates FVa and FVIIIa and thus limits thrombin generation directly; it promotes fibrinolysis through the activation of plasminogen activator inhibitor type 1 (PAI-1) and seemingly has the ability to modulate inflammation via inhibition of cytokine production in leucocytes. Interestingly, trials of APC treatment have shown that patients with severe sepsis treated with APC had a reduction of almost 20% in the relative risk of 28-day mortality. The patients receiving APC had significantly lower IL-6 activity compared with patients who received placebo, and it seems that the beneficial effect of this treatment is related to its anti-inflammatory properties, possibly through regulation of NFκB expression.

Summary

The pathophysiology and clinical laboratory manifestations of DIC are complex, and only by understanding these complicated interactions can the clinician appreciate the conflicting and extensive variety of clinical and laboratory findings that are typical of patients with DIC. Many of the diagnostic and therapeutic decisions that must be made are controversial and lack evidence. Nevertheless, therapy should be individualized depending on the nature of DIC, including consideration of: the aetiology; site and severity of haemorrhage or thrombosis; haemodynamic changes; and other clinical parameters that may be relevant for the individual case. Aggressive treatment of the underlying cause with supportive treatment, together with blood components as indicated, now seems to be the most rational therapy.

References and further reading

Bakhtiari K, Meijers JC, de Jonge E *et al.* (2004) Prospective validation of the International Society of Thrombosis and Haemostasis scoring system for disseminated intravascular coagulation. *Critical Care Medicine* **32**(12), 2416–2421

Bateman SW, Mathews KA, Brams-Ogg AC *et al.* (1999) Diagnosis of disseminated intravascular coagulation in dogs admitted to an intensive care unit. *Journal of the American Veterinary Medical Association* **215**(6), 798–804

Bick RL (2003) Disseminated intravascular coagulation current concepts of etiology, pathophysiology, diagnosis, and treatment. *Hematology/Oncology Clinics of North America* **17**(1), 149–176

Bick RL, Arun B and Frenkel EP (1999) Disseminated intravascular coagulation. clinical and pathophysiological mechanisms and manifestations. *Haemostasis* **29**(2–3), 111–134

Boisvert AM, Swenson CL and Haines CJ (2001) Serum and plasma latex agglutination tests for detection of fibrin(ogen) degradation products in clinically ill dogs. *Veterinary Clinical Pathology* **30**(3), 133–136

Bull BS and Bull MH (1994) Hypothesis: disseminated intravascular inflammation as the inflammatory counterpart to disseminated intravascular coagulation. *Proceedings of the National Academy of Science of the United States of America* **91**(17), 8190–8194

Caldin M, Furlanello T and Lubas G (1998) Sensitivity and specificity of citrated plasma FDPs and D-dimer in the diagnosis of disseminated intravascular coagulation (DIC) in dogs. *Journal of Veterinary Internal Medicine* **12**(3), 236–236

Cauchie P, Cauchie CH, Boudjeltia KZ *et al.* (2006) Diagnosis and prognosis of overt disseminated intravascular coagulation in a general hospital – meaning of the ISTH score system, fibrin monomers, and lipoprotein-C-reactive protein complex formation. *American Journal of Hematology* **81**(6), 414–419

Esmon CT, Fukudome K, Mather T *et al.* (1999) Inflammation, sepsis, and coagulation. *Haematologica* **84**(3), 254–259

Feldman BF., Madewell BR and O'Neill S (1981) Disseminated intravascular coagulation: antithrombin, plasminogen, and coagulation abnormalities in 41 dogs. *Journal of the American Veterinary Medical Association* **179**(2), 151–154

Gando S (2010) Microvascular thrombosis and multiple organ dysfunction syndrome. *Critical Care Medicine* **38**(2 Suppl), S35–S42

Giles AR, Nesheim ME and Mann KG (1984) Studies of Factors V and VIII:C in an animal model of disseminated intravascular coagulation. *Journal of Clinical Investigation* **74**(6), 2219–2225

Griffin A, Callan MB, Giger U *et al.* (2003) Evaluation of a canine D-dimer point-of-care test kit for use in samples obtained from dogs with disseminated intravascular coagulation, thromboembolic disease, and hemorrhage. *American Journal of Veterinary Research* **64**(12), 1562–1569

Kienast J, Juers M, Wiedermann CJ *et al.* (2006) Treatment effects of high-dose antithrombin without concomitant heparin in patients with severe sepsis with or without disseminated intravascular coagulation. *Journal of Thrombosis and Haemostasis* **4**(1), 90–97

Kim HK, Hong KH and Toh CH (2010) Application of the international normalized ratio (INR) in the scoring system for disseminated intravascular coagulation (DIC). *Journal of Thrombosis and Haemostasis* **8**(5), 1116–1118

Machida T, Kokubu H and Matsuda K (2010) clinical use of D-dimer measurement for the diagnosis of disseminated intravascular coagulation in dogs. *The Journal of Veterinary Medical Science* **72**(10), 1301–1306

Mischke, R, Fehr M and Nolte I (2005) Efficacy of low molecular weight heparin in a canine model of thromboplastin-induced acute disseminated intravascular coagulation. *Research in Veterinary Science* **79**(1), 69–76

Nelson OL and Andreasen C (2003) The utility of plasma D-dimer to identify thromboembolic disease in dogs. *Journal of Veterinary Internal Medicine* **17**(6), 830–834

Olrik Berthelsen L, Thuri Kristensen A, Wiinberg B *et al.* (2009) Implementation of the ISTH classification of non-overt DIC in a thromboplastin induced rabbit model. *Thrombosis Ressearch* **124**(4), 490–497

Shimura M, Wada H, Nakasaki T *et al.* (1999) Increased truncated form of plasma tissue factor pathway inhibitor levels in patients with disseminated intravascular coagulation. *American Journal of Hematology* **60**(2), 94–98

Stokol T, Brooks MB, Erb HN *et al.* (2000) D-dimer concentrations in healthy dogs and dogs with disseminated intravascular coagulation. *American Journal of Veterinary Research* **61**(4), 393–398

Taylor FB, Toh CH, Hoots WK *et al.* (2001) Towards definition, clinical and laboratory criteria, and a scoring system for disseminated intravascular coagulation. *Thrombosis and Haemostasis* **86**(5), 1327–1330

ten Cate H, Schoenmakers SH, Franco R *et al.* (2001) Microvascular coagulopathy and disseminated intravascular coagulation. *Critical Care Medicine* **29**(7 Suppl), S95–S97

ten Cate H (2003) Thrombocytopenia: one of the markers of disseminated intravascular coagulation. *Pathophysiology of Haemostasis and Thrombosis* **33**(5–6), 413–416

Thachil J, Fitzmaurice DA and Toh CH (2010) Appropriate use of D-dimer in hospital patients. *American Journal of Medicine* **123**(1), 17–19

Toh CH and Downey C (2005) Performance and prognostic importance of a new clinical and laboratory scoring system for identifying non-overt disseminated intravascular coagulation. *Blood Coagulation and Fibrinolysis* **16**(1), 69–74

Toh CH and Hoots WK (2007) The scoring system of the Scientific and Standardisation Committee on Disseminated Intravascular Coagulation of the International Society on Thrombosis and Haemostasis: a 5-year overview. *Journal of Thrombosis and Haemostasis* **5**(3), 604–606

Wiinberg B, Jensen AL, Johansson PI *et al.* (2008) Thromboelastographic evaluation of hemostatic function in dogs with disseminated intravascular coagulation. *Journal of Veterinary Internal Medicine* **22**(2), 357–365

Wiinberg B, Jensen AL, Johansson PI *et al.* (2010) Development of a model based scoring system for diagnosis of canine disseminated intravascular coagulation with independent assessment of sensitivity and specificity. *The Veterinary Journal* **185**, 292–298

31

Thrombosis

Stephanie A. Smith

Introduction

Thrombosis is the formation of a blood clot within the cardiovascular system, while thromboembolism describes a thrombus that has travelled through the vasculature and caused partial or complete obstruction of a vascular lumen. Thrombosis and thromboembolism occur as a consequence of derangements in the haemostatic system. These derangements can be inherited or acquired. Because normal haemostasis requires a complex interaction between platelets, the vascular wall and the proteins of the coagulation and fibrinolytic systems, abnormalities in any of these components may lead to hypercoagulability.

Pathophysiology

Thrombus formation may result from alterations of the vascular wall, blood flow or the composition of blood. This concept, known as Virchow's triad, provides the cornerstone for understanding the pathophysiological factors that predispose patients to thrombosis and thromboembolism.

Alterations of the vascular wall

Under normal physiological conditions, the intact vascular wall provides an environment that prevents thrombus formation. Resting endothelium has a neutral membrane surface that is incapable of supporting coagulation reactions. Resting endothelium also expresses inhibitors of coagulation: heparan sulphated proteoglycans are the physiological cofactors for inhibition of coagulation enzymes by antithrombin (AT); thrombomodulin supports activation of protein C; and tissue factor pathway inhibitor (TFPI) acts as an inhibitor of factor (F) Xa and tissue factor (TF)/FVIIa. Activation of, or damage to, the endothelium changes the surface properties from antithrombotic to prothrombotic. Activated endothelium secretes von Willebrand factor (vWF), expresses adhesion molecules that interact with platelets and leucocytes and provides a procoagulant membrane surface.

The intact resting endothelium also provides a barrier that prevents exposure of blood to the reactive subendothelial molecules TF and collagen. TF is the sole physiological initiator of coagulation, and acts as the regulatory subunit of the TF–FVIIa complex. Exposure of TF to blood will lead to thrombin formation. Collagen binds to vWF, allowing for adhesion of platelets to the site of injury.

Damage to the vascular wall may occur as a consequence of trauma (including catheterization), local or systemic inflammation, invasion by tumours, intravascular parasites, or atherosclerotic plaque formation.

Alterations in blood flow

Most interactions between the endothelium and the flowing blood occur in capillaries, where the ratio of endothelial cell surface to blood volume is extremely high. Continuous flow serves to deliver blood to inhibitory molecules on the capillary endothelial surface, allowing for efficient inhibition of any coagulation enzymes that are generated. Stasis of blood results in inefficiency of inhibition, because interaction of enzymes with endothelial cell surface inhibitors is minimized. Stasis may occur with hypoperfusion, hypovolaemia, immobility, vessel or cardiac chamber dilatation, or vascular compression.

Laminar flow also limits the interaction of blood cells with the endothelial wall, with platelets focused into the central lumen and away from the vascular wall under normal flow conditions. Turbulent flow increases shear, which activates endothelial cells and platelets, and increases the likelihood of interactions between platelet and endothelial adhesion molecules. Turbulence occurs with vessel or cardiac chamber dilatation, vascular compression, hyperviscosity and changes in blood cellular contents such as polycythaemia or leukaemia.

Alterations in blood composition

Hypercoagulability of blood can be a function of increased platelet reactivity, excessive generation of thrombin, changes in fibrin structure or hypofibrinolysis.

Increased platelet reactivity

Increased platelet reactivity is a function of increased activity of platelet agonists, decreased activity of platelet inhibitors or changes in platelet responses. Platelets can be primed for reactivity as a result of exposure to inflammatory cytokines, cell-mediated release of platelet agonists or upregulation of the arachidonic acid pathway. Endothelium normally produces prostacyclin, nitric oxide and ADPase, all of which inhibit platelet function.

Impairment of endothelial function results in loss of normal platelet inhibition.

Abnormal thrombin generation

An abnormality in either the speed or the quantity of thrombin generation may occur as a result of inherited or acquired factors, and this will have a direct effect on both platelet activation and fibrin formation. Thrombin generation may be excessive with increased TF exposure, elevations of procoagulant factors or deficiency of normal inhibitory systems.

Exposure of the blood to TF is increased with vasculitis, vascular injury or up-regulation of TF expression on circulating monocytes or neoplastic cells. Elevations in procoagulant factors (such as the increased levels of prothrombin associated with a mutation in the prothrombin promoter in humans) may also cause an increased risk for thrombosis.

Antithrombin (AT) is a serine protease inhibitor that targets a variety of coagulation enzymes, but it is inefficient unless complexed with an appropriate glycosaminoglycan (such as endothelial cell heparan sulphated proteoglycans or pharmaceutical heparin). Inherited AT deficiency is a thrombotic risk factor in humans, but has not been reported in canine or feline patients. Acquired AT deficiency may result from decreased synthesis (hepatic synthesis failure), increased loss (protein-losing nephropathy, protein-losing enteropathy, vascular leak syndromes) or increased consumption (any condition that causes increased thrombin generation, or disseminated intravascular coagulation (DIC)).

The protein C pathway involves a complex interplay among several endothelial cell-surface molecules, thrombin, protein C and protein S. Activated protein C is an essential regulator of thrombin generation; negative feedback occurs via inactivation of cofactors FVa and FVIIIa. In humans, an inherited deficiency of protein C is a major risk factor for thrombosis, and a mutation in the gene for human FV that renders it resistant to cleavage by activated protein C is the most common hereditary risk factor for thrombosis. Mutations that affect the protein C pathway have not been reported in dogs or cats. Acquired protein C deficiency may result from decreased synthesis (hepatic synthesis failure or vitamin K deficiency), increased loss (protein-losing nephropathy, protein-losing enteropathy, vascular leak syndromes) or increased consumption (any condition causing increased thrombin generation or DIC).

TFPI on endothelial surfaces is a critical inhibitor of the extrinsic pathway. Only a small amount of TFPI is normally present in the plasma, making assessment of the *in vivo* function of TFPI challenging. TFPI is released into the circulating plasma in response to administration of pharmaceutical heparin. The exact role of abnormalities of TFPI in thrombotic disorders (if any) has not yet been elucidated clearly.

Changes in fibrin structure

The factors that govern the structure of the fibrin clot that is formed when thrombin encounters fibrinogen are many and extremely complex. These factors include the rate of thrombin generation, the nature of the interaction of thrombin with fibrinogen, the quantity of fibrinogen, the exact amino acid sequence of the fibrinogen and cross-linking of fibrin by FXIIIa. Various mutations identified in the fibrinogen molecule are specific risk factors for thrombosis in humans, while elevated levels of fibrinogen are a risk factor for thrombosis in humans and other animals. Because fibrinogen is an acute phase reactant, hyperfibrinogenaemia is common in inflammatory disorders.

Hypofibrinolysis

Hypofibrinolysis results in prolonged survival of a fibrin clot once it has formed. Deficiency of plasminogen, potentially causing decreased fibrinolysis, has been reported in dogs. Decreased lysis is often a function of an increased plasma concentration of plasminogen activator inhibitor 1 (PAI-1), which is the primary regulatory inhibitor that affects the generation of plasmin. PAI-1 is an acute phase reactant, release of which is elevated in inflammatory conditions.

Causes of thrombosis: specific disorders with increased risk of thrombosis or thromboembolism

Systemic inflammatory response syndrome (SIRS)/sepsis

Systemic inflammation, with or without sepsis, is well described as a cause of microvascular thrombosis and DIC, but macrovascular thrombosis/thromboembolism may also occur. Thrombosis may be either arterial or venous in location. Coagulation activation occurs through complex mechanisms related to the massive cross-talk between the inflammatory and haemostatic systems. Proinflammatory cytokines up-regulate TF exposure, and alter the behaviour of platelets, leucocytes and endothelial cells. The acute phase response alters the balance of protein synthesis, resulting in changes in plasma concentrations of a variety of procoagulant, anticoagulant, profibrinolytic and antifibrinolytic factors.

Reported specific laboratory findings that support the presence of hypercoagulability include AT deficiency and protein C deficiency. Thrombocytopenia may develop as a result of platelet consumption, and increased fibrin degradation products (FDPs) or D-dimers indicate increased fibrinolysis.

Pancreatitis

Pancreatitis often results in systemic inflammation, and the associated haemostatic derangements. Local injury to the pancreas may expose TF, and consumption of α_2-macroglobulin is common. Given that this protein is an important inhibitor for a variety of haemostatic enzymes, normal inhibition of coagulation and fibrinolysis may be compromised. Experimental studies in animals and clinical studies in humans indicate the presence of platelet hyperreactivity, hyperfibrinogenaemia and hypofibrinolysis.

Arterial or venous thrombosis (particularly at catheterization sites) may occur in animal patients with pancreatitis.

Canine immune-mediated haemolytic anaemia (IMHA)

Venous thrombosis and pulmonary thromboembolism (PTE) are common sequelae of IMHA, and appear to be a major cause of mortality. The precise pathophysiology has not been defined, but may be similar to that which occurs with systemic inflammation. Hyperfibrinogenaemia is common in canine IMHA, and platelet hyper-reactivity, as indicated by increased expression of P-selectin, has been reported. Laboratory evidence of hypercoagulability includes AT deficiency, protein C deficiency, and increased FDPs or D-dimers indicating ongoing fibrinolysis.

Neoplasia

Venous thrombosis and thromboembolism are major causes of morbidity and mortality in human cancer patients, but appear to be less important in veterinary patients. Specific reported venous sites in dogs and cats include portal, splenic, caudal vena cava and pulmonary vessels. Arterial thromboembolism has also been reported to occur in dogs and cats in association with neoplastic disorders, in particular with pulmonary tumours, which have ready access to the arterial vasculature by way of invasion into the pulmonary venous system. Note, however, that arterial occlusion with pulmonary tumours may be a function of tumour embolism rather than true thromboembolism.

Pathophysiological mechanisms of thrombosis in neoplasia are related to the expression of TF by neoplastic cells and production of proinflammatory mediators. Some cancer cells also produce 'cancer procoagulant', a thrombin-generating enzyme. Acquired protein C resistance and AT or protein C deficiency may also develop. Neoplastic invasion of vessels, immobilization, repeated or indwelling catheterization and the use of procoagulant chemotherapeutics may be contributory.

Protein-losing disorders

Many proteins involved in coagulation and fibrinolysis are of relatively low molecular weight, similar to albumin. If disease severity is profound enough to result in hypoalbuminaemia, then it is likely that haemostatic proteins are deficient as well. In particular, loss of AT is likely to be of clinical consequence. Thrombosis is well recognized as a consequence of nephrotic syndrome in particular. In addition to loss of AT, nephrotic syndrome is generally associated with platelet hyper-reactivity, hyperfibrinogenaemia, hypercholesterolaemia and hypofibrinolysis. Thrombosis may be arterial or venous in location.

Cardiac disease

In dogs, cardiac disorders that lead to thrombosis are generally limited to infective endocarditis and heartworm disease. Both of these disorders cause disruption of the normal endothelial barrier, and can be associated with a significant inflammatory response. Laboratory markers indicative of hypercoagulability have been described in dogs with valvular dysfunction or cardiac insufficiency, but clinically relevant thrombosis is rare with these diseases.

In cats, cardiomyopathy is by far is the most common cause of thrombosis. Thrombi develop within the enlarged left atrium (Figure 31.1), and embolize to the peripheral arterial system, with aortic trifurcation (Figure 31.2) or femoral artery locations being most common. The pathogenesis is not well defined. Stasis associated with atrial enlargement is clearly a risk factor for thrombosis, but the degree of enlargement does not appear to be related directly to the risk of thrombosis. Endothelial damage may play a role, and laboratory markers of hypercoagulability have been reported.

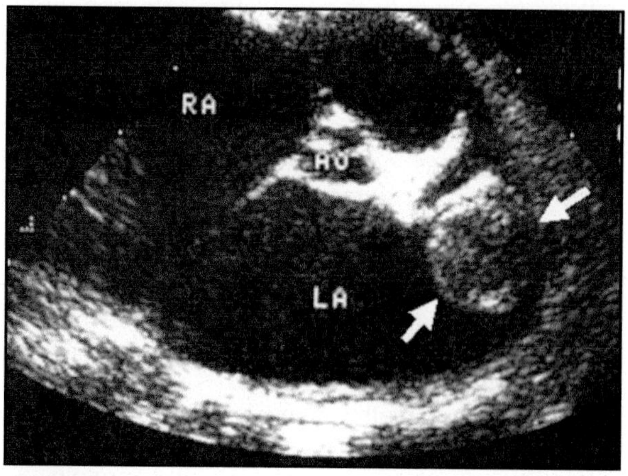

31.1 Echocardiographic image from a cat with cardiac disease. Note the ball thrombus (arrows) within the enlarged left atrium (LA).

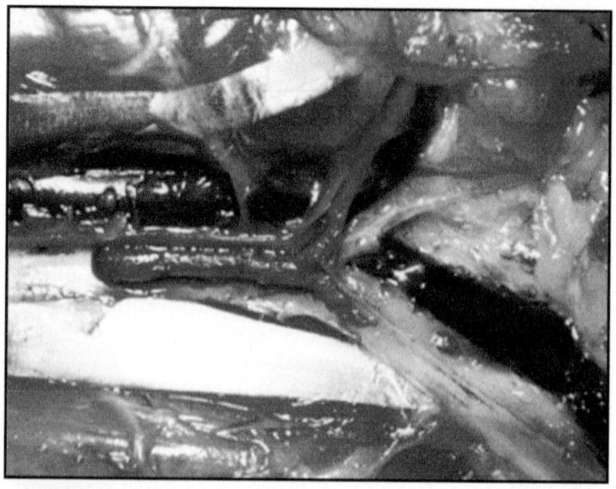

31.2 Post-mortem specimen from a cat with hypertrophic cardiomyopathy that died during an acute arterial thromboembolic episode. Note the large thrombus located at the aortic trifurcation.

Endocrinopathies

Hypercortisolism caused by corticosteroid therapy or hyperadrenocorticism is considered to be a risk factor for the development of venous thrombosis or

PTE in dogs. The exact risk is difficult to establish owing to the frequency of concomitant prothrombotic disorders. The mechanisms are ill-defined, but may be related to hypertension, hypercholesterolaemia, hyperfibrinogenaemia and increased PAI-1. Note that invasion of the vasculature by an adrenal tumour may result in local thrombus development.

Hypothyroidism has been reported to be a risk factor for the development of thrombosis as a function of atherosclerotic plaque development in dogs. An association between diabetes mellitus and thrombosis is not well defined in animals, but is clear in humans. Platelet hyper-reactivity, altered lipid metabolism, atherosclerosis, changes in endothelial function and decreased fibrinolysis have been implicated as mechanisms.

Arterial thromboembolism may occur in cats with thyrotoxic cardiomyopathy or in previously hyperthyroid cats that are currently euthyroid and have echocardiographically normal hearts.

Clinical signs

A clinical diagnosis of thrombosis/thromboembolism is based on a combination of the appropriate clinical signs and associated laboratory changes. Specialized imaging techniques may be applied for specific confirmation (Figure 31.3).

The clinical signs associated with thrombosis and thromboembolism are entirely dependent on the vascular location of the thrombus. Non-occlusive thrombi are often clinically silent. If located within a left cardiac chamber, the thrombus may cause intermittent peripheral signs due to showering of fragments and the resulting downstream occlusion of the arterial vasculature.

Occlusive arterial thrombi or thromboemboli cause ischaemia of the tissues supplied by the affected artery. Limbs and abdominal viscera are affected most commonly by thromboemboli in dogs and cats, but smaller thrombi may embolize to the cardiac or cerebral vasculature. Embolism of large thrombi to the limbs generally results in acute consequences such as extreme pain and loss of limb function. Embolism to the abdominal vasculature will result in acute loss of function of the supplied organ. Non-specific abdominal pain may be the only abnormality. Embolism to a coronary or cerebral artery may result in acute collapse, death or the sudden onset of neurological signs.

The clinical signs associated with occlusive venous thrombi tend to be more insidious in onset. Clinically apparent deep venous thrombosis of the limbs, while very common in humans, appears to be rare in animal patients. Venous thrombi are more commonly reported to affect the portal or central abdominal vasculature, potentially leading to ascites.

There is potential for central or deep venous thrombi to embolize to the pulmonary arterial vasculature, causing PTE. PTE appears to be particularly common in canine IMHA, and results in an acute onset of respiratory difficulty.

Clinical signs	Laboratory markers	Imaging results
Limb arterial thromboembolism (ATE)		
In the affected limb(s): paralysis or paresis; pain and distress; cold or cool limb; firm or rigid musculature; limb discoloration; weak or absent pulses; lack of detection of arterial flow using Doppler. Auscultable murmur, arrhythmia or history of cardiac disease	Elevated TAT [a,c]; elevated FDPs/D-dimers [a,b]; elevated aspartate aminotransferase and/or creatine kinase [a,b]; venous glucose in affected limb – central venous glucose [a]; venous lactate in affected limb – central venous lactate [a]	Contrast arteriogram indicative of intravascular space-occupying lesion [c]. Ultrasound examination findings indicative of intravascular space-occupying lesion. Nuclear scintigraphy indicative of abnormal perfusion to the limb [c]
Central venous thrombosis (CVT)		
Presence of an underlying disease known to predispose; abdominal pain; ascites	Elevated TAT [a,c]; elevated FDPs/D-dimers [a,b]	Contrast venogram indicative of intravascular space-occupying lesion [c]. Ultrasound examination findings indicative of intravascular space-occupying lesion
Pulmonary thromboembolism (PTE)		
Presence of an underlying disease known to predispose; respiratory distress; cyanosis	Elevated TAT [a,c]; elevated FDPs/D-dimers [a,b]; arterial hypoxaemia [a]; increased alveolar–arterial oxygen tension gradient [b]	Thoracic radiographs: mild radiographic changes disproportionate for degree of dyspnoea; pulmonary infiltrates (alveolar, interstitial or mixed pattern) [d]; main pulmonary artery segment enlargement [d]; generalized cardiomegaly [d]; oligaemia of caudal lung fields [d]; pleural effusion [d]. Echocardiography: dilation of the right atrium, ventricle and/or pulmonary artery [d]; right-sided hypertension [d]; paradoxical septal wall motion; visualization of space-occupying mass [d]. Helical CT [c]: intraluminal filling defect; abrupt termination of pulmonary artery; absence of pulmonary arterial branches. Pulmonary scintigraphy: hypoperfusion with concomitant ventilation

31.3 Clinical signs and diagnostic testing of thrombosis and thromboembolism in the most common presentations in small animals. FDPs, fibrin degradation products; TAT, thrombin–antithrombin complex. [a] Supportive only. [b] Normal findings make a diagnosis of thrombosis unlikely. [c] Rarely performed. [d] May or may not be present.

Diagnosis

The diagnosis requires a high index of clinical suspicion, based on the presence of a likely risk factor and appropriate clinical signs. Laboratory abnormalities may be supportive of the presence of increased thrombin generation or active fibrinolysis, but are generally not specifically diagnostic. Imaging is required for a definitive diagnosis, but it is often not able to be performed because of the status of the patient or limited access to sophisticated imaging modalities (see Figure 31.3).

Laboratory assessment

Laboratory indicators of hypercoagulability may be supportive of the likelihood of thrombosis/thromboembolism, but are generally not specific enough to allow for a definitive diagnosis.

Standard coagulation assays such as the prothrombin time (PT), activated partial thromboplastin time (aPTT), thrombin time (TT) and fibrinogen concentration are often performed in patients at risk of thrombosis, but are usually unremarkable. The PT and aPTT in particular tend to be insensitive to hypercoagulability and are usually within the reference range. If the underlying cause of hypercoagulability is inflammatory in nature (such as in canine IMHA or sepsis), fibrinogen may be elevated and/or TT may be decreased.

FDPs and D-dimers are present in the plasma as a result of plasmin-mediated degradation of fibrin. D-dimers in particular indicate that fibrin was cross-linked prior to lysis. Elevations in either FDPs or D-dimers are indicative of increased formation of fibrin (and therefore increased formation of thrombin) in association with lysis of that fibrin by plasmin. Increased FDPs and D-dimers are associated with a variety of disorders, including trauma, sepsis, DIC, anticoagulant rodenticide intoxication and other causes of internal haemorrhage. As such, elevation in FDPs or D-dimers is not specific for a diagnosis of thrombosis. Rather, elevation is an indicator of the *in vivo* presence of increased thrombin generation and increased plasmin lysis of fibrin. In humans, normal levels of D-dimers are used to rule-out thrombosis definitively.

A decrease in the inhibitory activity of AT relates directly to the risk of thrombosis in humans. Low levels of AT have been reported in a variety of animal disease conditions (protein-losing disorders, vascular leak syndromes and consumptive coagulopathies) and may cause an increased risk of thrombosis, but the specific relationship between the degree of AT deficiency and development of thrombosis has yet to be elucidated.

Thrombin has an extremely short-half-life *in vivo*, so plasma concentrations cannot be measured reliably. Given that AT is the primary inhibitor of thrombin *in vivo*, increased generation of thrombin results in increased formation of thrombin–AT (TAT) complexes. Consequently, the plasma TAT concentration is used to reflect the quantity of thrombin being generated *in vivo*. Elevated TAT levels indicate increased thrombin generation *in vivo*, but the increase may be either physiological (as an appropriate response to injury) or pathological in nature. TAT is therefore not a specific indicator of thrombosis.

Similarly, deficiency of protein C also relates directly to the thrombotic risk in humans. Low levels of protein C have been reported in dogs with IMHA, DIC, sepsis and other inflammatory diseases and may pose a risk factor for thrombosis. In SIRS, the risk of thrombosis may be more specifically a function of a decrease in the ability to activate protein C *in vivo*, as opposed to a deficiency of zymogen protein C.

Thromboelastography and thromboelastometry measure the viscoelastic properties of blood or plasma as a clot develops over time. The theoretical advantages over standard plasma-based tests include the ability to use a whole blood sample, the incorporation of the contributions of cells to clot formation, the sensitivity to both hyper- and hypocoagulability, and the potential to visualize lysis. The results of viscoelastic testing may be subject to artefacts due to the methodology used, and the presence of abnormalities of red cell mass. Use of viscoelastic testing has been reported in a wide variety of animal disease conditions, but the clinical utility of such technologies has yet to be proven definitively for most clinical circumstances in both human and veterinary medicine.

Diagnostic imaging

Imaging techniques may provide useful information that supports a clinical diagnosis of thrombosis/thromboembolism. Routine radiography is usually not helpful, although the absence of abnormalities on thoracic radiographs of a dyspnoeic patient is supportive of a diagnosis of PTE.

Contrast imaging has been used to identify space-filling lesions within cardiac chambers or the vasculature. In humans, selective pulmonary angiography is commonly performed to confirm PTE, but this approach is rarely used in animal patients owing to the requirement for general anaesthesia. Non-selective pulmonary angiography tends to be insensitive for the identification of PTE.

Ultrasonography and echocardiography are often used to visualize probable thrombi. In addition, echocardiography is indicated to investigate the presence of concomitant cardiac disease as an underlying cause of arterial thrombosis, or to provide supporting evidence for the possibility of a PTE via identification of right-sided cardiac changes (see Figure 31.3).

Helical computed tomography (CT) is the current gold standard for the identification of PTE in humans. CT was previously impractical in animals for confirming a diagnosis of PTE, owing to the requirement for general anaesthesia in a patient with respiratory compromise. As this technology improves with regard to speed and resolution, wider application in veterinary medicine is likely.

Nuclear scintigraphy may be used to identify the ventilation/perfusion mismatch that occurs with PTE (Figure 31.4a), and as a prognostic indicator for the return of perfusion in ischaemic limbs (Figure 31.4b). The application of nuclear scintigraphy is limited because of regulatory issues.

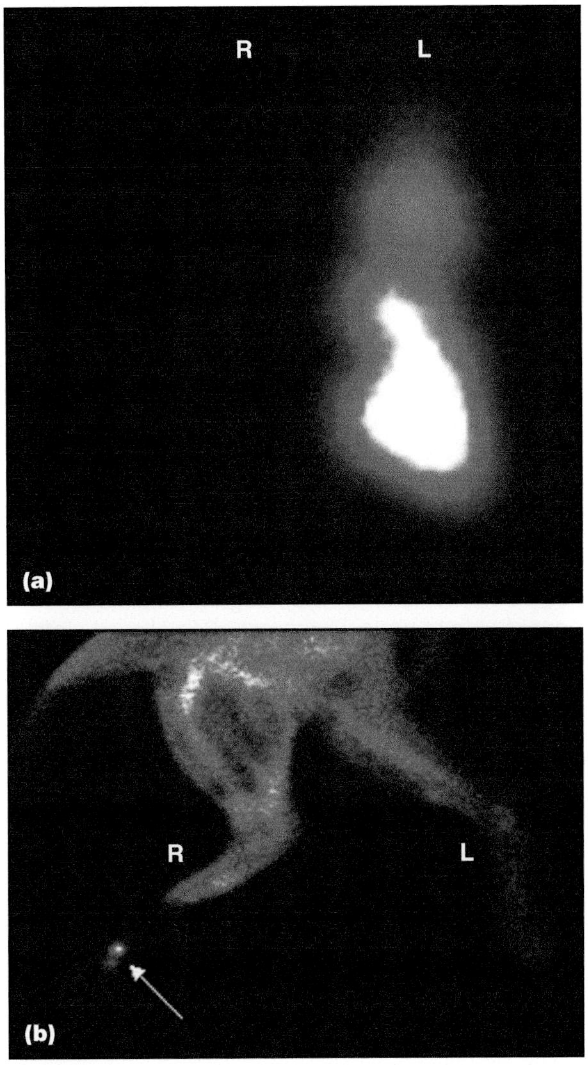

31.4 Nuclear scintigraphy can be used to evaluate perfusion in patients suspected of having thrombosis or thromboembolism. **(a)** A perfusion scan evaluating pulmonary perfusion in a cat with an acute onset of dyspnoea. The associated ventilation scan indicated normal ventilation in both lungs. Note the complete absence of perfusion to the right lung. **(b)** A perfusion scan evaluating flow to the limbs of a cat with hypertrophic cardiomyopathy and acute onset paralysis of the right rear limb with paresis of the left rear limb. The dot marked with the arrow indicates the location of the end of the toes. Note the loss of perfusion to the distal portion of the right rear limb.

Therapy

Supportive therapy

Supportive measures are an important component of the therapeutic approach to thrombosis. Treatment of the underlying disease is also vital for the successful management of the causative hypercoagulability.

Arterial thromboembolism often results in marked systemic effects, including abnormalities of perfusion, electrolyte dyscrasias and pain. Appropriate fluid therapy and analgesia are indicated. Central venous thrombosis may also affect systemic perfusion, owing to third space losses and the impact on venous return. Abdominocentesis may be indicated to improve perfusion. Patients with PTE may have significantly abnormal oxygen exchange that requires oxygen therapy and/or ventilatory support.

Thrombolysis

Thrombolysis may be accomplished with systemic or direct application of a lytic agent such as recombinant tissue-type plasminogen activator or streptokinase. Lysis of a central venous thrombosis is generally not indicated. In dogs with acute life-threatening PTE, lysis may improve survival, but while thrombolytic agents are commonly employed in experimental canine models of PTE, direct evidence supporting their use in clinical patients is lacking. Successful lysis of peripheral arterial thrombi using streptokinase in dogs has been described.

In cats with ATE, thrombolysis with either streptokinase or tissue-type plasminogen activator is associated with significant adverse events (sudden death, electrolyte dyscrasias, neurological signs, acid–base disorders or haemorrhage) and mortality rates similar to or higher than those with conservative approaches. Reperfusion injury, caused by the large tissue mass affected by ischaemia, is likely to be a serious problem in cats treated with thrombolytic agents, making their application difficult to justify.

Thromboprophylaxis

Heparins

Agents used for prevention of the development of thrombi in dogs and cats include unfractionated heparin (UFH), low molecular weight heparins (LMWH) and platelet inhibitors (primarily aspirin and clopidogrel). Heparins improve the inhibitory efficiency of AT. Aspirin is a cyclo-oxygenase inhibitor that decreases platelet thromboxane production. Clopidogrel is an inhibitor of the platelet receptor for ADP.

Heparins are of proven efficacy with reasonable safety in human thrombotic disorders, but in animals, evidence-based medicine is extremely limited regarding indications for the use of heparins, which heparins are best, and the appropriate dosing protocols.

UFH is a heterogeneous mixture of heparin molecules derived generally from porcine intestinal mucosa. Its advantages over other anticoagulants include low cost, ease of administration, more extensive clinical experience and the availability of a reversal agent (protamine). The disadvantages include inconsistent bioavailability (especially in inflammatory conditions), which results in variability in dose–response relationships, and a significant potential for adverse effects.

LMWHs are also heterogeneous preparations.

Different LMWHs are not interchangeable because of variations in potency, bioavailability and the tendency to accumulate. As a group, LMWHs all enhance AT inhibition of FXa more than AT inhibition of thrombin. Bioavailability and pharmacokinetics are more predictable than for UFH, and they tend to require less frequent dosing. LMWHs tend to have a lower incidence of adverse effects than does UFH. The major disadvantage of LWMH is cost.

The primary relevant adverse effects of UFH or LMWH in animals are bleeding (attributable to over-anticoagulation) or recurrent thrombosis (due to under anticoagulation). As such, appropriate dose protocols are important, but not well defined. Several studies have evaluated the pharmacokinetics of UFH, enoxaparin and dalteparin in normal dogs and cats, but no published studies have directly evaluated their pharmacokinetics in populations of sick animals.

Studies in normal dogs that used UFH at 200 IU/kg as a single subcutaneous injection indicated adequate anticoagulation with a duration of up to 6 hours. The results using UFH with repeated subcutaneous injection of 500 IU/kg either q8h or q12h suggested an initial dose of 500 IU/kg followed by reduced doses q12h. Dalteparin administered by repeated subcutaneous injection at 150 IU/kg q8h gave adequate levels of heparin.

Studies in normal cats using UFH at 250 IU/kg q6h produced therapeutic anticoagulation. Enoxaparin at 1 mg/kg s.c. q12h failed to induce sustainable anticoagulant activity according to the anti-FXa assay, but may have reduced *in vivo* thrombus formation in a TF-induced model of venous thrombosis. Dalteparin at 100 IU/kg s.c. q12h failed to induce sustainable anticoagulant activity.

Canine patients with IMHA developed thromboembolism despite treatment with UFH at 100–200 IU/kg s.c. q8h. Two recent clinical studies have indicated that individually adjusting the dose (up to 566 IU/kg) improved the outcome markedly. Although LMWHs are in widespread use in dogs with IMHA, published protocols are lacking.

No outcome-based studies have evaluated any dose of heparin for cats with ATE, and recommendations are highly variable. In cats with ATE, there is wide individual variation in heparin pharmacokinetics with some cats requiring high doses (up to 475 IU/kg) to maintain plasma concentrations within the therapeutic range. Dalteparin at 100 IU/kg q6 or 12h in cats with previous ATE was associated with some haemorrhagic complications, and similar survival times and frequency of recurrence to those for other therapies.

Antiplatelet agents

Aspirin has been prescribed as an antiplatelet therapy for decades in both dogs and cats at anti-inflammatory doses (5–20 mg/kg) and more recently at endothelial-sparing doses (0.5–1 mg/kg).

Use of low-dose aspirin (0.5 mg/kg q6 or 12h) in dogs with IMHA has been advocated based on a single retrospective study that reported lower mortality with this approach. Use of low-dose aspirin has become common owing to its low cost and ease of administration. However, heparins are markedly preferred over aspirin for the prevention of venous thrombosis or PTE in human patients, and several studies in normal dogs have failed to show relevant *in vivo* anti-platelet effects of aspirin in normal dogs at the low dose. One retrospective comparison with individually adjusted heparin indicated higher mortality in the groups receiving low-dose aspirin. The results of a prospective comparison of low-dose aspirin to heparin in dogs with IMHA are pending.

In dogs with protein-losing nephropathy and nephrotic syndrome, use of aspirin at 0.5–5 mg/kg q6 or 12h is employed widely. Direct evidence supporting its efficacy has not been reported.

Aspirin has been prescribed for decades for cats at risk for ATE at 81 mg/cat orally every 3 days, but no evidence supports its efficacy, and aspirin at this dose may result in significant gastrointestinal side effects. A dose of 5 mg/cat every 3 days was associated with similar or lower rates of ATE recurrence when compared with other therapies, and adverse effects were minimal, but *in vivo* effects on platelet function in normal or diseased cat populations have not been evaluated. Clopidogrel administered to normal cats at up to 75 mg/cat q24h altered platelet function and was not associated with adverse effects. The results of a prospective trial evaluating clopidogrel for the prevention of ATE in cats with cardiac disease are pending.

Prognosis

The prognosis for patients with thrombosis or thromboembolism is in large part dependent on the underlying disease process that predisposes to thrombus formation. Development of PTE in particular may compromise a patient with serious illness significantly, and may adversely affect short-term outcome.

ATE in cats (Figure 31.5) is associated with a poor prognosis, although recent reports suggest that aggressive supportive care can improve the short-

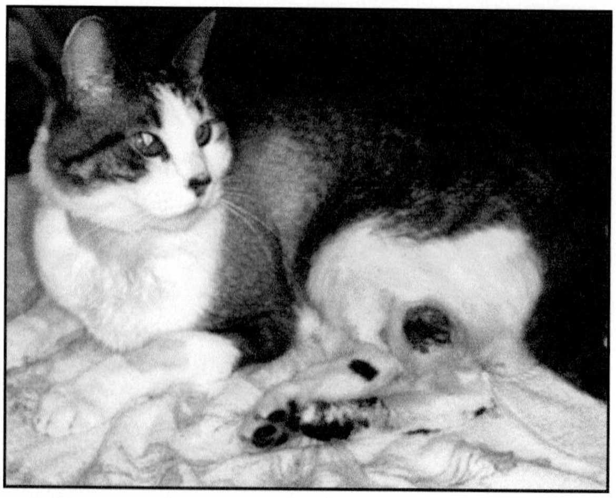

31.5 Tissue necrosis in a cat with a femoral arterial thromboembolism.

term outcome. Reported rates of survival to discharge are 33–49%. Hypothermia is a negative indicator: a model predicts a 50% probability of survival in cats with a rectal temperature on admission of 37.2°C. In most surviving cats the affected limbs return to function, although necrosis (Figure 31.5) or limb contracture may develop. Recurrent episodes of ATE are common (24–45%) and are often fatal, but progression of cardiac disease is a more significant contributor to morbidity and mortality. Concurrent congestive heart failure markedly worsens the long-term survival.

References and further reading

Boswood A, Lamb CR and White RN (2000) Aortic and iliac thrombosis in six dogs. *Journal of Small Animal Practice* **41**, 109–114

Breuhl EL, Moore G, Brooks MB and Scott-Moncrieff JC (2009) A prospective study of unfractionated heparin therapy in dogs with primary immune-mediated hemolytic anemia. *Journal of the American Animal Hospital Association* **45**, 125–133

Burns MG, Kelly AB, Hornof WJ and Howerth EW (1981) Pulmonary artery thrombosis in three dogs with hyperadrenocorticism. *Journal of the American Veterinary Medical Association* **178**, 388–393

Carr AP, Panciera DL and Kidd L (2002) Prognostic factors for mortality and thromboembolism in canine immune-mediated hemolytic anemia: a retrospective study of 72 dogs. *Journal of Veterinary Internal Medicine* **16**, 504–509

Hackner SG and Schaer BD (2010) Thrombotic disorders. In: *Schalm's Veterinary Hematology*, 6th edn, ed. DJ Weiss and KJ Wardrop, pp.668–678. Wiley-Blackwell, Ames, Iowa

Helmond SE, Polzin DJ, Armstrong PJ, Finke M and Smith SA (2010) Treatment of immune-mediated hemolytic anemia with individually adjusted heparin dosing in dogs. *Journal of Veterinary Internal Medicine* **24**, 597–605

Johnson LR, Lappin MR and Baker DC (1999) Pulmonary thromboembolism in 29 dogs: 1985–1995. *Journal of Veterinary Internal Medicine* **13**, 338–345

LaRue MJ and Murtaugh RJ (1990) Pulmonary thromboembolism in dogs: 47 cases (1986–1987). *Journal of the American Veterinary Medical Association* **197**, 1368–1372

Laste NJ and Harpster NK (1995) A retrospective study of 100 cases of feline distal aortic thromboembolism: 1977–1993. *Journal of the American Animal Hospital Association* **31**, 492–500

Laurenson MP, Hopper K, Herrera MA and Johnson EG (2010) Concurrent diseases and conditions in dogs with splenic vein thrombosis. *Journal of Veterinary Internal Medicine* **24**, 1298–1304

Palmer KG, King LG and Van Winkle TJ (1998) Clinical manifestations and associated disease syndromes in dogs with cranial vena cava thrombosis: 17 cases (1989–1996). *Journal of the American Veterinary Medical Association* **213**, 220–224

Ramsey CC, Burney DP, Macintire DK and Finn-Bodner S (1996) Use of streptokinase in four dogs with thrombosis. *Journal of the American Veterinary Medical Association* **209**, 780–785

Rush JE, Freeman LM, Fenollosa NK and Brown DJ (2002) Population and survival characteristics of cats with hypertrophic cardiomyopathy: 260 cases (1990–1999). *Journal of the American Veterinary Medical Association* **220**, 202–207

Schermerhorn T, Pembleton-Corbett JR and Kornreich B (2004) Pulmonary thromboembolism in cats. *Journal of Veterinary Internal Medicine* **18**, 533–535

Schoeman JP (1999) Feline distal aortic thromboembolism: a review of 44 cases (1990–1998). *Journal of Feline Medicine and Surgery* **1**, 221–231

Scott-Moncrieff JC, Treadwell NG, McCullough SM and Brooks MB (2001) Hemostatic abnormalities in dogs with primary immune-mediated hemolytic anemia. *Journal of the American Animal Hospital Association* **37**, 220–227

Smith CE, Rozanski EA, Freeman LM, Brown DJ, Goodman JS and Rush JE (2004) Use of low molecular weight heparin in cats: 57 cases (1999–2003). *Journal of the American Veterinary Medical Association* **225**, 1237–1241

Smith SA (2010) Overview of hemostasis. In: *Schalm's Veterinary Hematology*, 6th edn, ed. DJ Weiss and KJ Wardrop, pp.635–653, Wiley-Blackwell, Ames, Iowa

Smith SA and Tobias AH (2004) Feline arterial thromboembolism: an update. *Veterinary Clinics of North America: Small Animal Practice* **34**, 1245–1271

Smith SA, Tobias AH, Jacob KA, Fine DM and Grumbles PL (2003) Arterial thromboembolism in cats: acute crisis in 127 cases (1992–2001) and long-term management with low-dose aspirin in 24 cases. *Journal of Veterinary Internal Medicine* **17**, 73–83

Stokol T, Brooks M, Rush JE *et al.* (2008) Hypercoagulability in cats with cardiomyopathy. *Journal of Veterinary Internal Medicine* **22**, 546–552

Sykes JE, Kittleson MD, Chomel BB, Macdonald KA and Pesavento PA (2006) Clinicopathologic findings and outcome in dogs with infective endocarditis: 71 cases (1992–2005). *Journal of the American Veterinary Medical Association* **228**, 1735–1747

Van Winkle TJ and Bruce E (1993) Thrombosis of the portal vein in eleven dogs. *Veterinary Pathology* **30**, 28–35

Weinkle TK, Center SA, Randolph JF *et al.* (2005) Evaluation of prognostic factors, survival rates, and treatment protocols for immune-mediated hemolytic anemia in dogs: 151 cases (1993–2002). *Journal of the American Veterinary Medical Association* **226**, 1869–1880

Welch KM, Rozanski EA, Freeman LM and Rush JE (2010) Prospective evaluation of tissue plasminogen activator in 11 cats with arterial thromboembolism. *Journal of Feline Medicine and Surgery* **12**, 122–128

32

Canine blood groups and blood typing

Anne Hale

Introduction

Historically, transfusion compatibility in dogs was of limited concern until a canine patient had undergone a second transfusion or there was potential exposure to neoantigens secondary to immune-mediated disease. When evaluating the clinical significance of blood group systems or antigens, the clinician should consider the prevalence of the antigen and the prevalence of naturally occurring antibodies to it. For example, mismatch of the major antigen system of dog erythrocyte antigen (DEA) 1.0 (DEA 1.1.) occurs 24% of the time in untyped dogs, using current population indices. Routine survey of dogs with no previous transfusion history submitted for determination of DEA type (DEA 1.1, 3, 5 and 7) indicates an incidence of anti-DEA antibody of 8%. Together, these findings suggest that transfusion of untyped uncross-matched red blood cells (RBCs) carries a 32% risk of immunological transfusion reaction. If risk exists in one third of the transfusion events investigated for immunological transfusion reactions, compatibility should be an issue at the time of the first transfusion in canine patients. The importance of minimizing immunological transfusion reactions and maximizing the efficiency of transfusion support the extra expense of compatibility testing prior to transfusion.

Blood group systems in dogs have been defined since the early 1950s, when the dog was used as an animal model in human transfusion medicine. The DEA system was first developed through serological evaluation of a randomly selected dog population. Young *et al.* (1949) described 13 blood group specificities. Eight DEA systems were determined, through studies of the survival of transfused RBCs labelled with chromium 51, to have the potential to cause acute or delayed immunological transfusion reactions. Validation of the serological identification of these eight blood group systems was confirmed by the Second International Workshop on DEA held by the International Society of Animal Genetics (ISAG) in 1976. During the Third International Workshop on DEA in 1987, DEA nomenclature was switched from an alphanumerical to a numerical system. Figure 32.1 gives the current nomenclature for the canine RBC antigen systems. At this time, antisera are available for only six of these antigens commercially. DEA 6 and 8 are no longer recognizable owing to a lack of available antibody.

Clinicians should be aware that each of these blood group systems is inherited independently, which allows them all to coexist on the surface of the RBC. The current designation for DEA or blood type uses the numeral to indicate positive status, for example DEA 1.1,4 indicates that erythrocytes from the dog express DEA 1.1 and DEA 4, but do not express DEA 3, DEA 5 and DEA 7. When typing for DEA 1.1 only, the DEA status is indicated as DEA 1.1-positive or DEA 1.1-negative.

Canine blood groups

Dog erythrocyte antigen (DEA) 1.0

The DEA 1.0 system describes three antigens and a

Canine blood group system	Antigen phenotypes	Population prevalence	Incidence of naturally occurring antibody	Comments
1.0	1.1, 1.2, 1.3 [a], null	62%, 2%, 0.1%	< 2%	
3	3, null	5%	8–15%	
4	4, null	98%	Rare	
5	5, null	15%	8–12%	
6	6, null	96%	Unknown	No available typing system
7	7 [b], null	40–55%	10–40%	
8	8, null	20–40%	Unknown	No available typing system
Dal [c]	Dal, null	99%	Rare	No commercial typing system

32.1 Summary of dog erythrocyte antigens. [a] The 1.3 antigen was identified after the Third International Canine Immunogenetics meeting. [b] A 7' antigen has been identified after the Third International Canine Immunogenetics meeting. [c] Published in peer-reviewed journal, but not standardized by the International Society of Animal Genetics (ISAG).

null phenotype. A null phenotype means that the dog does not carry genes for expression of the antigen. This antigen system is most often associated with acute immunological transfusion reactions in dogs. DEA 1.1 is the most common antigen in this system and is expressed by the RBCs of 62% of dogs in different countries. DEA 1.2 and 1.3 are rarely identified. Inheritance of this system is Mendelian, with 1.1 > 1.2 > 1.3 > null representing the dominance hierarchy.

Identification of this system is based on serological testing. Polyclonal antisera exist that recognize all of the subtypes in this system. Monoclonal antibodies produced by immunizing mice with canine RBCs typically recognize only DEA 1.1.

The subtypes of this blood group system are likely to be the result of a difference in the number of molecules on the surface of the RBC and slight differences in the biochemical composition of the antigen. Dogs designated as DEA 1.2 by the use of polyclonal antisera will develop antibodies to DEA 1.1 upon exposure to DEA 1.1-positive cells. For that reason, DEA 1.2- and 1.3-positive dogs should receive DEA 1.1-negative cells when transfused.

Most of the point-of-care blood typing systems may recognize 'weak' expression of DEA 1.1, and when these results are compared with other methods (e.g. flow cytometry and tube agglutination) the cells are proven to have fewer molecules on their surface. As with the A subtypes in the human ABO system, 'weak' reactors will form antibody to the antigen when they are exposed to it by transfusion of RBCs bearing that antigen. 'Weak reacting' DEA 1.1 recipients are therefore capable of forming antibody to DEA 1.1 and should be transfused with DEA 1.1-negative cells to avoid alloimmunization.

Originally, canine neonatal isoerythrolysis was described when DEA 1.1-negative bitches that had been transfused previously with DEA 1.1-positive blood were bred with DEA 1.1-positive dogs. Recent work suggests that the incidence of this condition is less than 8% in the dog population in the United States (Blais *et al.*, 2009a).

DEA 3

The DEA 3 system describes one antigen and a null phenotype. This antigen is rare in the general canine population. A higher incidence of DEA 3 in American-bred Greyhounds and Japanese-bred dogs has been reported. Currently the only polyclonal antisera able to detect DEA 3 are used in a tube agglutination assay performed by an immunohaematology reference laboratory. Point-of-care typing is not available for this antigen.

Naturally occurring alloantibody to DEA 3 has been identified in 20% of the US canine population. This antibody has not been documented to cause acute transfusion reactions, but has caused delayed transfusion reactions (Young *et al.*, 1951). This delayed reaction leads to abrupt removal of cells from the circulation 5–7 days after transfusion. The significance of this delayed removal is seen in the management of patients with non-regenerative anaemia that are dependent upon blood transfusions.

DEA 4

The DEA 4 system also has one antigen and a null phenotype. DEA 4 is expressed commonly, with up to 98% of all dogs in some studies being DEA 4-positive. Because of its high prevalence, dogs that express DEA 4 only are often referred to as 'universal donors'. A universal donor is defined as a blood type that does not contain antigens likely to cause a reaction in random recipients. In humans, 'universal donor' refers to those with blood type O who are Rhesus factor-negative. The incidence of canine donor dogs with no appreciable antigen is 1 in 10,000. Therefore, donor dogs with only high-incidence antigens have been referred to as 'universal donors'. The DEA 4 antigen is currently defined by the use of polyclonal antisera in a tube agglutination technique as performed by a specialist laboratory, and testing for DEA 4 is not available in a point-of-care assay. Both acute and delayed transfusion reactions have been identified when DEA 4-negative recipients have antibody to DEA 4 and are transfused with DEA 4-positive blood (Melzer *et al.*, 2003). Fortunately, < 2% of the population is at risk of this event on the basis of the prevalence statistics cited above.

DEA 5

This system is relatively rare except in US-bred Greyhounds and Japanese-bred dogs. The prevalence in the general population, including purebred and mixed-breed dogs, is 10–15%. The DEA 5 system has one antigen and a null phenotype. Recognized through polyclonal antisera in a tube agglutination assay, this typing is only available through reference laboratories.

The prevalence of antibody to DEA 5 in the general population of dogs that have not received a blood transfusion previously is 10%. Mismatch of this antigen leads to delayed transfusion reactions in which RBCs are removed prematurely from circulation (Young *et al.*, 1951). Therefore, as with DEA 3, concern about this potential mismatch is only an issue in the management of non-regenerative anaemia.

DEA 7

The blood group system for DEA 7 includes two antigens, DEA 7 and DEA 7', and a null phenotype. The significance of this system has been widely debated by experts. Unlike the other DEA blood group systems, DEA 7 is not an integral erythrocyte membrane antigen. This antigen is found in the circulation and it attaches passively to the surface of the RBCs. There are three important aspects related to the DEA 7 system:

- The DEA 7 antigen can be found in the plasma unassociated with RBCs and can diffuse into the saliva
- DEA 7-positive individuals do not change their

status after experimental bone marrow transplantion with DEA 7- negative donor cells
- The passive attachment of the antigen to the erythrocyte makes consistent identification in classical typing systems difficult. Only polyclonal antiserum exists for the identification of DEA 7, which limits testing to reference laboratories.

Antibody to DEA 7 is present in 20–40% of the general canine population. Therefore, the potential for transfusion reaction related to DEA 7 is relatively high. However, because the antigen is not integral to erythrocytes, a low incidence of reaction has been documented. Antibody–antigen interaction causes a delayed transfusion reaction with accelerated removal of RBCs from circulation. Acute reactions have not been demonstrated. The DEA 7 status has more importance when considering compatibility for transplantation or massive blood transfusion.

Additional antigens of transfusion significance

Other blood group systems are likely to exist that have transfusion significance but have not yet been standardized by the ISAG. Often these are demonstrated in tightly bred populations of dogs. The Dal system is a single antigen system of high prevalence in dogs of the Dalmatian breed (Blais *et al.*, 2009b). However, this antigen appears to be lacking in some families of Dalmatians. Antibody to Dal is capable of producing an acute transfusion reaction. To date, antiserum to this antigen is of limited availability, and so the expression of Dal has not been evaluated widely. This system may be similar to the previously described DEA 6 but, owing to the lack of anti-DEA 6 antibody, any relationship cannot be confirmed. Several antigens have been described in the Japanese literature, suggesting that there may be undefined canine blood group antigens that have transfusion significance. As closer attention is paid to the importance of compatibility in canine transfusion, other antigens will be identified. The clinician must be aware of this potential, and utilize point-of-care and reference laboratory resources correctly to identify and manage these antigens.

Blood typing methods

Compatibility involves two components: blood type, and whether or not circulating antibody specific for blood types that are not expressed by the patient's RBCs is present. Blood type can be determined by several different methods and indicates the actual antigens present on the surface of the erythrocyte. The presence of antibody is determined by major and minor cross-matches. Both are important when predicting the outcome of a transfusion.

Originally, tube haemagglutination and haemolysis were used to determine blood type. This method is quite laborious, requires the production of antisera and demands the practice of good laboratory technique. For this reason, tube agglutination is only performed in reference laboratories. Most reference laboratories offer typing services for DEA 1.1. However, a few offer a full DEA identification including DEA 1.0, 3, 4, 5 and 7. Typically, this method of full DEA identification is reserved for advanced donor screening and not typing of a recipient at the time of transfusion. The use of gel columns (see below) has made the tube agglutination assays easier, which may lead to more widespread availability of full DEA typing.

Two point-of-care assays exist. One technique uses a card style agglutination test that relies on operator evaluation of agglutination (Rapid Vet H; DMS Laboratories New Jersey, USA). The other technique uses a membrane diffusion technique that allows colorimetric evaluation (DME 1.1; Alvedia, Lyon, France). Both tests offer rapid access to DEA 1.1 status in dogs. Additional point-of-care assays are under development that will provide even more options for the clinician in the future.

With these assays available cage-side, how should the clinician determine the most compatible donor–recipient pair using the available blood typing techniques? Figures 32.2 and 32.3 describe routine criteria to use when selecting a donor–recipient pair. DEA 1.1 compatibility will decrease the risk of acute transfusion reaction by 24%. It should also be noted that, by using DEA 1.1 compatible donor–recipient pairs, the clinician increases the usable donor pool by 64%. Blood typing for DEA 1.1 assists the clinician significantly in providing safe and effective transfusion medicine for his or her patients.

Decreasing exposure to other DEA systems can reduce the risk of acute and delayed transfusion reactions by an additional 8%. Full DEA typing may play an important role in the management of transplant patients and patients with non-regenerative anaemia, but may not be cost-effective for general transfusion needs.

Donor used for routine RBC transfusion
1. Check DEA 1.1 status. 2. Exclude 'weak' reactors. Weak reactors are those with faint lines or faint agglutination. These dogs may be DEA 1.2 or DEA 1.3 positive. 3. Cross-match potential donor with three or four random healthy dogs. 4. Exclude donors demonstrating a positive cross-match.
Donor used for potential transplant patient, transfusion dependent recipient or non-regenerative erythrocyte disorder
1. Perform full DEA testing (1.1, 1.2, 1.3, 3, 4, 5 and 7). 2. Exclude if positive for DEA 3, 5 and/or 7. 3. Perform major cross-match with 10 healthy dogs. 4. Exclude donors demonstrating a positive cross-match.

32.2 Recommendations for blood typing for maximum compatibility: donor identification.

Routine RBC transfusion
1. Check DEA 1.1 status. 2. Selected donor based on DEA 1.1 status of the recipient. Use DEA 1.1 negative donor for 'weak' reactors. Weak reactors are those with faint lines or faint agglutination. These dogs may be DEA 1.2 or DEA 1.3 positive. To avoid possible alloimmunization use a DEA 1.1 negative donor. 3. Perform cross-match between DEA 1.1 compatible donor and recipient. Minor cross-match is not required if recipient is receiving packed red blood cells only. 4. Exclude donor if cross-match is positive.
Potential transplant patient, transfusion dependent recipient or non-regenerative erythrocyte disorder
1. Check DEA 1.1 status. 2. Selected donor based on full DEA type (1.1, 1.2, 1.3, 4, 5 and 7). Use DEA 1.1 positive, 4 positive donors for DEA 1.1 positive recipients. Use DEA 1.1 negative, 4 positive donors for DEA 1.1 negative recipients and weak reacting DEA 1.1 positive recipients. Weak reactors are those with faint lines or faint agglutination. 3. Perform cross-match between type compatible donor and recipient. Minor cross-match is not required if recipient is receiving packed red blood cells only. 4. Exclude donors demonstrating a positive cross-match.

32.3 Recommendations for blood typing for maximum compatibility: recipient identification.

References and further reading

Andrews GA and Penedo MCT (2010) Erythrocyte antigens and blood groups. In: *Schalm's Veterinary Hematology, 6th edn*, ed. D Weiss and J Wardrop, pp.711–716. Blackwell Publishing Ltd., Ames, Iowa

Blais MC, Berman L, Oakley DA *et al.* (2009b) A red cell antigen lacking in some Dalmatians. *Journal of Veterinary Internal Medicine* **21**, 281–286

Blais MC, Rozanski EA, Hale AS *et al.* (2009a) Lack of evidence of pregnancy induced alloantibody in dogs. *Journal of Veterinary Internal Medicine* **23**, 462–465

Callan MB, Jones LT and Giger U (1995) Hemolytic transfusion reaction in a dog with an alloantibody to a common antigen. *Journal of Veterinary Internal Medicine* **9**, 277–280

Corrato A, Mazza G, Hale AS *et al.* (1997) Biochemical characterization of canine blood group antigens: immunoprecipitation of DEA 1.2, 4 and 7 and identification of a dog erythrocyte membrane antigen homologous to human Rhesus. *Veterinary Immunology and Immunopathology* **59**, 213–223

Frattali AL, Silberstein LE and Spitalnik SL (1996) Human blood group antigens and antibodies. In: *Principles of Transfusion Medicine, 2nd edn*, ed. EC Rossi, TL Simon, GS Moss and SA Gould, pp. 67–87. Williams and Wilkins, Baltimore

Giger U, Gelens CJ, Callan MB *et al.* (1995) An acute hemolytic transfusion reaction caused by dog erythrocyte antigen 1.1 incompatibility in a previously sensitized dog. *Journal of the American Veterinary Medical Association* **201**, 1358–1362

Giger U, Stieger K and Palos H (2005) Comparison of various canine blood typing methods. *Journal of the American Veterinary Medical Association* **66**, 1386–1392

Hale AS and Werfelmann J (2006) Incidence of canine serum antibody to known dog erythrocyte antigens in potential donors. *Journal of Veterinary Internal Medicine* **20**, 800

Lanevschi A and Wardrop KJ (2004) Principles of transfusion medicine in small animals. *Canadian Veterinary Journal* **42**, 4447–4454

Melzer KJ, Wardrop KJ, Hale AS and Wong VM (2003) A hemolytic transfusion reaction due to DEA 4 alloantibodies in a dog. *Journal of Veterinary Internal Medicine* **17**(6), 931–933

Rozanski E and Laforcade AM (2004) Transfusion medicine in veterinary emergency and critical care medicine. *Topics in Companion Animal Medicine* **19**, 83–87

Symons M and Bell K (1991) Expansion of the canine A blood group system. *Animal Genetics* **22**, 227–235

Young LE, Ervin DM and Yuile CL (1949) Hemolytic reactions produced in dogs by transfusion of incompatible dog blood and plasma: Serologic and hematologic aspects. *Blood* **4**, 1218–1231

Young LE, O'Brien WA, Swisher SN *et al.* (1951) Erythrocyte isoantibody reactions in dogs. Transfusion section. *New York Academy of Science* **13**, 209

33

Feline blood groups and blood typing

Michael J. Day†

Introduction

The basis of the feline blood group system was defined many years ago, and the clinical importance of these molecules in mediating blood transfusion reactions and neonatal isoerythrolysis (NI) in cats has long been recognized (Griot-Wenk and Giger, 1995). Recent developments in this area include: the recognition of a new blood group antigen; the molecular characterization of the regulation of expression of the A and B blood group antigens; and the wide commercial availability of simple in-practice tests for the determination of feline blood group. This has enabled the publication of numerous studies that define the prevalence of blood groups in different feline breeds and geographical populations (Figures 33.1 and 33.2). These discoveries are reviewed here.

Country	Group A (%)	Group B (%)	Group AB (%)	Reference
Australia (n = 187)	62	36	1.6	Malik *et al.*, 2005
Brazil (n = 172)	94.8	2.9	2.3	Medeiros *et al.*, 2008
Germany (n = 372)	98.7	1.1	0.2	Weingart *et al.*, 2006
Greece	78.3	20.3	1.4	Mylonakis *et al.*, 2001
Hungary	100	0	0	Bagdi *et al.*, 2001
Portugal (n = 132 DSH)	90.2	3.8	6.0	Silvestre-Ferreira *et al.*, 2004
Portugal (n = 5 DLH)	80	6.7	13.3	Silvestre-Ferreira *et al.*, 2004
United Kingdom (n = 105)	67.6	30.5	1.9	Forcada *et al.*, 2007

33.1 Blood groups in Domestic Shorthair (DSH) and Domestic Longhair (DLH) cats by geographical area 2000–2009. Data prior to 2000 (including information for other countries) are reviewed in Malik *et al.*, 2005.

The feline blood group system

The feline AB blood group system is relatively simple. Cats may be of blood group A, B or AB. The type A antigen is *N*-glycolyl-neuraminic acid (NeuGc) and the B antigen is *N*-acetyl-neuraminic acid (NeuAc). Type A cats have a dominance of NeuGc with small quantities of NeuAc, whereas type B cats have only NeuAc expression. Type AB cats have an equal amount of both molecules on the surfaces of their red blood cells (RBCs). Type B cats appear to lack the enzyme (cytidine monophospho-*N*-acetylneuraminic acid hydroxylase (CMAH)) that converts NeuAc to NeuGc.

The feline *CMAH* gene has now been sequenced and single nucleotide polymorphism (SNP) haplotypes have been associated with the A and B blood types (Bighignoli *et al.*, 2007). There are three alleles that control the AB blood type. The *A* allele is dominant over the *b* allele and the phenotype AB is the result of a third allele (a^{ab}) that allows co-dominant expression of both A and B. The a^{ab} allele is recessive to the *A* allele but dominant over the *b* allele. A cat of type A phenotype may therefore be of genotype *AA*, Aa^{ab} or *Ab*. A cat of type B phenotype must be of genotype *bb*, whereas a type AB cat may be of genotype $a^{ab}b$ or $a^{ab}a^{ab}$.

The inheritance of AB blood groups is now well understood by breeders, who will request that their cats are tested in order to identify animals at risk of neonatal isoerythrolysis (NI) (see below). Mating two type A cats may potentially produce type B kittens. If both type A cats are of genotype *AA*, then all kittens will also be *AA*. Where one parent is genotype *AA* and the other *Ab*, then 50% of the kittens will be *AA* and 50% *Ab*, but all will be of phenotype A. Similarly, an *AA* to Aa^{ab} mating will produce type A kittens of either parental genotype. Where both parents are genotype *Ab*, 50% of the kittens will be *Ab* but 25% will be *AA* and 25% *bb*. By similar reasoning, mating of two Aa^{ab} parents might give rise to 25% $a^{ab}a^{ab}$ kittens of AB phenotype.

Mating two type B cats (genotype *bb*) will always give rise to *bb* kittens. Mating an A to a B cat will have variable outcome. Where a genotype *AA* cat is mated to a *bb* cat, all offspring will be genotype *Ab* (phenotype A). Where a genotype *Ab* cat is mated to a *bb* cat, 50% of offspring will be *Ab* (phenotype A) and 50% *bb* (phenotype B). Mating of an Aa^{ab} to a *bb* cat should lead to an equal proportion of *Ab* (phenotype A) and $a^{ab}b$ (phenotype AB) kittens.

Blood group B is more prevalent amongst particular purebred cats, including the British Shorthair,

Breed	Group A (%)	Group B (%)	Group AB (%)	Number of cats	Country	Reference
Abyssinian	100	0	0	36	Australia	Barrs *et al.*, 2009
	89	11	0	30	Australia	Malik *et al.*, 2005
	100	0	0		Hungary	Bagdi *et al.*, 2001
Bengal	100	0	0	100	UK	Gunn-Moore *et al.*, 2009
	86	14	0	7	UK	Forcada *et al.*, 2007
Burmese	100	0	0	5	UK	Forcada *et al.*, 2007
	93	3	3	30	Australia	Malik *et al.*, 2005
Carthusian/Chartreux	77.8	18.5	3.7	27	Germany	Weingart *et al.*, 2006
Persian	80	20	0	5	UK	Forcada *et al.*, 2007
	67	22	11	9	Australia	Malik *et al.*, 2005
	100	0	0	7	Portugal	Silvestre-Ferreira *et al.*, 2004
	66.6	33.3	0		Hungary	Bagdi *et al.*, 2001
Ragdoll	80	20	0	5	Australia	Malik *et al.*, 2005
Russian Blue	80	20	0	5	Australia	Malik *et al.*, 2005
Siamese	100	0	0	13	UK	Forcada *et al.*, 2007
	100	0	0	12	Australia	Malik *et al.*, 2005
	100	0	0	19	Portugal	Silvestre-Ferreira *et al.*, 2004
	100	0	0		Hungary	Bagdi *et al.*, 2001
Somali	100	0	0	24	Australia	Barrs *et al.*, 2009
	71.4	23.8	4.8	21	Germany	Weingart *et al.*, 2006
Turkish Angora	53.6	46.4	0	28	Turkey	Arikan *et al.*, 2003
Turkish Van	42.3	57.7	0	78	Turkey	Arikan and Akkan, 2004
	40	60	0	85	Turkey	Arikan *et al.*, 2003

33.2 Feline blood groups: breed and geographical prevalence 2000–2009. Data presented are for groups of at least five cats. Data prior to 2000 (including information for other countries) are reviewed in Malik *et al.*, 2005.

Birman, Devon and Cornish Rex, Abyssinian, Persian, Somali, Turkish Angora and Turkish Van. All Siamese, Burmese and Tonkinese cats that have been tested are reported to be blood group A (see Figure 33.1). There are geographical differences in the prevalence of blood group antigens amongst purebred populations, and the prevalence may also change when the same breed groups in an area are sampled some time apart. Most Domestic Short- and Longhair cats throughout the world are of blood group A, but there are geographical differences and in some populations there is a greater prevalence of types B and AB (see Figure 33.1).

Cats of blood group A uncommonly have anti-B alloantibody in their serum and if present this is invariably of low titre. Conversely, type B cats usually have high-titred anti-A alloantibody in the circulation. This may be haemagglutinating (generally IgM) or haemolytic (IgG or IgM) antibody. These alloantibodies are not present at birth but appear within the first few months of life after degradation of maternally derived (colostral) antibody. It is thought that they are induced by exposure to cross-reactive environmental antigens. Type AB cats have neither alloantibody. The titre of alloantibodies may vary with geographical area. Various calculations of the risk of incompatible transfusion or the occurrence of NI can be made on the basis of the known prevalence of feline blood group antigens and expected titres of alloantibodies within a geographical area. In general terms the likelihood of incompatible first unmatched blood transfusion in a cat is much greater than for a dog (Knottenbelt *et al.*, 1999b; Malik *et al.*, 2005).

A new feline blood group antigen, *Mik*, has been identified recently (Weinstein *et al.*, 2007). Some type A cats lack expression of *Mik* and therefore have serum alloantibody specific for this antigen. In these cats, even an AB matched blood transfusion may potentially lead to a reaction, and so cross-matching would be required to detect this incompatibility.

Feline haemolytic transfusion reactions

Immunological transfusion reactions are classical type I or type II hypersensitivity phenomena and involve alloantibody binding, complement fixation and activation of inflammatory pathways (Day and Mackin, 2008). In whole blood transfusion, plasma proteins are more likely to induce type I reactions, while antigens associated with blood cells would trigger type II hypersensitivity. Transfusion reactions may therefore be acute or delayed in onset. Transfusion reactions are uncommon in cats where pre-transfusion blood typing and cross-matching is practised (Weingart *et al.*, 2004; Klaser *et al.*, 2005). Feline acute transfusion reactions may occur within seconds of a type B cat receiving type A or AB blood. These have an initial phase (lasting for several minutes) that may include restlessness, vocalization, salivation, urination, vomiting, diarrhoea, collapse, mydriasis, hypotension, bradycardia, arrhythmia, apnoea/hypopnoea or seizures. There is then a second phase of tachycardia and tachypnoea, arrhythmia and hypertension with a gradual return to normality in around an hour. Haemoglobinaemia and haemoglobinuria may occur if there is acute intravascular haemolysis.

Delayed reactions may occur 3–21 days after transfusion and relate to haemolysis of transfused cells (usually extravascular, without haemoglobinaemia or haemoglobinuria) with mild pyrexia and anorexia. Mismatched transfused RBCs will have a much shorter survival period (minutes to days, depending upon the titre of alloantibody in the recipient) than the 30–38 days that is standard for matched transfusions.

Feline neonatal isoerythrolysis

Haemolytic disease of the newborn (neonatal isoerythrolysis, NI) is of clinical significance in cats (Day and Mackin, 2008). Cat breeders are very aware of this disease and will often ask to have their breeding stock blood-typed in order to calculate the risk of NI occurring in any particular mating. The disease occurs where a type B queen gives birth to type A or AB kittens and it is therefore more likely to be a problem in those breeds with a high prevalence of type B. The high concentrations of anti-A alloantibody that may be present in type B cats will be transferred in colostrum, leading to the development of classical haemolytic anaemia at around 48 hours of life. Affected kittens may have severe clinical disease characterized by jaundice, haemoglobinuria, pallor and weakness, and may die. Alternatively, there is a subclinical form of disease in which kittens may simply display tail-tip necrosis at around 3 weeks of age. These kittens will be Coombs' test-positive. NI is a major cause of the 'fading kitten syndrome'.

Blood typing of breeding stock can help to ensure that such high-risk mating does not take place. The likelihood of NI affecting a litter can be determined before birth by testing serum from the queen against RBCs from the tom in a cross-matching procedure, and determining the titre of anti-A alloantibody present. At-risk kittens should not be allowed to suck from the mother during the period that colostrum can be absorbed and ideally would be fostered on to a type A queen, or be given a colostrum substitute such as milk from a type A queen. This latter approach is less than ideal, because feline milk is not as rich in immunoglobulins as colostrum.

Feline blood typing

Some diagnostic clinical pathology laboratories will offer feline blood typing, but many of these will simply utilize the commercial systems described below.

Agglutination tests

The 'gold standard' for feline blood typing remains the tube or microplate agglutination test, the principle of which is similar to the Coombs' test described in Chapter 5. A washed suspension of patient RBCs is incubated with reagents for the detection of blood group antigens A and B, and in a negative control well containing phosphate buffered saline only. In the microplate test, the reagents may be diluted serially and multiple control wells included. The standard reagent for detection of the A antigen is serum from a type B cat known to contain anti-A alloantibodies. The standard reagent for detection of the B antigen is the lectin from *Triticum vulgaris*, which at low concentration will only agglutinate RBCs that express the type B antigen. Agglutination with one or both reagents defines the blood type of the cat.

Recently, monoclonal antibodies specific for feline blood group antigens A and B have been developed (Green *et al.*, 2000; Kaoru and Kyo, 2001) and these are incorporated into a commercially produced tube-based agglutination test (Shigeta Animal Pharmaceuticals Inc., Oyabe City, Japan; Stieger *et al.*, 2005).

Card systems

The first in-practice technology to be developed was a card-based system (DMS rapidVet-H (feline); DMS Laboratories Ltd., Flemington, New Jersey). These cards are simple to use, and provide a rapid and accurate result. The typing cards have been validated against the gold standard microplate test (Knottenbelt *et al.*, 1999a). The cards have three 'wells' containing reagents for detection of A and B, and a negative control well to check for autoagglutination of the patient RBCs (Figure 33.3). The reagent for detection of the A antigen was initially serum from type B cats, but this has been replaced more recently with a monoclonal antibody specific for A. The anti-B reagent is *T. vulgaris* lectin. A diluent is added to each well, followed by the test blood. After mixing and a brief incubation with gentle rocking, the test is read by determining the presence of agglutination. Reactions for the B blood group antigen can be relatively weak, and it is generally recommended that where the card system suggests a type B or AB cat, the result should be confirmed using a second methodology.

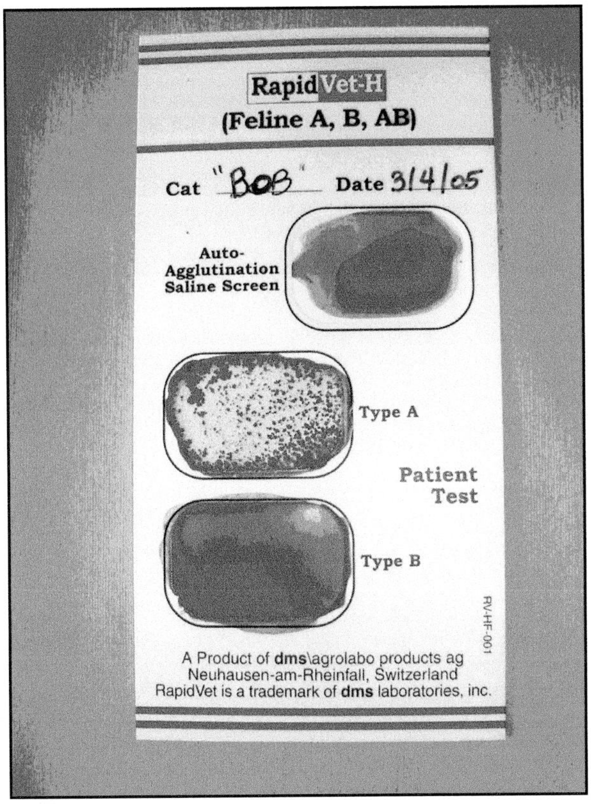

33.3 The DMS Laboratories feline blood typing card. In this test the three wells in the card are first 'activated' by the addition of diluent and then patient blood is added to each. After mixing and incubation the result is determined by inspection. In this card the presence of agglutination in the anti-A well indicates that the cat is of blood group A. (Reproduced from *BSAVA Manual of Emergency and Critical Care).*

Other methods

Further commercially based systems are now available that utilize either gel-based or immunochromatography technologies.

Gel-based

The gel-based test (DiaMed-VET Gel Test Anti A + B; DiaMed AG, Cressier sur Morat, Switzerland) has been evaluated, and it performs well when compared with standard laboratory technology (Stieger *et al.*, 2005). In the DiaMed Gel Test system the typing reagents (polyclonal anti-A serum and anti-B lectin) are impregnated into a gel set within a microcolumn formed in a plastic card (Figure 33.4). A volume of diluted whole blood or washed RBCs is added to the reservoir above the column, and the card is then centrifuged in a purpose-designed machine. The RBCs are gently forced against the gel. Where the RBCs carry the antigen corresponding to the reagent within the gel, they will not be able to migrate through the gel and remain as a band at the upper surface. Where the RBCs lack the antigen corresponding to the reagent within the gel, they pass through the gel to collect at the base of the column. A negative control column is included with each test.

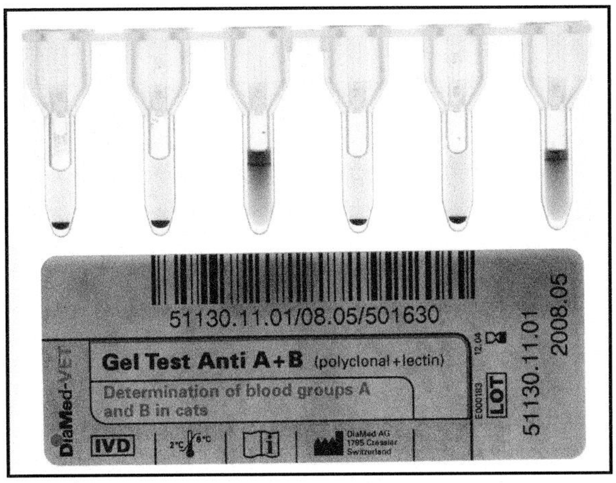

33.4 The DiaMed Gel Test system for feline blood typing. The six columns formed in this plastic card allow typing of two cats. From left to right the columns are negative control, B blood group antigen and A blood group antigen, and then a repeat of these for the second sample. A suspension of washed feline RBCs has been added to the reservoir above each column and the card has then been centrifuged. For both of the cats tested here, red cells have passed through the gel matrix to collect at the base of columns 1 (control) and 2 (anti-B reagent). The RBCs have collected at the top of the gel matrix in column 3 (anti-A reagent). This identifies both cats as being of blood group A.

Immunochromatography

The immunochromatographic test (DMEVET Quick Test A + B; Alvedia, Lyon, France) involves an initial dilution of blood and then insertion of a membrane strip impregnated with reagents into the diluted sample. The RBCs migrate through the strip to interact with the reagents, including a terminal positive control. Once the reaction is completed, the presence of discrete bands will indicate the presence of either or both of the A and B antigens (Figure 33.5).

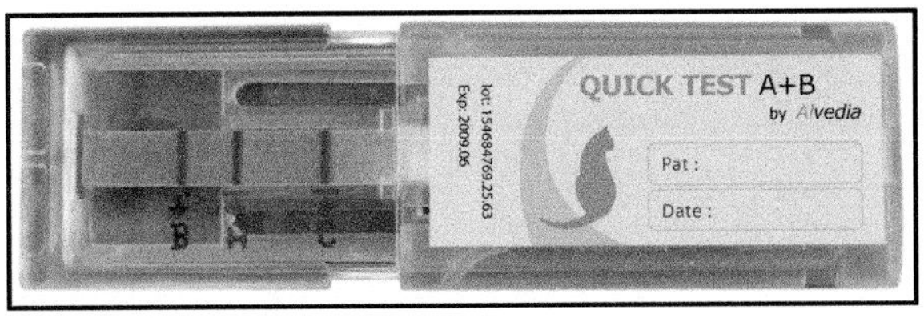

33.5 The Alvedia Quick Test system for feline blood typing. The left-hand end of this immunochromatographic strip has been inserted previously into a suspension of feline blood cells, and these have migrated through the strip matrix to interact at specific points with typing reagents (positions B and A). A control (C) reaction is also included. This test is validated by the presence of the control line and shows that the cat is of blood type AB.

Genetic testing

Most recently, the studies of the *CMAH* gene described above have opened the way to determining blood type by molecular testing using the polymerase chain reaction (PCR) (Bighignoli *et al.*, 2007). Such testing has the advantage of not necessarily requiring a blood sample (e.g. a buccal swab may be used). There is generally good correlation reported between the results of PCR and traditional blood typing methods, although some discordant results occur. PCR testing for feline blood type is not yet widely available, and the discovery of additional *CMAH* mutations may confuse the genotyping results in some individuals.

References and further reading

Andrews GA, Chavey PS, Smith JE *et al.* (1992) N-glycolylneuraminic acid and N-acetylneuraminic acid define feline blood group A and group B antigens. *Blood* **79**, 2485–2491

Arikan S and Akkan HA (2004) Titres of naturally occurring alloantibodies against feline blood group antigens in Turkish Van cats. *Journal of Small Animal Practice* **45**, 289–292

Arikan S, Duru SY, Gurkan M *et al.* (2003) Blood type A and B frequencies in Turkish Van and Angora cats in Turkey. *Journal of Veterinary Medicine A: Physiology, Pathology and Clinical Medicine* **50**, 303–306

Bagdi N, Magdus M, Leidinger E *et al.* (2001) Frequencies of feline blood types in Hungary. *Acta Veterinaria Hungarica* **49**, 369–375

Barrs VR, Giger U, Wilson B *et al.* (2009) Erythrocytic pyruvate kinase deficiency and AB blood types in Australian Abyssinian and Somali cats. *Australian Veterinary Journal* **87**, 39–44

Bighignoli B, Niini T, Grahn RA *et al.* (2007) Cytidine monophospho-N-acetylneuraminic acid hydroxylase (CMAH) mutations associated with the domestic cat AB blood group. *BMC Genetics* **8**, 27

Day MJ and Mackin AJ (2008) Immune-mediated haematological disease. In: *Clinical Immunology of the Dog and Cat, 2nd edn*, ed. MJ Day, pp.94–21. Manson Publishing, London

Forcada Y, Guitian J and Gibson G (2007) Frequencies of feline blood types at a referral hospital in the south east of England. *Journal of Small Animal Practice* **48**, 570–573

Green JL, Chavey PS, Andrews GA *et al.* (2000) Production and characterization of murine monoclonal antibodies to feline erythrocyte A and B antigens. *Comparative Haematology International* **10**, 30–37

Griot-Wenk ME, Callan MB, Casal ML *et al.* (1996) Blood type AB in the feline AB blood group system. *American Journal of Veterinary Research* **57**, 1438–1442

Griot-Wenk M and Giger U (1995) Feline transfusion medicine: blood types and their clinical importance. *Veterinary Clinics of North America: Small Animal Practice* **25**, 1305–1322

Griot-Wenk M, Pahlsson P, Chisholm-Chait A *et al.* (1993) Biochemical characterization of the feline AB blood group system. *Animal Genetics* **24**, 401–407

Gunn-Moore DA, Simpson KE and Day MJ (2009) Blood types in Bengal cats in the UK. *Journal of Feline Medicine and Surgery* **11**, 826–828

Kaoru A and Kyo K (2001) Determination of canine and feline blood types using monoclonal antibodies. *Provet* **10**, 12–16

Klaser DA, Reine NJ and Hohenhaus AE (2005) Red blood cell transfusions in cats: 126 cases (1999). *Journal of the American Animal Hospital Association* **226**, 920–923

Knottenbelt CM, Addie DD, Day MJ *et al.* (1999a) Determination of the prevalence of feline blood groups in the United Kingdom. *Journal of Small Animal Practice* **40**, 115–118

Knottenbelt CM, Day MJ, Cripps PJ *et al.* (1999b) Measurement of titres of naturally occurring alloantibodies against feline blood group antigens in the United Kingdom. *Journal of Small Animal Practice* **40**, 365–370

Malik R, Griffin DL, White JD *et al.* (2005) The prevalence of feline A/B blood types in the Sydney region. *Australian Veterinary Journal* **83**, 38–44

Medeiros MAS, Soares AM, Alviano DS *et al.* (2008) Frequencies of feline blood types in the Rio de Janeiro area of Brazil. *Veterinary Clinical Pathology* **37**, 272–276

Mylonakis ME, Koutinas AF, Saridomichelakis M *et al.* (2001) Determination of the prevalence of blood types in the non-pedigree feline population in Greece. *Veterinary Record* **149**, 213–214

Silvestre-Ferreira AC, Pastor J, Almeida O *et al.* (2004) Frequencies of feline blood types in northern Portugal. *Veterinary Clinical Pathology* **33**, 240–243

Stieger K, Palos H and Giger U (2005) Comparison of various blood-typing methods for the feline AB blood group system. *American Journal of Veterinary Research* **66**, 1393–1399

Weingart C, Arndt G and Kohn B (2006) Prevalence of feline blood types A, B and AB in non-pedigree and purebred cats in Berlin and Brandenburg. *Kleintierpraxis* **51**, 189

Weingart C, Giger U and Kohn B (2004) Whole blood transfusions in 91 cats: a clinical evaluation. *Journal of Feline Medicine and Surgery* **6**, 139–148

Weinstein NM, Blais M-C, Harris K *et al.* (2007) A newly recognized blood group in domestic shorthair cats: the Mik red cell antigen. *Journal of Veterinary Internal Medicine* **21**, 287–292

34

Canine transfusion medicine

Gillian Gibson and Anthony Abrams-Ogg

Introduction

Transfusion therapy, the transfer of blood or its components from a donor to a recipient, has been recorded in history as far back as the 17th century. However, it was not until the 20th century that human transfusion medicine made significant advancements – with the identification of blood type incompatibilities, improved methods of collecting and storing blood, and the development of volunteer donor blood-banking programmes driven by the demands of war-related injuries and bloodshed.

Canine transfusion medicine practices have been growing rapidly over the past few decades, reflecting knowledge and practices in human transfusion medicine, as well as the advancing capabilities of general practitioners and referral hospitals in managing critically ill patients and emergency situations. Historically, whole blood (drawn directly from the donor with the use of anticoagulant) has been used in veterinary medicine, usually administered to the recipient within hours of donation. As the need for and use of blood increases, so must its supply, which is dependent on the availability of healthy donors.

The practice of component therapy, the administration of specific blood components (packed red cells, plasma), is a more economical use of this limited resource. Storage of these products (blood-banking) facilitates their use.

Changes in guidance provided by the Royal College of Veterinary Surgeons note that the taking of blood from donors for immediate or anticipated clinical need is a recognized veterinary practice, and the UK Veterinary Medicines Directorate now permits authorization of blood banks for non-food animals following application for a specific manufacturer's licence. These combined changes in legislation and guidance have provided the opportunity for the development of in-house and commercial blood-banking within the UK, which has dramatically advanced the way in which veterinary surgeons may now practise transfusion medicine.

Knowledge and practice of appropriate blood collection, processing, storage and administration methods is essential for ensuring the safety of the donor and recipient, as well as maximizing the use of limited clinical resources.

Canine blood donors

Sources

Most canine blood donors in the UK are recruited as part of voluntary schemes in which donor animals provide blood for emergency situations or have scheduled routine donations for blood-banking purposes. Although many of the dogs belong to veterinary surgeons, nurses or other practice staff, it is also common to recruit client-owned dogs. Larger blood donor programmes host blood drives and may enlist working service dogs or visit rehoming kennels for retired Greyhounds. All of these donor sources are suitable, provided that informed owner consent is given and the donor screening protocol ensures that the dog is an eligible donor.

An alternative source of donors includes maintaining one or more practice-owned dogs on the premises for the purpose of providing in-house blood donations. However, in the UK this requires Home Office approval. Although having in-house blood donors ensures a reliable supply of blood, the costs associated with maintenance of donors are typically not recovered by transfusion charges and should be considered prior to entering into such an arrangement. Furthermore, the welfare of the donor must be protected, because there are ethical considerations regarding the lifestyle of the hospitalized donor. Successful blood donor programmes in North America that utilize in-house donors often use dogs that would otherwise have been euthanased (retired racing Greyhounds, dogs from overcrowded shelters, etc.). These programmes provide the necessary shelter, food and exercise for these dogs, and after a limited period of service as a blood donor, the dogs are rehomed as pets within the community.

Donor considerations

Canine blood donors should be healthy, good-tempered dogs that are between 1 and 8 years of age. Older donors should only be used at the discretion of the supervising veterinary surgeon, and only under exceptional circumstances. When using standard 450 ml human blood collection bags, a minimum bodyweight of 25 kg for a donor is required. The donor should be receiving appropriate preventive veterinary care, including vaccination, according to practice protocols. They should not be receiving any medication at the time of the donation with the exception of ectoparasite preventatives, routine worming medication or heartworm prophylaxis. Donation should not take place within 10–14 days of having received a vaccination. Any dog that has received a transfusion previously may have developed alloantibodies against different blood types and is unsuitable as a donor. In the past it has been advised not to use bitches that have whelped previously, owing to the potential risk of the bitch becoming sensitized to different red cell antigens during pregnancy. However, a recent study has found that there is no evidence of pregnancy-induced alloantibodies in dogs (Blais *et al.*, 2009). To prevent the possible untoward effects of stress on a bitch and her fetuses/puppies, a currently pregnant or recently whelped bitch should not be used as a blood donor. A further consideration when choosing a donor is breed conformation, with respect to venous access. Blood is collected routinely from the jugular vein in an aseptic manner, and the conformation of some breeds may hinder venepuncture and the maintenance of an aseptic phlebotomy site. The temperament of the donor should be such that it would be amenable to remaining still for the duration of the donation (approximately 10 minutes), with minimal restraint. The use of sedation is not recommended for canine donors, and the exclusion of potential donors that would require sedation is advised unless under exceptional circumstances.

Health assessment

The health of the donor should be assessed by the supervising veterinary surgeon by careful review of the clinical history, thorough physical examination and pre-donation screening blood tests. Predonation tests include determination of blood type (at a minimum DEA 1.1 status, see Chapter 32), annual haematology and comprehensive serum biochemistry profile, as well as infectious disease screening for infectious diseases endemic to their current or previous geographical location.

The risk of infection in any given donor depends on the infectious disease prevalence, and exposure of the potential donor to the infectious agent. Infectious disease agents that have the potential to be transmitted by blood transfusion include *Babesia*, *Leishmania*, *Ehrlichia*, *Anaplasma*, *Neorickettsia*, *Brucella canis*, *Trypanosoma cruzi*, *Bartonella vinsonii* and haemotropic *Mycoplasma* spp. Screening for infectious agents that may have an impact on the health of the donor is also an important consideration, and *Dirofilaria immitis* screening is routine in donors that live in endemic regions. In the UK, an emerging infectious agent of importance is *Angiostrongylus vasorum*. In addition to being a threat to the general health of the dog, occult coagulation abnormalities associated with *Angiostrongylus vasorum* infection may not become apparent until significant tissue trauma (e.g. injury, surgery) is induced. In an affected blood donor, there would be an increased risk of jugular vein haematoma formation, or failure of cessation of haemorrhage from the donor venepuncture site. Although there have been endemic pockets of infection in Wales, Ireland and Southern England for some time, the geographical range of the parasite is expanding rapidly. Given that current testing methods for this parasite are limited and may fail to identify an affected dog, routine prophylactic licensed treatment may be considered.

As knowledge develops, other infectious disease agents may be added to this list. Many of these infectious agents are vector-borne, and are not currently endemic in the UK. As such, many UK-based canine blood donor programmes exclude dogs that have travelled outside the UK as potential donors, as a cautious substitute for infectious disease screening. However with changing global climates and increased pet travel, veterinary surgeons must constantly review their infectious disease screening protocols to suit their population of donors (Wardrop *et al.*, 2005).

In addition to the annual comprehensive health examination, a complete donor history, physical examination and assessment of adequate red blood cell (RBC) mass (e.g. packed cell volume (PCV), haematocrit (Hct) or haemoglobin (Hb) level) should be performed prior to every donation to safeguard the health and assess the suitability of the donor.

Blood groups and typing

The RBC types are determined by species-specific, inherited antigens present on the cell surface. There have been at least 12 antigens identified using the dog erythrocyte antigen (DEA) system (see Chapter 32).

The relevance of blood type is related to its antigenic potential. When a dog receives a blood transfusion, antibodies against donor RBC antigens may result in a haemolytic reaction. There are no clinically significant naturally occurring alloantibodies in the dog (with the possible exception of DEA 7); therefore, most dogs will not experience a severe transfusion reaction if they receive incompatible blood on their first transfusion. However sensitization, via exposure to 'foreign' antigen in a red cell transfusion, elicits an alloantibody response sometimes as early as 4 days following transfusion.

The most significant blood group in this regard is DEA 1.1. Dogs negative for DEA 1.1 that are exposed to DEA 1.1-positive blood will produce a potent alloantibody response, which is likely to invoke an acute haemolytic transfusion reaction following repeat exposure. Therefore DEA 1.1-negative dogs should receive DEA 1.1-negative blood, and DEA 1.1-positive dogs may receive either 1.1-negative or 1.1-positive blood for their first transfusion. All subsequent transfusions should be of the appropriate DEA 1 type, as well as cross-matched to assess *in vitro* incompatibility that may have resulted from sensitization and antibody production.

The significance of transfusion incompatibility associated with red cell antigens DEA 3, 5 and 7 is variable. Sensitization to these antigens or the presence of naturally occurring alloantibodies may result in a delayed transfusion reaction involving sequestration and loss of transfused RBCs. Clinically this may be recognized as a decline in PCV several days after the transfusion, although in many cases resolution of the underlying cause of anaemia and the recipient red cell regenerative response may hide this potential decline.

Most dogs are DEA 4-positive. There is no known natural alloantibody to this antigen, and in many instances its transfusion significance is minor. However a report of a DEA 4-negative dog, sensitized by previous transfusion, experiencing an acute haemolytic transfusion reaction after administration of DEA 4-positive blood suggests that more investigation into the significance of this antigen may be warranted. The situation is similar for the recently described Dal antigen (Blais *et al.*, 2007). Most dogs are Dal-positive, but a Dal-negative dog transfused with Dal-positive blood will be sensitized and at risk for a haemolytic transfusion reaction. The Dal-negative blood type was first identified in some Dalmatians, but it has now been identified in Dobermanns, Shi Tzus and mixed-breed dogs (Blais, unpublished data). Another transfusion reaction in a sensitized dog missing a common red cell antigen was reported earlier (Callan *et al.*, 1995). These reactions emphasize the importance of performing a cross-match for any dog that has been transfused previously.

Blood typing is based on an agglutination reaction. Most antigens are detected by visualizing haemagglutination following incubation with polyclonal or monoclonal antibodies. When using these antibodies, agglutination detects the presence of the particular RBC antigen being tested, and the dog is then considered positive for that antigen. Lack of haemagglutination in response to the antibody indicates that the dog is negative for the test antigen.

DEA 1.1 testing can be performed readily by a variety of methods (reference laboratory and in-house testing), and should be performed on all donors, and ideally recipients (Figure 34.1). Given that the typing methods yield a result based on an agglutination reaction, autoagglutination of canine red blood cells may prevent accurate typing from being performed. In this case, if the autoagglutination persists despite washing the red blood cells with saline, the dog is considered to be DEA 1.1-negative until the underlying cause of agglutination can be resolved and typing repeated. This prevents misclassification of a DEA 1.1-negative dog as DEA 1.1-positive, which is important when choosing the blood donor for the agglutinating recipient. If a DEA 1.1-negative dog were to receive DEA 1.1-positive blood, it would then be sensitized against the DEA 1.1 antigen.

On occasion, weak positive DEA 1.1 results may be noted, and should be interpreted with caution. These may represent DEA 1.2-positive dogs (which are DEA 1.1-negative) and in the case of a weak positive, the typing should be performed by another method to confirm the result. Typing of severely anaemic dogs may be complicated by the relatively

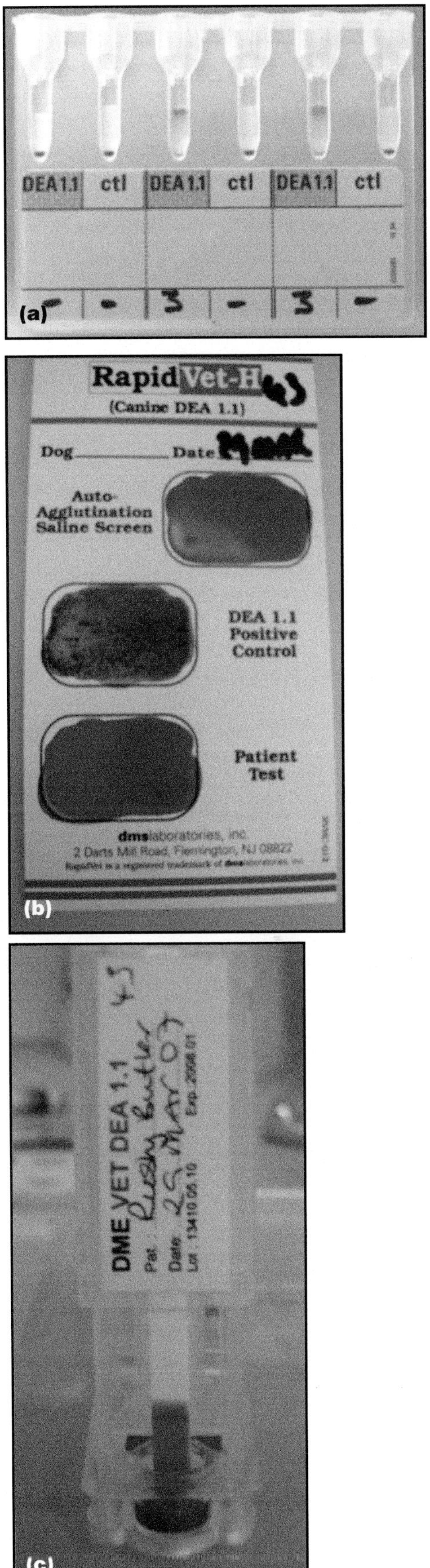

34.1 Dog erythrocyte antigen (DEA) 1.1 blood typing methods: **(a)** DiaMed, Cressier, Switzerland; **(b)** DMS Laboratories, Flemington, NJ, USA; **(c)** Alvedia DME, Lyon, France.

low concentration of RBC antigen present compared with the test antibody concentration. A prozone effect may be created that prevents the agglutination of RBCs needed to achieve a result. In some cases this may be overcome by first separating the plasma from the RBCs of the test sample, removing a drop of plasma, and then resuspending the test RBCs in the remaining test plasma prior to performing the test, thereby increasing the relative concentration of RBC antigen in the test sample. Furthermore, dogs that have received a transfusion previously may yield a 'mixed field' reaction because the test may detect the antigens of the donor RBCs; in this case the accurate blood type may not be identifiable. If it is not possible to blood type the patient prior to an emergency transfusion, a pre-transfusion sample of whole blood should be obtained to permit retrospective typing.

Typing for other antigens is possible through specialized laboratories; however, the necessity of extended type screening of donors is controversial given the low risk of significant first transfusion reactions related to these antigens. Subsequent potential incompatibilities with repeated transfusion, caused by recipient exposure to known or yet undetermined RBC antigens, would mostly be identified by cross-match. As noted previously, following the first transfusion it is highly recommended to perform a cross-match prior to every subsequent transfusion, even when using DEA 1.1 compatible blood, and even if the same donor has been used successfully in the past.

Cross-matching

Cross-matching determines the serological compatibility between the patient and donor blood, based on an agglutination reaction, and allows detection of naturally occurring alloantibodies or alloantibodies produced as a consequence of sensitization. It is still possible for a patient to experience a haemolytic or non-haemolytic transfusion reaction despite a compatible cross-match; therefore, recipient monitoring during and after administration of the product is essential.

- The **major cross-match** is an assessment of the compatibility between donor RBCs and patient plasma/serum.
- The **minor cross-match** is an assessment of the compatibility between donor plasma/serum and patient RBCs.

Minor cross-match incompatibilities are mostly of concern when large volumes of plasma are to be administered (also of note if using whole blood), or where any potential immunological transfusion reaction would be detrimental to the recipient. Patient autoagglutination or haemolysis may mimic an incompatibility reaction between dogs, and therefore a control sample, evaluating the compatibility of the patient RBCs and patient plasma/serum, should be assessed concurrently.

Cross-matching in dogs should be performed:

- Prior to repeat transfusion (> 4 days)
- If there has been a history of a transfusion reaction
- If the recipient's transfusion history is not known.

Techniques

Cross-match techniques are described in many textbooks. They may be performed by reference laboratories, and some in-house kits for the major cross-match are available. Examples of a rapid slide method and a standard tube cross-match procedure are described in Figure 34.2. If a recipient and donor are found to be incompatible via cross-matching, transfusion should not proceed and an alternative donor should be sourced and cross-matched.

A complete cross-match typically performed at an experienced reference laboratory would include a similar procedure to that described in Figure 34.2, but would be conducted at 4°C, room temperature and 37°C, and would also include complement and an antiglobulin test (indirect Coombs' test). This is more time-consuming and is typically not available on an emergency basis. The main value of a complete cross-match over the simplified tube procedure described in Figure 34.2b is that it will reveal incompatibilities that may cause delayed haemolysis. However, a simplified cross-match may be performed rapidly and is likely to detect incompatibilities that will cause a severe acute haemolytic reaction. It is better to perform a simplified tube cross-match, or even a rapid slide method cross-match, than to omit a cross-match on the grounds that it is incomplete.

Interpretation

Interpretation of cross-match results depends on an understanding of and sufficient level of experience in examining RBC suspensions for haemolysis and agglutination (both macroscopic and microscopic). Following completion of the cross-match procedure, the tube is held against a light source to evaluate for haemolysis (light pink to dark red discoloration of the plasma) or agglutination (Figure 34.3).

If macroscopic agglutination is suspected, further microscopic evaluation is necessary to confirm RBC agglutination rather than rouleaux formation (Figure 34.4). With rouleaux, RBCs align to resemble a standing or fallen stack of coins. This type of formation is often normal, and is not indicative of the presence of alloantibody. Rouleaux may be more pronounced in animals with altered protein composition (e.g. hyperglobulinaemia). With agglutination, RBCs aggregate in 'grape-like' clusters. In some cases it may be difficult to distinguish between agglutination and rouleaux, in which case further RBC dilution may assist in clarification.

Some dogs may have alloantibodies present at levels that are too low to be detected by cross-match procedures, and they may experience a mild haemolytic transfusion reaction despite an apparently compatible cross-match result. Vigilant monitoring of the recipient during and following blood product

(a) Rapid slide method

1. Collect blood into an EDTA tube from recipient and donor. Alternatively, for the donor sample, a segment of anticoagulated blood from the donor blood tubing may be used.
2. Centrifuge tubes to settle the red blood cells (RBCs), remove the supernatant and transfer to a clean, labelled glass or plastic tube.
3. Label four glass slides as:
   - Donor control = donor RBCs and donor plasma [a]
   - Major cross-match = donor RBCs and recipient plasma [a]
   - Minor cross-match = recipient RBCs and donor plasma [a]
   - Recipient control = recipient RBCs and recipient plasma [a].
4. On to each slide place 1 drop of undiluted RBCs [b] and 2 drops of plasma [a]. Rapidly mix together with an applicator stick.
5. Gently rock the slides back and forth and observe for macroscopic agglutination within 2 minutes. Place a coverslip and observe for microscopic agglutination (with a ×40 objective or ×100 oil immersion lens) within 5 minutes.

(b) Tube method

1–2. Complete steps 1–2 as above.

3. Wash the RBCs three times with normal saline solution, discarding the supernatant after each wash. To wash RBCs: add approximately 4 ml saline, mix well and centrifuge for 1–2 minutes. The saline is removed from the supernatant, leaving a packed RBC pellet at the bottom of the tube.
4. Resuspend the washed RBCs to create a 3–5% solution by adding 0.2 ml of RBCs to 4.8 ml normal saline (or 1 drop RBC to 20 drops saline).
5. For each donor prepare three tubes labelled 'major', 'minor' and 'recipient control'.
6. Add to each tube 1 drop of the appropriate 3–5% RBCs and 2 drops of plasma according to the following:
   - Donor control = donor RBCS and donor plasma [a]
   - Major cross-match = donor RBCs and recipient plasma [a]
   - Minor cross-match = recipient RBCs and donor plasma [a]
   - Recipient control = recipient RBCs and recipient plasma [a].
7. Incubate the tubes for 15 minutes at room temperature [b].
8. Centrifuge the tubes for approximately 15 seconds to allow the cells to settle.
9. Examine and the samples for haemolysis (reddening of the solution).
10. Gently tap the tubes to resuspend the cells, examine and score the tubes for agglutination as follows:
    - 4+ one solid aggregate of cells
    - 3+ several large clumps/aggregates of cells
    - 2+ medium-sized clumps/aggregates of cells, clear background
    - 1+ small/microscopic aggregates of cells, turbid reddish background
    - +/– microscopic aggregates.

    If macroscopic agglutination is not observed, transfer a small amount of the tube contents to a labelled glass slide and examine for microscopic agglutination (take care not to confuse with rouleaux formation).
11. Recipient control:
    - If there is no haemolysis or agglutination noted in the recipient control tube, the results are valid and incompatibilities can be interpreted
    - If there is haemolysis or agglutination present in equal scoring to the donor test samples, the compatibility and suitability of the donor cannot be accurately assessed.

34.2 Cross-matching. **(a)** Rapid slide method. [a] Serum may also be used and may cause less rouleaux formation. [b] If the results are equivocal, the test may be repeated using diluted RBCs. To dilute RBCs add 0.2 ml of packed RBCs to 4.8 ml normal saline (or 1 drop packed RBC to 20 drops saline). **(b)** Tube method. [a] Serum may also be used and may cause less rouleaux formation. [b] Ideally the cross-match procedure would also be performed at 4 and 37°C.

administration for early detection and treatment of possible transfusion reactions is therefore always recommended.

Blood collection systems

All whole blood collection should take place in an aseptic manner and use an appropriate anticoagulant.

Closed systems

A closed system is one in which the only exposure of the bag or its contents to air prior to patient administration is when the needle is uncapped for venepuncture. Following production of the blood collection system, there must be no exposure of the system components to the external environment, and the entire system must be sterilized by an approved method as per human blood transfusion service guidelines. Examples of closed systems are

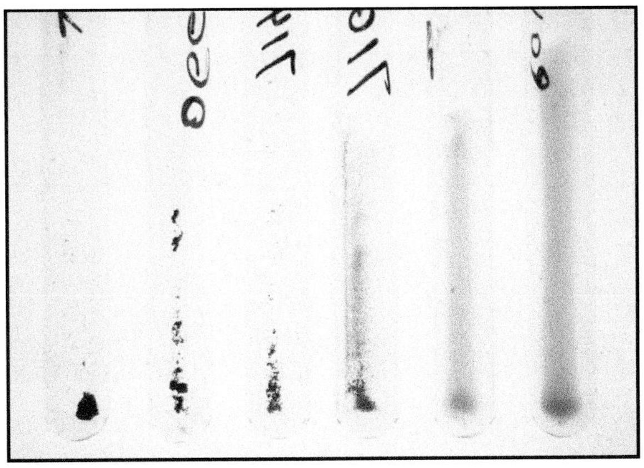

34.3 Grading of agglutination reactions in a canine cross-match. From left to right: 4+, one solid aggregate of red cells; 3+, several large aggregates; 2+, medium aggregates, clear background; 1+, small aggregates, turbid reddish background; ±, tiny or microscopic aggregates, turbid reddish background; negative.

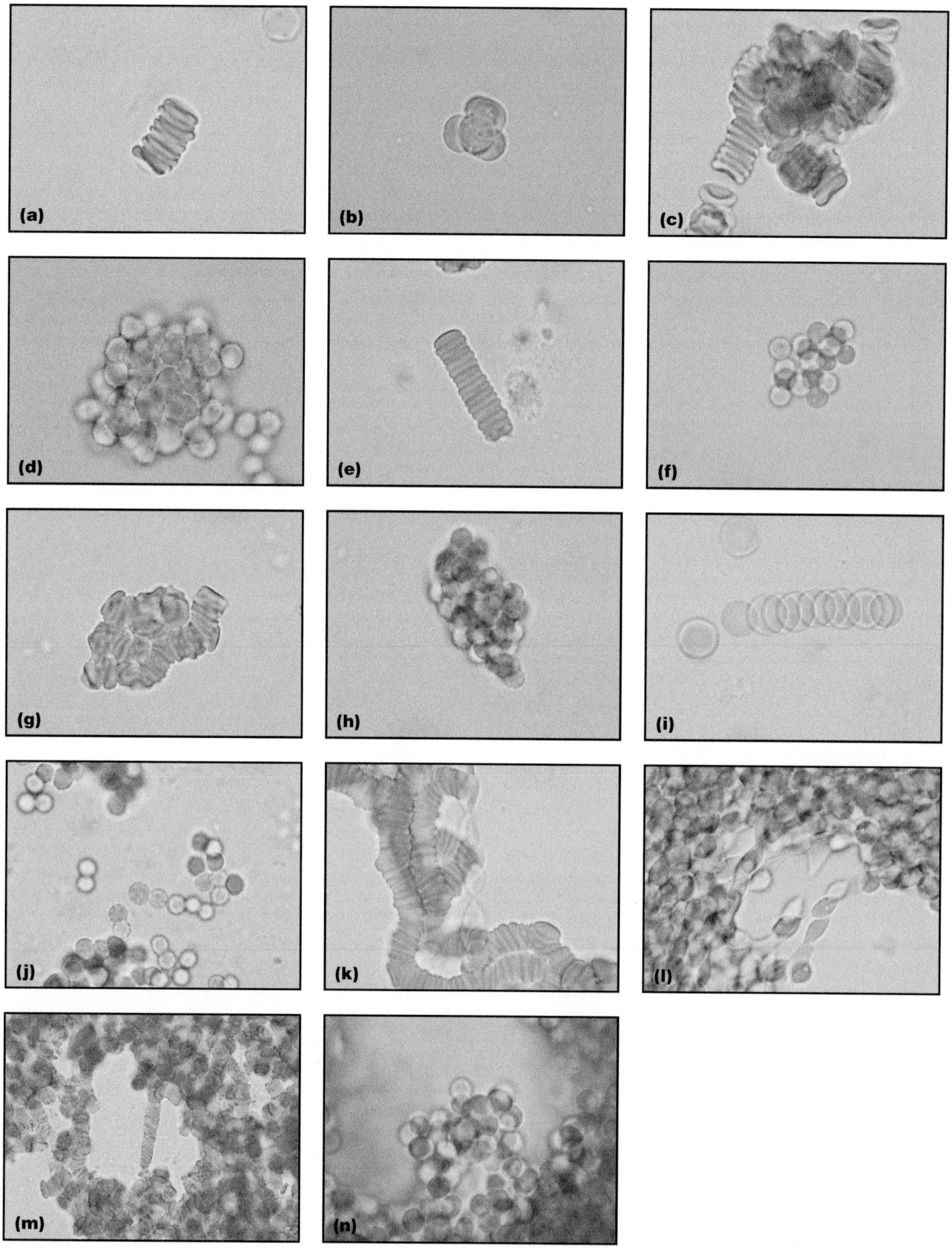

34.4 Microscopic agglutination and pseudoagglutination. All micrographs were obtained using a x100 oil immersion objective unless otherwise indicated. **(a)** Canine single rouleau formation. **(b)** Tiny canine aggregate. **(c)** Small canine rouleaux network. **(d)** Small canine aggregate. **(e)** Feline single rouleau formation. **(f)** Feline medium density aggregate. **(g)** Small feline rouleaux network. **(h)** Small high-density feline aggregate. **(i)** Canine single rouleau formation with the appearance of a fallen-over stack of coins. Such formations occur in thin layer wet mounts. **(j)** Low density feline aggregate resulting in a 'string of beads' effect. Red cell crenation is also present. **(k)** Medium-sized feline rouleaux network pulling apart to form a 'chain of lemons'. **(l)** Large feline aggregate pulling apart to form several 'chains of lemons'. **(m)** Large canine rouleaux networks bridged by a single rouleau formation (x40 high-power objective). **(n)** Large high-density feline aggregate. Close inspection of the edge of such formations aids in distinguishing between rouleaux and aggregates.

commercially available collection bags (from human and veterinary medical suppliers) that already contain anticoagulant and a swaged-on phlebotomy needle and are sterilized, sealed and protected in a plastic or foil overwrap (Figure 34.5a). Most of the standard human collection bag systems contain one or multiple bags (for component processing) to collect 450 ml into 63 ml of citrate–phosphate–dextrose (CPD), citrate–phosphate–dextrose–adenine-1 (CPDA-1), or similar anticoagulant–preservative solution, using a 16 gauge needle. The volume of blood that may be collected safely from canine donors is approximately 20% of their blood volume, every 3–4 weeks. A recommended upper volume collection limit is 18 ml/kg for dogs, and extension of the donor interval to every 8 weeks avoids the need for iron supplementation. For this reason, to ensure the safety of the donor when collecting this volume of blood, the standard human collection systems are most often used for canine donors weighing more than 25 kg.

Collection of a smaller volume may be desirable when collecting blood or preparing blood products for a recipient of low body weight, or when a donor weighing less than 25 kg must be used. Some smaller volume (250 ml and 350 ml) closed collection systems have become available in the past few years and may be used for this purpose. Alternatively, an appropriate volume of anticoagulant–preservative solution may be poured out of the collecting bag through the needle. Finally, as with feline donations, collection of a small volume of blood may be performed using a butterfly needle attached to a syringe to which anticoagulant–preservative has been added. However, systems that do not already contain anticoagulant, or that require needle attachment prior to phlebotomy/donation, are considered to be open systems.

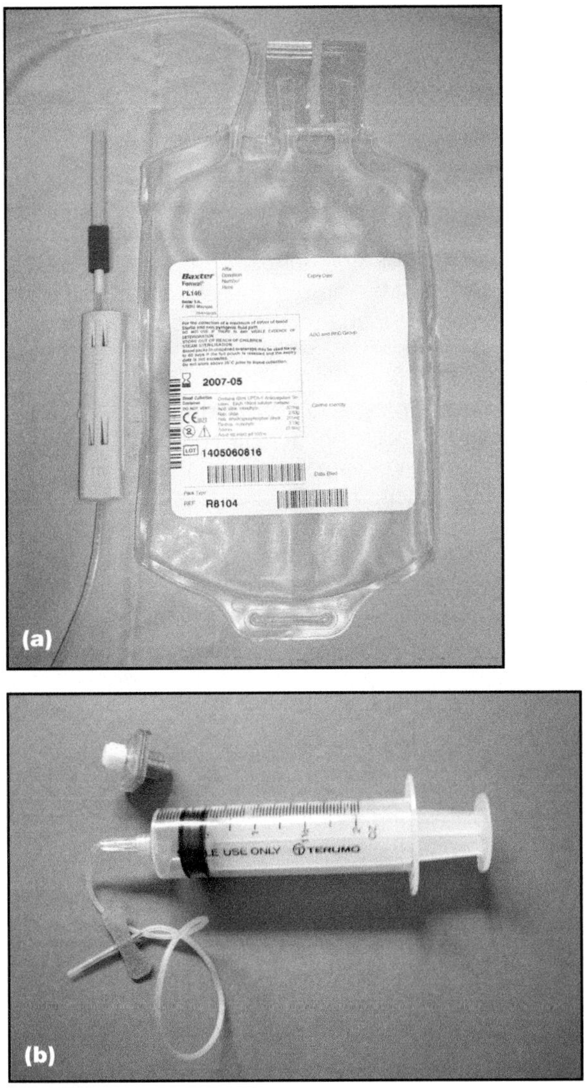

34.5 **(a)** Closed collection system. **(b)** Open collection system.

Open systems

An open system is one in which there is one or more additional sites of potential bacterial contamination during blood collection or processing. Blood collection using syringes or empty collection or transfer bags with anticoagulant added at the time of donation are all classified to be open systems (Figure 34.5b).

All blood collected in an open system must be used within 4 hours of collection, or if stored in a refrigerator (1–6°C) within 24 hours of collection, or it must be discarded. By comparison, whole blood collected in a closed collection system has a storage life of 21–28 days depending on the anticoagulant–preservative used. Blood components prepared from whole blood collected in a closed system have a variable storage life depending on the product, anticoagulant–preservative used and storage method.

Anticoagulant–preservation solutions

An anticoagulant is required to prevent the blood from clotting during and after the donation. Sodium citrate is used most commonly, because the citrate chelates calcium, thereby inhibiting several calcium-dependent steps of the coagulation cascade. Sodium heparin is not a suitable anticoagulant for transfusion purposes. Added preservatives help to maintain RBC viability for variable lengths of storage. Mammalian erythrocytes are living cells that require energy to remain viable and functional for their purpose of transporting oxygen to tissues. Storage conditions must maintain the appropriate balance of pH, glucose, ATP and diphosphoglycerate (2,3-DPG) to maintain adequate RBC viability.

The citrate-containing anticoagulant–preservative solutions most often used are ACD (acid–citrate–dextrose or anticoagulant–citrate–dextrose), CPD or CPDA-1. Most commercially available collection systems contain CPD or CPDA-1. ACD is used more often in open systems when collecting smaller volumes of blood. The dextrose component provides a source of nutrition for the RBCs so that they may continue to support ATP generation through glycolytic pathways. Phosphate serves to optimize the pH for RBC survival, and is a substrate for 2,3-DPG production. Maintaining adequate 2,3-DPG levels is important for maximizing oxygen release from haemoglobin to tissues.

Adenine supplementation provides an adequate nucleotide substrate pool for ATP synthesis by the RBCs.

The volume of anticoagulant used and the duration of time for which the blood product can be stored depend on the composition of the anticoagulant, the collection method and the product type. For whole blood collection ACD is used at a ratio of 1 ml anticoagulant to 7–9 ml of blood, and CPD and CPDA-1 are usually used in ratio of 1 ml anticoagulant to 7 ml of blood. Whole blood in CPD or CPDA-1 may be stored for 21 or 28 days respectively (Wardrop *et al.*, 1994; Callan, 2000).

Human blood-banking standards have set the requirements for storage of transfusion products, and for RBCs this includes a minimum of 75% cell viability for 24 hours post transfusion. *In vivo* studies of viability indicate that canine packed RBCs (PRBCs) stored in CPDA-1 maintain adequate viability for only 20 days of storage. The addition of nutrient additive solutions may extend the storage life of canine PRBCs to 35 days (Nutricel, Optisol) or 37 days (Adsol), depending on the particular solution used. Glass bottles, used several decades ago, have been replaced completely by plastic blood bags. The standard material used for the production of RBC storage bags is polyvinyl chloride with a plasticizer. The extractable plasticizer has been found to improve RBC storage by reducing haemolysis and membrane loss. Use of bags allows for easier component production, storage and transport of transfusion components, and, for some components, permits the necessary gas exchange required to maintain cellular viability.

Blood donation

Health check

Prior to every donation the donor file is reviewed and a thorough history is taken from the owner; some donor programmes find it useful to have the owner complete a specially designed questionnaire. The age and general good health of the donor is confirmed. Many aspects of the health check will have been covered through the donor selection procedure; however, it is important to assess any changes in the donor status for a repeat donor. Relevant questions posed to the owner include: any significant change in the dog's health status; any recent vaccinations or recent/current medications, treatments or surgery since the last donation; and information regarding the timing of oestrous cycles, breeding or pregnancy if appropriate. A full physical examination is performed and noted in the donor file. A small sample of blood for measurement of the PCV or Hb concentration is obtained to ensure the safety of the donor, and the result is recorded in the donor file. Variable recommendations exist as to the necessity for fasting donors for up to 12 hours prior to blood collection, in an attempt to minimize nausea, which may be associated occasionally with the procedure, and to prevent lipaemia in the collected blood. Although lipaemia per se does not appear to affect the quality of whole blood or PRBCs, it may contribute to increased rouleaux formation (complicating cross-match testing), platelet activation and RBC haemolysis (which would be noted in harvested plasma products).

Blood collection

Preparation

All equipment should be prepared and arranged prior to starting the donation procedure, and it is frequently helpful to habituate the donor to the room and the equipment, especially to the noise of the suction machine if used, beforehand.

The donation session usually requires the participation of three people – one phlebotomist and two adequately trained personnel to restrain and monitor the donor, as well as to assist with handling of the collection equipment during the donation. The decision as to whether or not the owner of the donor dog should be present or absent is decided on an individual basis, with consideration of whether the compliance of the donor will be improved or adversely affected by the presence of their owner.

Collection site

The jugular vein is the recommended venepuncture site owing to its size and accessibility. Venepuncture should be performed with a rapid, uninterrupted single stick to avoid cell damage or excessive activation of coagulation factors. Strict aseptic technique and the use of sterile equipment minimizes the possibility of bacterial contamination. Hair can be clipped from over the jugular groove and EMLA cream applied at the time of the pre-donation health check to allow adequate time for the topical anaesthetic to take effect.

Patient positioning and monitoring

Most dogs are able to donate without the use of sedation, and it is preferable to train a donor to accept the procedure. Placing the dog in lateral recumbency, on a comfortable blanket on a table (Figure 34.6), facilitates comfortable restraint (for donor and veterinary personnel) for the approximate

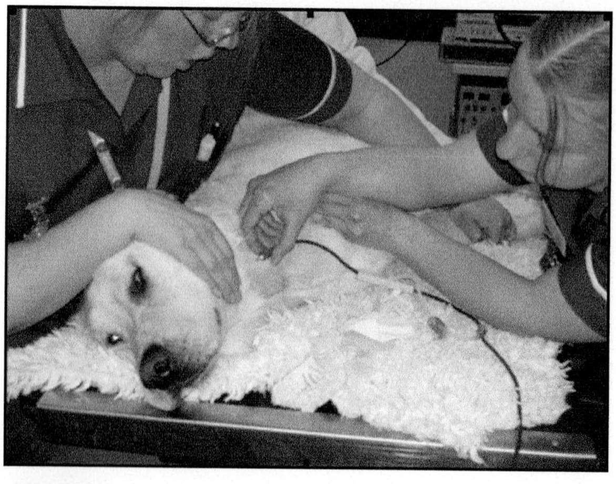

34.6 Canine blood donor in lateral recumbency.

10 minutes required for blood collection. There is less chance of trauma to the jugular vein in this position, because small movements of the head are less likely to occur during collection. Furthermore, adequate digital pressure may be applied to the venepuncture site for haemostasis while the animal maintains a recumbent position post donation. Other positions, in decreasing order of author preference, include sitting, standing and sternal recumbency.

All donors must be monitored closely for hypotension during blood collection by assessing their mucous membrane colour, pulse rate and quality, and respiratory rate and effort. If any concerns develop, the donation should be aborted.

Collection systems

Collection of whole blood from dogs using a commercial blood bag may be accomplished via gravity alone; however, the use of a specialized vacuum chamber may decrease the donation time and therefore the amount of time for which the donor must be restrained. This simple cylindrical acrylic plastic chamber houses the collection bag during the donation, with the donor tubing passing out of a notch at the top of the chamber. A vacuum source that can be regulated at low vacuum pressures (less than –10 inches of mercury or –254 mmHg) is attached to the chamber, and the entire chamber with the collection bag inserted is placed on a gram scale (Figure 34.7). The scale is used to monitor the weight of the bag during collection, to ensure that an adequate and not excessive amount of blood is collected in order to preserve the appropriate ratio of anticoagulant to blood.

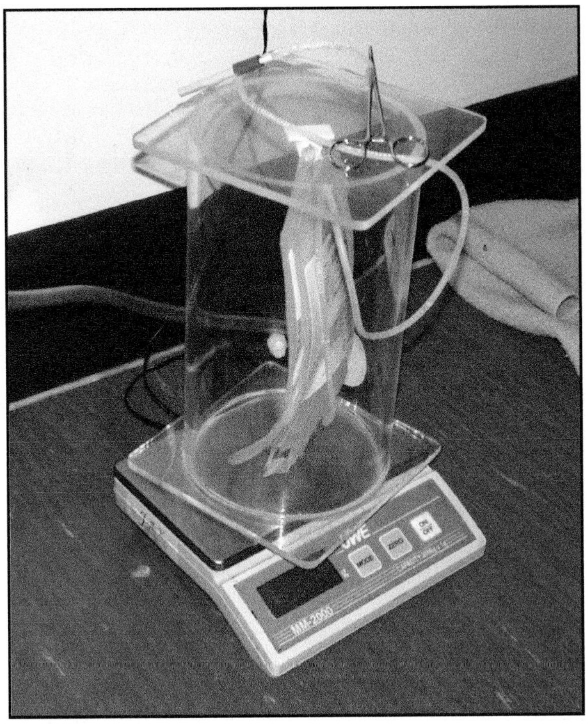

34.7 Vacuum-assisted blood collection chamber, and scale used to determine collection volume by weight.

When collecting blood via gravity alone, the bag should be placed on the scale and the weight of the bag and anticoagulant set to zero (tare) prior to venepuncture; as before, the bag is weighed during donation to confirm collection of the correct blood volume. The volume of blood collected into a commercial blood bag is 450 ml, with an allowable 10% variance (405–495 ml). The weight of 1 ml of canine blood is approximately 1.053 g; therefore, an acceptable unit collected using one of these bags weighs approximately 426–521 g. The donor tubing is clamped to prevent any air from entering the system prior to removing the needle from the jugular vein. Digital pressure is applied to the venepuncture site to prevent haematoma formation and to assist in rapid haemostasis.

Procedure

1. The dog is restrained securely and comfortably (lateral recumbency on a table is recommended; see Figure 34.6).
2. The venepuncture site is prepared aseptically.
3. The phlebotomist applies pressure at the thoracic inlet to raise the jugular vein and facilitate palpation and visualization of the vessel, taking care to avoid contamination of the venepuncture site. If this is difficult to prevent, sterile gloves should be worn. A guarded haemostat or clamp provided with the collection bag is engaged on the donor tubing to prevent air from entering the bag when the needle is exposed.
4. When using vacuum-assisted collection the vacuum chamber is placed on a gram scale (see Figure 34.7).
5. The collection bag is then placed into the chamber, hanging the bag from the clip on the chamber.
6. The donor tubing is placed in the notch at the top of the chamber to allow the tube to exit the chamber, ensuring that enough tube length remains within the cylinder to prevent occlusion during collection.
7. The lid is placed on the chamber and the suction turned on to –2 inches of mercury (–50.8 mmHg). The lid of the chamber is lifted gently to ensure that a tight seal has formed. If whistling is heard, or if the seal is not tight, a small piece of moistened cotton wool is placed at the notch where the tubing exits the chamber to improve the vacuum seal. The suction machine is turned off prior to performing venepuncture.
8. The needle cap is removed and venepuncture performed using a 16 G needle attached to the collection bag. In some dogs it is helpful first to puncture the skin adjacent to the jugular vein and then advance the needle into the vein. The clamp or haemostat on the donor tubing is removed and the phlebotomist checks for a flashback of blood. If no flashback is seen, the donor tubing should be checked for any occlusion and the needle may require repositioning.
9. Once successful blood flow is established, the bag should be positioned lower than the donor to aid in gravitational flow. If using vacuum-assisted

collection the suction is turned on at this point, using a recommended vacuum pressure of –2 to –7 inches of mercury (–50.8 to –177.8 mmHg).

10. The collection bag is inverted gently periodically to mix the blood and anticoagulant. If using a vacuum chamber this gentle mixing is typically not required. If the chamber must be entered during the collection (slowing or cessation of blood flow, checking tube for occlusion) suction must be discontinued in order to remove the lid and make such adjustments.
11. Once the blood donation is complete, any blood remaining in the tubing is stripped into the bag either mechanically (preferably; Figure 34.8) or using the fingers. The bag is gently rocked back and forth to ensure adequate mixing and is then gently compressed by hand to refill the tubing.

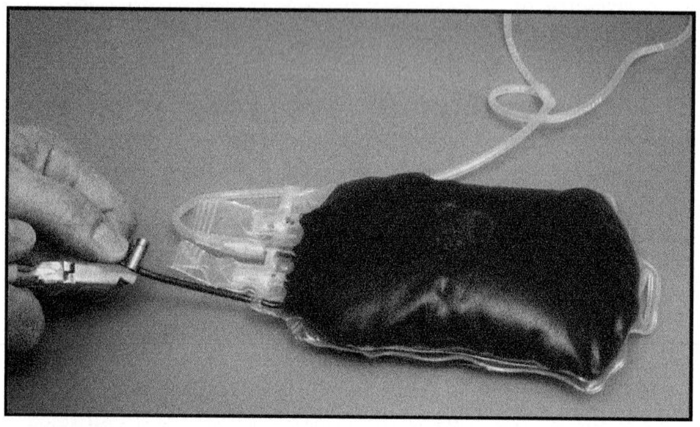

34.8 Upon completion of the transfusion, any blood remaining in the tubing is stripped into the bag.

Storage and labelling

If the collected blood is to be used or stored as whole blood, the tubing should be refilled with the anticoagulated blood and clamped at the distal (needle) end with a hand sealer clip or heat sealer (Figure 34.9a). Subsequently, the tubing is clamped in segments 10 cm in length (marked by 'X's on the tubing), with a double clamp between segments, to be used for cross-match testing (Figure 34.9).

If the blood is collected in a multiple bag system to be used for blood component preparation, the donation tubing line should not be refilled and clamped (see 'Blood product preparation and storage' for how to prepare the whole blood bag for centrifugation. The bag should be labelled with the product type, donor identification, date of collection, date of expiration, donor blood type, donor PCV (or Hct or Hb) and phlebotomist identification prior to use and storage.

Smaller volumes of blood may be collected following feline collection procedures (see Chapter 35).

Following donation

Once adequate haemostasis at the venepuncture site has been achieved, the donor dog is slowly allowed to rise and walk around the donation room. Food and water are offered. Adverse effects associated with donation are uncommon but may include hypotension, bruising or bleeding from the venepuncture site, or dermatitis/skin irritation following the use of clippers and surgical scrub. Evidence of hypotension is typically observed within the first few minutes following donation and may include pale mucous membranes, weakness, lethargy, weak pulses or refusal of food in some cases. Bruising or re-bleeding from the venepuncture site may be an immediate or delayed observation, and skin reaction may be detected a few days following donation. Activity should be restricted to lead-controlled walks only for at least 24 hours after donation. Use of a harness or a lead that is passed under the chest to avoid pressure on the jugular venepuncture site is recommended.

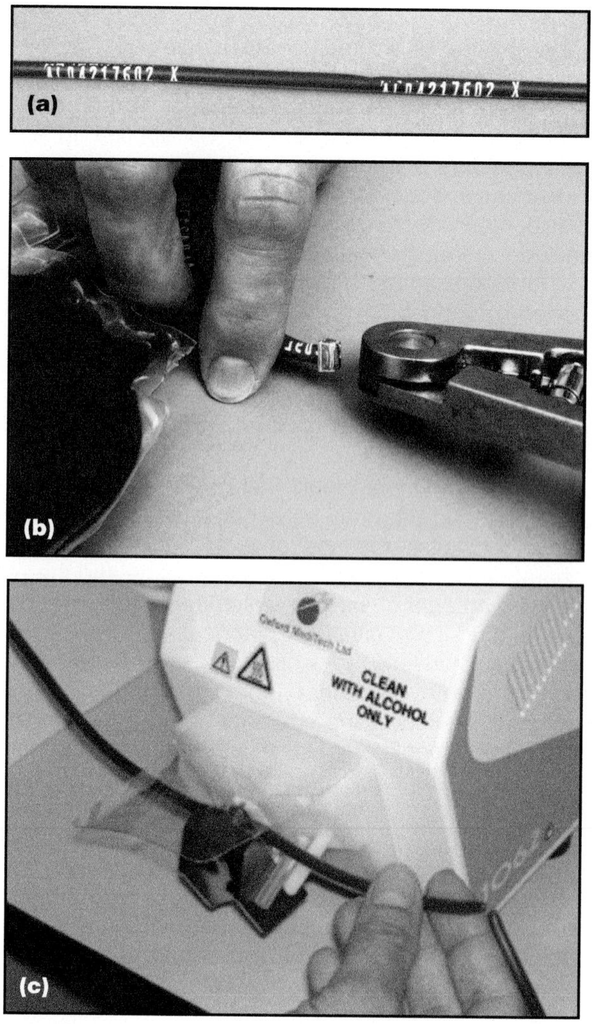

34.9 **(a)** Segments of tubing 10 cm long (marked by 'X' on the tubing) are made for later use as cross-match segments. **(b)** Aluminium sealer clips are most cost-efficient for the quantity of blood bags processed by most veterinary clinics. **(c)** Thermal sealers are more time efficient when large quantities of blood are being processed. If a sealing system is not available, firm knots may be tied, but these do not provide as secure a barrier against leakage and contamination.

The donor record should be completed with information regarding the success or complications of the donation, the volume of blood collected, which jugular vein was used, and calculation of the next available donation date.

Blood product preparation and storage

Initial blood collection yields fresh whole blood. Whole blood may be either stored or separated into red cell (PRBCs) and plasma components (fresh plasma, stored plasma, or platelet-rich plasma concentrates) (Figures 34.10 and 34.11). In larger veterinary centres with a greater emergency and critical care caseload, preparation of blood components is essential to extend the resource. Blood component therapy permits options for smaller volume, specific replacement therapy and reduces the frequency of transfusion reactions.

For preparation of most of the components described, blood processing requires variable-speed, large-capacity, temperature-controlled centrifuges as well as some other ancillary equipment. To prevent microbial contamination a closed collection system must be used for the initial blood collection, and the transfer of components to satellite bags must be contained within the system by integral tubing. Components produced in this manner have variable shelf life depending on the product and storage method. If blood collected into open systems is processed into components, these components must be used within 4 hours, or refrigerated and used within 24 hours of collection.

Many blood banks have facilities to prepare smaller than standard volumes of component products, either by using multi-bag collection systems with more numerous, small satellite transfer bags or by the use of a specialized tube welder to attach an additional satellite bag to the collection system in a closed, sterile manner.

Red blood cell products

Fresh whole blood

Fresh whole blood (FWB) is collected following strict aseptic technique as described above. If not refrigerated, transfusion must be carried out within 8 hours of collection. All blood components (RBCs, platelets, labile and stable coagulation factors, plasma proteins) are present and functional. FWB is the product used most commonly in private veterinary practices; however, if components were always available, the administration of FWB would be restricted to those anaemic patients with concurrent haemostatic defects.

Stored whole blood

Fresh whole blood not used within 8 hours of collection may be stored in a refrigerator at 1–6°C for approximately 21–28 days, depending on the anticoagulant–preservative used. The unit is then classified as stored whole blood (SWB), which will differ only from FWB by the functional reduction of labile clotting factors and platelets. When available, SWB may be useful in anaemic animals with concurrent hypoproteinaemia or loss of circulating blood volume due to haemorrhage.

1. The blood centrifuge is set at the appropriate temperature, speed and time as described in the component processing section and by the centrifuge manufacturer.
2. If a multibag system including a leucocyte reduction filter was used, the collection bag is hung from a hook approximately 2 m above the ground. The tubing seal is broken, allowing the whole blood to run through the filter and into the next empty satellite bag.
3. Once filtration is complete, the tubing is sealed above the filter and then in progressive segments along the length from the filter to the blood bag. In a bag without a pre-storage leucocyte reduction filter, the donor tubing segment is filled with anticoagulated whole blood, and sealed in a similar fashion. These tubing segments provide cross-match samples that can be stored with the red cell product and allow sampling of the donor blood without compromising the closed collection system.
4. The filter and initial collection bag, including the donor tubing and needle, are removed above the sterile seal and disposed of in accordance with health and safety regulations. When using collection sets without a filter, the needle only is removed, below a seal, and discarded.
5. The blood bag and remaining satellite bags are placed in a centrifuge bucket, with the tubing end of the bag pointing upwards. The loose segments of tubing are tucked inside the bucket.
6. The bucket containing the bags is weighed, and a counterweight bucket is created using an empty centrifuge bucket filled with water to a matching weight. Alternatively, a second unit of blood to be processed can be used, with small foam weights or pieces of plastic tubing used to equalize the weights of the two buckets.
7. The buckets are placed in the centrifuge, the lid replaced, outer lid locked and the centrifuge is started.
8. At the end of centrifugation the bucket is removed carefully and taken to the processing area. A plasma extractor, gram scale, guarded haemostats, sealing mechanism and scissors are required.
9. The spring-loaded plasma extractor is placed on the laboratory bench area, and the lever is pulled down and locked under the locking hook.
10. The blood bag is removed gently from the centrifuge bucket and examined for gross evidence of adequate plasma separation. In some cases improper balancing of the centrifuge or centrifuge failure may result in incomplete plasma separation, and repeated centrifugation may be required.
11. The lever is released gently, allowing the front panel of the plasma extractor to gently press the blood bag. The seal at the top of the bag is gently rocked open, and the plasma will begin to flow into the first satellite bag. When the plasma has been extracted almost completely, the tubing just above the plasma bag may be clamped and the lever on the plasma extractor pulled down and locked in an open position.
12. If using a bag system with preservative solution, the seal of the preservative solution bag is now opened and the solution bag raised to allow the preservative to flow among the packed red blood cells. Once the preservative has been transferred completely to the packed red cell bag the red cell bag may be sealed.
13. The clamp on the plasma bag is released slowly, and any air in the unit is gently expressed out into the tubing and into the empty preservative bag. The plasma bag is then sealed.
14. The extra tubing and preservative bag are removed and discarded appropriately.
15. Both the separated plasma and packed red blood cell bags are labelled with product type, donor identification, date of collection, date of expiration, donor blood type, donor PCV (or Hct or Hb), and phlebotomist identification prior to use and storage. This information is usually kept in a log outside the storage refrigerator/freezer for stock control and to minimize the opening and closing of the storage appliances.

34.10 Processing of whole blood for the preparation of components.

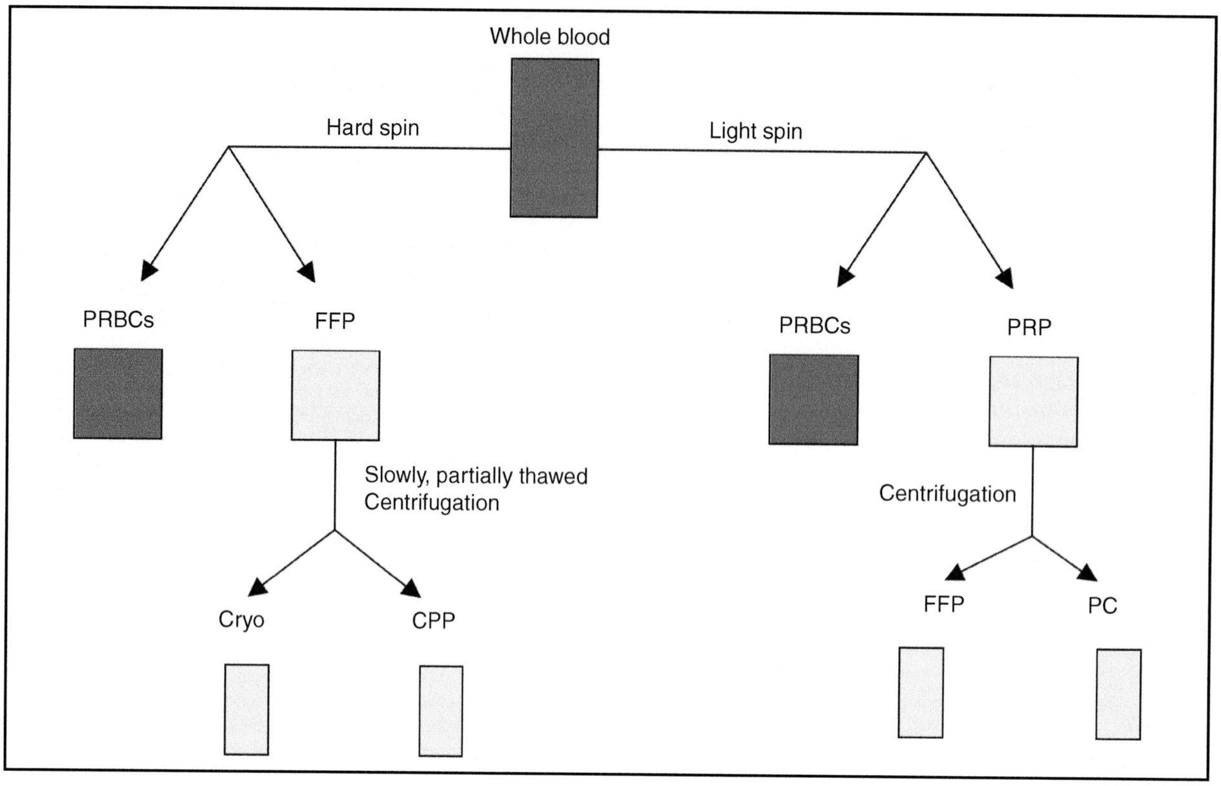

34.11 Processing of blood components. CPP, cryoprecipitate poor plasma; Cryo, cryoprecipitate; FFP; fresh frozen plasma; PC, platelet concentrate; PRBCs, packed red blood cells; PRP, platelet-rich plasma.

Packed red cells

The PRBCs are separated from the plasma by centrifugation. The unit must be collected in a bag with attached satellite bags to allow extraction and transfer of plasma within a closed system. The remaining PRBC unit provides the same RBC properties as a unit of whole blood. PRBC transfusion is indicated in severely anaemic animals, especially those that are normovolaemic, to provide additional oxygen-carrying support. The PCV of the unit is greater than that of the whole blood because it will have been greatly concentrated, and is usually in the range of 70–80% (without added nutrient solution), with the volume yield dependent on the donor Hct. PRBCs collected initially into CPDA-1 may be stored at 4°C for 20 days, with an extension to 35 days if a nutrient additive solution is added. PRBC units without added nutrient solution should be re-suspended or co-administered with 100 ml of physiological saline to reduce the viscosity and improve the flow of the red cell solution.

Plasma products

Fresh frozen plasma

Fresh frozen plasma (FFP) is separated from PRBCs and frozen within 8 hours of collection, according to human blood-banking standards. FFP provides maximum quantities of the labile coagulation factors (F) V and VIII and von Willebrand factor, as well as all other coagulation factors and plasma proteins. Plasma that is refrozen after thawing, or plasma prepared and frozen later than 8 hours after collection, has reduced quantities of labile coagulation factors and von Willebrand factor. Typically, the separated plasma must be placed in the freezer within 6 hours of collection to ensure adequate hard freezing within the 8-hour interval.

FFP is indicated for use in animals with acquired or inherited coagulopathies (inherited factor deficiencies, vitamin K deficiency or antagonism, disseminated intravascular coagulation (DIC), severe liver disease), and may be used prophylactically in patients with known coagulopathies, either perioperatively or at the time of active bleeding. As FFP contains other plasma proteins, it may be used in animals with hypoproteinaemia; however, large volumes and repeated transfusions are required to produce a clinically significant and sustained improvement. FFP may be stored for up to 1 year when frozen below –20°C.

Stored frozen plasma

Stored frozen plasma (SFP) is FFP > 1 year of age, plasma not frozen quickly enough to fully protect labile factors, or FFP that has been thawed and refrozen without opening the bag. Some loss of clotting factors and anti-inflammatory proteins will have occurred, however SFP can be used for colloidal support (in hypoproteinaemia) and still provides vitamin K-dependent factors (which are not labile) to treat vitamin K deficiency or vitamin K antagonist poisoning. SFP may be stored frozen at –20°C for 5 years from the date of collection.

Platelet-rich plasma and platelet concentrate

Platelet-rich plasma (PRP) and platelet concentrate (PC) may be prepared from FWB; however, these products are some of the most challenging to prepare owing to the nature of platelets. To enhance survival and function of the platelets in the resulting product, extreme care and attention must be given to the unit during all phases of handling. Leucocyte reduction filters will also reduce platelets, and blood collected for the production of canine platelet products should use a collection bag without an in-line pre-storage leucocyte reduction filter.

FWB is centrifuged on a 'light' spin – the actual rate and time of which is dependent on the particular centrifuge, with the aim to produce a platelet unit containing at least 5 × 10^{10} platelets. An example of a protocol is 2000 *g* for 2.5 minutes at 20–24°C. The speed and time of centrifugation are lower than those typically used to separate PRBCs and plasma, and the product is not refrigerated. The PRP is separated from the PRBCs, and may either be administered to the recipient, stored (see below) or processed further into PC and FFP.

To prepare PC, PRP, with an attached empty satellite bag, is centrifuged at 5000 *g* for 5 minutes. All but approximately 35–70 ml of the supernatant plasma is transferred into the empty bag and frozen (FFP), leaving the PC in a small volume of liquid plasma in the second bag. The PRP and PC may be stored at 20–24°C, with gentle continuous or intermittent agitation, for 5 days when collected using a closed system. Given that the storage temperature is higher than that used for other blood products, platelet products are more susceptible to bacterial contamination, and if collected in an open system, they should be used within 4 hours of collection. These products are used when there is uncontrollable, severe or life-threatening bleeding (e.g. intracranial haemorrhage) caused by thrombocytopenia or thrombocytopathia, although the difficulties associated with their production often results in the use of more readily available FWB.

Cryoprecipitate

Preparation of cryoprecipitate (Cryo) provides a source of concentrated von Willebrand factor, FVIII, FXIII, fibrinogen and fibronectin from a unit of FFP. Cryo may be prepared from FFP within 12 months of collection. A unit of FFP is slowly thawed until only approximately 10% of the plasma remains frozen, and then centrifuged at 5000 *g* and 4°C for 5 minutes. The Cryo-poor plasma, or the Cryosupernatant, is expressed, leaving behind the Cryo in a small volume of plasma (10–15 ml). The Cryo-poor plasma contains many clotting factors (including vitamin K-dependent factors II, VII, IX and X), as well as other anticoagulant and fibrinolytic factors, albumin and globulin, which had been present in the unit of FFP. The Cryo and remaining Cryo-poor plasma are refrozen immediately and should be used within 1 year of the original collection. The use of desmopressin (DDAVP) at 0.6 µg/kg body weight, diluted in 15 ml of physiological saline, administered by slow intravenous injection 30–60 minutes prior to donation, may increase the amount of von Willebrand factor in the donor FFP and increase the yield of cryoprecipitate (Johnstone, 1999). Cryoprecipitate is used in the management of patients with bleeding caused by deficiency or dysfunction of FVIII (haemophilia A), von Willebrand factor or fibrinogen. Cryo-poor plasma may be used for other coagulopathies that do not require supplementation of the Cryo components, or for patients with hypoproteinaemia.

Storage of blood products

Red cell products should be stored in a refrigerator maintained at 1–6°C, in an upright position. The shelf life of the product is based on the anticoagulant–preservative solution used in collection. Specialized blood storage refrigerators with built-in temperature alarms are available, or a dedicated regular household refrigerator with low in-and-out traffic may be used. A refrigerator thermometer should be checked daily to ensure appropriate storage conditions.

Almost all of the plasma products are stored frozen at −20°C or below. Regular household freezers may suffice, however the temperature should be checked daily using a thermometer, and opening and closing of the freezer minimized. Furthermore, some household freezers have variable temperature sections, as well as automatic thaw–freeze cycles that may be inappropriate for plasma storage. In addition to monitoring freezer temperature, simple procedures at the time of initial freezing of plasma assist in improving plasma stability. One method is to place an elastic band around the plasma bag prior to freezing. Once the plasma is hard frozen the elastic band is removed, and a 'waist' is visible (Figure 34.12). Disappearance of the 'waist' during storage would suggest that the unit

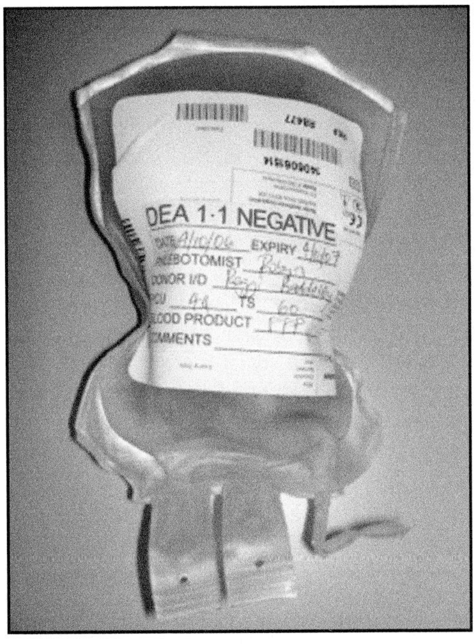

34.12 A unit of frozen plasma showing the 'waist' created by freezing with a rubber band in place.

has thawed and refrozen, signifying compromise of storage conditions and plasma quality. Alternatively, the bag may be frozen horizontally and stored vertically to detect a change in position of an air bubble. The frozen plasma unit is vulnerable to cracking if dropped, and should be handled with care. Cardboard storage boxes are available for individual plasma units to provide additional protection against damage to hard-frozen plasma products.

Indications for transfusion

Blood products are used to treat a variety of conditions, including those associated with anaemia (haemorrhage, haemolysis or reduced erythropoiesis), coagulopathies, sepsis, DIC and specific factor deficiencies.

RBC products increase the oxygen-carrying capacity of the blood, and thus improve oxygen delivery to peripheral tissues in patients with acute or chronic anaemia. Adequate tissue oxygenation is a balance between oxygen consumption and oxygen delivery. Tissue oxygen delivery is dependent on the blood haemoglobin concentration and cardiac output.

Anaemia

With peracute blood loss anaemia, the effects of anaemia need to be considered separately from those of hypovolaemia. Signs of hypovolaemia may be present (prolonged capillary refill time, dry mucous membranes, poor peripheral pulses, tachycardia, decreased central venous pressure) with an apparently normal PCV as fluid shifts have not yet occurred. The site of haemorrhage is typically grossly apparent. Crystalloids or synthetic colloids should be used for initial rapid acute volume replacement, with an anticipated need for a subsequent RBC transfusion. A whole blood transfusion or PRBC with plasma or synthetic colloids would be appropriate.

Dogs with chronic anaemia tend to maintain a normal intravascular volume, but with a reduced RBC mass, therefore PRBC is the component of choice. Chronic anaemia is better tolerated than acute anaemia owing to inherent adaptive mechanisms, including an increase in 2,3-DPG (and an accompanying shift in the oxygen dissociation curve) and increased cardiac output. For many animals with chronic anaemia the clinical signs depend on the level of activity of the patient, as well as the presence of coexisting disease. In humans with chronic anaemia the cardiac output at rest is usually not increased until the Hb is < 7 g/l (approximate PCV < 21%), although in patients with concurrent cardiac disease the threshold is likely to be higher. Transfusion of RBC may be indicated when signs of weakness, fatigue and increased respiratory rate at rest become apparent.

The goal of an RBC transfusion is not to cure the disease, but temporarily to provide haemoglobin to the patient to allow stabilization, prevent the onset of or reduce tissue hypoxia, and permit time for diagnosis and treatment of the underlying disease.

The decision to transfuse RBCs is based therefore on several factors, including the Hb concentration (or PCV), onset of anaemia (acute versus chronic), presence of ongoing losses and most importantly the clinical signs shown by the patient. Tachypnoea, tachycardia, bounding peripheral pulses, collapse, lethargy and weakness are all signs that would prompt the consideration of a red cell transfusion. Infusion of Oxyglobin may also be considered if available (see Chapter 36). There is not a precise PCV below which a transfusion is required, although any patient with a PCV < 20% should be considered a potential candidate, and almost all canine patients will benefit once the PCV is ≤ 12%.

Coagulopathies

Plasma products are a source of coagulation factors and various plasma proteins, and deficiencies of these factors or selected proteins are potential indications for their use.

Correct diagnosis and identification of the type of haemostatic abnormality (e.g. primary or secondary haemostatic defect) is important for appropriate planning and therapy. Deficiency of von Willebrand factor, manifested as a primary haemostatic defect, may be controlled with Cryo or FFP transfusion. These would also be suitable products for use in a dog with haemophilia A (FVIII deficiency). FFP may be indicated in acquired bleeding disorders such as liver disease or DIC. Either FFP or SFP is suitable for treatment of vitamin K antagonism (rodenticide toxicity).

Historically, FFP has been advocated for use in dogs with sepsis or systemic inflammatory response syndrome (SIRS), for example in dogs with severe pancreatitis, because theoretically the provision of protease inhibitors present in plasma may be beneficial. However, this practice is under clinical review and to date the evidence has not been overwhelmingly supportive.

Hypoproteinaemia

Hypoproteinaemia may result from haemorrhage, intestinal or glomerular loss, or decreased production associated with liver failure. The benefit of plasma transfusion to a hypoproteinaemic patient is limited – the circulation time of transfused albumin in hypoproteinaemic states is potentially very short, and with protein-losing diseases several units of plasma would be required to correct the albumin deficit. Other modes of therapy (hyperalimentation, synthetic colloids) are suggested for longer-term management of hypoproteinaemia. In general, plasma transfusion for the treatment of hypoproteinaemic patients is restricted to those with concurrent anaemia or coagulation abnormalities.

Other uses

Occasionally, plasma transfusions will be used for their short-term effect prior to surgical exploration or tissue biopsy. An alternative to plasma is lyophilized canine albumin, which is available from some commercial veterinary blood banks. Human albumin may also be used if there is no other option, but carries the risk of Type I and Type III hypersensitivity reactions.

Administration of blood products

Blood products are usually administered intravenously, but may also be given via an intraosseous route if required (e.g. kittens, puppies). They should not be given intraperitoneally.

Equipment

An in-line blood filter (170–260 μm) is required for all blood products (including plasma) and is incorporated in standard blood infusion sets. A paediatric filter with reduced dead space (Figure 34.13) or microaggregate filters of 18–40 μm are useful for infusing smaller volumes of products and blood collected in syringes. The purpose of the in-line filter is to eliminate blood clots and other large cellular particles that could produce emboli in the recipient.

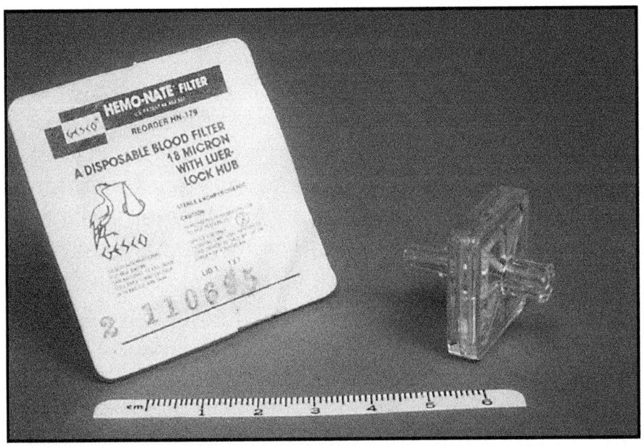

34.13 Paediatric filter used for administration of small volumes of blood products.

Preparation

Visual inspection of the product is necessary, especially when using stored products. Discoloration of red cells (brown, purple), the presence of clots or haemolysis may indicate bacterial contamination, or other storage lesions, and that the blood should not be used. Plasma bags must be examined for evidence of thawing and refreezing, in which case the product may have decreased efficacy with respect to coagulation factor activity. Given that frozen plasma products are hard solid, if the bag is torn or cracked the closed system has been breached and there is a risk of microbial contamination.

Stored RBC products do not need to be warmed prior to use, unless they are being given to neonates, other very small animals, hypothermic animals, or if they are administered rapidly in large volumes. Warming may lead to structural damage (e.g. haemolysis) of the RBCs as well as providing favourable conditions for proliferation of any microbial contaminant. If there is a valid indication for warming of a RBC product this can be accomplished most safely and easily by leaving the unit at room temperature for approximately 30 minutes or placing the entire sealed unit (covered in a protective sealed plastic bag) in a warm water bath (temperature < 37°C) for approximately 15 minutes prior to administration. Alternatively, a segment of intravenous administration tubing can be run through a warm water bath or infusion warmer during the transfusion. Microwave warming of RBCs is contraindicated.

FP products are thawed gently in a warm water bath to return them to a liquid state prior to administration. The entire plasma bag should be enclosed in a sealed plastic bag, which remains in place during thawing of the plasma in a warm water bath to protect the injection ports from contamination.

Procedure

Once the selected component unit is ready for administration, the appropriate administration set is attached to the bag – and in doing so for the first time since collection the closed collection system is breached. Most often the products are administered with the aid of gravitational flow. Fluid pumps should not be used for RBC transfusions unless they have been validated appropriately for such use by the manufacturer, because they could induce red cell haemolysis. Packed RBCs stored without nutrient additive solution may be re-suspended in or co-administered with 100 ml physiological saline to decrease their viscosity and improve flow.

The amount of blood product to be administered depends on the specific product, desired effect and patient's response. A general rule-of-thumb is that 2 ml of transfused whole blood per kg recipient weight will raise the PCV by 1%. Most patients will receive between 10 and 22 ml/kg, and a suggested formula to calculate the amount of whole blood required for transfusion in dogs is:

$$\text{volume (ml)} = 85 \times \text{bodyweight (kg)} \times \frac{\text{desired PCV} - \text{actual PCV}}{\text{donor PCV}}$$

For PRBC or FFP the average volume for infusion is 6–12 ml/kg.

The rate of administration depends on the cardiovascular status of the recipient. In general, the rate should only be 0.25–1.0 ml/kg/h for the first 20 minutes to observe for immediate transfusion reactions; if well tolerated the rate may then be increased to deliver the remaining product within 4 hours. Blood products should not be infused over a period of time greater than 4 hours (in keeping with the general rule for open collection systems) owing to the increasing risk of bacterial proliferation within the product held at room temperature. In an animal with an increased risk of volume overload (cardiovascular disease, impaired renal function) the rate of administration should not exceed 3–4 ml/kg/h. If it is likely to take more than 4 hours to deliver the desired volume, the product may be divided so that a portion remains refrigerated for later use (within 24 hours). In emergency situations, such as haemorrhagic shock, whole blood or PRBCs can be administered as rapidly as is necessary.

An animal should not receive food or medications during a transfusion, and the only fluid that may be administered through the same catheter is 0.9% saline.

The dose listed for Oxyglobin in a normovolaemic dog is 10–30 ml/kg at rate $\leq$ 10ml/kg/h. An in-line filter is not required with use of this solution.

Recording and monitoring transfusions

The following parameters should be measured prior to (baseline), every 15–30 minutes during, and 1, 12 and 24 hours after transfusion:

- Attitude
- Rectal temperature
- Pulse rate and quality
- Respiratory rate and character
- Mucous membrane colour
- Capillary refill time.

The PCV, total protein and plasma colour (to assess for the development of haemolysis) should be assessed prior to and usually 12 and 24 hours following transfusion. Urine coloration may also be a useful indicator of haemolysis.

It is helpful to design a transfusion monitoring sheet, with time points and monitoring parameters noted, to prompt the observer during transfusion. Careful monitoring will allow for prompt recognition and treatment of transfusion reactions, as well as evaluation of transfusion efficacy. In the case of plasma transfusion for correction of haemostatic abnormalities, reassessment of coagulation parameters following transfusion is required to assist in evaluating the efficacy of therapy.

Transfusion reactions

Any undesired side effect noted as a consequence of a blood product transfusion is considered to be a 'transfusion reaction'. The reported frequency of transfusion reactions is variable, as is their severity. Treatment for any suspected transfusion reaction is to discontinue the transfusion immediately, and to treat the clinical signs accordingly. The types of transfusion reaction recognized may be classified as immunological (haemolytic or non-haemolytic) and non-immunological, as well as acute or delayed.

Immunological transfusion reactions

Acute haemolytic reaction

The type of transfusion reaction of most concern is an acute haemolytic reaction with intravascular haemolysis. This is an antigen–antibody, type II hypersensitivity reaction, primarily mediated by IgG. This type of reaction is seen in DEA 1.1-negative dogs sensitized to DEA 1.1 upon repeated exposure, as well as other sensitized alloantibody-mediated incompatibilities. Clinical signs may include fever, tachycardia, dyspnoea, muscle tremors, vomiting, weakness, collapse, haemoglobinaemia and haemoglobinuria. These reactions may lead to shock, and uncommonly DIC and renal damage.

If such a reaction is suspected, the transfusion should be discontinued immediately, and intravenous access must be maintained with administration of a crystalloid solution, or colloid when required, while carefully monitoring the patient for development of fluid overload (by measuring central venous pressure and heart rate, and by lung auscultation). Blood pressure and urine output should be monitored because hypotension may follow, and pressor agents and diuretics may be administered as required (e.g. low dose dopamine infusion, furosemide).

Acute febrile non-haemolytic transfusion reactions and reactions to bacteria-contaminated blood products may have similar signs to acute haemolytic reactions. The donor and recipient blood type should be confirmed and a cross-match performed, if not already performed pre-transfusion. The product type, date of expiration, volume and rate of administration should be checked. A sample of donor and recipient blood should be examined for evidence of haemolysis, and saved for microbial culture and further infectious disease screening if needed. A Gram or haematological stain of a smear of donor blood may be helpful initially to investigate contamination of the unit, and if bacterial contamination is suspected, broad-spectrum intravenous antibiotic therapy should be initiated. Given that DIC and renal failure may occur, monitoring the animal's coagulation profile, BUN, creatinine and electrolytes is advisable.

Non-haemolytic reactions

Non-haemolytic immunological reactions are those of acute type I hypersensitivity reactions (allergic or anaphylactic), most often mediated by IgE and mast cells. These patients show a range of clinical signs from urticaria to pulmonary oedema, which may include pruritus, erythema, oedema, vomiting and dyspnoea. If this type of reaction occurs, the transfusion should be stopped and the patient examined for evidence of haemolysis and shock. Antihistamines (diphenhydramine 1–2 mg/kg i.m. or chlorphenamine 2.5–5 mg i.m. for a small to medium-sized dog, or 5–10 mg i.m. for a medium to large dog) and steroid medication (dexamethasone 0.5–1.0 mg/kg i.v.) may be required. If the reaction subsides, the transfusion may be restarted at 25–50% of the previous rate. If there is evidence of anaphylactic shock, adrenaline, intravenous fluids, antihistamines, H2 blockers (e.g. cimetidine, ranitidine), colloids, dopamine and aminophylline may also be administered at standard dosages as needed, in addition to the above treatment measures.

Reactions to leucocytes and platelets may occur, manifested by a febrile non-haemolytic transfusion reaction, which may last up to 20 hours post transfusion. These are recognized as an increase in body temperature by > 1°C without an obvious underlying cause. The risk of these types of reaction may be minimized by the use of leucocyte reduction filters in the preparation of blood components.

Delayed reactions

A delayed haemolytic reaction with extravascular haemolysis may be recognized 2–21 days after transfusion, and some signs may be similar to those of an acute haemolytic reaction (e.g. hyperbilirubinaemia/bilirubinuria), but they are usually less severe. The owner may notice jaundice or anorexia, and on examination the animal may be febrile or have an unexpected decline in PCV (Kerl and Hohenhaus, 1993). This type of reaction requires intervention less frequently, other than perhaps administration of anti-pyretics.

Other delayed immune-mediated transfusion reactions that may occur include post-transfusion purpura (thrombocytopenia noted within the first week after blood transfusion), neonatal isoerythrolysis, and immunosuppression of the recipient.

Non-immunological transfusion reactions

These include anaphylactoid reactions, which often result from too rapid an infusion rate and may subside after discontinuation of the transfusion or reduction of the infusion rate. They may be clinically indistinguishable from urticarial and anaphylactic reactions. If an apparent allergic reaction is mild and subsides, the transfusion may be continued at a slower rate. If a reaction does not recur, the reaction was probably anaphylactoid. Continuing the transfusion is not recommended if the reaction was moderate to severe. Circulatory overload may occur in any patient receiving excessive volumes of blood products, especially those with cardiac or renal disease, and treatment with diuretics may be required. A potential consequence following administration of large volumes of plasma or whole blood is citrate intoxication causing hypocalcaemia, which is of greater risk in patients with impaired liver function. Clinical signs of hypocalcaemia may be noted (e.g. vomiting, muscle tremors, tetany, changes on the ECG), but routine serum calcium levels will be normal. The ionized calcium level, if available, will be low. Treatment includes calcium gluconate (50–150 mg/kg i.v. of a 10% solution) or calcium chloride (5–10 mg/kg i.v. of a 10% solution) by slow infusion.

Other non-immunological reactions include polycythaemia and hyperproteinaemia (typically as a consequence of excessive product administration), hypothermia, dilutional coagulopathy (from treatment of major haemorrhage with large volumes of stored whole blood), thrombosis, microbial contamination, hyperammonaemia, hypophosphataemia, hyperkalaemia, acidosis, pre-transfusion (*in vitro*) haemolysis, haemosiderosis, air embolus, and infectious disease transmission. Many of the potential contributors to a non-immunological transfusion reaction occur as a result of processing or storage lesions. Hypothermia, uncommonly encountered following transfusion of refrigerated or frozen products to neonates or very small dogs, would be noted and should be addressed by routine patient monitoring during and following transfusion.

Preventive measures necessary to minimize the risk of transfusion reactions include appropriate donor screening, collection, preparation, storage and administration of products. Adherence to standard protocols helps to ensure safety and efficacy of transfusions in practice.

Autologous transfusion

The term autologous transfusion refers to a transfusion in which the blood donor and recipient are identical. There are three basic types of autologous transfusion used to reduce the requirement for allogenic transfusion products:

- Collection and storage of the patient's blood at some time prior to a surgical procedure that is likely to be associated with blood loss (e.g. orthopaedic surgery), so that the patient's own blood may be transfused when needed at the time of surgery
- Immediate preoperative donation and isovolaemic haemodilution with crystalloid fluids, with subsequent reinfusion of the donated fresh whole blood that has been held at room temperature for less than 6 hours to maintain platelet function
- Cell salvage and reinfusion of blood from the thoracic or abdominal cavity subsequent to trauma or intraoperative or postoperative haemorrhage (most common in veterinary medicine).

The advantages offered by autologous transfusion include: decreased recipient exposure to allogenic blood, thereby avoiding the risk of alloimmunization; reduced potential for transmission of infectious agents; fewer immunosuppressive effects of allogenic transfusions; and a reduction in the occurrence of non-haemolytic immunological transfusion reactions. The demand for allogenic transfusion products, a limited resource, is also reduced and the autologous product is available immediately.

Cell salvage

Specially designed cell salvage devices exist that include a collection container of variable volume capacity, aspiration method, anticoagulation system and red cell washing mechanism; they produce concentrated autologous red cells ready for reinfusion. The washing stage removes red cell debris, free haemoglobin, platelets, anticoagulant cytokines, clotting factors and plasma. These processes all occur within a closed system. Not surprisingly the cost of these devices prevents their routine use in veterinary medicine. Other devices and systems involve collection of the shed blood into sterile containers containing anticoagulant, but without the washing process, in which case filtration of the blood prior to administration is of utmost importance.

There are descriptions of less sophisticated cell salvage procedures in many emergency and critical care texts. These all utilize some form of blood aspiration (sterile vacuum suction tip or syringe and tubing), with an attached collection reservoir (bag, syringe or sterilized canister), after which the blood is reinfused into the patient. Filtration of the blood during the collection, as well as during patient transfusion, with a 40 μm filter is recommended to minimize the risk of microembolization. The addition of anticoagulant is dependent on the nature of the haemorrhage. Blood that has been in contact with serosal surfaces in the pleural or peritoneal cavities for greater than 1 hour becomes defibrinized; therefore blood collected from slow haemorrhage into these cavities is unlikely to require anticoagulant. However, blood collected from a site of rapid, fresh haemorrhage will require anticoagulation. Use of CPD at a dose of 25–30 ml per 500 ml of autotransfused blood has been recommended. Blood collected in this manner should be used within 4–6 hours of initiating collection.

Recovery and reinfusion of shed blood is most often appropriate in cases where haemorrhage occurs from a clean wound (e.g. open heart surgery, vascular surgery, orthopaedic procedures) and the blood may be removed and collected by aspiration at a rate that does not induce undue haemolysis. Knowledge of the potential complications of autologous transfusion, described below, aid further in assessing the risks and benefits and achieving a decision regarding the appropriate use of autotransfusion on an individual patient basis.

Complications

The potential complications associated with autologous transfusion are divided broadly into haematological and non-haematological effects. Haematological complications include haemolysis, thrombocytopenia and coagulation abnormalities. Non-haematological problems include microembolization, air embolism, hypocalcaemia, parenteral infusion of topically administered agents, dissemination of malignancy and microbial contamination.

Haematological complications

Haemolysis of RBCs leads to an increase in the free Hb, which with increasing concentration in the reinfusate carries the risk of acute tubular necrosis. Haemolysis may occur as a consequence of RBC contact with traumatized serosal surfaces, as well as secondary to the collection method (e.g. too high aspiration/suction pressure, air exposure) or during reinfusion. For these reasons use of vacuum suction at a level of –10 to –15 mmHg (–0.39 to –0.59 inches of mercury) for a closed-chest drainage system or –40 to –60mmHg (–1.57 to –2.36 inches of mercury) intraoperatively, limiting collection of intracavitary haemorrhage to that of less than 4–6 hours' duration, and ensuring that the blood aspiration device (needle, suction tip) is kept below the surface of the blood to prevent air interface damage, are all recommended.

Reductions in platelet number and function have been seen in dogs receiving autotransfusion, as well as recipients of stored blood products; however, the clinical significance of these findings is not clear and is likely to be of most relevance in massive transfusions.

Salvaged blood is also deficient in coagulation factors and other proteins, as well as containing increased fibrin degradation products and D-dimers, as a result of the clotting activation and fibrinolysis that occurs during haemorrhage and blood pooling within the body cavity. The risk of clinical coagulation abnormalities induced by transfusion of hypocoagulable salvaged blood is increased when large volume transfusions are administered, and patient monitoring via laboratory assessment of coagulation is advised because intervention with other transfusion products (e.g. FFP, cryoprecipitate) may be necessary.

Non-haematological complications

Transfusion of microemboli, containing cellular elements or proteins, may result in pulmonary or renal dysfunction. This risk is minimized by the use of filtration methods, either by the washing process with automated cell-salvage devices, or the use of in-line filters during collection or reinfusion of salvaged blood. Air emboli, introduced to the patient during reinfusion of salvaged blood, are limited when a gravity flow infusion system is used and the risk is minimized by close monitoring during reinfusion. With appropriate precautions, the risks of either microembolization or air embolization are no greater in autotransfusion than in allogenic transfusion.

The development of hypocalcaemia is a risk when reinfusing blood with excessive citrate anticoagulant (e.g. unwashed salvaged cells), especially in patients with underlying liver disease. Monitoring ionized calcium levels, and for clinical signs of hypocalcaemia, during and following autologous transfusion are recommended. Inadvertent infusion of topically applied preparations, such as antimicrobial agents, cleaning agents, clotting agents (sponge/fabric materials) may cause systemic adverse effects in the recipient, and avoidance of collection of blood from areas of product application is advisable.

Microbial contamination of the reinfused blood is certainly possible, given the nature of the emergency collection and non-standardized collection systems employed, especially with collection from the abdominal cavity. The risk of sepsis associated with reinfusion of bacterially infected blood is much greater in a compromised patient (e.g. one in shock) than in a healthy dog. Minimizing the risk of microbial contamination is achieved by using sterile collection and reinfusion equipment, avoiding the use of blood with possible enteric contamination, and discarding any unused harvested blood 4–6 hours after collection.

A concern that often arises is the use of blood that may contain malignant cells (e.g.

from haemoabdomen following a ruptured splenic haemangiosarcoma) – and whether the use of this blood would be contraindicated. Currently there is little evidence to suggest that the practice of autotransfusion in these patients would be likely to contribute to dissemination of malignancy when using cell salvage devices that include washing of RBCs before reinfusion, or additional post-collection treatments such as blood irradiation. However there are few data to support or refute the possibility of tumour dissemination when using direct patient reinfusion techniques, as most commonly employed in veterinary medicine, and as such the use of blood possibly contaminated by malignant cells should be considered contraindicated unless under extreme, life-saving circumstances. In addition the infusion of such blood may aggravate pre-existing DIC.

Conclusion

Recommendations and protocols for canine transfusion medicine have been based on human blood-banking standards and transfusion guidelines, and have been followed by numerous veterinary surgeons who practice transfusion medicine worldwide. Clinical experience reported and published by veterinary colleagues has continued to promote the safe practice of transfusion therapy. While these standards should be maintained wherever possible, and following less than ideal standards may increase the risk of adverse reactions or complications associated with transfusion, a potentially life-saving transfusion should not be withheld in emergency circumstances when these standards cannot be met fully.

References and further reading

Blais MC, Berman L, Oakley DA *et al.* (2007) Canine *Dal* blood type: a red cell antigen lacking in some Dalmatians. *Journal of Veterinary Internal Medicine* **21**, 281–286

Blais MC, Rozanski EA, Hale AS *et al.* (2009) Lack of evidence of pregnancy-induced alloantibodies in dogs. *Journal of Veterinary Internal Medicine* **23**, 462–465

British Committee for Standards in Haematology (BCSH), Blood Transfusion Task Force (2001) Guidelines for the clinical use of red cell transfusions. *British Journal of Haematology* **113**, 24–31

British Committee for Standards in Haematology (BCSH), Blood Transfusion Task Force (2004)

Guidelines for the use of fresh-frozen plasma, cryoprecipitate and cryosupernatant. *The British Society for Haematology* **126**, 11–28

Brooks M (2000) Transfusion of plasma and plasma derivatives. In: *Schalm's Veterinary Hematology 5th edn*, ed. BF Feldman, JG Zinkl and NC Jain, pp.838–843. Lippincott Williams and Wilkins, Philadelphia

Callan MB (2000) Red blood cell transfusions in the dog and cat. In: *Schalm's Veterinary Hematology 5th edn*, ed. BF Feldman, JG Zinkl and NC Jain, pp.833–837. Lippincott Williams and Wilkins, Philadelphia

Callan MB, Jones LT, Giger U *et al.* (1995) Hemolytic transfusion reactions in a dog with an alloantibody to a common antigen. *Journal of Veterinary Internal Medicine* **9**, 277–279

Chan DL (2009) Autotransfusions using cell-saver devices. *Proceedings International Veterinary Emergency and Critical Care Symposium*, pp.663–665.

Couto CG and Iazbik MC (2005) Effects of blood donation on arterial blood pressure in retired racing greyhounds. *Journal of Veterinary Internal Medicine* **19**, 845–848

D'Alessandro A, Liumbruno G, Grazzini G *et al.* (2010) Red blood cell storage: the story so far. *Blood Transfusion* **8**, 82–88

Feldman B (2000) Blood transfusion guidelines. In: *Kirk's Current Veterinary Therapy XIII: Small Animal Practice*, ed. JD Bonagura, pp.400–403. WB Saunders, Philadelphia

Giger U (2000) Blood typing and crossmatching to ensure compatible transfusions. In: *Kirk's Current Veterinary Therapy XIII: Small Animal Practice*, ed. JD Bonagura, pp.396–399. WB Saunders, Philadelphia

Giger U and Blais MC (2005) Ensuring blood compatibility: update on canine typing and crossmatching. *Proceedings of the American College of Veterinary Internal Medicine*, pp.721–723

Giger U, Gelens CJ, Callan MB *et al.* (1995) An acute hemolytic transfusion reaction caused by dog erythrocyte antigen 1.1 incompatibility in a previously sensitized dog. *Journal of the American Veterinary Medical Association* **206**, 1358–1362

Hale AS (1995) Canine blood groups and their importance in veterinary transfusion medicine. *Veterinary Clinics of North America: Small Animal Practice* **25**, 1323–1332

Harrell KA and Kristensen AT (1995) Canine transfusion reactions and their management. *Veterinary Clinics of North America: Small Animal Practice* **25**, 1333–1364

Hohenhaus AE (2000a) Blood banking and transfusion medicine. In: *Textbook of Veterinary Internal Medicine, Diseases of the Dog and Cat, 5th edn*, ed. SJ Ettinger and EC Feldman, pp.348–356. WB Saunders, Philadelphia

Hohenhaus A (2000b) Transfusion reactions. In: *Veterinary Hematology, 5th edn*, ed. BF Feldman, JG Zinkl and NC Jain, pp.864–868. Lippincott Williams and Wilkins, Philadelphia

Johnstone I (1999) Desmopressin enhances the binding of plasma von Willebrand factor to collagen in plasmas from normal dogs and dogs with Type I von Willebrand's disease. *Canadian Veterinary Journal* **40**, 645–648

Kerl ME and Hohenhaus AE (1993) Packed red blood cell transfusions in dogs: 131 cases (1989). *Journal of the American Veterinary Medical Association* **202**, 1495–1499

National Blood Service (2005) *Guidelines for the Blood Transfusion Services in the United Kingdom*, 7th edn. The Stationery Office, Norwich

Prittie JE (2003) Triggers for use, optimal dosing, and problems associated with red cell transfusions. *Veterinary Clinics of North America: Small Animal Practice* **33**, 1261–1275

Purvis D (1995) Autotransfusion in the emergency patient. *Veterinary Clinics of North America: Small Animal Practice* **25**, 1291–1304

Schneider A (2000) Principles of blood collection and processing. In: *Schalm's Veterinary Hematology 5th edn*, ed. BF Feldman, JG Zinkl and NC Jain, pp.827–832. Lippincott Williams and Wilkins, Philadelphia

Stowell CP, Giordano GF, Kiss J *et al.* (1997) Guidelines for blood recovery and reinfusion in surgery and trauma. *American Association of Blood Banks Autologous Transfusion Committee*, 1996–1997. American Association of Blood Banks, Bethesda, MD

Wardrop KJ (1995) Selection of anticoagulant-preservatives for canine and feline blood storage. *Veterinary Clinics of North America: Small Animal Practice* **25**, 1263–1276

Wardrop KJ, Owen TJ and Meyers KM (1994) Evaluation of an additive solution for preservation of canine red blood cells. *Journal of Veterinary Internal Medicine* **8**, 253–257

Wardrop KJ, Reine N, Birkenheuer A *et al.* (2005) Canine and feline blood donor screening for infectious disease. *Journal of Veterinary Internal Medicine* **19**, 135–142

Wardrop KJ, Tucker RL and Anderson EP (1998) Use of an in vitro biotinylation technique for determination of posttransfusion viability of stored canine packed red blood cells. *American Journal of Veterinary Research* **59**, 397–400

Wardop KJ, Tucker RL and Mugnai K (1997) Evaluation of canine red blood cells stored in a saline, adenine, and glucose solution for 35 days. *Journal of Veterinary Internal Medicine* **11**, 5–8

Wardrop KJ, Young J and Wilson E (1994) An in vitro evaluation of storage media for the preservation of canine packed red blood cells. *Veterinary Clinical Pathology* **23**, 83–88

35

Feline transfusion medicine

Barbara Kohn and Christiane Weingart

Introduction

Blood transfusions have become an important component of feline intensive medical and surgical care. The number of blood transfusions given at the Small Animal Clinic of the Freie Universität Berlin has increased steadily: from September 1998 to August 1999, a total of 20 cats were transfused; 2 years later this number was 37 cats; and in 2009 a total of 58 cats received blood transfusions. Feline blood transfusions are now often given in first-opinion practice. Traditionally, cats were transfused with fresh whole blood (WB); however, component therapy is increasingly available at university hospitals and available from commercial blood banks. This chapter reviews the practical aspects of transfusion medicine in cats.

Feline blood donors

Donor cats should be healthy large adults, with no history of previous blood transfusion, with a pleasant demeanour and easily accessible jugular veins. Donor cats should not be on any medication other than those that prevent endo- and ectoparasites. Arthropod control is essential because fleas and ticks are the vectors of agents potentially transmitted by transfusion. Blood donors should be up-to-date with core vaccinations (feline calicivirus, herpesvirus and panleucopenia). Cats that have outdoor access should not be used as blood donors; indoor cats guarantee restricted access to other cats, which minimizes the risk of disease transmission. Pregnant queens should not be used as donors, because donation poses an undesirable stress on the donor and the fetuses.

Blood donors may be obtained from several sources, such as closed colonies owned by the hospital, voluntary donor programmes or cats owned by staff and students. An advantage of closed colonies is the ready availability of donors in emergency situations. However, the additional costs incurred for care, vaccination and deworming of these animals must be considered. Cat owners can be 'on call' if fresh blood is required, and/or their animals can donate blood regularly if the hospital practises blood banking. Volunteer donors require more labour-intensive procedures that include physical examination and blood collection for diagnostic tests and blood typing. All this must be done prior to transfusion, which makes it more difficult to use these animals in emergency situations. Moreover, donors might not be acceptable because of seropositivity to feline leukaemia virus (FeLV) or feline immunodeficiency virus (FIV), abnormalities in the complete blood count (CBC) or serum biochemical profile, or physical abnormalities (e.g. cardiac murmurs).

Clinical evaluation

A complete history of the donor animal should be taken before each blood collection. Annual laboratory evaluation consisting of a CBC and serum biochemistry profile is recommended in cats that donate regularly. Before beginning the blood draw, the current bodyweight, temperature, pulse and respiration must be measured. Before each blood donation a clinical examination and a CBC should be performed and important biochemical parameters (e.g. electrolytes, creatinine) should be measured. Donor cats must have a haematocrit (Hct) of > 0.30 l/l, and preferably of > 0.35 l/l.

Infections and parasites

A consensus statement providing veterinary surgeons with guidelines for screening canine and feline donors for infectious diseases has been produced by the American College of Veterinary Internal Medicine (ACVIM; Wardrop *et al.*, 2005). The following recommendations are included in this statement:

- Infectious agents such as FeLV and FIV should be evaluated by standard enzyme-linked immunosorbent assay (ELISA) techniques to detect antigen and antibody, respectively.
- Haemotropic *Mycoplasma* spp. (*Mycoplasma haemofelis*, '*Candidatus* Mycoplasma haemominutum', '*Candidatus* Mycoplasma turicensis') should be evaluated by polymerase chain reaction (PCR). Although blood smear examination for the organisms on the surface of erythrocytes has been used to detect active infections, the organisms are unlikely to be apparent in chronically infected, asymptomatic cats. Cats that recover from haemoplasma infections can remain chronic carriers and

should be excluded from blood donation.
- Natural transmission of bartonellosis (e.g. *Bartonella henselae*, *B. clarridgeiae* or *B. koehlerae*) by blood transfusion is possible, because the organism is an intraerythrocytic bacterium. Controversy surrounds whether routine screening of blood donors by immunofluorescent antibody test (IFAT), PCR or culture should be recommended, and whether seropositive cats should be used as blood donors.
- Testing for *Cytauxzoon felis*, *Ehrlichia* and *Babesia* spp., *Anaplasma phagocytophilum*, *Dirofilaria immitis* and *Neorickettsia risticii* should be considered if cats have been in endemic areas and have been exposed to ticks or other vectors.
- An aliquot of blood should be stored from each donated unit of blood, to allow retrospective testing in cases of suspected transfusion-associated disease transmission. Absolute safety with regard to transmission of infectious diseases can never be guaranteed.

Other pre-transfusion tests

To ensure efficient and safe transfusions, blood from both donor and recipient should be typed. A universal feline blood donor does not exist. Owing to their naturally occurring alloantibodies, cats with blood type A should only receive type A blood, and cats with blood type B should only receive type B blood. Type AB cats, which have no alloantibodies, may be transfused with blood of type AB or A. Given that anti-B alloantibodies in type A cats occur in only small amounts, significant clinical transfusion reactions are not expected if whole type A blood is given to an AB cat. Type AB cats are considered AB-universal red blood cell (RBC) recipients; they can receive RBCs of types A, B and AB. Owing to the existence of blood groups outside the AB system (e.g. the *Mik* antigen) the cross-match has become an important pre-transfusion test, because blood cross-matching demonstrates the serological compatibility between donor and recipient. Unlike the situation in dogs, in cats not only RBC-compatible but also blood type-compatible plasma must be given, because plasma from a type A cat may contain anti-B alloantibodies and type B plasma contains anti-A antibodies.

Blood groups and typing

The feline blood groups and the principles of blood typing are discussed in Chapter 33. Contrary to the situation in dogs, blood typing or cross-matching should be performed on all cats at the time of the first blood transfusion, owing to the frequency of naturally occurring alloantibodies.

Cross-matching

The cross-matching test is discussed in detail in Chapter 34. In cats a simplified slide cross-match procedure allows the detection of AB incompatibilities associated with strong anti-A agglutinins. In contrast to dogs, in cats the initial cross-match test may be incompatible as a result of the presence of naturally occurring alloantibodies. Furthermore, based on the cross-match results and knowledge of the donor's blood type, it may be possible to predict the blood type of the patient. If the major cross-match is strongly incompatible, the recipient is probably a type B cat, and the donor has type A or AB blood. If the minor cross-match is strongly incompatible, the recipient is likely to be a type A (or AB) cat, and the donor has type B blood. If both cross-matches are compatible, the donor and the recipient have the same AB blood type. Other incompatibilities (e.g. with *Mik* antigens) might not be detectable with the slide test, so the tube test is the preferred method.

Anticoagulant–preservative solutions

The goal of blood preservation is to provide viable and functional blood components for patients that require blood transfusion. The function and viability of feline erythrocytes depend mainly on the ability to generate adenosine triphosphate (ATP) through anaerobic glycolysis.

If blood is administered within a day of collection, 3.13% sodium citrate (1 ml 3.13% sodium citrate per 9 ml of blood) may be used as an anticoagulant solution. Some of the disadvantages of using heparin as an anticoagulant are that it activates platelet adhesion and aggregation and inhibits thrombin formation and factor IX activation. Furthermore, heparin has no preservative function. For these reasons heparin is not recommended for routine blood collection and storage. Anticoagulants for storage of feline blood include acid–citrate–dextrose (ACD), citrate–phosphate–dextrose (CPD) and citrate–phosphate–dextrose–adenine (CPDA-1). Dextrose is a substrate for glycolysis. Citrate prevents coagulation by inhibiting the calcium-dependent steps of the coagulation cascade. The addition of phosphate results in a high ATP concentration during storage. CPDA-1 (1.2 ml CPDA-1 per 8.8 ml of blood) is the preservative solution of choice; the anticoagulant can be withdrawn from a blood bag port using a syringe. The addition of adenine improves the synthesis of ATP (Abrams-Ogg, 2000).

The American Association of Blood Banks defines the shelf life as the number of days after collection, assuming proper collection (closed system) and storage, at which 75% RBC viability is maintained. This viability is measured 24 hours after the transfusion is given. After 35 days of storage in CPDA-1 the 24-hour post-transfusion viability has been reported to be 85% for feline erythrocytes (Bücheler and Cotter, 1994).

Additive solutions have been used to prepare

RBCs in cats and may provide longer storage, but there have been no studies yet on the resulting storage time (Abrams-Ogg, 2000).

Blood donation

Sedation

Sedation is necessary in most cases (e.g. ketamine 5–6 mg/kg bodyweight mixed with midazolam 0.5 mg per cat i.m. or ketamine 2 mg/kg and midazolam 0.1 mg/kg mixed together, i.v.). The main disadvantages of ketamine-based protocols are the prolonged post-anaesthetic effect and the possibility of arrhythmogenesis in cats with undiagnosed hypertrophic cardiomyopathy. For these reasons, some veterinary surgeons prefer to use regimens based on neuroleptanalgesia (e.g. butorphanol 0.1–0.2 mg/kg + diazepam 0.5 mg/kg, mixed together, i.v.). If sedation is insufficient, propofol (4 mg/kg i.v. induction dose) can be added (Abrams-Ogg, 2000). Inhalation anaesthesia with isoflurane, using mask induction, has also been described.

An oxygen mask may be placed over the cat's face during donation, and an endotracheal tube should be available in case ventilatory support is required.

Venepuncture and blood collection

The sedated cat is positioned in sternal or lateral recumbency (Figures 35.1 and 35.2). Blood is best taken from cats from the jugular vein after clipping and disinfection. Blood can be taken via syringes containing 1 ml 3.13% sodium citrate per 9 ml of blood and connected to a 19-gauge butterfly needle ('open system'). Three people are required for blood collection: a restrainer, a phlebotomist and a third person to aspirate the blood and rock the syringe gently during blood collection, mixing the blood with the anticoagulant. Only gentle suction is applied to avoid collapsing the vein or haemolysing the blood.

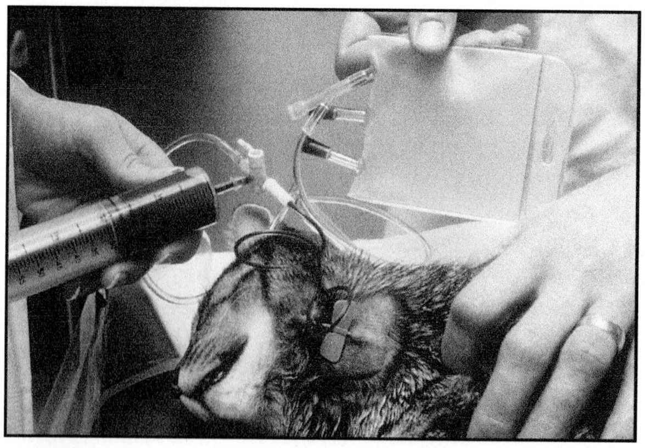

35.2 Feline blood donation. A 19-gauge butterfly needle is attached to a 60 ml syringe into which the anticoagulant–preservative solution has been drawn.

At the University of Pennsylvania, a closed small bag system has been developed for cats, which consists of two paediatric blood bags sealed to a 19-gauge butterfly catheter. It allows closed blood collection, separation of plasma and packed cell components, and storage (Springer *et al.*, 1998). In closed collection systems the blood does not come into contact with the environment at any time, either during collection or during separation into blood components, thus minimizing the risk of bacterial contamination and allowing for storage of the blood products.

A semi-closed sterile system with on-site addition of CPDA-1 through an injection port has been designed by commercial blood banks in the USA. This consists of a three-way stopcock, placed between a butterfly catheter and a syringe, and single or double storage bags. After collecting the blood into the syringe, the stopcock is turned, and the blood is injected slowly into the storage bag (Figure 35.3; Abrams-Ogg, 2000).

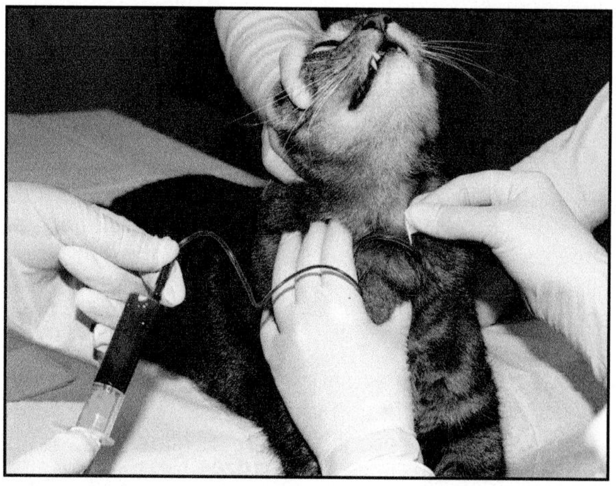

35.1 Feline blood donation. Blood is collected by jugular venepuncture with the cat in sternal recumbency. Blood is taken via a plastic syringe that contains 1 ml of 3.13% sodium citrate per 9 ml of blood and which is connected to a 19-gauge butterfly needle. The syringe is rocked gently during blood collection.

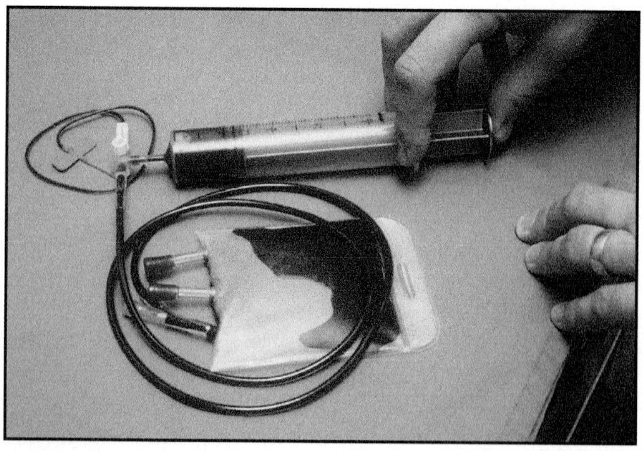

35.3 For blood-banking purposes, a three-way stopcock is placed between the butterfly and the syringe, and a storage bag of 100 ml capacity is attached. After collecting the blood into the syringe, the stopcock is turned, and the blood is injected slowly into the storage bag.

Volume and frequency

The entire blood volume of the (non-obese) cat amounts to approximately 66 ml/kg; 10% of the blood volume can be collected from healthy cats without any side effects. In order to reduce the stress and risks associated with donation, only 10% of the total blood volume should be withdrawn from volunteer donors two to three times a year. Over a 3-year period 134 cats donated blood at the Small Animal Clinic of the University of Berlin. No adverse side effects occurred in 133 cats. One cat died 2 days after blood collection as the result of an occult dilated cardiomyopathy, confirmed by necropsy examination. Thus, blood collection is not without potentially serious risks to the donor, and informed client consent should be obtained prior to collection (Weingart *et al.*, 2004).

According to other authors the maximum acceptable donation volume amounts to 11 ml/kg, referred to as 'one feline unit'. Cats can donate once every 3–4 weeks, or can be bled again after 2 weeks in times of emergency if the Hct is acceptable.

Aftercare of the donor/complications

Side effects after blood donation can occur, especially in cats suffering from diseases such as occult cardiomyopathy or renal insufficiency (Griot-Wenk and Giger, 1995). Therefore, a careful clinical and laboratory examination before donation is important. The collection of a unit of blood (50 ml) from a healthy lean donor cat weighing more than 5 kg is usually safe, but can lead to a decrease in arterial blood pressure, packed cell volume (PCV), and heart rate (because of a delay in the baroreflex effector response due to anaesthesia) (Iazbik *et al.*, 2007).

After blood donation, cats should be monitored (mucous membrane colour, pulse rate and strength, respiratory rate), and infused subcutaneously with approximately 20 ml/kg lactated Ringer's solution. Intravenous volume replacement is recommended after donation of more than 10% of the blood volume. If cats have to donate regularly every 3–4 weeks, an oral iron supplement (ferrous sulphate, 10 mg/kg orally) is recommended.

Preparation and storage of blood products

The small blood volume collected and the difficulties in separation of blood elements make fresh whole blood (WB) transfusions still the norm in feline patients, but component therapy has become available both at teaching hospitals and in commercial animal blood banks. Optimally, transfusion therapy is performed by selection of the most appropriate blood component and administration of that component in the manner most likely to avoid transfusion reactions. The principle of component therapy consists of dividing whole blood into its single elements, mainly packed RBCs and plasma, by centrifugation. The preparation of components for cats is a technical challenge because the units are too small for the standard-size centrifuge buckets. A detailed description of the preparation of feline packed RBCs and fresh frozen plasma (FFP) has been published (Lucas *et al.*, 2004).

Blood component therapy has several advantages: two cats can be treated with one unit of WB, the different blood products have different storage times, and only the component needed can be administered. This helps to prevent hypervolaemia, immune-mediated reactions and RBC sensitization. In cats with primary heart disease or chronic anaemia, packed RBCs are preferable to WB transfusions to reduce the risk of hypervolaemia and lung oedema.

Only blood products taken with the closed system described above should be stored longer than 24 hours in the refrigerator. The open collection system has been used in the Small Animal Clinic of the University of Berlin and the blood products obtained have been stored successfully without microbial growth (Weingart *et al.*, 2004); it must be noted, however, that all blood banking is done by experienced staff.

The most important blood products for cats are WB, packed RBCs and (fresh) frozen plasma (FP). WB and packed RBCs are stored in a refrigerator at 4°C. The refrigerator chosen for storage should be one of the least frequently opened ones available, in order to maintain as consistent a temperature as possible. The recommended maximum storage time for packed RBCs and whole blood in CPDA-1 is 20 days. Bags should be stored horizontally to ensure a better distribution of the anticoagulant. In addition, gentle mixing of the blood bags twice weekly is recommended to maximize exposure to the preservative solutions.

The FFP (separated from RBCs within 8 hours after collection) and FP (separated from RBCs more than 8 hours after collection) should ideally be stored at −30°C for no longer than 1 and 5 years, respectively. Canine FFP contains albumin, globulins, all coagulation factors and von Willebrand factor, whereas FP contains albumin, globulins and therapeutic levels of coagulation factors II, VII, IX and X (Hohenhaus, 2000a). No studies have been done yet for feline plasma.

Platelet transfusions are rarely necessary in feline medicine. If indicated, platelets are usually administered as a fresh WB transfusion, because manufacture of platelet-rich plasma is very difficult as a result of the small amounts of blood that can be withdrawn from cats. Leucocyte transfusions are not generally practised in human or in veterinary medicine because of the very short half-life of granulocytes.

In order to avoid degeneration of the blood in storage, the temperature, packaging and appropriate handling during holding and transport periods are very important. To ensure high-quality blood components the blood-banking process should be checked regularly (i.e. for bacterial culture, temperature of refrigerator/freezer and hygiene control).

Availability and use of (commercial) blood banks

The advantage of blood banking and preserving blood is obvious, because it guarantees immediate availability in an emergency situation. In addition, it reduces the burden of blood donor recruitment and collection for the on-call veterinary clinician and technician. Commercial small animal blood banks, which supply selected blood products, exist in some countries. University and large private small animal hospitals may have their own blood banks.

Indications for blood transfusions

Transfusion for anaemia

The most common reason for blood transfusion in the cat is anaemia caused by blood loss (mostly acute, rarely chronic), ineffective erythropoiesis or haemolysis (Figure 35.4). The transfusion is performed to increase oxygen-carrying capacity.

Adequate transfusion practices result in a successful patient outcome. The survival rate of 88 anaemic cats at 1 and 10 days after transfusion was 84 and 64%, respectively. None of the deaths appeared to be related to transfusion reactions (Weingart *et al.*, 2004).

Whether a blood transfusion is indicated depends in part on the haematocrit. A transfusion of RBCs is recommended for critically ill cats if the Hct falls below 0.10–0.15 l/l. However, even more important is the general condition of the patient: parameters such as tachycardia, weak pulse, prolonged capillary refill time, lethargy and weakness are indicators for the need of a transfusion. In general, cats with chronic anaemia tolerate a low Hct better than those with an acute anaemia. In cases of (per-)acute anaemia or if the animal needs surgery, blood transfusions are given at higher Hct values. A packed cell volume (PCV) of 20% is often used as the transfusion trigger in patients with anaemia caused by acute haemorrhage. However, animals with peracute blood loss will not show a drop in Hct for hours following haemorrhage, until intercompartmental fluid shifts occur or fluid therapy is instituted.

Therefore, the factors that determine whether a transfusion is required are variable and include the perfusion status, the ability of the lungs to oxygenate the blood, the chronicity of the anaemia and the regenerative capacity of the bone marrow. Blood transfusions should only be used with a proper indication and assessment of the prognosis (Giger, 2009a).

Transfusion for other indications

In contrast to dogs, there is a minor need for blood products in cats to treat coagulopathies or thrombocytopenia. FP or FFP contains clotting factors, immunoglobulins and albumin, and its administration is beneficial in cats with coagulopathies, and in those in whom transfer of passive immunity has failed. Nineteen cases treated with FFP at the Animal Medical Center in New York for coagulation disorders have been described (Hohenhaus, 2000b). The underlying diseases in these cats were liver disease (six cats), lymphoma (six cats) and various miscellaneous disorders (seven cats). Disseminated intravascular coagulation (DIC) was the most common coagulopathy. Thirteen of the nineteen cats received FFP prior to an invasive procedure (e.g. exploratory laparotomy, ultrasound-guided liver biopsy). In another report, DIC was the reason for 30 of 46 cats (65%) being transfused with blood products (Estrin *et al.*, 2006). These cats received FFP alone (11), FFP and packed RBCs (10), packed RBCs alone (2), and 7 cats received a haemoglobin-based oxygen carrying solution (Oxyglobin) in combination with FFP and RBCs.

(Fresh frozen) plasma should not be used as a source of albumin (e.g. in protein-losing nephropathy or enteropathy), for volume expansion or nutritional support. Calculations suggest that 45 ml/kg of plasma would need to be given to increase serum albumin concentration by 1 g/dl (Hohenhaus, 2006). Moreover, the effect on oncotic pressure is

Number of cats	Blood loss	Haemolysis	Ineffective erythropoiesis	Other indications (number)	Blood products used (number)	Reference
91	40	13	35	Coagulopathy (2), hypoproteinaemia (2)	WB (163)	Weingart *et al.*, 2004
81	18		18	Presurgical preparation (23), neoplasia (17), coagulopathy (10), liver disease (7)	WB (49) PRBCs (44) FFP (19)	Castellanos *et al.*, 2004
126	66	12	48		WB (127) PRBCs (21)	Klaser *et al.*, 2005
27	14	-	8	Acute renal failure (3), lymphoma (1), haematemesis/bone marrow disorder (1)	WB (47) PRBCs (63)	Roux *et al.*, 2008
19	-	-	-	Coagulopathies	FFP	Hohenhaus, 2000b
30	-	-	-	Disseminated intravascular coagulation	PRBCs (27) FFP (26)	Estrin *et al.*, 2006

35.4 Indications for blood transfusion in cats. FFP, fresh frozen plasma; PRBCs, packed red blood cells; WB, whole blood.

minimal at the dosages used clinically when compared with synthetic hyperoncotic agents (Giger, 2009a).

Another indication for transfusion is thrombocytopenia. Transfusion of platelets is very effective if the platelets have a normal survival time. Transfusion is less effective if there is an increased utilization or sequestration of platelets, or in cases of immune-mediated thrombocytopenia, because the transfused platelets are destroyed as quickly as the body's own platelets. Nonetheless, administration of platelets may be indicated as a life-saving measure in cases of acute bleeding from severe thrombocytopenia or if surgery is necessary. A volume of 10 ml/kg fresh whole blood results in an approximate increase of 10 $\times 10^9$/l platelets in the recipient (Abrams-Ogg, 2003). This can be enough to stop a life-threatening haemorrhage (Wondratschek *et al.*, 2010).

Administration of whole blood and blood components

Warming

In normothermic cats, refrigerated blood does not need to be warmed routinely before administration. In hypothermic patients or in specific clinical situations, such as transfusion of neonates or resuscitation of trauma patients necessitating rapid massive transfusion, the blood should be warmed in a 37°C water bath or incubator immediately before administration. In-line warming of blood may be achieved by passing the intravenous tubing through a warm water bath ($\leq$ 37°C). Excessive heat should not be used because of the risk of RBC membrane damage and haemolysis, or bacterial growth if contamination is present. Frozen plasma products must be thawed in a 37°C water bath or incubator. Higher temperatures may result in denaturation of proteins. Plasma must be used within 4 hours of thawing.

Venous access

Blood is administered into the cephalic, medial femoral or jugular vein. Sterility must be maintained when connecting the blood component bag to the infusion set and the tubing to the catheter. If no venous access is available the intraosseous route can be used successfully for the administration of blood and plasma. This route is useful for emergency administration of blood products to animals in which rapid vascular access is difficult owing to vascular collapse or small body size. Over 90% of RBCs administered this way are found in the circulation within 5 minutes. The intravenous catheter should be as large as possible; forcing red cells rapidly through a small gauge catheter may result in haemolysis. Neonates can also be transfused by peritoneal injection. About 50% of transfused RBCs will be absorbed into the circulation from the peritoneal space in 24 hours, and 70% within 48–72 hours, but they will have a shorter lifespan, and therefore the intraperitoneal administration of RBC is not recommended. In emergency situations the administration of plasma is possible, but it is absorbed slowly (Hohenhaus, 2006).

Administration

Blood that is collected in syringes can be transferred into transfer or storage bags or into empty physiological saline infusion bottles using aseptic techniques (Figures 35.5 and 35.6). The transfusion is administered with a special transfusion set with an incorporated microfilter (size of pores approximately 170 µm), which removes blood clots and debris that could cause embolism (Figure 35.6). Another method is transfusion with an infusion pump using a syringe with a paediatric filter (Figure 35.7). An advantage is the individual regulation of the transfusion rate. There is also no need for transfer of the blood into a transfer bag, therefore the risk of contamination is reduced.

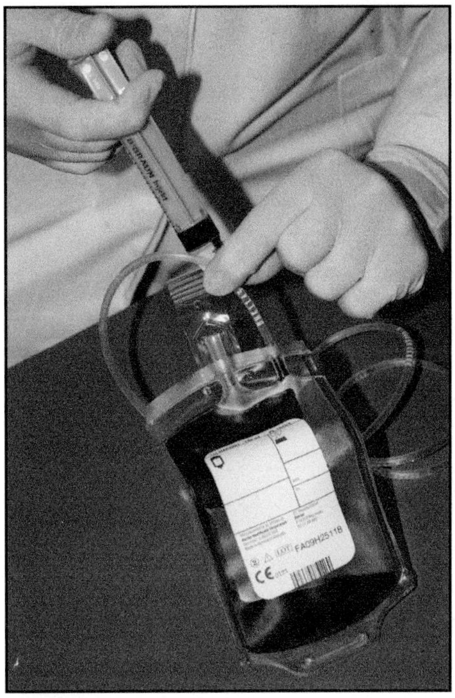

35.5 Blood that is collected in syringes can be transferred into 150 ml transfer bags.

Stored whole blood should be mixed gently before transfusion. Dilution of the packed RBCs with 20–30 ml of saline facilitates passage through small filters; this regulates the velocity of the transfusion more exactly and it also washes the small amount of blood entirely out of the bag. Only physiological saline may be used to dilute the blood. Fluids containing calcium (e.g. lactated Ringer's solution) may overcome the anticoagulant properties of citrate, resulting in coagulation of the blood. Solutions such as 5% dextrose in water are hypotonic and may induce haemolysis (Hohenhaus, 2000a).

Partially used or opened blood bags should be used within 24 hours because of the risk of contamination and damage to blood products.

Patients receiving a blood transfusion should be monitored. Even if AB compatible blood is

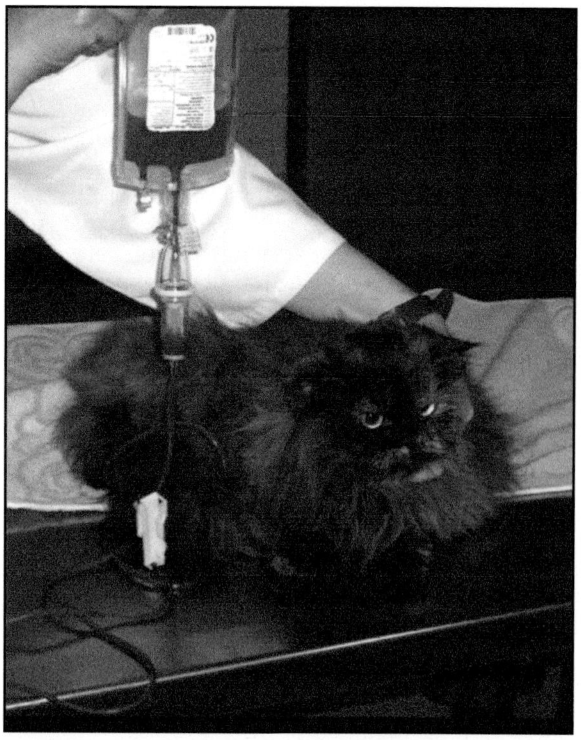

35.6 Feline blood transfusion. The transfusion is being administered with a special transfusion set with an incorporated microfilter, which removes blood clots and debris that could cause embolism.

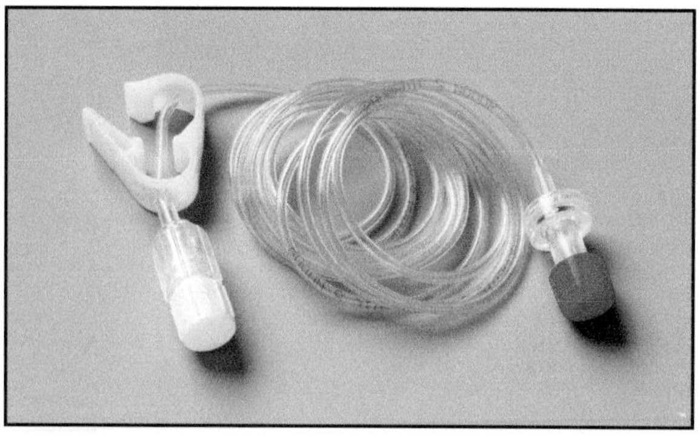

35.7 Human paediatric filter incorporating a 200 μm filter for transfusion of small volumes. In emergency cases an intravenous bolus injection with a syringe is possible (connected with a filter).

administered and the cross-match is negative, there is a small risk of transfusion reactions. Therefore, rectal temperature, heart rate, respiratory rate, colour of the mucous membranes and capillary refill time should be determined every 10 minutes during the first 30 minutes and then every 30 minutes thereafter.

Transfusion rate and volume

Initially, the blood should be transfused very slowly (1–3 ml over 5 minutes as a 'test dose'); the patient needs to be monitored for signs of incompatibility. Subsequently, depending on the status of the recipient, the transfusion rate can be increased. Normovolaemic cats can receive up to 5–10 ml/kg/h. In cats suffering from cardiac disease, there is a high risk of life-threatening circulatory overload at higher transfusion rates. The transfusion rate in cats with heart disease must be very slow (< 4 ml/kg/h). However, in case of massive haemorrhage, the transfusion should be given as rapidly as possible. The transfusion should be completed within 4 hours of initiation because of the risk of bacterial growth.

The transfusion volume depends on the Hct and the general condition of the patient; in cats, however, it is often dictated by the amount of blood that is available. Based on a donor Hct of 0.37 l/l, the Hct of the recipient can be increased by approximately 0.01 l/l with a transfusion of 3 ml whole blood per kg bodyweight, provided that there is no further blood loss. The following formula can be used to calculate the transfusion volume:

$$\underset{\text{blood (ml)}}{\text{Volume of whole}} = \underset{(\%)}{\text{PCV rise}} \times \underset{(\text{kg})}{\text{bodyweight}} \times 2$$

Cats with a coagulopathy should receive plasma at a recommended starting dosage of about 5–10 ml/kg. Multiple doses may be required to control bleeding because of the short half-life of clotting factors. Transfusion of fresh plasma and FFP should be completed within 4 hours.

Record keeping

Records should be kept of all transfusions, documenting both the donor unit used and the recipient of the transfusion.

Transfusion reactions and management

Adverse effects of transfusion or transfusion reactions mostly appear during or shortly after the transfusion; they can be caused by any blood component. However, transfusion reactions are rare and often mild (reactions occurred in 1.2% of 163 whole blood transfusions at the Small Animal Clinic of University of Berlin). The reported frequencies of transfusion reactions in cats are illustrated in Figure 35.8. By following the transfusion guidelines with reference to donor selection, blood typing, blood storage and administration, most transfusion reactions can be prevented.

Transfusion reactions can be divided into immunological and non-immunological reactions, which may be acute or delayed (Figure 35.9). Acute transfusion reactions occur during or within a few hours after a transfusion, and delayed reactions occur after completion of the transfusion. The delay may be weeks or even years.

Immunological reactions

Acute immunological transfusion reactions occur because antibodies that can elicit an immune response are present in the plasma of the donor or the recipient.

An acute haemolytic transfusion reaction caused by destruction of the donor's erythrocytes through

Number of cats (%)	Clinical signs (number)	Blood product	Reference
2/91 (1.2)	Fever (2), bradycardia (1), hyperbilirubinaemia (AB compatibility) (1), retching (1), tachypnoea (1)	WB	Weingart *et al.*, 2004
3/81 (3.7)	Mild fever (2), acute haemolysis (incompatible transfusion)	WB, PRBCs	Castellanos *et al.*, 2004
11/126 (8.7)	Fever (5), face rubbing and angioedema (2), vomiting (1), salivation (1), pulmonary oedema (1), acute haemolysis (1, incompatible transfusion)	WB, PRBCs	Klaser *et al.*, 2005
12/133 (9.0)	Fever (4), facial oedema (1), circulatory overload (2), haemolysis over 2 days (3), acute haemolysis with fever (1), death (1)	WB, PRBCs	Henson *et al.*, 1994
1/27 (3.7)	Pulmonary oedema	WB, PRBCs	Roux *et al.*, 2008

35.8 Transfusion reactions in cats. WB, whole blood; PRBCs, packed red blood cells.

	Immunological	Non-immunological
Acute	Acute haemolytic reaction (haemoglobinuria, haemoglobinaemia, fever, vomiting, tachycardia, tachypnoea), urticaria, oedema, febrile non-haemolytic reaction, anaphylaxis	Fever, vomiting, electrolyte disturbances (hypocalcaemia, hyperkalaemia, hypomagnesaemia), hyperammonaemia, embolism (air, clots), endotoxic shock (sepsis, fever), circulatory overload (coughing, dyspnoea, vomiting), physical damage of RBCs, hypothermia
Delayed	Delayed haemolytic reaction, transfusion-induced immunosuppression, post-transfusion purpura, graft-*versus*-host disease	Transmission of infectious agents, haemosiderosis

35.9 Classification of transfusion reactions.

naturally occurring antibodies during or shortly after the transfusion is the most severe transfusion reaction. Such reactions have been described for AB-incompatible blood transfusions. Prior to blood transfusion in cats, blood typing of donor and recipient is strongly recommended because naturally occurring alloantibodies can lead to these severe incompatibility reactions. While the half-life of transfused feline erythrocytes is approximately 35–38 days for compatible transfusions, the half-life is shortened to approximately 1–2 hours if a type B cat is transfused with type A erythrocytes and to approximately 2 days in case of a transfusion of type B erythrocytes into a type A cat (Giger and Bücheler, 1991). Cats with blood type B that receive type A blood may develop a severe acute haemolytic transfusion reaction with clinical signs such as lethargy, bradycardia, dyspnoea, cardiac arrhythmia, salivation, vomiting, defecation and urination, together with neurological disorders. Death may occur during this phase. If the cats survive they develop tachycardia, tachypnoea, fever, haemoglobinaemia and haemoglobinuria. Given that the anti-B alloantibodies in type A blood are generally of low titre, significant clinical transfusion reactions are not to be expected. If type A cats receive blood from type B cats, only mild incompatibility reactions such as restlessness, tachycardia and tachypnoea occur. However, the transfusion is not efficient because of the rapid destruction of erythrocytes, which will occur within 5 days. Therefore, type A cats may only receive type A blood and type B cats must only receive type B blood. Type AB cats, which have no antibodies, may be transfused with blood of types AB or A.

Recently the feline blood group *Mik* was discovered. The absence of this novel *Mik* RBC antigen can be associated with naturally occurring anti-*Mik* alloantibodies and may cause an acute haemolytic transfusion reaction after an AB-matched blood transfusion. Cross-matching of any cat to be transfused with AB-matched blood may be the recommendation in the near future (Giger, 2009b).

Other immunologically mediated acute transfusion reactions include urticaria and facial oedema caused by reactions of the recipient to donor leucocytes or plasma proteins. Most of these reactions are mild and self-limiting. Anaphylactic shock is very rare and the clinical presentation may include hypotension, tachycardia, bronchoconstriction, vomiting and diarrhoea.

Febrile non-haemolytic reactions are caused by sensitivity to white cell or platelet antigens. Such antibodies cannot be discovered by blood typing or cross-matching; therefore, these reactions cannot be prevented. A transfusion-associated fever is defined as an increase in body temperature of more than 1°C over the pre-transfusion temperature. These reactions have a good prognosis, but may be confused with a haemolytic transfusion reaction (Beutler, 2006).

In delayed haemolytic transfusion reactions, development of previously undetected alloantibodies occurs approximately 4–14 days after transfusion of apparently compatible blood. The patient has usually been alloimmunized by a previous transfusion or pregnancy, and the concentration of antibody is below the level of serological detection at the time of transfusion. If the transfused blood contains the corresponding antigen, an anamnestic immune response occurs with the formation of antibodies that lead to haemolysis. Fever is the most common sign in humans. The Coombs' test can be positive and an immune-mediated haemolytic anaemia may be suspected (Beutler, 2006). Other delayed transfusion reactions described in humans are transfusion-induced immunosuppression, post-transfusion purpura and graft-versus-host disease. Delayed transfusion reactions are not preventable by blood typing or cross-matching. Such transfusion reactions are likely to occur not only in humans but also in cats, although they have not been described thus far.

Non-immunological reactions

Fever is one of the most common transfusion reactions. If the fever occurs together with haemolysis, it might be caused by blood type incompatibility or bacterial contamination. However, in most cases fever is neither due to haemolysis nor to sepsis, so the transfusion may be continued slowly.

Vomiting is mostly a consequence of a high transfusion rate, or it can be caused by feeding the patient before or during the transfusion. If other causes (e.g. an acute haemolytic reaction) are excluded, the transfusion may be continued but at a slower rate.

Hypocalcaemia can be caused by transfusing large volumes of the anticoagulant citrate, which binds calcium. Citrate is metabolized quickly by the liver, so citrate intoxication is only to be expected in patients with liver failure, in case of massive transfusion, or in case of an incorrect anticoagulant–blood ratio. Hypomagnesaemia can also result from citrate toxicity (Abrams-Ogg, 2000).

Given that blood is a colloid, blood transfusions can cause signs of hypervolaemia and pulmonary oedema. Therefore, cats with cardiac insufficiency, lung or renal disease or chronic anaemia must be monitored carefully during and after the transfusion.

Microbial contamination with *Serratia marcescens* or *Pseudomonas fluorescens* in feline units has been described. The transfusion of *S. marcescens*-contaminated whole blood was described in 14 cats. Blood was collected with an open system with ACD anticoagulant and stored for 4–26 days at 4°C. Six cats developed clinical signs of a transfusion reaction: vomiting (four cats), collapse (four), diarrhoea (three), icterus (two), panting (two) and pyrexia (one), and four cats died. Three units were recorded as being discoloured. An investigation of the outbreak identified *S. marcescens* in a jar of alcohol-soaked cotton balls and in a bag of saline solution used during venepuncture. Cats that did not develop adverse reactions had received units with a short storage time, associated with a low level of endotoxin (Hohenhaus *et al.*, 1997). *P. fluorescens* is capable of growing in RBC units stored both at refrigerated and at room temperatures. Contamination with *P. fluorescens* can result in colour changes and haemolysis of RBC products. In general, discoloration of blood indicates deoxygenation, haemolysis and formation of methaemoglobin, which may be a result of bacterial contamination. Screening of blood products for colour change, estimating bacterial concentration by microscopy, microbial culture and/or 16S rRNA PCR testing are ways to detect bacteria in stored blood. Aseptic collection, temperature-controlled storage, and regular visual monitoring of stored units are strongly recommended in order to prevent bacterial growth (Kessler *et al.*, 2009).

Further causes for haemolysis are physical (i.e. overheating or freezing of the blood bag or mixing the blood with hypotonic solutions). During transfusion the patient may exhibit haemoglobinaemia and haemoglobinuria without other signs of an acute haemolytic transfusion reaction.

During storage, the ATP content of RBCs decreases and some cells undergo haemolysis, resulting in leakage of potassium into the storage medium. Therefore, a large-volume transfusion of stored blood might cause hyperkalaemia, mainly in patients with renal failure. Owing to damage to RBCs and leucocytes during storage, patients at risk of DIC, sepsis or thrombosis (e.g. cats with immune-mediated haemolytic anaemia (IMHA)) should preferably receive fresh RBC products.

Ammonia builds up during storage of RBCs, resulting in hyperammonaemia. Therefore, fresh RBC products or products stored for no longer than 2 weeks should be given to cats with liver disease.

The risk of transferring infectious agents (e.g. FeLV, FIV, feline coronavirus, haemotropic *Mycoplasma* spp., *Bartonella* spp.) is greater in cats than in dogs. It can be minimized by thorough donor screening, but it cannot be eliminated completely.

Massive transfusions

In human medicine massive transfusion is associated with high mortality rates. Complications described in humans include hypothermia, acid–base derangements, electrolyte abnormalities (hypocalcaemia, hypomagnesaemia, hypokalaemia, hyperkalaemia), citrate toxicity and transfusion-associated acute lung injury.

Massive transfusion and multiple red cell transfusions have been described in 27 cats (Roux *et al.*, 2008). Massive transfusion was defined by transfusion of 60 ml/kg or more over 24 hours, or transfusions of 30 ml/kg over 3 hours. Multiple transfusions were defined by three or more transfusions with packed RBCs or whole blood during a single stay at the hospital. 16 cats survived to discharge and 11 died or were euthanased. No acute transfusion reactions were recorded. One cat developed signs of fluid overload and six cats became hypocalcaemic, but this was not associated with clinical signs. The authors concluded that multiple transfusions are well tolerated in cats and may be associated with a favourable outcome.

Management of acute transfusion reactions

If an acute transfusion reaction is suspected, the transfusion should be stopped. A clinical examination should be performed, including blood pressure measurement. Samples of patient blood and urine should be taken for baseline evaluation of haematological, biochemical and coagulation values. The serum and urine should be examined for haemoglobinaemia and haemoglobinuria. A stained blood smear of the RBC product should be examined for microorganisms. If electrolytes cannot be measured, certain electrocardiographic changes suggest hyperkalaemia (decreased height of P waves, loss of P waves, widening of the QRS complex and large T waves) or hypocalcaemia (long QT interval with a normal heart rate). If transfusion of a contaminated unit is suspected, a microbiological culture (and 16S rRNA PCR) of the donor (and recipient) blood should be performed. Repeating the blood typing of donor and recipient and repeating the cross-match might be indicated (Hohenhaus, 2006).

Venous access and blood pressure should be maintained by an infusion with a crystalloid solution such as lactated Ringer's solution. Severe transfusion reactions with signs of shock may be treated with short-acting glucocorticoids (e.g. methylprednisolone succinate 10 mg/kg slowly i.v. once). Glucocorticoids may suppress mediators of acute haemolytic transfusion reactions, but their efficacy has not been evaluated in animal patients (Hohenhaus, 2006). If anaphylactic shock has occurred, adrenaline (1:10,000 solution, 0.1 ml/kg i.v.) is administered. Persistent hypotension can be treated with a bolus of a synthetic colloid (5 ml/kg hetastarch i.v. over 15 minutes). Bradycardia may be treated with atropine (0.04 mg/kg i.v.).

If bacterial contamination of the blood product is suspected, empirical antibiotic therapy should be given. High fever can be treated with cooling and antipyretics (e.g. dipyrone/metamizol 10–20 mg/kg slowly i.v.). In case of erythema or urticaria, antihistamines (e.g. diphenhydramine 2 mg/kg slowly i.v.) and/or anti-inflammatory doses of glucocorticoids (i.e. prednisolone 0.5 mg/kg) should be given. In the case of vomiting, anti-emetics (e.g. metoclopramide 0.2–0.3 mg/kg s.c.; maropitant 0.5–1 mg/kg s.c.) are recommended. If circulatory overload is suspected, cats are treated with oxygen supplementation and furosemide (2 mg/kg i.v.) to reduce intravascular volume by diuresis (Hohenhaus, 2000a).

Treatment of citrate intoxication involves slowing or stopping the transfusion and slowly infusing calcium gluconate (0.5–1.5 ml/kg of 10% calcium gluconate over 10–20 minutes). A second intravenous line is needed for concurrent administration of calcium gluconate. The heart rate and electrocardiogram should be monitored during calcium infusion (Abrams-Ogg, 2000).

If the transfusion reactions subside and if there is no haemolysis, the transfusion may be restarted at a slower rate and the recipient must be observed carefully.

Autotransfusion and preoperative autologous blood donation

In human medicine, preoperative autologous blood donation is commonly used to reduce the incidence of allogenic transfusion and the associated risks of blood-borne diseases, transfusion and allergic reactions, and postoperative infection. Autologous blood donation means that the patient's own blood is collected a few weeks before the operation and transfused postoperatively as needed. In feline transfusion medicine, preoperative autologous blood donation is described in association with complications in patients undergoing partial craniectomy for removal of an intracranial mass (Fusco *et al.*, 2000).

Autotransfusion may also be an option in situations where blood is not available. In this case blood lost into either the thoracic or abdominal cavity is collected, filtered and re-infused. Blood is collected into either sterile fluid administration bags or blood collection bags. An anticoagulant is not necessary. Autotransfusion is contraindicated if contamination with urine, bacteria, bile or neoplastic cells is possible (Hackett, 2000).

References and further reading

Abrams-Ogg AC (2000) Practical blood transfusion. In: *Manual of Canine and Feline Haematology and Transfusion Medicine,* ed. M Day *et al.* pp.261–303. BSAVA Publications, Gloucester

Abrams-Ogg AC (2003) Triggers for prophylactic use of platelet transfusions and optimal platelet dosing in thrombocytopenic dogs and cats. *Veterinary Clinics of North America: Small Animal Practice* **33**, 1401–1418

Beutler E (2006) Preservation and clinical use of erythrocytes and whole blood. In: *Williams Hematology,* ed. MA Lichtman, E Beutler, TJ Kipps *et al.*, pp.2159–2173. The McGraw-Hill Companies, New York

Bücheler J and Cotter SM (1994) Storage of feline and canine whole blood in CPDA-1 and determination of the posttransfusion viability. *Journal of Veterinary Internal Medicine* **8**, 172

Castellanos I, Couto CG and Gray TL (2004) Clinical use of blood products in cats: a retrospective study (1997–2000). *Journal of Veterinary Internal Medicine* **18**, 529–532

Estrin MA, Wehausen CE, Jessen CR *et al.* (2006) Disseminated intravascular coagulation in cats. *Journal of Veterinary Internal Medicine* **20**, 1334–1339

Fusco JV, Hohenhaus AE, Aiken SW *et al.* (2000) Autologous blood collection and transfusion in cats undergoing partial craniectomy. *Journal of the American Veterinary Medical Association* **216**, 1584–1588

Giger U (2009a) Transfusion medicine. In: *Small Animal Critical Care Medicine*, ed. DC Silverstein, K Hopper, pp.281–286. WB Saunders Company, Philadelphia

Giger U (2009b) Blood-typing and crossmatching. In: *Kirk's Current Veterinary Therapy XIV Small Animal Practice*, ed. JD Bonagura, pp.260–265. WB Saunders Company, Philadelphia

Giger U and Bücheler J (1991) Transfusion of type-A and type-B blood to cats. *Journal of the American Veterinary Medical Association* **198**, 411–418

Griot-Wenk ME and Giger U (1995) Feline transfusion medicine. Blood types and their clinical importance. *Veterinary Clinics of North America: Small Animal Practice* **25**, 1305–1322

Hackett T (2000) Autologous transfusion. In: *Schalm's Veterinary Hematology*, ed. BF Feldman, JG Zinkl and NC Jain, pp.861–863. Lippincott Williams and Wilkins, Baltimore

Henson MS, Kristensen AT, Armstrong PJ *et al.* (1994) Feline blood component therapy: retrospective study of 246 transfusions. *Journal of Veterinary Internal Medicine* **8**, 169

Hohenhaus AE (2000a) Blood banking and transfusion medicine. In: *Textbook of Veterinary Internal Medicine*, ed. SJ Ettinger and EC Feldman, pp.348–356. WB Saunders, Philadelphia

Hohenhaus AE (2000b) Feline coagulopathies. *WSAVA/FECAVA World Congress 2000*, Amsterdam, Proceedings, pp.197–199

Hohenhaus AE (2006) Blood transfusion and blood substitutes. In: *Fluid, Electrolyte, and Acid-base Disorders in Small Animal Practice*, ed. SP DiBartola, pp.567–583. Saunders Company, Philadelphia

Hohenhaus AE, Drusin MD and Garvey MS (1997) *Serratia marcescens* contamination of feline whole blood in a hospital blood bank. *Journal of the American Veterinary Medical Association* **210**, 794–798

Iazbik MC, Ochoa PG, Westendorf N *et al.* (2007) Effects of blood collection for transfusion on arterial blood pressure, heart rate, and PCV in cats. *Journal of Veterinary Internal Medicine* **21**, 1181–1184

Kessler RJ, Rankin S, Young S *et al.* (2009) *Pseudomonas fluorescens* contamination of a feline packed red blood cell unit and studies of canine units. *Veterinary Clinical Pathology* **39**, 29–38

Klaser DA, Reine NJ, Hohenhaus AE (2005) Red blood cell transfusion in cats: 126 cases (1999). *Journal of the American Veterinary Medical Association* **226**, 920–923

Lucas RL, Lentz KD and Hale AS (2004) Collection and preparation of blood products. *Clinical Techniques in Small Animal Practice* **19**, 55–62

Roux AF, Deschamps JY, Blais MC *et al.* (2008) Multiple red cell transfusion in 27 cats (2003–2006): indications, complications and outcomes. *Journal of Feline Medicine and Surgery* **10**, 213–218

Springer T, Hatchett WL, Oakley DA *et al.* (1998) Feline blood storage and component therapy using a closed collection system. *Proceedings 16th ACVIM Forum,* San Diego, p.738

Wardrop KJ, Reine N, Birkenheuer A *et al.* (2005) Canine and feline blood donor screening for infectious disease. *Journal of Veterinary Internal Medicine* **19**, 135–142

Weingart C, Giger U and Kohn B (2004) Whole blood transfusions in 91 cats: a clinical evaluation. *Journal of Feline Medicine and Surgery* **6**, 139–148

Wondratschek C, Weingart C and Kohn B (2010) Primary immune-mediated thrombocytopenia in cats. *Journal of the American Animal Hospital Association* **46**, 12–19

36

Blood substitutes

Virginia Rentko

Introduction

The designation 'blood substitute' is a misnomer, because no solution developed to date possesses all of the properties of blood. 'Substitute' products for some of the properties of blood, including the oxygen-carrying ability, volume-expanding property and clotting capability, have been developed and used in animals.

Haemoglobin-based oxygen-carrying fluid

The primary function of blood is to transport oxygen and carbon dioxide, so the first 'substitute' to consider is a haemoglobin-based oxygen-carrying solution (HBOC), belonging to a family of drugs called oxygen therapeutics. Haemoglobin glutamer-200 or Oxyglobin (OPK Biotech, Cambridge, MA, USA) is cell-free, bovine-derived, polymerized haemoglobin (Hb) in lactated Ringer's solution (Figure 36.1). It is isosmotic in a balanced electrolyte solution. The polymers range in size from 65 kilodaltons (kD) to 500 kD with an average molecular weight of 200 kD. It has good buffering capacity with a pH of 7.8. The viscosity is closer to that of a crystalloid solution than that of blood. It is stable at room temperature for 3 years and requires no preparation for its use.

Property	Figure for Oxyglobin
Glutaraldehyde-polymerized bovine haemoglobin	13 g/dl
Sodium	146–160 mEq/l
Chloride	10–20 mEq/l
Potassium	3.5–5.5 mEq/l
Osmolality	300 mOSm/kg
pH	7.8
Molecular size	~50% 65–130 kD ~45% > 130 kD < 5% unstabilized tetramer
P_{50}	37 mmHg
Colloid osmotic pressure	43 mmHg
Viscosity	1.5 centipoise
Plasma half-life	15–50 hours, dose dependent

36.1 Physicochemical properties of Oxyglobin.

At the time of writing/editing this chapter Oxyglobin is not available. However, it is expected that it will become available again, from a new manufacturer, during 2012.

The Hb is stored in a deoxygenated state, and Oxyglobin is packaged in a foil overwrap to protect it from oxygen. Once the bag is opened, any unused portion should be discarded after 24 hours to avoid bacterial contamination and oxidation to methaemoglobin. No cross-matching is required, because the product is acellular. The colloid osmotic pressure is 43 mmHg, higher than that of blood and synthetic colloids such as hetastarch. Therefore, Oxyglobin exerts a significant colloidal effect and expands vascular volume. The potential for overexpansion of the vascular volume is an important consideration during its use in normovolaemic patients. As is true of the use of other colloids in the cat, this species is more sensitive to the volume-expanding property of Oxyglobin when compared with the dog. One early report of the use of Oxyglobin in cats reported adverse effects associated with the colloidal effects of the solution. Of 44 cats with adverse effects, 29 had pulmonary oedema or pleural effusion (Gibson *et al.*, 2002).

The P_{50} (the partial pressure of oxygen (PO_2) at which the Hb is 50% saturated) is a measure of oxygen affinity for Hb. The Hb–oxygen equilibrium (or dissociation) curve for the Hb in Oxyglobin is 'right-shifted' as compared with native red blood cell (RBC) Hb (Figure 36.2). This right-shifting or higher P_{50} results in Hb that binds oxygen less tightly than native Hb. Therefore, at similar oxygen pressures the Hb in Oxyglobin releases its oxygen more readily to tissues than native Hb, thus facilitating delivery of oxygen to tissue beds. Also of note is the difference in saturation between RBCs and Oxyglobin. The Hb–oxygen dissociation 'curve' for plasma is almost flat. This is due to the fact that normally only 2–3% of the oxygen carried in the blood is dissolved in the plasma. The remaining 97–98% is bound to Hb in the RBCs. Thus, an increase in inspired oxygen

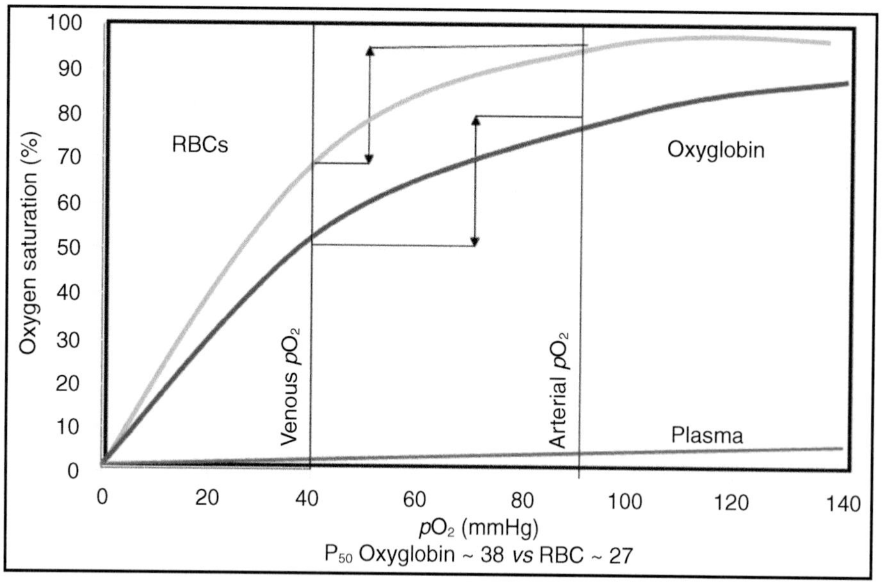

36.2 Haemoglobin–oxygen equilibrium. Oxyglobin's haemoglobin has a lower affinity for oxygen (right-shifted curve) compared with RBCs. The arterio-venous difference in oxygen saturation is similar between RBCs and Oxyglobin. Plasma is poorly saturated with oxygen.

(F_iO_2) provides little increase in the amount of oxygen dissolved in the plasma, and therefore provides little benefit to an anaemic patient with a deficit in RBC mass but normal RBC saturation.

Oxyglobin is of bovine origin and this is relevant to its oxygen affinity, which is dependent on chloride ions that are abundant in the plasma of mammals. Bovine Hb has pronounced Bohr (pH) and Haldane (CO_2) effects, which allow more efficient uptake, transport and release of oxygen to tissues compared with whole blood (Horn *et al.*, 1997; Page *et al.*, 1998). Furthermore, the fact that Oxyglobin is acellular allows it to be distributed uniformly throughout the plasma. Unlike native, tetrameric Hb, which after being released by RBCs during haemolysis is cleared rapidly, the Hb of Oxyglobin is chemically modified and polymerized to slow its clearance from the vascular space.

In contrast to these beneficial effects, concerns have been raised regarding the potential of Oxyglobin to increase arterial blood pressure (Rohlfs *et al.*, 1998), and even to increase mortality rates (Grundy and Barton, 2001). In a study in dogs with hypovolaemia, systemic vascular resistance increased after administration of Oxyglobin, when compared with baseline and infusion of autologous blood. However, despite the resultant decrease in cardiac output, systemic and regional tissue oxidative metabolism were restored (Driessen *et al.*, 2001). The combination of its colloidal properties, plasma oxygen-carrying capacity and low viscosity has triggered interest in the use of Oxyglobin in hypoperfused patients. Case reports have described its use in heatstroke, haemoabdomen and perioperatively (Day *et al.*, 2001).

Indications

Oxyglobin is indicated for the treatment of anaemia, independent of its cause. Its most effective use is as a temporary oxygen bridge. If the cause of blood loss or haemolysis can be treated effectively, repeated use of Oxyglobin or RBC transfusions can be avoided. Because of its relatively short half-life compared with that of RBCs, Oxyglobin is not the ideal choice for the treatment of anaemia caused by ineffective erythropoiesis. However, it can be life-saving in these patients when used as an oxygen bridge until compatible RBCs are available.

Haemolytic anaemia is a common indication for RBC transfusion. Conflicting retrospective data exist on the association of survival and the choice of oxygen-carrying support, RBC transfusion *versus* Oxyglobin (Grundy and Barton, 2001; Rentko *et al.*, 2002). Circumstances in which Oxyglobin may be the best choice in patients with haemolytic anaemia are persistent agglutination in a previously transfused patient, and rapid destruction of transfused RBCs resulting in negligible effects on packed cell volume (PCV). A recent randomized, prospective study comparing the use of packed RBC transfusion and Oxyglobin for oxygen-carrying support in the treatment of dogs with babesiosis showed similar overall improvements (Zambelli and Leisewitz, 2009). Blood gas and acid–base parameters and blood pressure were similar, but subjective parameters such as appetite and wellbeing were significantly better 8–48 hours following infusion in the dogs that received packed RBCs. By 72 hours, no difference was noted between the groups. The dogs entered into the study had non-agglutinating anaemia (10–20%). 11 of 12 dogs survived the study.

Dose rates in dogs

The recommended dose in dogs is 15–30 ml/kg at a rate of up to 10 ml/kg/h. In choosing the dosage and rate of administration of Oxyglobin, several factors should be considered. Most important is the estimated blood volume of the animal. Animals with anaemia caused by haemolysis or ineffective erythropoiesis are typically euvolaemic unless compromised by dehydration. Often, animals with chronic anaemia may have a slightly expanded blood volume to maintain adequate oxygen delivery as compensation for a reduced RBC mass. In these patients, a conservative rate of administration should be chosen, ≤ 5 ml/kg/h in the dog and 0.5–3 ml/kg/h in the cat, to avoid potential complications of overexpansion of the vascular volume. In clinical situations in which the need for oxygen-carrying support would be anticipated for more than a day, a continuous rate infusion could be considered. Such a method of administration may be useful in cases of haemolytic anaemia in which there is a rapid decline in RBC mass and a need for oxygen-carrying support is anticipated until the haemolysis is controlled. Figure 36.3 describes the guidelines for achieving a constant, desired plasma concentration of Hb by using a loading dose and a constant rate infusion in dogs.

The plasma half-life of Oxyglobin is dose-dependent (Figure 36.4). Oxyglobin is metabolized by the reticuloendothelial system. There is renal excretion of unstabilized tetramers, which make up < 5% of the product. In clinical situations where rapid volume expansion may be a concern, pharmacokinetic data can be used to guide administration to maintain a constant therapeutic concentration while decreasing the likelihood of circulatory overload (Rentko *et al.*, 2003). A loading dose based on the volume of distribution, followed by a constant rate of infusion based on clearance, will provide a constant therapeutic level of plasma Hb. The desired plasma Hb concentration is dependent on the severity of the anaemia and the related clinical signs.

The choice of rate of administration varies with the indication for use. In dogs with anaemia secondary to haemorrhagic or hypovolaemic shock, initial boluses of 10 ml/kg with regular reassessment for adjustment of the rate can be used to restore haemodynamic stability. As with other resuscitative strategies, care should be taken with use of the product in patients with uncontrolled haemorrhage, to avoid exacerbation of blood loss. Oxyglobin should not be considered a resuscitative fluid in cats owing to the potential for circulatory overload. Administration of a large volume of Oxyglobin (30 ml/kg) will cause haemodilution of the PCV by up to 25% immediately following the infusion. The PCV will not reflect the plasma Hb concentration. A point-of-care haemoglobinometer can be used to measure plasma Hb accurately (Jahr *et al.*, 2000).

Monitoring

Monitoring changes in oxygenation is an essential clinical assessment. A patient in need of additional oxygen-carrying support shows signs of anaemia or poor perfusion: lethargy, weakness, decreased appetite, tachycardia, decreased pulse quality, pallor, a change in respiratory pattern, and increased or decreased capillary refill time. Improvement in these clinical signs following an infusion in a normovolaemic patient is indication of restoration of oxygenation. The monitoring of oxygenation in a hypovolaemic patient via heart rate and arterial blood pressure is confounded by the vasopressive effects of Oxyglobin. Indirect measures such as acid–base status (pH and PCO_2) and metabolism (lactate) can be used.

Repeated use of Oxyglobin raises the possibility of immunological sensitization of the recipient to the foreign bovine protein. Hamilton *et al.* (2001) administered Oxyglobin experimentally to dogs repeatedly without any anaphylactic or other hypersensitivity reactions. Over 50 weeks, antibodies to the Hb solution developed, but the antibodies showed no effect on the oxygen-carrying ability of the solution. No immune complexes or serum sickness developed.

Use of Oxyglobin in cats

In two retrospective studies conducted in cats, 72 cats received 80 infusions and 48 cats received 70 infusions, respectively (Gibson *et al.*, 2002; Weingart and Kohn, 2008). Anaemia was the indication for use in all but two cats. Interestingly, although blood loss was the primary cause of anaemia that directed the use of Oxyglobin in both studies, Gibson *et al.* (2002) reported more common use in cats with anaemia associated with ineffective erythropoiesis than Weingart and Kohn (2008) (Figure 36.5). Overall, chronic anaemia (ineffective erythropoiesis)

Baseline PCV (%)	Desired plasma Hb concentration (g/l)	Loading dose (ml/kg)	Hours to achieve loading dose at 6 ml/kg/h	Constant rate infusion (ml/kg/h)
> 15	10	6	1	0.2
10–15	20	12	2	0.4
< 10	30	18	3	0.6

36.3 Guidelines for constant rate infusion of Oxyglobin in canine patients.

Dose (ml/kg)	Immediate post-infusion plasma haemoglobin concentration (g/dl)	Duration (hours) of plasma haemoglobin concentration > 1 g/dl	Terminal half-life (hours)	Cleared from plasma (days)
10	1.5–2.0	11–23	18–26	4–5
15	2.0–2.5	23–39	19–30	4–6
21	3.4–4.3	66–70	25–34	5–7
30	3.6–4.8	74–82	22–43	5–9

36.4 Pharmacokinetic parameters after a single infusion of Oxyglobin. (Source: Oxyglobin package insert)

Factor compared	Reference	Blood loss	Haemolysis	Ineffective erythropoiesis
Reason for use	Gibson *et al.*, 2002	41%	16%	34%
	Weingart and Kohn, 2008	52%	27%	17%
Dosage (median)	Gibson *et al.*, 2002	12.5 ml/kg		
	Weingart and Kohn, 2008	9.6 ml/kg	12.3 ml/kg	8.5 ml/kg
Hourly rate of administration (median)	Gibson *et al.*, 2002	3.7 ml/kg/h		
Use of other blood products	Gibson *et al.*, 2002	54%		
	Weingart and Kohn, 2008	72%	54%	63%
Survival to discharge	Gibson *et al.*, 2002	32%		
	Weingart and Kohn, 2008	56%	69%	38%

36.5 Oxyglobin use in cats with anaemia associated with different causes.

was a slightly more common indication than haemolysis in both studies. This may be related to the greater incidence of chronic anaemia versus haemolytic anaemia in cats. The reasons cited for the use of Oxyglobin related to the difficulty in obtaining compatible feline blood. Prior to discharge from the hospital, 56% of cats in the Gibson study and 63% of cats in the Weingart and Kohn study had also received blood or blood products. Cats with anaemia associated with blood loss received adjunctive blood products most commonly. The median dosage was also similar between the studies (Figure 36.5). The median rate of administration used in the two studies was similar (≤ 5 ml/kg/h), although the exact rate was not reported in the Weingart and Kohn study. Complications related to circulatory overload (pulmonary oedema and pleural effusion) occurred in 15% and 35%, respectively, of all cats infused. Notably, 40% of these cats in one study showed these signs prior to infusion (Gibson *et al.*, 2002), and all of the cats in the other study had pre-existing heart disease (Weingart and Kohn, 2008). The overall rate of survival to discharge was 32% and 43%, respectively. Survival rates at 24 hours were markedly different between the studies (Figure 36.5). One study examined survival with regard to the cause of the anaemia and showed marked differences between causes, with the greatest survival rate in cats with haemolysis (Weingart and Kohn, 2008). Care must be given not to over-interpret the differences in complications of circulatory overload and survival rates between the studies, given their retrospective nature and the limited number of cats in each group. One possible explanation may be that the greater survival rate and fewer complications in the study of Weingart and Kohn (2008) could be attributed to greater clinical experience using Oxyglobin because this study was reported 5 years after the other study.

The use of Oxyglobin to treat deceased perfusion in cats was reported in a retrospective study of 46 cats with disseminated intravascular coagulation (DIC; Estrin *et al.*, 2006). Seven cats received Oxyglobin treatment in combination with other blood products, including packed RBCs and fresh-frozen plasma. No difference in outcome was noted between cats that received Oxyglobin with or without blood products and those given blood products alone. The most important clinical considerations for the use of Oxyglobin in cats are estimation of the blood volume of the cat, assessment for pre-existing cardiac disease, and the rate of administration. Given that cats are sensitive to circulatory overload, very slow rates of infusion (0.5–2 ml/kg/h) are recommended (Adamantos *et al.*, 2005).

Effects on clinical pathology

The plasma or serum of patients administered Oxyglobin appears red, and this may cause artefactual increases or decreases in the results of some serum biochemistry tests. This coloration cannot be distinguished from haemolysis, but the typical interference caused by haemolysis is not the same for Oxyglobin. In general, measurements of electrolytes and blood urea nitrogen are valid on any analyser. However, the nature of the interference varies by type of analyser and reagents used. Any assay that uses colorimetric methods is affected. Likewise, optical methods used to measure prothrombin time and activated partial thromboplastin time are affected, while measurements made using mechanical (fibrometer), magnetic or light-scattering techniques are valid. A good resource for detailed information on potential interference is www.HBOClab.com.

Most haematology parameters (e.g. white blood cells (WBCs), RBCs and platelet counts, and WBC differentials) are not affected by the presence of Oxyglobin. However, techniques that depend on the direct measurement of Hb may be affected because the measurement of Hb uses the combination of RBC Hb plus that in the Oxyglobin. Mean corpuscular haemoglobin concentration (MCHC) and mean corpuscular haemoglobin (MCH) will be increased because the plasma haemoglobin is included in the calculation of these parameters. The results of pulse oximetry are considered to be valid following administration of Oxyglobin, but cautious interpretation of the readings should be made if a large volume of Oxyglobin is administered to a severely anaemic animal because the result reflects the relative ratio of plasma and red cell haemoglobin. Given the right-shift of the Hb–oxygen dissociation curve of Oxyglobin, a lower value for saturation could be obtained in this circumstance.

Erythropoietin

Erythropoietin (EPO) is a haemopoietic growth factor, synthesized in the kidney, that stimulates RBC production. Recombinant human EPO (rHuEPO) has been administered, as an off-label use, for the treatment of anaemia associated with chronic renal failure in dogs and cats. rHuEPO increases haematocrit directly in proportion to dose. Its use is generally reserved for patients with moderate to severe anaemia, owing to the high incidence of the development of antibodies to rHuEPO. Because the anti-rHuEPO antibodies cross-react with native EPO, the resultant anaemia can be life-threatening. Adverse effects in dogs and cats include refractory anaemia/erythroid hypoplasia, hypertension, polycythaemia, seizures, vomiting, iron deficiency, fever and other less common effects. Langston *et al.* (2003) have written a complete review of the use of erythropoietin in dogs and cats.

Factor VIIa and anti-fibrinolytics

Recombinant factor VIIa (rFVIIa) is used widely in human patients as a global haemostatic agent for bleeding disorders caused by haemophilia, thrombocytopenia, surgical blood loss and trauma. Its potential uses in veterinary patients have been reviewed, but no reports of its clinical use in dogs or cats have been published (Kristensen *et al.*, 2003). Similarly, the use of anti-fibrinolytics in human patients to decrease bleeding and reduce post-operative inflammation holds interest for veterinary patients. Aprotinin, a serine protease inhibitor, and the lysine analogues epsilon aminocaproic acid (EACA) and tranexamic acid (TEA) have been used effectively in human patients. The safety profile of the lysine analogues has been superior to that of aprotinin. One brief communication regarding the use of EACA and TEA in three dogs with uncontrolled bleeding reported promising results (Cooper, 2008).

Conclusion

As the field of transfusion medicine has grown and the use of blood products has become routine over the past 20 years, the desire for the use of substitutes to lessen the strain on limited blood resources has also developed. A haemoglobin-based oxygen-carrying solution has the most widespread clinical use in dogs and cats. Other strategies to substitute the properties of blood, including the clotting capability, are gaining wider interest, but clinical applications may be limited owing to cost and antigenicity.

References and further reading

Adamantos S, Boag A and Hughes D (2005) Clinical use of a haemoglobin-based oxygen carrying solution in dogs and cats. *In Practice* **27**, 399–405

Cooper E (2008) Antifibrinolytics: A role in veterinary medicine. *Proceedings of the International Veterinary Emergency and Critical Care Symposium*, pp.405–407

Day TK, Duffy TC, Kirby R *et al.* (2001) Tissue perfusion and oxygenation – clinical cases. *Compedium on Continuing Education for the Practicing Veterinarian* **23**(7A), 2–16

Driessen B, Jahr JS, Lurie F *et al.* (2001) Inadequacy of low-volume resuscitation with hemoglobin-based oxygen carrier hemoglobin glutamer-200 (bovine) in canine hypovolemia. *Journal of Veterinary Pharmacology and Therapeutics* **86**, 683–692

Estrin M, Wehausen CE, Jessen CR and Justine AL (2006) Disseminated intravascular coagulation in cats. *Journal of Veterinary Internal Medicine* **20**, 1334–1339

Gibson GR, Callan MB, Hoffman V and Giger U (2002) Use of hemoglobin-based oxygen carrying solution in cats: 72 cases (1998–2000). *Journal of the American Veterinary Medical Association* **221**, 96–102

Grundy SA and Barton C (2001) Influence of drug treatment on survival of dogs with immune-mediated hemolytic anemia: 88 cases (1989–1999). *Journal of the American Veterinary Medical Association* **218**, 543–546

Hamilton RG, Kelly N, Gawryl MS and Rentko VT (2001) Absence of immunopathology associated with repeated IV administration of bovine Hb-based oxygen carrier in dogs. *Transfusion* **41**, 219–25

Horn EP, Standl T, Wilhelm S *et al.* (1997) Bovine hemoglobin increases skeletal muscle oxygenation during 95% artificial arterial stenosis. *Surgery* **121**, 411–418

Jahr JS, Lurie F, Driessen B *et al.* (2000) Validation of oxygen saturation measurements in a canine model of hemoglobin-based oxygen carrier (HBOC) infusion. *Clinical and Laboratory Science* **13**, 173–179

Kristensen AT, Edwards ML and Devey J (2003) Potential uses of recombinant human factor VIIA in veterinary medicine. *Veterinary Clinics of North America: Small Animal Practice* **33**, 1437–1451

Langston CE, Reine NJ and Dittrell D (2003) The use of erythropoietin. *Veterinary Clinics of North America: Small Animal Practice* **33**, 1245–1260

Page T, Light WR, McKay CB *et al.* (1998) Oxygen transport by erthyrocyte/hemoglobin solution mixtures in an in vitro capillary as a model of hemoglobin-based oxygen carrier performance. *Microvascular Research* **55**, 54–64

Rentko VT, Handler SR and Hanson BJ (2002) Influence of oxygen carrying support on survival of dogs with immune-medicated hemolytic anemia: 143 cases. *Proceedings of the International Veterinary Emergency and Critical Care Symposium*, p.210

Rentko VT, Pearce LB, Moon-Massat PF *et al.* (2003) Pharmacokinetics of low doses of a hemoglobin-based oxygen carrier in dogs [abstract]. *Journal of Veterinary Internal Medicine* **17**, 407

Rohlfs RJ, Bruner E, Chiu A *et al.* (1998) Arterial blood pressure responses to cell-free hemoglobin solutions and the reaction with nitric oxide. *Journal of Biological Chemistry* **273**, 12128–12134

Weingart C and Kohn B (2008) Clinical use of a haemoglobn-based oxygen carrying solution (Oxyglobin®) in 48 cats (2002–2006). *Journal of Feline Medicine and Surgery* **10**, 431–438

Zambelli AB and Leisewitz AL (2009) A prospective, randomized comparison of Oxyglobin (Hb-200) and packed red blood cell transfusion for canine babesiosis. *Journal of Veterinary Emergency and Critical Care* **19**, 102–112

Appendix 1

Reference values for haematology and haemostasis

The reference ranges given in these tables are those used in the clinical pathology laboratories of the Editors. The ranges given in individual chapters may vary because of the geographical spread of the authors. It should always be remembered that any table of reference values of this kind is for guidance only. Whenever a sample is sent to a laboratory for analysis, the laboratory should provide a reference value for that specific laboratory, the specific test and the specific patient type so that interpretation of the results can be done reliably.

Laboratory results: complete blood count

Parameter	Reference range		SI unit
	Dog	*Cat*	
White blood cells (WBCs)	6–15	6–18	x 10^9/l
Segmented neutrophils	3.0–9.0	3.0–11.0	x 10^9/l
Band neutrophils	0–0.5	0–0.6	x 10^9/l
Lymphocytes	1.0–3.6	1.0–4.0	x 10^9/l
Monocytes	0.04–0.5	0.05–0.5	x 10^9/l
Eosinophils	0.04–0.6	0.04–0.6	x 10^9/l
Basophils	0–0.1	0–0.1	x 10^9/l
Red blood cells (RBCs)	5.5–8.5	5.0–10.0	x 10^{12}/l
Haemoglobin (Hb)	132–190	90–150	g/l
Haematocrit	0.40–0.56	0.29–0.45	l/l
Mean corpuscular volume (MCV)	60–77	40–55	fl
Mean corpuscular haemoglobin concentration (MCHC)	320–360	310–360	g/l
Platelets	180–500	180–550	x 10^9/l

Haemostasis

Parameter	Reference range		SI unit
	Dog	*Cat*	
Buccal mucosal bleeding time (BMBT)	< 4	< 2.4	min
Activated coagulation time (ACT)	60–110	50–75	s
Fibrinogen	1–3	1–3	g/l

Appendix 2

List of abbreviations

AAG	α1 acid glycoprotein
AATP	acquired amegakaryocytic thrombocytopenia
Ab	antibody
ACT	activated clotting time
ACTH	adrenocorticotropic hormone
ADP	adenosine diphosphate
AIHA	autoimmune haemolytic anaemia
AIN	anaemia of inflammation and neoplasia
AINP	autoimmune neutropenia
AITP	autoimmune thrombocytopenia
ALL	acute lymphoblastic leukaemia
ALP	alkaline phosphatase
ALT	alanine aminotransferase
AML	acute myeloid leukaemia
APC	active protein C
APP	acute phase protein
aPTT	activated partial thromboplastin time
AST	aspartate transaminase
AT	antithrombin
ATE	aortic thromboembolism
ATP	adenosine triphosphate
AZT	zidovudine (azidothymidine)
BALF	bronchiolar–alveolar lavage fluid
BFU	burst-forming unit
BFU-E	burst-forming unit – erythroid
BM	bone marrow
BMBT	buccal mucosal bleeding time
BUN	blood urea nitrogen
cAMP	cyclic adenosine monophosphate
CBA	collagen binding assay
CBC	complete blood count
CBNP	circulating blood neutrophil pool
CCNU	lomustine
CD	cluster of differentiation
CE	canine ehrlichiosis
CEL	chronic eosinophilic leukaemia
CFU	colony-forming unit
CFU-E	colony-forming unit – erythroid
CFU-M	colony-forming unit – macrophage
CH	cell haemoglobin mean
CHCM	cell haemoglobin concentration mean
CKCS	Cavalier King Charles Spaniel
CKD	chronic kidney disease
CLAD	canine leucocyte adhesion deficiency
CLL	chronic lymphocytic leukaemia
CMAH	cytidine monophospho-*N*-acetylneuraminic acid hydroxylase
CME	canine monocytic ehrlichiosis
CML	chronic myeloid leukaemia
CNS	central nervous system
cPCR	conventional non-quantitative polymerase chain reaction
CPD	citrate phosphate dextrose
CPDA	citrate phosphate dextrose adenine-1
CRD	chronic renal disease
CRP	C-reactive protein
CSF	cerebrospinal fluid
CV	coefficient of variation
cWBC	corrected white blood cell count
DAT	direct antiglobulin test
DDAVP	1-desamino-8-D-arginine vasopressin (desmopressin)
DEA	dog erythrocyte antigen
DIC	disseminated intravascular coagulation
DLH	Domestic Longhair (cat)
2,3-DPG	2,3-diphosphoglycerate
DSH	Domestic Shorthair (cat)
DVT	deep vein thrombosis
EACA	epsilon aminocaproic acid
EBP	eosinophilic bronchopneumopathy
ECG	electrocardiogram
EDTA	ethylenediamine tetra-acetic acid
EL	eosinophilic leukaemia
ELISA	enzyme-linked immunosorbent assay
EPCR	endothelial cell protein C receptor
EPO	erythropoietin
ESA	erythropoiesis stimulating agents
Fc	immunoglobulin heavy chain (fragment crystallizable)
FDPs	fibrin(ogen) degradation products
FeLV	feline leukaemia virus
FFP	fresh frozen plasma
FGF	fibroblast growth factor
FIV	feline immunodeficiency virus
FP	frozen plasma
FWB	fresh whole blood
GAG	glycosaminoglycan
GC–MS	gas chromatography–mass spectrometry
G-CSF	granulocyte colony-stimulating factor
GEF	guanine nucleotide exchange factor

GI	gastrointestinal
GM-CSF	granulocyte–monocyte colony-stimulating factor
GP	glycoprotein
GWAS	genome-wide association study/ studies
Hb	haemoglobin
HBOC	haemoglobin-based oxygen-carrying (solution)
Hct	haematocrit
HDW	haemoglobin concentration distribution width
HES	hypereosinophilic syndrome
HIF	hypoxia-inducible factor
HIV	human immunodeficiency virus
HMWK	high molecular weight kininogen
HPLC	high performance liquid chromatography
HRE	hypoxia response element
HUS	haemolytic–uraemic syndrome
IDA	iron deficiency anaemia
IFAT	immunofluorescent antibody test
IFN-γ	interferon gamma
Ig	immunoglobulin (IgG, IgM, IgA, IgE)
IL	interleukin (e.g. IL-1 to IL-18)
IMHA	immune-mediated haemolytic anaemia
IMNP	immune-mediated neutropenia
IMTP	immune-mediated thrombocytopenia
ISAG	International Society of Animal Genetics
ITAM	immunoreceptor tyrosine-based activation motif
IVIG	intravenous human immunoglobulin
LGL	large granular lymphocyte
LHGL	leukaemic phase of high-grade lymphoma
LMWH	low molecular weight heparin
LPD	lymphoproliferative disease
LPS	lipopolysaccharide
LR	leukaemoid reaction
MA	maximum amplitude
MBNP	marginating blood neutrophil pool
MCH	mean corpuscular haemoglobin
MCHC	mean corpuscular haemoglobin concentration
MCV	mean corpuscular volume
MDS	myelodysplastic syndrome
MHC	major histocompatibility complex
MODS	multiple organ dysfunction syndrome
MPD	myeloproliferative disease
MPV	mean platelet volume
NBT	nitroblue tetrazolium
NI	neonatal isoerythrolysis
NK	natural killer (cell)
nRBC	nucleated red blood cell
NRIMHA	non-regenerative immune-mediated haemolytic anaemia
PAI-1	plasminogen activator inhibitor type 1
PAP	plasmin–anti-plasmin (complex)
PARR	PCR detection of antigen receptor rearrangements
PC	platelet concentrate
PC	protein C
PCR	polymerase chain reaction
PCV	packed cell volume
PDGF	platelet-derived growth factor
PDW	platelet distribution width
PF3	platelet factor 3
PF4	platelet factor 4
PFA	platelet function analyser
PFK	phosphofructokinase
PIVKA	proteins induced by vitamin K absence
PK	pyruvate kinase
PRBCs	packed red blood cells
PRCA	pure red cell aplasia
PRP	platelet-rich plasma
PS	protein S
PT	prothrombin time
PTE	pulmonary thromboembolism
PTH	parathyroid hormone
PWM	pokeweed mitogen
QBC	quantitative buffy coat (analysis)
qPCR	quantitative polymerase chain reaction
RA	refractory anaemia
RAEB	refractory anaemia with an excess of blasts
RBC	red blood cell
RCMD	refractory cytopenias with multilineage dysplasia
RDW	red cell distribution width
rHuEPO	recombinant human erythropoietin
rHuG-CSF	recombinant human granulocyte colony-stimulating factor
rHuGM-CSF	recombinant human granulocyte–monocyte colony-stimulating factor
RIM	rapid immunomigration
rMCV	reticulocyte mean cell volume
RMSF	Rocky Mountain spotted fever
ROTEM	rotation thromboelastometry
rRNA	ribosomal ribonucleic acid
RT-PCR	reverse transcriptase polymerase chain reaction
SCID	severe combined immunodeficiency
SCT	stem cell transplantation
SFP	stored frozen plasma
SIRS	systemic inflammatory response syndrome
SLE	systemic lupus erythematosus
SLL	small lymphocytic lymphoma
SLS	sodium lauryl sulphate
SWB	stored whole blood
TAFI	thrombin activatable fibrinolysis inhibitor
TAT	thrombin–antithrombin complex
TBNP	total blood neutrophil pool
TCR	T cell receptor

TCT	thrombin clotting time
TEA	tranexamic acid
TEG	thromboelastography
TF	tissue factor
TFPI	tissue factor pathway inhibitor
TIBC	total iron binding capacity
TM	thrombomodulin
TNCC	total nucleated cell count
TNF	tumour necrosis factor
TSAT	transferrin saturation
TT	thrombin time
UFH	unfractionated heparin
uPA	urokinase-type plasminogen activator
UPC	urine protein:creatinine ratio
USG	urine specific gravity
vWD	von Willebrand's disease
vWf	von Willebrand factor
WB	whole blood
WBC	white blood cell

Index

Page numbers in *italic* refer to figures.

Index